AF323161

New Developments in Biomedical Engineering

New Developments in Biomedical Engineering

Edited by

Domenico Campolo

New Developments in Biomedical Engineering

Edited by Domenico Campolo

CBS, Edition **2017**

Published by InTech

Janeza Trdine 9, 51000 Rijeka, Croatia

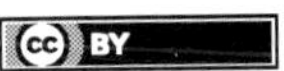

Notice
Statements and opinions expressed in the chapters are these of the individual contributors and not necessarily those of the editors or publisher. No responsibility is accepted for the accuracy of information contained in the published chapters. The publisher assumes no responsibility for any damage or injury to persons or property arising out of the use of any materials, instructions, methods or ideas contained in the book.

Additional hard copies can be obtained from orders@intechopen.com

New Developments in Biomedical Engineering,
Edited by Domenico Campolo
p. cm.
ISBN 978-953-7619-57-2

Preface

Biomedical Engineering is a highly interdisciplinary and well established discipline spanning across Engineering, Medicine and Biology. A single definition of Biomedical Engineering is hardly unanimously accepted but it is often easier to identify what activities are included in it.

This volume collects works on recent advances in Biomedical Engineering and provides a bird-view on a very broad field, ranging from purely theoretical frameworks to clinical applications and from diagnosis to treatment.

The 35 chapters composing this book can be grouped into five major domains:

I.   *Modeling*: chapters 1 - 4 propose advanced approaches to model physiological phenomena which are, in general, nonlinear, non-stationary and non-deterministic;

II. *Data Analysis*: chapters 5 - 14 relate to the analysis and processing of data which originate from the human body and which incorporate spatial or temporal patterns indicative for diagnostic purposes;

III. *Physiological Measurements*: chapters 15 - 24 describe a variety of biophysical methods for assessing physiological functions, for use in research as well as in clinical practice;

IV. *Biomedical Devices and Materials*: chapters 25 - 30 highlight aspects behind design and characterization of biomedical instruments which include electromechanical transduction and control;

V.   *Recent Approaches to Behavioral Analysis*: finally, chapters 31 - 35 propose recent and novel approaches to the analysis of behavior in humans and animal models, with emphasis on home-care delivery and monitoring.

This book is meant to provide a small but valuable sample of contemporary research activities around the world in the field of Biomedical Engineering and is expected to be useful to a large number of researchers in different biomedical fields.

I wish to thank all the authors for their valuable contribution to this book as well as the IN-TECH editorial staff, in particular Dr Aleksandar Lazinica, for their timely support.

Singapore, December 2009

Domenico Campolo (Editor)
School of Mechanical & Aerospace Engineering
Nanyang Technological University Singapore 639798

Contents

Contents

Contents

Nonparametric Modeling and Model-Based Control of the Insulin-Glucose System[*]

Mihalis G. Markakis[1], Georgios D. Mitsis[2], George P. Papavassilopoulos[3]
and Vasilis Z. Marmarelis[4]
[1] *Massachusetts Institute of Technology, Cambridge, MA, USA*
[2] *University of Cyprus, Nicosia, Cyprus*
[3] *National Technical University of Athens, Athens, Greece*
[4] *University of Southern California, Los Angeles, CA, USA*

1. Introduction

Diabetes represents a major threat to public health with alarmingly rising trends of incidence and severity in recent years, as it appears to correlate closely with emerging patterns of nutrition/diet and behavior/exercise worldwide. The concentration of blood glucose in healthy human subjects is about 90 mg/dl and defines the state of normoglycaemia. Significant and prolonged deviations from this level may give rise to numerous pathologies with serious and extensive clinical impact that is increasingly recognized by current medical practice. When blood glucose concentration falls under 60 mg/dl, we have the acute and very dangerous state of hypoglycaemia that may lead to brain damage or even death if prolonged. On the other hand, when blood glucose concentration rises above 120 mg/dl for prolonged periods of time, we are faced with the detrimental state of hyperglycaemia that may cause a host of long-term health problems (e.g. neuropathies, kidney failure, loss of vision etc.). The severity of the latter clinical effects is increasingly recognized as medical science advances and diabetes is revealed as a major lurking threat to public health with long-term repercussions.

Prolonged hyperglycaemia is usually caused by defects in insulin production, insulin action (sensitivity) or both (Carson et al., 1983). Although blood glucose concentration depends also on the action of several other hormones (e.g. epinephrine, norepinephrine, glucagon, cortisol), the exact quantitative nature of this dependence remains poorly understood and the effects of insulin are considered the most important. So traditionally, the scientific community has focused on the study of this causal relationship (with infused insulin being the "input" and blood glucose being the "output" of a system representing this functional relationship), using mathematical modeling as the means of quantifying it. Needless to say, the employed mathematical model plays a critical role in achieving (or not) the goal of

* This work was supported by the Myronis Foundation (Graduate Research Scholarship), the European Social Fund (75%) and National Resources (25%) - Operational Program Competitiveness - General Secretariat for Research and Development (Program ENTER 04), a grant from the Empeirikion Foundation of Greece and the NIH Center Grant No P41-EB001978 to the Biomedical Simulations Resource at the University of Southern California.

effective glucose control. In addition, blood glucose concentration depends on many factors other than hormones, such as nutrition/diet, metabolism, endocrine cycles, exercise, stress, mental activity etc. The complexity of these effects cannot be modeled explicitly in a practical context at the present time and, thus, the aggregate effect of all these factors is usually represented for modeling purposes as a stochastic "disturbance" that is additive to the blood glucose level (or its rate of change).

Numerous studies have been conducted over the last 40 years to examine the feasibility of continuous blood glucose concentration control with insulin infusions. Since the achievement of effective glucose control depends on the quantitative understanding of the relationship between infused insulin and blood glucose, much effort has been devoted to the development of reliable mathematical and computational models (Bergman et al., 1981; Cobelli et al., 1982; Sorensen, 1985; Tresp et al., 1999; Hovorka et al., 2002; Van Herpe et al., 2006; Markakis et al., 2008a; Mitsis et al., in press). Starting with the visionary works of Kadish (Kadish, 1964), Pfeiffer et al. on the "artificial beta cell" (Pfeiffer et al., 1974), Albisser et al. on the "artificial pancreas" (Albisser et al., 1974) and Clemens et al. on the "biostator" (Clemens et al., 1977), the efforts for on-line glucose regulation through insulin infusions have ranged from the use of relatively simple linear control methods (Salzsieder et al., 1985; Fischer et al., 1990; Chee et al., 2003a; Hernjak & Doyle, 2005) to more sophisticated approaches including optimal control (Swan, 1982; Fisher & Teo, 1989; Ollerton, 1989), adaptive control (Fischer et al., 1987; Candas & Radziuk, 1994), robust control (Kienitz & Yoneyama, 1993; Parker et al., 2000), switching control (Chee et al., 2005; Markakis et al., in press) and artificial neural networks (Prank et al., 1998; Trajanoski & Wach, 1998). However, the majority of recent publications have concentrated on applying model-based control strategies (Parker et al., 1999; Lynch & Bequette, 2002; Rubb & Parker, 2003; Hovorka et al., 2004; Hernjak & Doyle, 2005; Dua et al., 2006; Van Herpe et al., 2007; Markakis et al., 2008b) for reasons that are elaborated below.

These studies have had the common objective of regulating blood glucose levels in diabetics with appropriate insulin infusions, with the ultimate goal of an automated closed-loop glucose regulation (the holy grail of "artificial pancreas"). Due to the inevitable difficulties introduced by the complexity of the problem and the limitations of proper instrumentation or methodology, the original grand goal has often been substituted by the more modest goal of "diabetes management" (Harvey et al., 1986; Berger et al., 1990; Deutsch et al., 1990; Salzsieder et al., 1990) and the use of man-in-the-loop control strategies with partial subject participation, such as meal announcement (Goriya et al., 1988; Fisher, 1991; Brunetti et al., 1993; Hejlesen et al., 1997; Shimoda et al., 1997; Chee et al., 2003b).

In spite of the immense effort and the considerable resources that have been dedicated to this task, the results so far have been modest, with many studies contributing to our better understanding of this problem but failing to produce an effective solution with potential clinical utility and applicability. Technological limitations have always been a major issue, but recent advancements in the technology of long-term glucose sensors and insulin micro-pumps (Laser & Santiago, 2004; Klonoff, 2005) removed some of these past roadblocks and presented us with new opportunities in terms of measuring, analyzing and controlling blood glucose concentration with on-line insulin infusions.

It is our view that the lack of a widely accepted model of the insulin-glucose system (that is accurate under realistic operating conditions) represents at this time the main obstacle in achieving the stated goal. We note that almost all efforts to date for modeling the insulin-glucose system (and consequently, for developing control strategies based on these models) have followed the "parametric" or "compartmental" route, which postulates a specific model structure (in the form of a set of differential/difference and algebraic equations) based on specific hypotheses regarding the underlying physiological mechanisms, in accordance with existing knowledge and current scientific understanding. The unknown parameters of the postulated model are subsequently estimated from the data, usually through least-squares or Bayesian fitting (Sorenson, 1980). Although this approach retains physiological relevance and interpretability of the obtained model, it presents the major limitation of being constrained *a priori* and, therefore, being subject to possible biases that may narrow the range of its applicability. This constraint becomes even more critical in light of the intrinsic complexity of physiological systems which includes the presence of nonlinearities, nonstationarities and patient-specific dynamics.

We propose that this modeling challenge be addressed by the so-called "nonparametric" approach, which employs models of the general form of Volterra functional expansions and their many variants (Marmarelis, 2004). The main advantage of this generic model form is that it remains valid for a very broad class of systems and covers most physiological systems under realistic operating conditions. The unknown quantities in these nonparametric models are the "Volterra kernels" (or their equivalent representations that are discussed below), which are estimated by use of the available data. Thus, there is no need for *a priori* postulation of a specific model and no problems with potential modeling biases. The estimated nonparametric models are "true to the data" and capable of predicting the system output for all possible inputs. The latter attribute of "universal predictor" makes them suitable for the purpose of model-based control of complex physiological systems, for which accurate parametric models are not available under broad operating conditions.

This book chapter begins with a brief presentation of the nonparametric modeling approach and its comparative advantages to the traditional parametric modeling approaches, continues with the presentation of a nonparametric model of the insulin-glucose system and concludes with demonstrating the feasibility of incorporating such a model in a model-based control strategy for the regulation of blood glucose.

2. Nonparametric Modeling

The modeling of many physiological systems has been pursued in the context of the general Volterra-Wiener approach, which is also termed nonparametric modeling. This approach views the system as a "black box" that is defined by its specific inputs and outputs and does not require any prior assumptions about the model structure. As mentioned before, the nonparametric approach is generally applicable to all nonlinear dynamic systems with finite memory and contains unknown kernel functions that are estimated in practice by use of the available input-output data. Although the seminal Wiener formulation of this problem required the use of long data-records of white-noise inputs (Marmarelis & Marmarelis, 1978), this requirement has been removed and nonparametric modeling is now feasible with arbitrary input-output data of modest length (Marmarelis, 2004). In this formulation, the dynamic relationship between the input $i(n)$ and output $g(n)$ of a causal, nonlinear system of order Q and memory M is described in discrete-time by the following general/canonical expression of the output in terms of a hierarchical series of discrete multiple convolutions of the input:

$$g(n) = \sum_{q=0}^{Q} \sum_{m_1=0}^{M} \cdots \sum_{m_q=0}^{M} k_q(m_1,\ldots,m_q) i(n-m_1)\ldots i(n-m_q) =$$

$$k_0 + \sum_{m=0}^{M} k_1(m) i(n-m) + \sum_{m_1=0}^{M} \sum_{m_2=0}^{M} k_2(m_1,m_2) i(n-m_1) i(n-m_2) + \ldots \qquad , \qquad (1)$$

where the qth convolution term corresponds to the effects of the qth order nonlinearities of the causal input-output relationship and involves the Volterra kernel $k_q(m_1,\ldots,m_q)$, which characterizes fully the qth order nonlinear properties of the system. The linear component of the model/system corresponds to the first convolution term and the respective first order kernel $k_1(m)$ corresponds to the traditional impulse response function of a linear system. The general model of Eq. (1) can approximate any causal and stable system with finite memory to a desired accuracy for appropriate values of Q (Boyd & Chua, 1984). This approach has been employed extensively for modeling physiological systems because of their intrinsic complexity (Marmarelis, 2004).

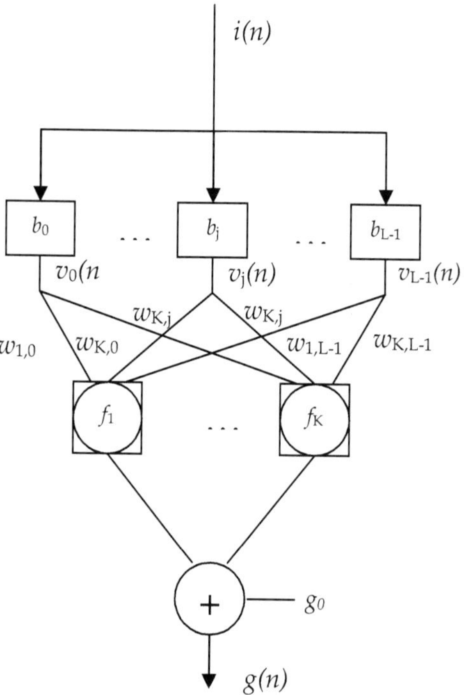

Fig. 1. The architecture of the Laguerre-Volterra network (LVN) that yields efficient approximations of nonparametric Volterra models in a robust manner using short data-records under realistic operating conditions (see text for description).

Among the various methods that have been developed for the estimation of the discrete Volterra kernels from input-output data, we select the method utilizing a Volterra-equivalent network in the form of a Laguerre-Volterra Network (LVN), which has been found to be efficient for the accurate representation of high-order systems in the presence of noise using short input-output records (Mitsis & Marmarelis, 2002). Therefore, it is well suited to the present application that typically relies on relatively short input-output records and is characterized by considerable measurement errors and systemic noise. The LVN model consists of an input layer of a Laguerre filter-bank and a hidden layer of K hidden units with polynomial activation functions (Figure 1). At each discrete time n, the input signal $i(n)$ is convolved with the Laguerre filters and the filter-bank outputs are subsequently transformed by the hidden units, the outputs of which form additively the model output. The unknown parameters of the LVN are the in-bound weights and the coefficients of the polynomial activation functions of the hidden units, along with the Laguerre parameter of the filter-bank and the output offset. These parameters are estimated from input-output data through an iterative procedure based on gradient descent. The filter-bank outputs v_j are the convolutions of the input $i(n)$ with the impulse response of the jth order discrete-time Laguerre function, b_j:

$$b_j(m) = \alpha^{(m-j)/2}(1-\alpha)^{1/2}\sum_{i=0}^{j}(-1)^i\binom{m}{i}\binom{j}{i}\alpha^{j-i}(1-\alpha)^i,\tag{2}$$

where the Laguerre parameter a in Eq. (2) lies between 0 and 1 and determines the rate of exponential decay of the Laguerre functions. As indicated in Figure 1, the weighted sums u_k of the filter-bank outputs v_j are subsequently transformed into z_k by the hidden units through polynomial transformations:

$$u_k(n) = \sum_{j=0}^{L-1} w_{k,j} v_j(n),\tag{3}$$

$$z_k(n) = \sum_{q=1}^{Q} c_{q,k} u_k^q(n).\tag{4}$$

The model output $g(n)$ is formed as the summation of the hidden-unit outputs z_k and a constant offset value g_0:

$$g(n) = \sum_{k=1}^{K} z_k(n) + g_0 = \sum_{k=1}^{K}\sum_{q=1}^{Q} c_{q,k} u_k^q(n) + g_0,\tag{5}$$

where L is the number of functions in the filter-bank, K is the number of hidden units, Q is the nonlinear order of the model and $w_{k,j}$ and $c_{q,k}$ are the in-bound weights and the polynomial coefficients of the hidden units respectively. The input and output time-series data are used to estimate the LVN model parameters ($w_{k,j}$, $c_{q,k}$, the offset g_0 and the Laguerre parameter a) with an iterative gradient-descent algorithm as (Mitsis & Marmarelis, 2002):

$$\delta^{(r+1)} = \delta^{(r)} + \gamma_\beta \varepsilon^{(r)}(n)\sum_{k=1}^{n} f_k^{'(r)}(u_k^{(r)}(n))\sum_{j=0}^{L} w_{k,j}[v_j(n-1)+v_{j-1}(n)],\tag{6}$$

$$w_{k,j}^{(r+1)} = w_{k,j}^{(r)} + \gamma_w \varepsilon^{(r)}(n) f_k^{\circledcirc(r)}(u_k^{(r)}(n))v_j(n),\tag{7}$$

$$c_{m,k}^{(r+1)} = c_{m,k}^{(r)} + \gamma_c \varepsilon^{(r)}(n)(u_k^{(r)}(n))^m \, , \tag{8}$$

where δ is the square root of the Laguerre parameter a, γ_β, γ_w and γ_c are positive learning constants, f denotes the polynomial activation function of Eq. (4), r denotes the iteration index and $\varepsilon^{(r)}(n)$ and $f_k^{'(r)}(u_k)$ are the output error and the derivative of the polynomial activation function of the kth hidden unit evaluated at the rth iteration, respectively.

The equivalent Volterra kernels can be obtained in terms of the LVN parameters as:

$$k_n(m_1,...,m_n) = \sum_{k=1}^{K} c_{n,k} \sum_{j_1=0}^{L-1} ... \sum_{j_n=0}^{L-1} w_{k,j_1}...w_{k,j_n} b_{j_1}(m_1)...b_{j_n}(m_n) \, , \tag{9}$$

which indicates that the Volterra kernels are implicitly expanded in terms of the Laguerre basis and the LVN represents a parsimonious way of parameterizing the general nonparametric Volterra model (Marmarelis, 1993; Marmarelis, 1997; Mitsis & Marmarelis, 2002; Marmarelis, 2004).

The structural parameters of the LVN model (L,K,Q) are selected on the basis of the normalized mean-square error (NMSE) of the output prediction achieved by the model, defined as the sum of squares of the model residuals divided by the sum of squares of the de-meaned true output. The statistical significance of the NMSE reduction achieved for model structures of increased order/complexity is assessed by comparing the percentage NMSE reduction with the *alpha*-percentile value of a chi-square distribution with p degrees of freedom (p is the increase of the number of free parameters in the more complex model) at a significance level *alpha*, typically set at 0.05.

The LVN representation is just one of the many possible Volterra-equivalent networks (Marmarelis & Zhao, 1997) and is also equivalent to a variant of the general Wiener-Bose model, termed the Principal Dynamic Modes (PDM) model. The PDM model consists of a set of parallel branches, each one of which is the cascade of a linear dynamic filter (PDM) followed by a static, polynomial nonlinearity (Marmarelis, 1997). This leads to model representations that are more parsimonious and facilitate physiological interpretation, since the resulting number of PDMs has been found to be small (2 or 3) in actual applications so far. The PDM model is formulated next for a finite memory, stable, discrete-time SISO system with input i and output g. The input signal $i(n)$ is convolved with each of the PDMs p_k and the PDM outputs $u_k(n)$ are subsequently transformed by the respective polynomial nonlinearities f_k to produce the model-predicted blood glucose output as:

$$\begin{aligned}
g(n) &= g_b + f_1[u_1(n)] + ... + f_K[u_K(n)] = \\
&= g_b + f_1[p_1(n)*i(n)] + ... + f_K[p_K(n)*i(n)]
\end{aligned} \tag{10}$$

where g_b is the basal value of g and the asterisk denotes convolution. Note the similarity between the expressions of Eq. (5) and Eq. (10), with the only difference being the basis of functions used for the implicit expansion of the Volterra kernels (i.e., the Laguerre basis versus the PDMs) that makes the PDM representation more parsimonious – if the PDMs of the system can be found.

3. A Nonparametric Model of the Insulin-to-Glucose Causal Relationship

In the current section, we present and briefly analyze a PDM model of the insulin-glucose system (Figure 2), which is a slightly modified version of a model that appeared in (Marmarelis, 2004). This PDM model has been obtained from analysis of infused insulin – blood glucose data from a Type 1 diabetic over an eight-hour period. In the subsequent computational study it will be treated as the putative model of the actual system, in order to examine the efficacy of the proposed model-predictive control strategy. It should be emphasized that this model is subject-specific and valid only for the specific type of fast-acting insulin analog that was used in this particular measurement. Different types of insulin analogs are expected to yield different models for different subjects (Howey et al., 1994). The PDM model employed in each case must be estimated with data obtained from the specific patient with the particular type of infused insulin. Furthermore, this model is expected to be generally time-varying and, thus, it must be adapted over time at intervals consistent with the insulin infusion schedule.

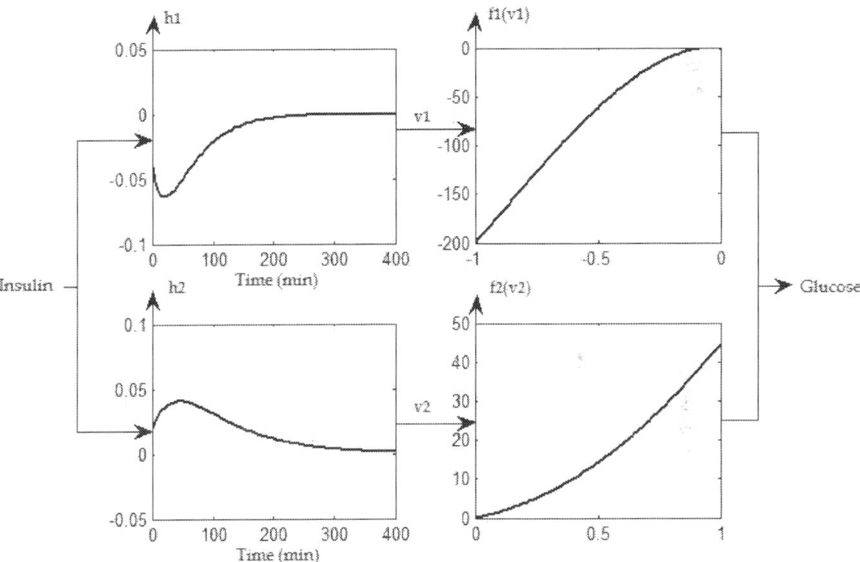

Fig. 2. The putative PDM model of the insulin–glucose system used in this computational study (see text for description of its individual components).

Firstly, we give a succinct mathematical description of the PDM model of Figure 2: the input $i(n)$, which represents the concentration of infused insulin at discrete time n (not the rate of infusion as in many computational studies), is transformed by the upper (h_1) and lower (h_2) branches through convolution to generate the PDM outputs $v_1(n)$ and $v_2(n)$. Subsequently, $v_1(n)$ and $v_2(n)$ are mapped by the cubic nonlinearities f_1 and f_2 respectively; their sum, $f_1(v_1)+f_2(v_2)$, represents the time-varying deviation of blood glucose concentration from its basal value g_0. The blood glucose concentration at each discrete time n is given by:

$$g(n) = g_0 + f_1[h_1(n)^*i(n)] + f_2[h_2(n)^*i(n)] + D(n), \tag{11}$$

where g_0 = 90 mg/dl is a typical basal value of blood glucose concentration and $D(n)$ represents a "disturbance" term that incorporates all the other systemic and extraneous influences on blood glucose (described in detail later).

Remarkably, the two branches of the model of Figure 2 appear to correspond to the two main physiological mechanisms by which insulin affects blood glucose according to the literature, even though no prior knowledge of this was used during its derivation. The first mechanism (modeled by the upper PDM branch) is termed *"glucolepsis"* and reduces the blood glucose level due to higher glucose uptake by the cells (and storage of excess glucose in the liver and adipose tissues) facilitated by the insulin action. The second mechanism (modeled by the lower PDM branch) is termed *"glucogenesis"* and increases the blood glucose level through production or release of glucose by internal organs (e.g. converting glycogen stored in the liver), which is triggered by the elevated plasma insulin. It is evident from the corresponding PDMs in Figure 2 that glucogenesis is somewhat slower and can be viewed as a counter-balancing mechanism of "biological negative feedback" to the former mechanism of glucolepsis. Since the dynamics of the two mechanisms and the associated nonlinearities are different, they do not cancel each other but partake in an intricate act of dynamic counter-balancing that provides the desired physiological regulation. Note also that both nonlinearities shown in the PDM model of Figure 2 are supralinear (i.e. their respective outputs change more than linearly relative to a change in their inputs) and of significant curvature (i.e. second derivative); intuitively, this justifies why linear control methods, based on linearizations of the system, will not suffice and, thus, underlines the importance of considering a nonlinear control strategy in order to achieve satisfactory regulation of blood glucose.

The glucogenic branch corresponds to the combination of all factors that counter-act to hypoglycaemia and is triggered by the concentration of insulin: although their existence is an undisputed fact (Sorensen, 1985) to the best of our knowledge, none of the existing models in the literature exhibits a strong glucogenic component. This emphasizes the importance of being "true to the data" and the dangers from imposing a certain structure *a priori*. Another consequence is that including a significant glucogenic factor complicates the dynamics and much more care should be taken in the design of a controller.

Unlike the extensive use of parametric models for the insulin-glucose system, there are very few cases to date where the nonparametric approach has been followed e.g. the Volterra model in (Florian & Parker, 2002) which is, however, distinctly different from the nonparametric model of Figure 2. A PDM model of the functional relation between spontaneous variations of blood insulin and glucose in dog was presented by Marmarelis et al. (Marmarelis et al., 2002) and exhibits some similarities to the model presented above. Driven by the fact that the Minimal Model (Bergman et al., 1981) and its many variations over the last 25 years is by far the most widely used model of the insulin-glucose system, the equivalent nonparametric model was derived computationally and analytically (i.e. the Volterra kernels were expressed in terms of the parameters of the Minimal Model) and was shown to differ significantly from the model of Figure 2 (Mitsis & Marmarelis, 2007). To emphasize the important point that the class of systems representable by the Minimal Model and its many variations (including those with pancreatic insulin secretion) can be also represented accurately by an equivalent nonparametric model, although the opposite is generally not true, we have performed an extensive computational study comparing the parametric and nonparametric approaches (Mitsis et al., in press).

4. Model - Based Control of Blood Glucose

In this section we formulate the problem of on-line blood glucose regulation and propose a model predictive control strategy, following closely the development in (Markakis et al., 2008b). A model-based controller of blood glucose in a nonparametric setting has also been proposed by Rubb & Parker (Rubb & Parker, 2003); however, both the model and the formulation of the problem are quite different than the ones presented here.

4.1 Closed - Loop System of Blood Glucose Regulation

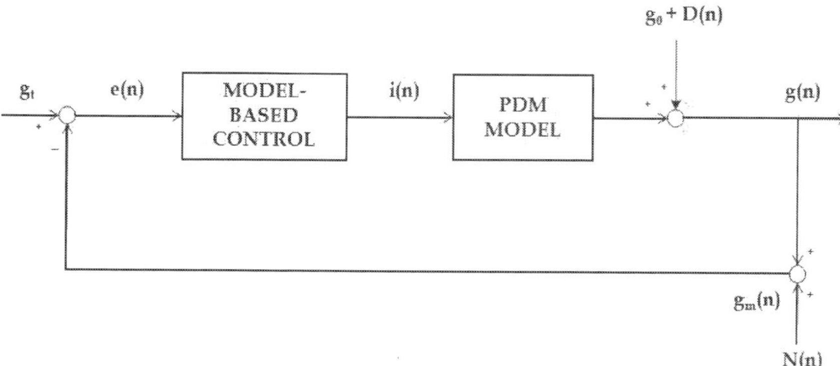

Fig. 3. Schematic of the closed-loop model-based control system for on-line regulation of blood glucose.

The block diagram of the proposed closed-loop control system for on-line regulation of blood glucose is shown in Figure 3. The PDM model presented in Section 3 plays the role of the real system in our simulations and defines the deviation of blood glucose from its basal value, in response to a given sequence of insulin infusions $i(n)$. The glucose basal value g_0 and the glucose disturbance $D(n)$ are superimposed on it to form the total value of blood glucose $g(n)$. Measurements of the latter are obtained in practice through commercially-available continuous glucose monitors (CGMs) that generate data-samples every 3 to 10 min (depending on the specific CGM). In the present work, the simulated CGM is assumed to make a glucose measurement every 5 min. Since the accuracy of these CGM measurements varies from 10% to 20% in mean absolute deviation by most accounts, we add to the simulated glucose data Gaussian "measurement noise" $N(n)$ of 15% (in mean absolute deviation) in order to emulate a realistic situation. Moreover, the short time lag between the concentration of blood glucose and interstitial fluids glucose is modeled as a pure delay of 5 minutes in the measurement of $g(n)$. A digital, model-based controller is used to compute the control input $i(n)$ to the system, based on the measured error signal $e(n)$ (the difference between the targeted value of blood glucose concentration g_t and the measured blood glucose $g_m(n)$). The objective of the controller is to attenuate the effects of the disturbance signal and keep $g(n)$ within bounds defined by the normoglycaemic region. Usually the targeted value of blood glucose g_t is set equal (or close) to the basal value g_0 and a conservative definition of the normoglycaemic region is from 70 to 110 mg/dl.

4.2 Glucose Disturbance

It is desirable to model the glucose disturbance signal D in a way that is consistent with the accumulated qualitative knowledge in a realistic context and similar to actual observations in clinical trials - e.g. see the patterns of glucose fluctuations shown in (Chee et al., 2003b; Hovorka et al., 2004). Thus, we have defined the glucose disturbance signal through a combination of deterministic and stochastic components:

1. Terms of the exponential form $n^3 \cdot exp(-0.19 \cdot n)$, which represent roughly the metabolic effects of Lehmann-Deutsch meals (Lehmann & Deutsch, 1992) on blood glucose of diabetics. The timing of each meal is fixed and its effect on glucose concentration has the form of a negative gamma-like curve, whose peak-time is at 80 minutes and peak amplitude is 100 mg/dl for breakfast, 350 mg/dl for lunch and 250 mg/dl for dinner;

2. Terms of the exponential form $n \cdot exp(-0.15 \cdot n)$, which represent random effects due to factors such as exercise or strong emotions. The appearance of these terms is modeled with a Bernoulli arrival process with parameter $p=0.2$ and their effect on glucose concentration has again the form of a negative gamma-like function with peak-time of approximately 35 minutes and peak amplitude uniformly distributed in [-10 , 30] mg/dl;

3. Two sinusoidal terms of the form $a_i \cdot sin(\omega_i \cdot n + \varphi_i)$ with specified amplitudes and frequencies (a_i and ω_i) and random phase φ_i, uniformly distributed within the range [-π/2 , π/2]. These terms represent circadian rhythms (Lee et al., 1992; Van Cauter et al., 1992) with periods 8 and 24 hours and amplitudes around 10 mg/dl;

4. A constant term B which is uniformly distributed within the range [50 , 80] and represents a random bias of the subject-specific basal glucose from the nominal value of g_0 that many diabetics seem to exhibit.

An illustrative example of the combined effect of these disturbance factors on glucose fluctuations can be seen in Figure 4.

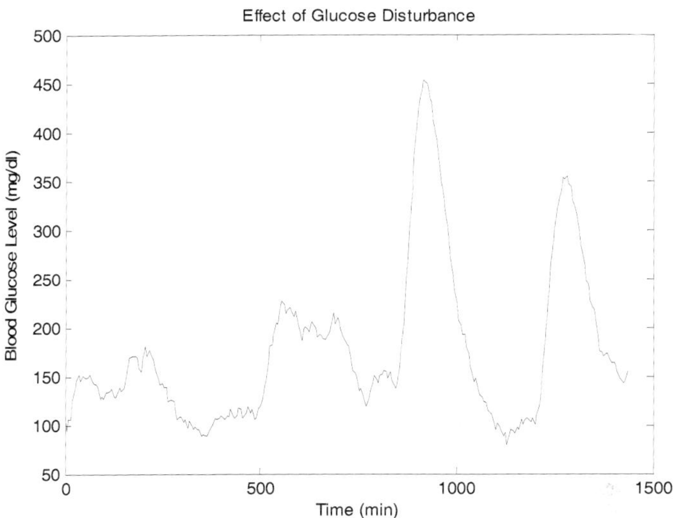

Fig. 4. Typical effect of glucose disturbance on the levels of blood glucose over a period of 24 hours.

The structure of the glucose disturbance signal described above is not known to the controller. However, in order to apply Model Predictive Control (MPC - the specific form of model-based control employed here) it would be desirable to predict the future values of the glucose disturbance term D(n) within some error bounds, so that we can obtain reasonable predictions of the future values of blood glucose concentration over a finite horizon. To achieve this, we hypothesize that the glucose disturbance signal D can be considered as the output of an Auto-Regressive (AR) model:

$$D(n) = D \cdot a + w(n), \tag{12}$$

where $D = [D(n-1)\ D(n-2)\ ...\ D(n-K)]$, $a = [a_1\ a_2\ ...\ a_K]^T$ is the vector of coefficients of the AR model, $w(n)$ is an unknown "innovation process" (usually viewed as a white sequence), and K is the order of the AR model. At each discrete-time instant n, the prediction task consists of estimating the coefficient vector a, which in turn allows the estimation of the future values of glucose disturbance: we use the estimated disturbance values as if they were actual values, in order to compute the glucose disturbance over the desired future horizon, using the AR model sequentially. The estimation of the coefficient vector can be performed with the least-squares method (Sorenson, 1980). Note, however, that we cannot know *a priori* whether the AR model is suitable for capturing the glucose disturbance presented above or if the least-squares criterion is appropriate in the AR context. What is most pertinent is the lack of correlation among the residuals. For this reason, we also compute the autocorrelation of the residuals and seek to make its values for all non-zero lags statistically insignificant, a fact indicating that all structured or correlated information in the glucose disturbance signal has been captured by the AR model. A critical part of this procedure is the determination of the best AR model order K at every discrete-time instant. In the present study, we use for this task the Akaike Information Criterion (Akaike, 1974).

4.3 Model - Based Control of Blood Glucose

Here we outline the concept of Model Predictive Control (MPC), which is at the core of the proposed control algorithm. Having knowledge of the nonlinear model and of all the past input-output pairs, the goal of MPC is to determine the control input value $i(n)$ at every time instant n, so that the following cost function is minimized:

$$J(n) = [g(n+p\,|\,n) - g_t]^{\mathrm{T}} \cdot \Gamma_y \cdot [g(n+p\,|\,n) - g_t] + \Gamma_u \cdot i(n)^2 , \tag{13}$$

where $g(n+p\,|\,n)$ is the vector of predicted output values over a future horizon of p steps using the model and the past input values, Γ_y is a diagonal matrix of weighting coefficients assigning greater importance to the near-future predictions, and Γ_u a scalar that determines how "expensive" is the control input. We also impose a "physiological" constraint to the above optimization problem in order to avoid large deviations of plasma insulin from its basal value and, consequently, the risk of hypoglycaemia: we limit the magnitude of $i(n)$ to a maximum of 1.5 mU/L. The procedure is repeated at the next time step to compute $i(n+1)$ and so on. More details on MPC and relevant control issues can be found in (Camacho & Bordons, 2007; Bertsekas, 2005).

In our simulations, we considered a prediction horizon of 40 min ($p = 8$ samples) and exponential weighting Γ_y with a time constant of 50 min. As measures of precaution against hypoglycaemia, we used a target value for blood glucose that is greater than the reference value ($g_t = 105$ mg/dl) and also applied asymmetric weighting to the predicted output vector, as in (Hernjak & Doyle, 2005), whereby we penalized 10 times more the deviations of the vector $g(n+p\,|\,n)$ that are below g_t. The scalar Γ_u was set to 0 throughout our simulations.

4.4 Results

Throughout this section we assume that MPC has perfect knowledge of the nonlinear PDM model. Figure 5 presents MPC in action: the top panel shows the blood glucose levels without any control, apart from the basal insulin infusion (blue line), called also the "No-Control" case, and after MPC action (green line). The mean value (MV), standard deviation (SD) and the percentage of time that glucose is found outside the normoglycaemic region of 70-110 mg/dl (PTO) are reported between the panels for MPC and "No-Control". The bottom panel shows the infused insulin profile determined by the MPC. Figure 6 presents the autocorrelation function of the estimated innovation process w. The fact that its values for all non-zero time-lags are statistically insignificant (smaller than the confidence bounds determined by the null hypothesis that the residuals are uncorrelated with zero mean) implies that the structure of the glucose disturbance signal is captured by the AR-Model. This result is important, considering that we have included a significant amount of stochasticity in the disturbance signal. In Figure 7 we show how the order of the AR model varies with time, as determined by the AIC, for the simulation case of Figure 5.

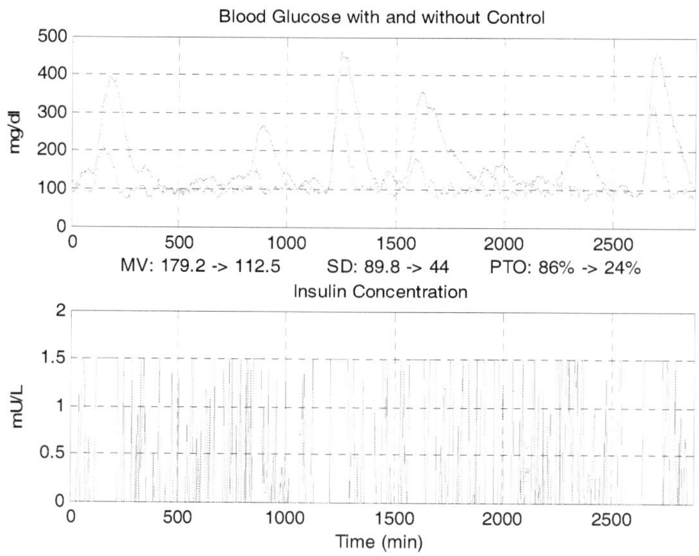

Fig. 5. Model Predictive Control of blood glucose concentration: The top panel shows the blood glucose levels corresponding to the general stochastic disturbance signal, with basal insulin infusion only (blue line) and after MPC action (green line). The mean value (MV), standard deviation (SD) and percentage of time that the glucose is found outside the normoglycaemic region of 70-110 mg/dl (PTO) are reported between the panels for MPC and without control action. The bottom panel shows the insulin profile determined by the MPC.

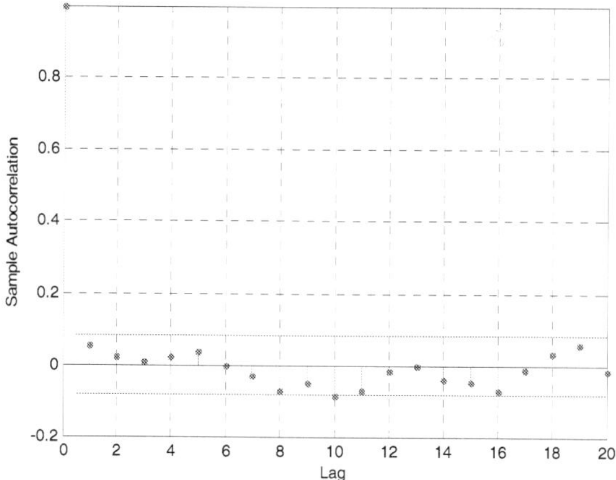

Fig. 6. Estimate of the autocorrelation function of the AR model residuals for the simulation run of Figure 5.

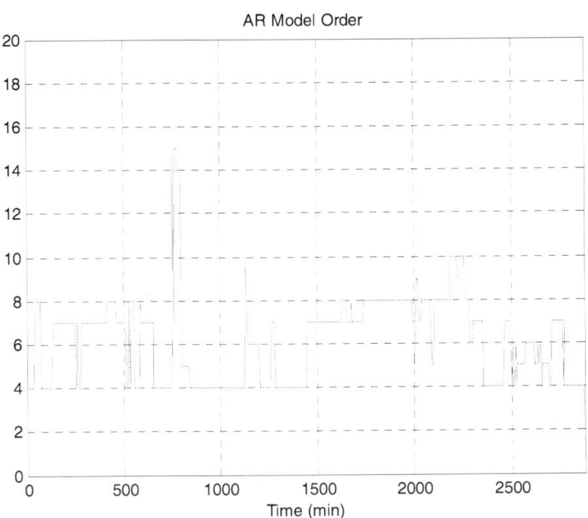

Fig. 7. The time-variations of the AR model order (as determined by AIC) for the simulation run of Figure 5.

Figure 8 provides further insight into how the attenuation of glucose disturbance is achieved by MPC: the controller determines the precise amount of insulin to be infused, given the various constraints, so that the time-varying sum of the outputs of glucolepsis (blue line) and glucogenesis (green line) cancel the stochastic disturbance (red line) in order to maintain normoglycaemia. A comment, however, must be made on the large values of the various signals of Figure 8: the PDM model presented in Section 3 aims primarily to capture the input-to-output dynamics of the system under consideration and not its internal structure (like parametric models do). So, even though the PDMs of Figure 2 seem intuitive and can be interpreted physiologically, we cannot expect that every signal will make physiological sense.

Finally, in order to average out the effects of stochasticity in glucose disturbance upon the results of closed-loop regulation of blood glucose, we report in Table 1 the average performance achieved by MPC over 20 independent simulation runs of 48 hours each. The evaluation of performance is done by comparing the standard indices (mean value, standard deviation, percent of time outside the normoglycaemic region) for the MPC and the "No-Control" case. The total number of hypoglycaemic events is also reported in the last row, since it is critical for patient safety. The results presented in this Table and in the Figures above indicate that MPC can regulate blood glucose quite well (as attested by the significant improvement in all measured indices) and, at the same time, does not endanger the patient.

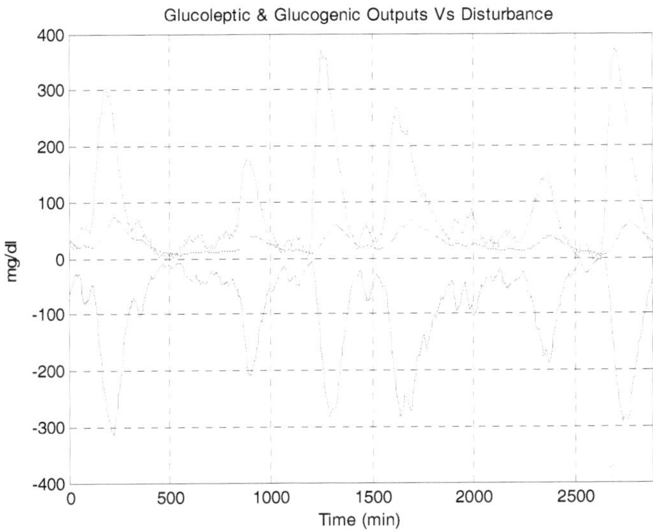

Fig. 8. MPC preserves normoglycaemia by cancelling out the effects of glucose disturbance (red line), the glucoleptic branch (blue line) and the glucogenic (green line) branch.

	NO CONTROL	MPC
MV	182.6	111.5
SD	89	42
PTO	87	25
HYPO	0	0

Table 1. Averages of 20 independent simulation runs of 48 hours each. Presented are the mean value (MV) and the standard deviation (SD) of glucose fluctuations, the percentage of time that glucose is found outside the normoglycaemic region 70-110 mg/dl (PTO) and the number of hypoglycaemic events, for the cases of no control action and MPC.

5. Discussion

This chapter is dedicated to the potential application of nonparametric modeling for model-based control of blood glucose through automated insulin infusions and seeks to:

1. Briefly outline the nonparametric modeling methodology and present a data-based nonparametric model, in the form of Principal Dynamic Modes (PDM), of the dynamics between infused insulin and blood glucose concentration. This model form provides an accurate, parsimonious and interpretable representation of this causal relationship for a specific patient and was obtained using a relatively short data-record. The estimation of nonparametric models (like the one presented here) is robust in the presence of noise and/or measurement errors and not liable to

model misspecification errors that are possible (or even likely) in the case of hypothesis-based parametric or compartmental models. More information on the performance of nonparametric models in the context of the insulin-glucose system can be found in (Mitsis et al., in press);

2. Show the efficacy of utilizing PDM models in Model Predictive Control (MPC) strategies for on-line regulation of blood glucose. The results of our computational study suggest that a closed-loop, PDM - MPC strategy can regulate blood glucose well in the presence of stochastic and cyclical glucose disturbances, even when the data are corrupted by measurement errors and systemic noise, without risking dangerous hypoglycaemic events;

3. Suggest an effective way for predicting stochastic glucose disturbances through an Auto-Regressive (AR) model, whose order is determined adaptively by use of the Akaike Information Criterion (AIC) or other equivalent statistical criteria. It is shown that this AR model is able to capture the basic structure of the glucose disturbance signal, even when it is corrupted by noise. This simple approach offers an attractive alternative to more complicated techniques that have been previously proposed -- e.g. utilizing a Kalman filter (Lynch & Bequette, 2002).

A comment is warranted regarding the procedure of insulin infusions, either intravenously or subcutaneously. Various studies have shown that in the case of fast acting, intravenously infused insulin the time-lag between the time of infusion and the onset of its effect on blood glucose is not significant, e.g. see (Hovorka, 2005) and references within. However, in the case of subcutaneously infused insulin, the considerably longer time-lag may compromise the efficacy of closed-loop regulation of blood glucose. Although this issue remains an open problem, the contribution of this study is that it demonstrates that the dynamic effects of infused insulin on blood glucose concentration may be "controllable" under the stipulated conditions, which seem realistic. Nonetheless, additional methodological improvements are possible, if the circumstances require them, which also depend on future technical advancements in glucose sensing and micro-pump technology, as well as the synthesis of even faster-acting insulin analogs.

There are numerous directions for future research, including improved methods for prediction of the glucose disturbance and the adaptability of the PDM model to the time-varying characteristics of the insulin-to-glucose relationship. From the control point of view, a critical issue remains the possibility of plant-model mismatch and its effect on the proposed MPC strategy (since the presented MPC results rely on the assumption that the controller has knowledge of an accurate PDM model). Last but not least, it is obvious that the clinical validation of the proposed control strategy, based on nonparametric models, is the ultimate step in adopting this approach.

6. References

Akaike, H. (1974). A new look at the statistical model identification. *IEEE Transactions on Automatic Control*, Vol. 19, pp. 716-723

Albisser, A.; Leibel, B.; Ewart, T.; Davidovac, Z.; Botz, C. & Zingg, W. (1974). An artificial endocrine pancreas. *Diabetes,* Vol. 23, pp. 389–404

Berger, M.; Gelfand, R. & Miller, P. (1990). Combining statistical, rule-based and physiologic model-based methods to assist in the management of diabetes mellitus. *Computers and Biomedical Research*, Vol. 23, pp. 346-357

Bergman, R.; Phillips, L. & Cobelli, C. (1981). Physiologic evaluation of factors controlling glucose tolerance in man. *Journal of Clinical Investigation*, Vol. 68, pp. 1456-1467

Bertsekas, D. (2005). *Dynamic Programming and Optimal Control*, Athena Scientific, Belmont, MA

Boyd, S. & Chua, L. (1985). Fading memory and the problem of approximating nonlinear operators with Volterra series. *IEEE Transactions on Circuits and Systems*, Vol. 32, pp. 1150-1161

Brunetti, P.; Cobelli, C.; Cruciani, P.; Fabietti, P.; Filippucci, F.; Santeusanio, F. & Sarti, E. (1993). A simulation study on a self-tuning portable controller of blood glucose. *International Journal of Artificial Organs*, Vol. 16, pp. 51–57

Camacho, E. & Bordons, C. (2007). *Model Predictive Control*, Springer, New York, NY

Candas, B. & Radziuk, J. (1994). An adaptive plasma glucose controller based on a nonlinear insulin/glucose model. *IEEE Transactions on Biomedical Engineering*, Vol. 41, pp. 116–124

Carson, E.; Cobelli, C. & Finkelstein, L. (1983). *The Mathematical Modeling of Metabolic and Endocrine Systems*, John Wiley & Sons, New Jersey, NJ

Chee, F.; Fernando, T.; Savkin, A. & Van Heerden, V. (2003a). Expert PID control system for blood glucose control in critically ill patients. *IEEE Transactions on Information Technology in Biomedicine*, Vol. 7, pp. 419-425

Chee, F.; Fernando, T. & Van Heerden, V. (2003b). Closed-loop glucose control in critically ill patients using continuous glucose monitoring system (CGMS) in real time. *IEEE Transactions on Information Technology in Biomedicine*, Vol. 7, pp. 43-53

Chee, F.; Savkin, A.; Fernando, T. & Nahavandi, S. (2005). Optimal H_∞ insulin injection control for blood glucose regulation in diabetic patients. *IEEE Transactions on Biomedical Engineering*, Vol. 52, pp. 1625-1631

Clemens, A.; Chang, P. & Myers, R. (1977). The development of biostator, a glucose controlled insulin infusion system (GCIIS). *Hormone and Metabolic Research*, Vol. 7, pp. 23–33

Cobelli, C.; Federspil, G.; Pacini, G.; Salvan, A. & Scandellari, C. (1982). An integrated mathematical model of the dynamics of blood glucose and its hormonal control. *Mathematical Biosciences,* Vol 58, pp. 27-60

Deutsch, T.; Carson, E.; Harvey, F.; Lehmann, E.; Sonksen, P.; Tamas, G.; Whitney, G. & Williams, C. (1990). Computer-assisted diabetic management: a complex approach. *Computer Methods and Programs in Biomedicine*, Vol. 32, pp. 195-214

Dua, P.; Doyle, F. & Pistikopoulos, E. (2006). Model-based blood glucose control for type 1 diabetes via parametric programming. *IEEE Transactions on Biomedical Engineering*, Vol. 53, pp. 1478-1491

Fischer, U.; Schenk, W.; Salzsieder, E.; Albrecht, G.; Abel, P. & Freyse, E. (1987). Does physiological blood glucose control require an adaptive strategy?, *IEEE Transactions on Biomedical Engineering*, Vol. 34, pp. 575-582

Fischer, U.; Salzsieder, E.; Freyse, E. & Albrecht, G. (1990). Experimental validation of a glucose insulin control model to simulate patterns in glucose-turnover. *Computer Methods and Programs in Biomedicine*, Vol. 32, pp. 249–258

Fisher, M. & Teo, K. (1989). Optimal insulin infusion resulting from a mathematical model of blood glucose dynamics. *IEEE Transactions on Biomedical Engineering*, Vol. 36, pp. 479–486

Fisher, M. (1991). A semiclosed-loop algorithm for the control of blood glucose levels in diabetics. *IEEE Transactions on Biomedical Engineering*, Vol. 38, pp. 57–61

Florian, J. & Parker, R. (2002). A nonlinear data-driven approach to type 1 diabetic patient modeling. *Proceedings of the 15th Triennial IFAC World Congress*, Barcelona, Spain

Furler, S.; Kraegen, E.; Smallwood, R. & Chisolm, D. (1985). Blood glucose control by intermittent loop closure in the basal model: computer simulation studies with a diabetic model. *Diabetes Care*, Vol. 8, pp. 553-561

Goriya, Y.; Ueda, N.; Nao, K.; Yamasaki, Y.; Kawamori, R.; Shichiri, M. & Kamada, T. (1988). Fail-safe systems for the wearable artificial endocrine pancreas. *International Journal of Artificial Organs*, Vol. 11, pp. 482–486

Harvey, F. & Carson, E. (1986). Diabeta - an expert system for the management of diabetes, In: *Objective Medical Decision- Making: System Approach in Disease*, Ed. Tsiftsis, D., Springer, New York, NY

Hejlesen, O.; Andreassen, S.; Hovorka, R. & Cavan, D. (1997). Dias-the diabetic advisory system: an outline of the system and the evaluation results obtained so far. *Computer methods and programs in biomedicine*, Vol. 54, pp. 49-58

Hernjak, N. & Doyle, F. (2005). Glucose control design using nonlinearity assessment techniques. *American Institute of Chemical Engineers Journal*, Vol. 51, pp. 544-554

Hovorka, R. (2005). Continuous glucose monitoring and closed-loop systems. *Diabetes*, Vol. 23, pp. 1-12

Hovorka, R.; Shojaee-Moradie, F.; Carroll, P.; Chassin, L.; Gowrie, I.; Jackson, N.; Tudor, R.; Umpleby, A. & Jones, R. (2002). Partitioning glucose distribution / transport, disposal, and endogenous production during IVGTT. *American Journal of Physiology*, Vol. 282, pp. 992–1007

Hovorka, R.; Canonico, V.; Chassin, L.; Haueter, U.; Massi-Benedetti, M.; Orsini-Federici, M.; Pieber, T.; Schaller, H.; Schaupp, L.; Vering, T. & Wilinska, M. (2004). Nonlinear model predictive control of glucose concentration in subjects with type 1 diabetes. *Physiological Measurements*, Vol. 25, pp. 905–920

Howey, D.; Bowsher, R.; Brunelle, R. and Woodworth, J. (1994). [Lys(B28), Pro(B29)]-human insulin: A rapidly absorbed analogue of human insulin. *Diabetes*, Vol. 43, pp. 396–402

Kadish, A. (1964). Automation control of blood sugar. A servomechanism for glucose monitoring and control. *American Journal of Medical Electronics*, Vol. 39, pp. 82-86

Kienitz, K. & Yoneyama, T. (1993). A robust controller for insulin pumps based on H-infinity theory. *IEEE Transactions on Biomedical Engineering*, Vol. 40, pp. 1133-1137

Klonoff, D. (2005). Continuous glucose monitoring: roadmap for 21st century diabetes therapy. *Diabetes Care*, Vol. 28, pp. 1231-1239

Laser, D. & Santiago, J. (2004). A review of micropumps. *Journal of Micromechanics and Microengineering*, Vol. 14, pp. 35-64

Lee, A.; Ader, M.; Bray, G. & Bergman, R. (1992). Diurnal variation in glucose tolerance. *Diabetes*, Vol. 41, pp. 750-759

Lehmann, E. & Deutsch, T. (1992). A physiological model of glucose-insulin interaction in type 1 diabetes mellitus. *Journal of Biomedical Engineering*, Vol. 14, pp. 235-242

Lynch, S. & Bequette, B. (2002). Model predictive control of blood glucose in type 1 diabetics using subcutaneous glucose measurements, *Proceedings of the American Control Conference*, pp. 4039-4043, Anchorage, AK

Markakis, M.; Mitsis, G. & Marmarelis, V. (2008a). Computational study of an augmented minimal model for glycaemia control, *Proceedings of the 30th Annual International EMBS Conference*, pp. 5445-5448, Vancouver, BC

Markakis, M.; Mitsis, G.; Papavassilopoulos, G. & Marmarelis, V. (2008b). Model predictive control of blood glucose in type 1 diabetics: the principal dynamic modes approach, *Proceedings of the 30th Annual International EMBS Conference*, pp. 5466-5469, Vancouver, BC

Markakis, M.; Mitsis, G.; Papavassilopoulos, G.; Ioannou, P. & Marmarelis, V. (in press). A switching control strategy for the attenuation of blood glucose disturbances. *Optimal Control, Applications & Methods*

Marmarelis, V. (1993). Identification of nonlinear biological systems using Laguerre expansions of kernels. *Annals of Biomedical Engineering*, Vol. 21, pp. 573-589

Marmarelis, V. (1997). Modeling methodology for nonlinear physiological systems. *Annals of Biomedical Engineering*, Vol. 25, pp. 239-251

Marmarelis, V. & Marmarelis, P. (1978). *Analysis of physiological systems: the white-noise approach*, Springer, New York, NY

Marmarelis, V. & Zhao, X. (1997). Volterra models and three-layer perceptrons. *IEEE Transactions on Neural Networks*, Vol. 8, pp. 1421-1433

Marmarelis, V.; Mitsis, G.; Huecking, K. & Bergman, R. (2002). Nonlinear modeling of the insulin-glucose dynamic relationship in dogs, *Proceedings of the 2nd Joint EMBS/BMES Conference*, pp. 224-225, Houston, TX

Marmarelis, V. (2004). *Nonlinear Dynamic Modeling of Physiological Systems*. IEEE Press & John Wiley, New Jersey, NJ

Mitsis, G. & Marmarelis, V. (2002). Modeling of nonlinear physiological systems with fast and slow dynamics. I. Methodology. *Annals of Biomedical Engineering*, Vol. 30, pp. 272-281

Mitsis, G. & Marmarelis, V. (2007). Nonlinear modeling of glucose metabolism: comparison of parametric vs. nonparametric methods, *Proceedings of the 29th Annual International EMBS Conference*, pp. 5967-5970, Lyon, France

Mitsis, G.; Markakis, M. & Marmarelis, V. (in press). Non-parametric versus parametric modeling of the dynamic effects of infused insulin on plasma glucose. *IEEE Transactions on Biomedical Engineering*

Ollerton, R. (1989). Application of optimal control theory to diabetes mellitus. *International Journal of Control*, Vol. 50, pp. 2503-2522

Parker, R.; Doyle, F. & Peppas, N. (1999). A model-based algorithm for blood glucose control in type 1 diabetic patients. *IEEE Transactions on Biomedical Engineering*, Vol. 46, pp. 148-157

Parker, R.; Doyle, F.; Ward, J. & Peppas, N. (2000). Robust H_∞ glucose control in diabetes using a physiological model. *American Institute of Chemical Engineers Journal*, Vol. 46, pp. 2537-2549

Pfeiffer, E.; Thum, C. & Clemens, A. (1974). The artificial beta cell—a continuous control of blood sugar by external regulation of insulin infusion (glucose controlled insulin infusion system). *Hormone and Metabolic Research*, Vol. 6, pp. 339–342

Prank, K.; Jürgens, C.; Von der Mühlen, A. & Brabant, G. (1998). Predictive neural networks for learning the time course of blood glucose levels from the complex interaction of counter regulatory hormones. *Neural Computation*, Vol. 10, pp. 941–953

Rubb, J. & Parker, R. (2003). Glucose control in type 1 diabetic patients: a Volterra model-based approach, *Proceedings of the International Symposium on Advanced Control of Chemical Processes*, Hong Kong

Salzsieder, E.; Albrecht, G.; Fischer, U. & Freyse, E. (1985). Kinetic modeling of the glucoregulatory system to improve insulin therapy. *IEEE Transactions on Biomedical Engineering*, Vol. 32, pp. 846–855

Salzsieder, E.; Albrecht, G.; Fischer, U.; Rutscher, A. & Thierbach, U. (1990). Computer-aided systems in the management of type 1 diabetes: the application of a model-based strategy. *Computer Methods and Programs in Biomedicine*, Vol. 32, pp. 215-224

Shimoda, S.; Nishida, K.; Sakakida, M.; Konno, Y.; Ichinose, K.; Uehara, M.; Nowak, T. & Shichiri, M. (1997). Closed-loop subcutaneous insulin infusion algorithm with a short-acting insulin analog for long-term clinical application of a wearable artificial endocrine pancreas. *Frontiers of Medical and Biological Engineering*, Vol. 8, pp. 197–211

Sorensen, J. (1985). A physiological model of glucose metabolism in man and its use to design and assess insulin therapies for diabetes. *PhD Thesis*, Department of Chemical Engineering, MIT, Cambridge, MA

Sorenson, H. (1980). *Parameter Estimation*, Marcel Dekker Inc., New York, NY

Swan, G. (1982). An optimal control model of diabetes mellitus. *Bulletin of Mathematical Biology*, Vol. 44, pp. 793-808

Trajanoski, Z. & Wach, P. (1998). Neural predictive controller for insulin delivery using the subcutaneous route. *IEEE Transactions on Biomedical Engineering*, Vol. 45, pp. 1122–1134

Tresp, V.; Briegel, T. & Moody, J. (1999). Neural network models for the blood glucose metabolism of a diabetic. *IEEE Transactions on Neural Networks*, Vol. 10, pp. 1204-1213

Van Cauter, E.; Shapiro, E.; Tillil, H. & Polonsky, K. (1992). Circadian modulation of glucose and insulin responses to meals—relationship to cortisol rhythm. *American Journal of Physiology*, Vol. 262, pp. 467–475

Van Herpe, T.; Pluymers, B.; Espinoza, M.; Van den Berghe, G. & De Moor, B. (2006). A minimal model for glycemia control in critically ill patients, *Proceedings of the 28th IEEE EMBS Annual International Conference*, pp. 5432-5435, New York, NY

Van Herpe, T.; Haverbeke, N.; Pluymers, B.; Van den Berghe, G. & De Moor, B. (2007). The application of model predictive control to normalize glycemia of critically ill patients, *Proceedings of the European Control Conference*, pp. 3116-3123, Kos, Greece

2

State-space modeling for single-trial evoked potential estimation

Stefanos Georgiadis, Perttu Ranta-aho, Mika Tarvainen and Pasi Karjalainen
Department of Physics, University of Kuopio, Kuopio
Finland

1. Introduction

The exploration of brain responses following environmental inputs or in the context of dynamic cognitive changes is crucial for better understanding the central nervous system (CNS). However, the limited signal-to-noise ratio of non-invasive brain signals, such as evoked potentials (EPs), makes the detection of single-trial events a difficult estimation task. In this chapter, focus is given on the state-space approach for modeling brain responses following stimulation of the CNS.

Many problems of fundamental and practical importance in science and engineering require the estimation of the state of a system that changes over time using a series of noisy observations. The state-space approach provides a convenient way for performing time series modeling and multivariate non stationary analysis. Focus is given on the determination of optimal estimates for the state vector of the system. The state vectors provide a description for the dynamics of the system under investigation. For example, in tracking problems the states could be related to the kinematic characteristics of the moving object. In EP analysis, they could be related to trend-like changes of some component of the potentials caused by sequential stimuli presentation. The observation vectors represent noisy measurements that provide information about the state vectors.

In order to analyze a dynamical system, at least two models are required. The first model describes the time evolution of the states, and the second connects observations and states. In the Bayesian state-space formulation those are given in a probabilistic form. For example, the state is assumed to be influenced by unknown disturbances modeled as random noise. This provides a general framework for dynamic state estimation problems. Often, an estimate of the state of the system is required every time that a new measurement is available. A recursive filtering approach is then needed for estimation. Such a filter consists of essentially two stages: prediction and update. In the prediction stage, the state evolution model is used to predict the state forward from one measurement time to the next. The update stage uses the latest measurement to modify the prediction. This is achieved by using the Bayes theorem, which can be seen as a mechanism for updating knowledge about the current state in the light of extra information provided from new observations. When all the measurements are available, that is, in the case of batch processing, then a smoothing strategy is preferable. The smoothing problem can also be treated within the same framework. For example, a forward-backward approach can be adopted, which gives the smoother estimates as corrections of the filter estimates with the use of an additional backward recursion.

A mathematical way to describe trial-to-trial variations in evoked potentials (EPs) is given by state-space modeling. Linear estimators optimal in the mean square sense can be obtained with the use of Kalman filter and smoother algorithms. Of importance is the parametrization of the problem and the selection of an observation model for estimation. Aim in this chapter is the presentation of a general methodology for dynamical estimation of EPs based on Bayesian estimation theory.

The rest of the chapter is organized as follows: In Section 2, a brief overview of single-trial analysis of EPs is given focusing on dynamical estimation methods. In Section 3, state-space mathematical modeling is presented in a generalized probabilistic framework. In Sections 4 and 5, the linear state-space model for dynamical EP estimation is considered, and Kalman filter and smoother algorithms are presented. In Section 6, a generic way for designing an observation model for dynamical EP estimation is presented. The observation model is constructed based on the impulse response of an FIR filter and can be used for different kind of EPs. This form enables the selection of observation model based on shape characteristics of the EPs, for instance, smoothness, and can be used in parallel with Kalman filtering and smoothing. In Section 7, two illustrative examples based on real EP measurements are presented. It is also demonstrated that for batch processing the use of the smoother algorithm is preferable. Fixed-interval smoothing improves the tracking performance and reduces greater the noise. Finally, Section 8 contains some conclusions and future research directions related to the presented methodology.

2. Single-trial estimation of evoked potentials

Electroencephalogram (EEG) provides information about neuronal dynamics on a millisecond scale. EEG's ability to characterize certain cognitive states and to reveal pathological conditions is well documented (Niedermeyer & da Silva, 1999). EEG is usually recorded with Ag/AgCl electrodes. In order to reduce the contact impedance between the electrode-skin interface, the skin under the electrode is abraded and a conducting electrode past is used. The electrode placement commonly conforms the international 10-20 system shown in Figure 1, or some extensions of it for additional EEG channels. For the names of the EEG channels the following letters are usually used: A = ear lobe, C = central, Pg = nasopharyngeal, P = parietal, F = frontal, Fp = frontal polar, and O = occipital.

Evoked potentials obtained by scalp EEG provide means for studying brain function (Niedermeyer & da Silva, 1999). The measured potentials are often considered as voltage changes resulted by multiple brain generators active in association with the eliciting event, combined with noise, which is background brain activity not related to the event. Additionally, there are contributions from non-neural sources, such as muscle noise and ocular artifacts. In relation to the ongoing EEG, EPs exhibit very small amplitudes, and thus, it is difficult to be detected straight from the EEG recording. Therefore, traditional research and analysis requires an improvement of the signal-to-noise ratio by repeating stimulation, considering unchanged experimental conditions, and finally averaging time locked EEG epochs. It is well known that this signal enhancement leads to loss of information related to trial-to-trial variability (Fell, 2007; Holm et al., 2006).

The term event-related potentials (ERPs) is also used for potentials that are elicited by cognitive activities, thus differentiate them from purely sensory potentials (Niedermeyer & da Silva,

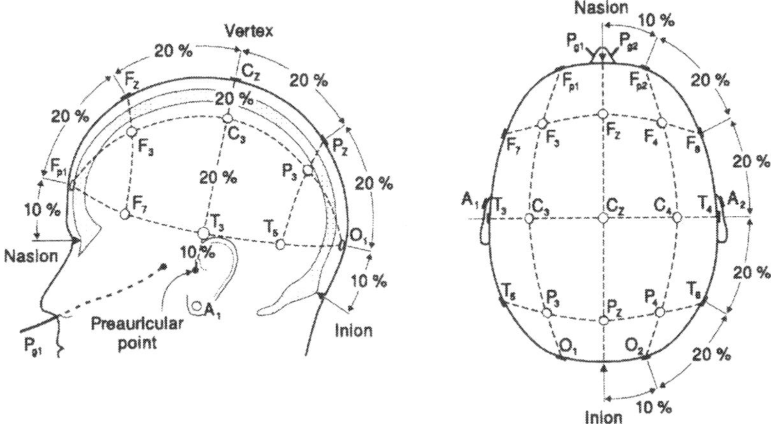

Fig. 1. The international 10-20 electrode system, redrawn from (Malmivuo & Plonsey, 1995).

1999). A generally accepted EP terminology denotes the polarity of a detected peak with the letter "N" for negative and "P" for positive, followed by a number indicating the typical latency. For example, the P300 wave is an ERP seen as a positive deflection in voltage at a latency of roughly 300 ms in the EEG. In practice, the P300 waveform can be evoked using a stimulus delivered by one of the sensory modalities. One typical procedure is the oddball paradigm, whereby a deviant (target) stimulus is presented amongst more frequent standard background stimuli. Elicitation of P300 type of responses usually requires a cognitive action to the target stimuli by the test subject. An example of traditional EP analysis, that is averaging epochs sampled relative to the two types of stimuli, here involving auditory stimulation, is presented in Figure 2. In Figure 2 (a) it is shown the extraction of time-locked EEG epochs from continuous measurements from an EEG channel. In this plot, markers (+) indicate stimuli presentation time. In Figure 2 (b), the average responses for standard and deviant stimuli are presented, and zero at the x-axis indicates stimuli presentation time. Notice, that often the potentials are plotted in reverse polarity.

Evoked potentials are assumed to be generated either separately of ongoing brain activity, or through stimulus-induced reorganization of ongoing activity. For example, it might be possible that during the performance of an auditory oddball discrimination task, the brain activity is being restructured as attention is focused on the target stimulus (Intriligator & Polich, 1994). Phase synchronization of ongoing brain activity is one possible mechanism for the generation of EPs. That is, following the onset of a sensory stimulus the phase distribution of ongoing activity changes from uniform to one which is centered around a specific phase (Makeig et al., 2004). Moreover, several studies have concluded that averaged EPs are not separate from ongoing cortical processes, but rather, are generated by phase synchronization and partial phase-resetting of ongoing activity (Jansen et al., 2003; Makeig et al., 2002). Though, phase coherence over trials observed with common signal decomposition methods (e.g. wavelets) can result both from a phase-coherent state of ongoing rhythms and from the presence of a phase-coherent EP which is additive to ongoing EEG (Makeig et al., 2004; Mäkinen et al., 2005). Furthermore, stochastic changes in amplitude and latency of different components of the EPs are able to explain the inter trial variability of the measurements (Knuth et al., 2006; Mäkinen et al., 2005; Truccolo et al., 2002). Perhaps both type of variability may be present in EP signals (Fell, 2007).

Several methods have been proposed for EP estimation and denoising, e.g. (Cerutti et al., 1987; Delorme & Makeig, 2004; Karjalainen et al., 1999; Li et al., 2009; Quiroga & Garcia, 2003; Ranta-aho et al., 2003). The performance and applicability of every single-trial estimation method depends on the prior information used and the statistical properties of the EP signals. In general, the exploration of single-trial variability in event related experiments is critical for the study of the central nervous system (Debener et al., 2006; Fell, 2007; Makeig et al., 2002). For example, single-trial EPs could be used to study perceptual changes or to reveal complicated cognitive processes, such as memory formation. Here, we focus on the case that some parameters of the EPs change dynamically from stimulus-to-stimulus. This situation could be a trend-like change of the amplitude or latency of some EP component.

The most obvious way to handle time variations between single-trial measurements is sub-averaging of the measurements in groups. Sub-averaging could give optimal estimators if the EPs are assumed to be invariant within the sub-averaged groups. A better approach is to use moving window or exponentially weighted average filters, see for example (Delorme & Makeig, 2004; Doncarli et al., 1992; Thakor et al., 1991). A few adaptive filtering methods have also been proposed for EP estimation, especially for brain stem potential tracking, e.g. (Qiu et al., 2006). The statistical properties of some moving average filters and different recursive estimation methods for EP estimation have been discussed in (Georgiadis et al., 2005b). Some smoothing methods have also been proposed for modeling trial-to-trial variability in EPs (Turetsky et al., 1989). Kalman smoother algorithm for single-trial EP estimation was introduced in (Georgiadis et al., 2005a), see also (Georgiadis, 2007; Georgiadis et al., 2007; 2008).

State-space modeling for single-trial dynamical estimation considers the EP as a vector valued random process with stochastic fluctuations from stimulus-to-stimulus (Georgiadis et al., 2005b). Then past and future realizations contain information of relevance to be used in the estimation procedure. Estimates for the states, that are optimal in the mean square sense, are given by Kalman filter and smoother algorithms. Of importance is the parametrization of the problem and the selection of an observation model for the measurements. For example, in (Georgiadis et al., 2005b; Qiu et al., 2006) generic observation models were used based on time-shifted Gaussian smooth functions. Furthermore, data based observation models can also be used (Georgiadis, 2007).

3. Bayesian formulation of the problem

In this chapter, sequential observations are considered to be available at discrete time instances t. The observation vector z_t is assumed to be related to some unobserved parameter vector (state vector) through some model of the form

$$z_t = h_t(\theta_t, v_t), \tag{1}$$

for every $t = 1, 2, \ldots$. The simplest non stationary process that can serve as a model for the time evolution of the states is the first order Markov process. This can be expressed with the following state equation:

$$\theta_t = f_t(\theta_{t-1}, \omega_t). \tag{2}$$

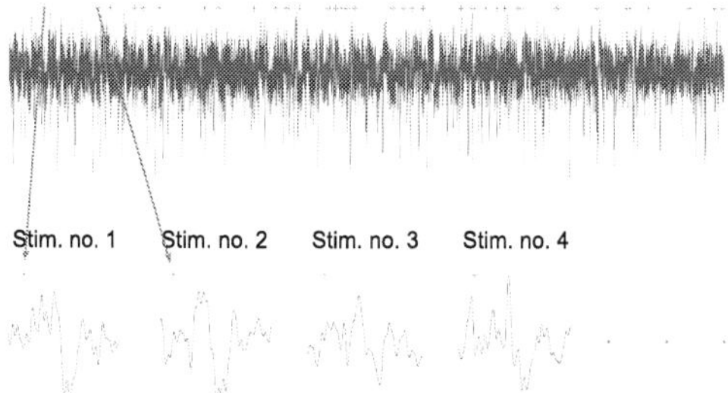

(a) Extracting EEG epochs.

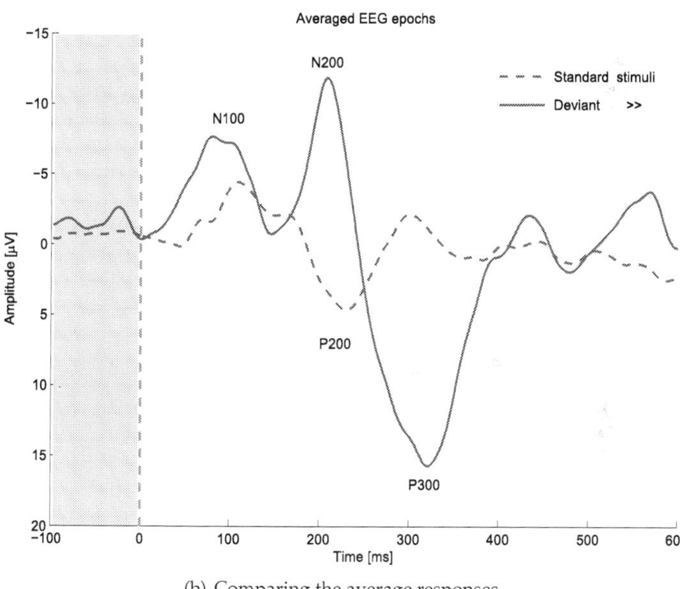

(b) Comparing the average responses.

Fig. 2. Traditional EP analysis for a stimuli discrimination task.

The last two equations form a state-space model for estimation. Other common assumptions made for the model are summarized bellow:

- f_t, h_t are well defined vector valued functions for all t.
- $\{\omega_t\}$ is a sequence of independent random vectors with different distributions, and represents the state noise process.
- $\{v_t\}$ is a white noise vector process, that represents the observation noise.

- The random vectors ω_t, v_t are mutually independent for every t.
- The distributions of ω_t, v_t are known or preselected.
- There is an initial state θ_0 with known distribution.

The previous estimation problem can also be described in a different way. The stochastic process $\{\theta_t\}, \{z_t\}$ are said to form a (first order) evolution-observation pair, if for some random starting point θ_0 and some evolution up to t the following properties hold (Kaipio & Somersalo, 2005):

- The process $\{\theta_t\}$ is a Markov process, that is,

$$p(\theta_t|\theta_{t-1}, \theta_{t-2}, \ldots, \theta_0) = p(\theta_t|\theta_{t-1}). \tag{3}$$

- The process $\{z_t\}$ has the memory-less property (3) with respect to the history of $\{\theta_t\}$, that is,

$$p(z_t|\theta_t, \theta_{t-1}, \theta_{t-2}, \ldots, \theta_0) = p(z_t|\theta_t). \tag{4}$$

- The process $\{\theta_t\}$ depends on the past observations only through its own history, that is,

$$p(\theta_t|\theta_{t-1}, z_{t-1}, z_{t-2}, \ldots, z_1) = p(\theta_t|\theta_{t-1}). \tag{5}$$

An evolution-observation pair can be illustrated with the following dependency scheme:

$$\theta_0 \longrightarrow \theta_1 \longrightarrow \theta_2 \longrightarrow \ldots \longrightarrow \theta_t \longrightarrow \ldots$$
$$\downarrow \qquad \downarrow \qquad \qquad \downarrow$$
$$z_1 \qquad z_2 \qquad \qquad z_t$$

Notice, that as soon as a state-space model is defined for an evolution-observation pair, then the assumptions of the model come in parallel with the above definitions (Kaipio & Somersalo, 2005). Assume that the stochastic processes $\{\theta_t\}, \{z_t\}$ form an evolution-observation pair. Then the following problems are under consideration:

- *Prediction*, that is, the determination of $p(\theta_t|z_{t-1}, z_{t-2}, \ldots, z_1)$.
- *Filtering*, that is, the determination of $p(\theta_t|z_t, z_{t-1}, \ldots, z_1)$.
- *Fixed interval smoothing*, that is, the determination of $p(\theta_t|z_T, \ldots, z_t, \ldots, z_1)$, when a complete measurement sequence is available for $t = 1, 2, \ldots, T$.

Based on the conditional or posterior densities, estimators for the states can be defined in a Bayesian framework. It can also be noticed, that all the above problems are computationally related to the prediction problem as an intermediate step.

4. Dynamical estimation of EPs with a linear state-space model

The sampled potential (from channel l) relative to the successive stimulus or trial t can be denoted with a column vector of length M, i.e. $z_t = (z_t(1), z_t(2), \ldots, z_t(M))^T$ for $t = 1, \ldots, T$, where T is the total number of trials, and $(\cdot)^T$ denotes transposition.

A widely used model for EP estimation is the additive noise model (Karjalainen et al., 1999), that is,

$$z_t = s_t + v_t. \tag{6}$$

The vector s_t corresponds to the part of the activity that is related to the stimulation, and the rest of the activity v_t is usually assumed to be independent of the stimulus. Single-trial EPs can be modeled as a linear combination of some pre-selected basis vectors. Then the model takes the form

$$z_t = H_t \theta_t + v_t, \tag{7}$$

where H_t is the observation matrix, which contains the basis vectors $\psi_{t,1}, \ldots, \psi_{t,k}$ of length M in its columns, and θ_t is a parameter vector of length k. The estimated EPs $\hat{s}_t$ can be obtained by using the estimated parameters $\hat{\theta}_t$ as follows:

$$\hat{s}_t = H_t \hat{\theta}_t. \tag{8}$$

The measurement vectors z_t can be considered as realizations of a stochastic vector process, that depend on some unobserved parameters θ_t (state vectors) through (7). For the time evolution of the hidden process θ_t a linear first order Markov model can be used (Georgiadis et al., 2005b), that is,

$$\theta_t = F_t \theta_{t-1} + \omega_t, \tag{9}$$

with some initial distribution for θ_0. Equations (7), (9) form a linear state-space model, where F_t, H_t are preselected matrices. Other assumptions of the model are that for every $i \neq j$ the observation noise vectors v_i, v_j and the state noise vectors ω_i, ω_j are mutually independent and independent of θ_0.

5. Kalman filter and smoother algorithms

Kalman filtering problem is related to the determination of the mean square estimator $\hat{\theta}_t$ for θ_t given the observations $z_1, \ldots, z_t$ (Kalman, 1960). This is equal to the conditional mean

$$\hat{\theta}_t = E\{\theta_t | z_1, \ldots, z_t\} = E\{\theta_t | Z_t\}. \tag{10}$$

The optimal linear mean square estimator can be obtained recursively by restricting to a linear conditional mean, or by assuming v_t and ω_t to be Gaussian (Sorenson, 1980). The Kalman filter algorithm can be written as follows:

- Initialization

$$C_{\tilde{\theta}_0} = C_{\theta_0} \tag{11}$$
$$\hat{\theta}_0 = E\{\theta_0\} \tag{12}$$

- Prediction step

$$\hat{\theta}_{t|t-1} = F_t \hat{\theta}_{t-1} \tag{13}$$
$$C_{\tilde{\theta}_{t|t-1}} = F_t C_{\tilde{\theta}_{t-1}} F_t^T + C_{\omega_t} \tag{14}$$

- Filtering step

$$K_t = C_{\tilde{\theta}_{t|t-1}} H_t^T (H_t C_{\tilde{\theta}_{t|t-1}} H_t^T + C_{v_t})^{-1} \tag{15}$$
$$\hat{\theta}_t = \hat{\theta}_{t|t-1} + K_t(z_t - H_t \hat{\theta}_{t|t-1}) \tag{16}$$
$$C_{\tilde{\theta}_t} = (I - K_t H_t) C_{\tilde{\theta}_{t|t-1}}, \tag{17}$$

for $t = 1, \ldots, T$. The matrix K_t is the Kalman gain, $\hat{\theta}_{t|t-1}$ is the prediction of θ_t based on $\hat{\theta}_{t-1}$, and $\hat{\theta}_{t-1} = E\{\theta_{t-1}|z_{t-1}, \ldots, z_1\}$ is the optimal estimate at time $t - 1$.

If all the measurements $z_t, t = 1, \ldots, T$ are available, then the fixed interval smoothing problem can be considered, that is,

$$\hat{\theta}_t^s = E\{\theta_t|z_1, \ldots, z_T\} = E\{\theta_t|Z_T\}. \tag{18}$$

The forward-backward method for the smoothing problem (Rauch et al., 1965), which gives the smoother estimates as corrections of the filter estimates is complete through the backward recursion:

- Smoothing

$$A_t = C_{\tilde{\theta}_t} F_{t+1}^T C_{\tilde{\theta}_{t+1|t}}^{-1} \tag{19}$$

$$\hat{\theta}_t^s = \hat{\theta}_t + A_t(\hat{\theta}_{t+1}^s - \hat{\theta}_{t+1|t}) \tag{20}$$

$$C_{\tilde{\theta}_t^s} = C_{\tilde{\theta}_t} + A_t(C_{\tilde{\theta}_{t+1}^s} - C_{\tilde{\theta}_{t+1|t}})A_t^T, \tag{21}$$

for $t = T - 1, T - 2, \ldots, 1$. For initialization of the backward recursion the filter estimates are used, i.e. $\hat{\theta}_T^s = \hat{\theta}_T$.

6. EP estimation based on a generic model

The following state-space model for dynamical estimation of evoked potentials is here considered:

$$\theta_t = \theta_{t-1} + \omega_t \tag{22}$$

$$z_t = H\theta_t + v_t, \tag{23}$$

with the selections $F_t = I, t = 1, \ldots, T$, i.e. a random walk model, and $H_t = H$ for all t.

The observation model can be formed from the impulse response of an FIR filter. Consider a linear (non-causal) finite response filter with impulse function defined by the sequence $\{h(n)\}$ over the interval $-M \leq n \leq M$. For a given input $z_t(n), n = 1, \ldots, M$ the output is given by

$$y_t(n) = \sum_{k=-\infty}^{\infty} h(n-k)z_t(k) = \sum_{k=1}^{M} h(n-k)z_t(k), \tag{24}$$

where $z_t(n) = 0$ for $n < 1$.

The output of the filter $y_t = (y_t(1), y_t(2), \ldots, y_t(n), \ldots, y_t(M))^T$ in terms of the input vector $z_t = (z_t(1), z_t(2), \ldots, z_t(n), \ldots, z_t(M))^T$, for $n = 1, \ldots, M$, is given in a compact matrix form by

$$y_t = \begin{bmatrix} h(0) & h(-1) & \cdots & h(1-M) \\ h(1) & h(0) & \cdots & h(2-M) \\ \vdots & \vdots & \vdots & \vdots \\ h(n-1) & h(n-2) & \cdots & h(n-M) \\ \vdots & \vdots & \vdots & \vdots \\ h(M-1) & h(M-2) & \cdots & h(0) \end{bmatrix} z_t, \tag{25}$$

where the filter operator P, i.e. $y_t = Pz_t$, contains time-shifted versions of the impulse function in its columns. The performance of the filter can be approximated by choosing less vectors to form an observation model H with k columns, selected for $i = 1, \ldots, k$ as

$$\psi_i = (h(-d_i), \ldots, h(M - 1 - d_i))^T, \tag{26}$$

where d_i can be selected based on the values $0, M/(k-1), 2M/(k-1), \ldots, M$. An approximation of the filter performance can be obtained, for example, through the matrix $H(H^T H)^{-1} H^T$ in the ordinary least squares sense. Different observation models, for example, the Gaussian basis (Georgiadis et al., 2005b; Qiu et al., 2006; Ranta-aho et al., 2003), here seen as a low pass filter, can be used.

For the covariances of the state and observation noise processes the choices $C_{\omega_t} = \sigma_\omega^2 I$, $C_{v_t} = \sigma_v^2 I$ for every trial t can be made. Then, the selection of the last variance term is not essential, since only the ratio $\sigma_v^2 / \sigma_\omega^2$ has effect on the estimates. A detailed proof can be found in (Georgiadis et al., 2007). Then the choice $C_{v_t} = I$ can be made, and care should be given to the selection of only one parameter σ_ω^2. In general, if it is tuned too small fast fluctuation of EPs are going to be lost, and if it is selected too big the estimates have too much variance. The selection can be based on experience and visual inspection of the estimates as a balance between preserving expected dynamic variability and greater noise reduction. Extensive discussion and examples related to the selection of this parameter can be found in (Georgiadis, 2007; Georgiadis et al., 2005b; 2007).

7. Examples

7.1 Amplitude variability

In this example, measurements were obtained from an EP experiment with visual stimulation. 310 fixed intensity flash stimuli (red squares) were presented to the subject through a monitor (screen 36.5 x 27.6 cm, distance 1 m). The stimuli were randomly presented every 1.5s (from 1.3s to 1.7s) and their duration was 0.3s. The measurement device was BrainAmp MR plus and the sampling rate was $Fs = 5000$Hz. Prior to the estimation procedure the EEG channels were band pass filtered with pass band 1-500Hz. Then epochs of 0.5s relative to the presentation of stimuli were sampled from channel Oz. All the epochs were kept for estimation.

The observation model was created based on a low pass FIR filter with impulse response obtained by truncating an ideal low pass filter (sinc function) with a Hanning window. The cut-off frequency was selected to be $f_c = 20$Hz and the number of vectors was selected to be $k = 21$. The empirical rule:

$$k = \left[\frac{f_c}{F_s/2} M \right] + 1, \tag{27}$$

where $[\cdot]$ denotes integer part, seemed to produce good values for k for different values of F_s, f_c, M. The selected observation model is illustrated in Figure 3, where the columns of the matrix H are represented as rows in an image plot.

Kalman filter and smoother estimates were computed for the model (22), (23) with the selection $\sigma_\omega^2 = 1$. The value was chosen empirically by visual examination of the estimates. For initialization of the algorithms, half of the measurements were used in a backward recursion with Kalman filter algorithm. The last (converged) estimates were used to initialize the Kalman filter forward run. For the initialization of the final backward recursion (Kalman smoother) the filter estimates were used.

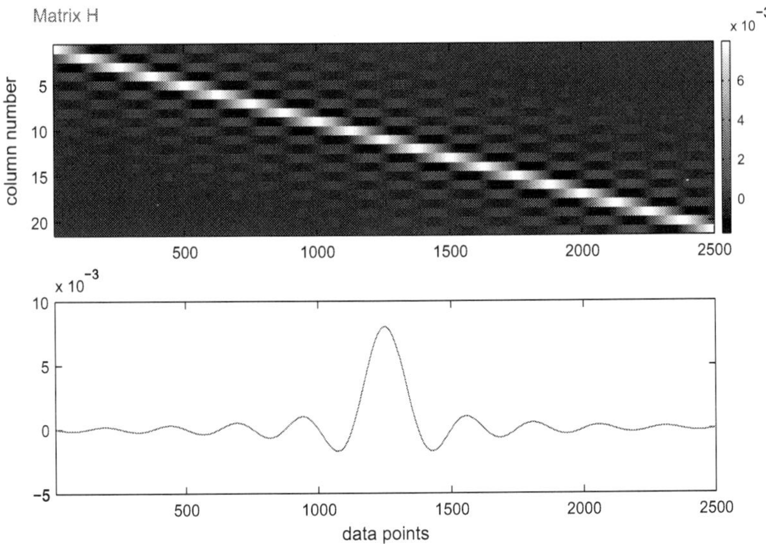

Fig. 3. The selected observation model. Up: the columns of the matrix H as rows in an image plot. Down: the 11th column.

Figure 4 (top, left) shows the noisy EP measurements as an image plot. The positive dominant peak, here occurring about 160 ms after visual stimulation, is visible at the center of the image. The obtained estimates are presented in the same figure for Kalman filter (top, right) and smoother (bottom left). The averaged EPs obtained from the raw measurements and from the estimates are also seen in the middle of the figure. The positive dominant peak can be observed from this plot. Clearly, the time variation of the EPs is revealed. A decrease in amplitude of the dominant positive peak is clearly observable, suggesting possible habituation to the stimuli presentation. The amplitude of the peak, estimated simply as the maximum value within the time interval 100-200ms after the presentation of the stimuli, is also plotted as a function of the successive stimulus t. Furthermore, the time-varying latency of the peak is presented. From these plots it can be easier observed the gradual decrease of the amplitude. Finally, the improvement due to the smoothing procedure is visible. The smoother algorithm cancels the time-lag of the filtering procedure. In parallel, it removes greater the noise, thus improving the latency estimation, especially for the very weak evoked potentials.

7.2 Latency variability

In this example, measurements related to the P300 event related potential were used. The P300 peak is one of the most extensively studied cognitive potential and there exist many studies where the trial-to-trial variability of the component is discussed, for example, (Holm et al., 2006).

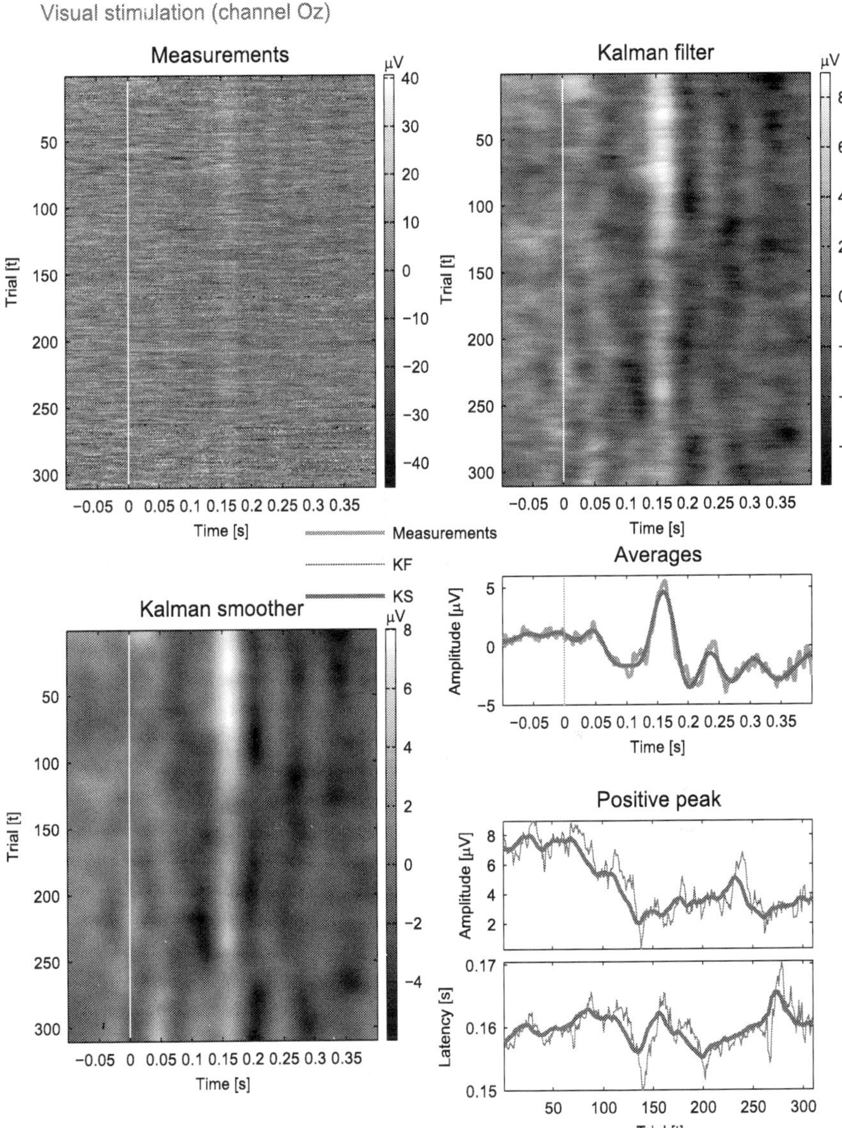

Fig. 4. Single-trial EP amplitude variability.

EEG measurements were obtained from a standard oddball paradigm with auditory stimulation. During the recording, 569 auditory stimuli were presented with an inter-stimulus interval of 1s, 85% of the stimuli at 800Hz and randomly presented 15% deviant tones at 560Hz. The subject was sitting in a chair and was asked to press a button every time he heard the deviant target tone. The sampling rate of the EEG was 500 Hz. From the recordings, channel Cz was selected for analysis, after bandpass filtering in the range 1-40Hz. Average responses from the two conditions are shown in Figure 2 (Section 2). For investigation of the single trial variability of the P300 peak, EEG epochs from -100 ms to 600 ms relative to the stimulus onset of each deviant stimulus were here used.

The model was designed as in section 7.1 but now for the slower P300 wave the selection $f_c = 10$Hz was made. The application of the empirical rule (27) gave in this case $k = 15$. Kalman smoother estimates were computed with the selection $\sigma_\omega^2 = 9$, with respect to the expected faster variability of the potential.

In Figure 5 (I) there are presented the EP measurements in the original stimulus order (trial-by-trial). In the same figure (II) the obtained estimates based on the measurements (I) are shown. Clearly, in the estimates, the dynamic variability of the P300 peak potential is revealed, suggesting that it cannot be considered as occurring at fixed latency from the stimuli presentation. At the same image (II), the estimated latency is also plotted as a function of the consecutive trial t. The latency of the peak was estimated from the Kalman smoother estimates based on the maximum value within the time interval 250-370ms after the presentation of the stimuli.

The estimated time-varying latency of the P300 peak was then used to order the single-trial measurements. The sorted single-trials (condition-by-condition) are shown at Figure 5 (III). The shorted latency estimates are plotted again over the image plot. This plot clearly demonstrates that the latency estimates obtained with Kalman smoother are of acceptable accuracy.

Finally, the algorithm was also applied to the sorted measurements (III). The value $\sigma_\omega^2 = 4$ was selected and new point estimates for the latency were obtained as before. Kalman smoother estimates and the new latency estimates are plotted in Figure 5 (IV). The linear trend of the sorted potentials allows the use of even smaller value for state-noise variance parameter (Georgiadis et al., 2005b), thus reducing even more the noise without reducing the variability of the peak. The last obtained estimates of the latencies were plotted over the original non sorted measurements (I). The similarities between the estimated latency fluctuations in (I) and (II) underline the robustness of the method.

8. Conclusion and Future Directions

EP research has to deal with several inherent difficulties. Traditional analysis is based on averaged data often by forming extra grand averages of different populations. Thus, trial-to-trial variability and individual subject characteristics are largely ignored (Fell, 2007). Therefore, the study of isolated components retrieved by averages might be misleading, or at least it is a simplification of the reality. For example, habituation may occur and the responses could be different from the beginning to the end of the recording session. Furthermore, cognitive potentials exhibit rich latency and amplitude variability that traditional research based on averaging is not able to exploit for studying complex cognitive processes. Latency variability could be used, for instance, for studying perceptual changes, quantifying stimulus classification speed or task difficulty.

In this chapter, state-space modeling for single-trial estimation of EPs was presented in its general form based on Bayesian estimation theory. This formulation enables the selection of different models for dynamical estimation. In general, the applicability of the proposed

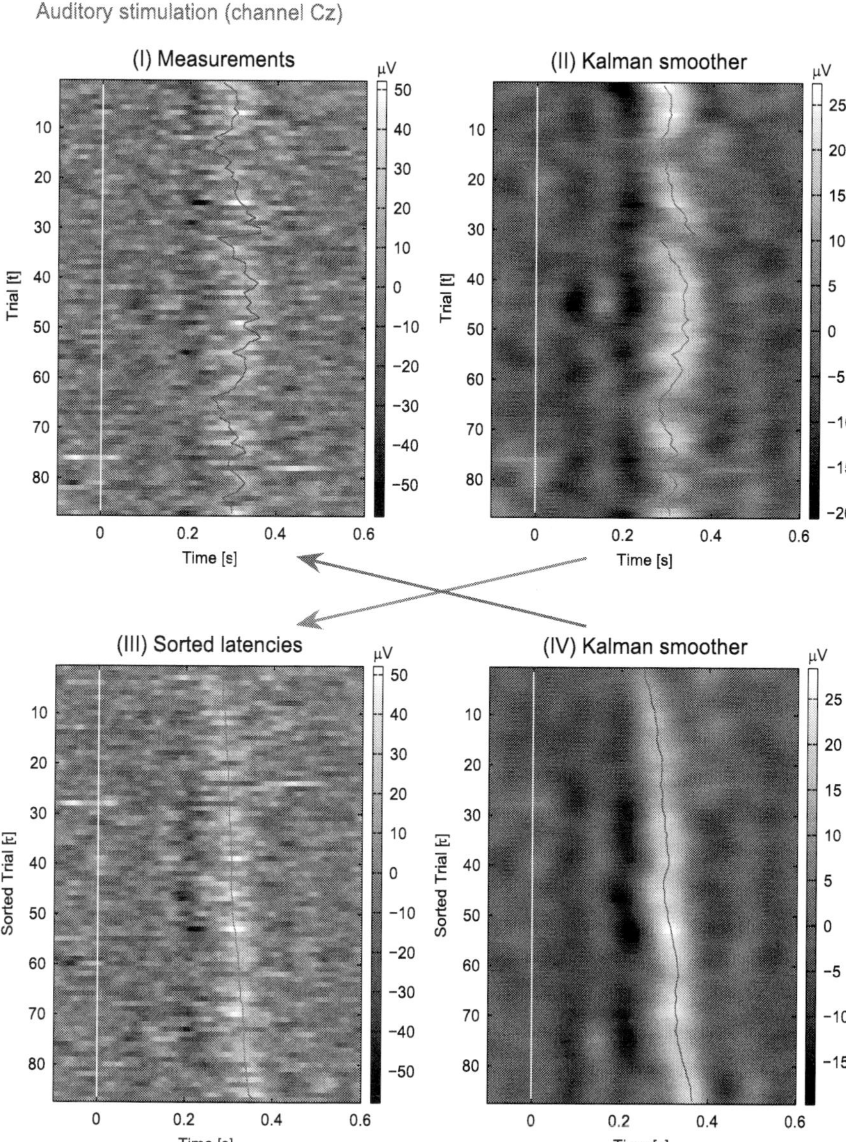

Fig. 5. Single-trial EP latency variability.

methodology primarily relates on the assumption of hidden dynamic variability from trial-to-trial or from condition-to-condition. A practical method for designing an observation model was also presented and its capability to reveal meaningful amplitude and latency fluctuations in EP measurements was demonstrated. In the approach, optimal estimates for the states are obtained with Kalman filter and smoother algorithms. When all the measurements are available (batch processing) Kalman smoother should be used.

EPs also contain rich spatial information that can be used for describing brain dynamics (Makeig et al., 2004; Ranta-aho et al., 2003). In this study, this important issue was not discussed and emphasis was given on optimal estimation of some temporal EP characteristics. Future development of the presented methodology involves the extension of the approach to multichannel and multimodal data sets, for instance, simultaneously measured EEG/ERP and fMRI/BOLD signals (Debener et al., 2006), for the study of dynamic changes of the central nervous system.

Acknowledgments

The authors acknowledge financial support from the Academy of Finland (project numbers: 123579, 1.1.2008-31.12.2011, and 126873, 1.1.2009-31.12.2011).

9. References

Cerutti, S., Bersani, V., Carrara, A. & Liberati, D. (1987). Analysis of visual evoked potentials through Wiener filtering applied to a small number of sweeps, *Journal of Biomedical Engineering* **9**(1): 3–12.

Debener, S., Ullsperger, M., Siegel, M. & Engel, A. (2006). Single-trial EEG-fMRI reveals the dynamics of cognitive function, *Trends in Cognitive Sciences* **10**(2): 558–63.

Delorme, A. & Makeig, S. (2004). EEGLAB: an open source toolbox for analysis of single-trial EEG dynamics including independent component analysis, *Journal of Neuroscience Methods* **134**(1): 9–21.

Doncarli, C., Goering, L. & Guiheneuc, P. (1992). Adaptive smoothing of evoked potentials, *Signal Processing* **28**(1): 63–76.

Fell, J. (2007). Cognitive neurophysiology: Beyond averaging, *NeuroImage* **37**: 1069–1027.

Georgiadis, S. (2007). *State-Space Modeling and Bayesian Methods for Evoked Potential Estimation*, PhD thesis, Kuopio University Publications C. Natural and Environmental Sciences 213. (available: http://bsamig.uku.fi/).

Georgiadis, S., Ranta-aho, P., Tarvainen, M. & Karjalainen, P. (2005a). Recursive mean square estimators for single-trial event related potentials, *Proc. Finnish Signal Processing Symposium - FINSIG'05*, Kuopio, Finland.

Georgiadis, S., Ranta-aho, P., Tarvainen, M. & Karjalainen, P. (2005b). Single-trial dynamical estimation of event related potentials: a Kalman filter based approach, *IEEE Transactions on Biomedical Engineering* **52**(8): 1397–1406.

Georgiadis, S., Ranta-aho, P., Tarvainen, M. & Karjalainen, P. (2007). A subspace method for dynamical estimation of evoked potentials, *Computational Intelligence and Neuroscience* **2007**: Article ID 61916, 11 pages.

Georgiadis, S., Ranta-aho, P., Tarvainen, M. & Karjalainen, P. (2008). Tracking single-trial evoked potential changes with Kalman filtering and smoothing, *30th Annual International Conference of the IEEE Engineering in Medicine and Biology Society*, Vancouver, Canada, pp. 157–160.

Holm, A., Ranta-aho, P., Sallinen, M., Karjalainen, P. & Müller, K. (2006). Relationship of P300 single trial responses with reaction time and preceding stimulus sequence, *International Journal of Psychophysiology* **61**(2): 244–252.

Intriligator, J. & Polich, J. (1994). On the relationship between background EEG and the P300 event-related potential, *Biological Psychology* **37**(3): 207–218.

Jansen, B., Agarwal, G., Hegde, A. & Boutros, N. (2003). Phase synchronization of the ongoing EEG and auditory EP generation, *Clinical Neurophysiology* **114**(1): 79–85.

Kaipio, J. & Somersalo, E. (2005). *Statistical and Computational Inverse Problems*, Applied Mathematical Sciences, Springer.

Kalman, R. (1960). A new approach to linear filtering and prediction problems, *Transactions of the ASME, Journal of Basic Engineering* **82**: 35–45.

Karjalainen, P., Kaipio, J., Koistinen, A. & Vauhkonen, M. (1999). Subspace regularization method for the single trial estimation of evoked potentials, *IEEE Transactions on Biomedical Engineering* **46**(7): 849–860.

Knuth, K., Shah, A., Truccolo, W., Ding, M., Bressler, S. & Schroeder, C. (2006). Differentially variable component analysis (dVCA): Identifying multiple evoked components using trial-to-trial variability, *Journal of Neurophysiology* **95**(5): 3257–3276.

Li, R., Principe, J., Bradley, M. & Ferrari, V. (2009). A spatiotemporal filtering methodology for single-trial ERP component estimation, *IEEE Transactions on Biomedical Engineering* **56**(1): 83–92.

Makeig, S., Debener, S. & Delorme, A. (2004). Mining event-related brain dynamics, *Trends in Cognitive Science* **8**(5): 204–210.

Makeig, S., Westerfield, M., Jung, T.-P., Enghoff, S., Townsend, J., Courchesne, E. & Sejnowski, T. (2002). Dynamic brain sources of visual evoked responses, *Science* **295**: 690–694.

Mäkinen, V., Tiitinen, H. & May, P. (2005). Auditory even-related responses are generated independently of ongoing brain activity, *NeuroImage* **24**(4): 961–968.

Malmivuo, J. & Plonsey, R. (1995). *Bioelectromagnetism*, Oxford university press, New York.

Niedermeyer, E. & da Silva, F. L. (eds) (1999). *Electroencephalography: Basic Principles, Clinical Applications, and Related Fields*, 4th edn, Williams and Wilkins.

Qiu, W., Chang, C., Lie, W., Poon, P., Lam, F., Hamernik, R., Wei, G. & Chan, F. (2006). Real-time data-reusing adaptive learning of a radial basis function network for tracking evoked potentials, *IEEE Transanctions on Biomedical Engineering* **53**(2): 226–237.

Quiroga, R. Q. & Garcia, H. (2003). Single-trial evoked potentials with wavelet denoising, *Clinical Neurophysiology* **114**: 376–390.

Ranta-aho, P., Koistinen, A., Ollikainen, J., Kaipio, J., Partanen, J. & Karjalainen, P. (2003). Single-trial estimation of multichannel evoked-potential measurements, *IEEE Transactions on Biomedical Engineering* **50**(2): 189–196.

Rauch, H., Tung, F. & Striebel, C. (1965). Maximum likelihood estimates of linear dynamic systems, *AIAA Journal* **3**: 1445–1450.

Sorenson, H. (1980). *Parameter Estimation, Principles and Problems*, Vol. 9 of *Control and Systems Theory*, Marcel Dekker Inc., New York.

Thakor, N., Vaz, C., McPherson, R. & Hanley, D. F. (1991). Adaptive Fourier series modeling of time-varying evoked potentials: Study of human somatosensory evoked response to etomidate anesthetic, *Electroencephalography and Clinical Neurophysiology* **80**(2): 108–118.

Truccolo, W., Mingzhou, D., Knuth, K., Nakamura, R. & Bressler, S. (2002). Trial-to-trial variability of cortical evoked responses: implications for the analysis of functional connectivity, *Clinical Neurophysiology* **113**(2): 206–226.

Turetsky, B., Raz, J. & Fein, G. (1989). Estimation of trial-to-trial variation in evoked potential signals by smoothing across trials, *Psychophysiology* **26**(6): 700–712.

3

Non-Stationary Biosignal Modelling

Carlos S. Lima, Adriano Tavares, José H. Correia,
Manuel J. Cardoso[1] and Daniel Barbosa
University of Minho
Portugal
[1]University College of London
England

1. Introduction

Signals of biomedical nature are in the most cases characterized by short, impulse-like events that represent transitions between different phases of a biological cycle. As an example hearth sounds are essentially events that represent transitions between the different hemodynamic phases of the cardiac cycle. Classical techniques in general analyze the signal over long periods thus they are not adequate to model impulse-like events. High variability and the very often necessity to combine features temporally well localized with others well localized in frequency remains perhaps the most important challenges not yet completely solved for the most part of biomedical signal modeling. Wavelet Transform (WT) provides the ability to localize the information in the time-frequency plane; in particular, they are capable of trading on type of resolution for the other, which makes them especially suitable for the analysis of non-stationary signals.

State of the art automatic diagnosis algorithms usually rely on pattern recognition based approaches. Hidden Markov Models (HMM's) are statistically based pattern recognition techniques with the ability to break a signal in almost stationary segments in a framework known as quasi-stationary modeling. In this framework each segment can be modeled by classical approaches, since the signal is considered stationary in the segment, and at a whole a quasi-stationary approach is obtained.

Recently Discrete Wavelet Transform (DWT) and HMM's have been combined as an effort to increase the accuracy of pattern recognition based approaches regarding automatic diagnosis purposes. Two main motivations have been appointed to support the approach. Firstly, in each segment the signal can not be exactly stationary and in this situation the DWT is perhaps more appropriate than classical techniques that usually considers stationarity. Secondly, even if the process is exactly stationary over the entire segment the capacity given by the WT of simultaneously observing the signal at various scales (at different levels of focus), each one emphasizing different characteristics can be very beneficial regarding classification purposes.

This chapter presents an overview of the various uses of the WT and HMM's in Computer Assisted Diagnosis (CAD) in medicine. Their most important properties regarding biomedical applications are firstly described. The analogy between the WT and some of the biological processing that occurs in the early components of the visual and auditory systems, which partially supports the WT applications in medicine is shortly described. The use of the WT in the analyses of 1-D physiological signals especially electrocardiography (ECG) and phonocardiography (PCG) are then reviewed. A survey of recent wavelet developments in medical imaging is then provided. These include biomedical image processing algorithms as noise reduction, image enhancement and detection of micro-calcifications in mammograms, image reconstruction and acquisition schemes as tomography and Magnetic Resonance Imaging (MRI), and multi-resolution methods for the registration and statistical analysis of functional images of the brain as positron emission tomography (PET) and functional MRI.

The chapter provides an almost complete theoretical explanation of HMMs. Then a review of HMMs in electrocardiography and phonocardiography is given. Finally more recent approaches involving both WT and HMMs specifically in electrocardiography and phonocardiography are reviewed.

2. Wavelets and biomedical signals

Biomedical applications usually require most sophisticated signal processing techniques than others fields of engineering. The information of interest is often a combination of features that are well localized in space and time. Some examples are spikes and transients in electroencephalograph signals and microcalcifications in mammograms and others more diffuse as texture, small oscillations and bursts. This universe of events at opposite extremes in the time-frequency localization can not be efficiently handled by classical signal processing techniques mostly based on the Fourier analysis. In the past few years, researchers from mathematics and signal processing have developed the concept of multiscale representation for signal analysis purposes (Vetterli & Kovacevic, 1995). These wavelet based representations have over the traditional Fourier techniques the advantage of localize the information in the time-frequency plane. They are capable of trading one type of resolution for the other, which makes them especially suitable for modelling non-stationary events. Due to these characteristics of the WT and the difficult conditions frequently encountered in biomedical signal analysis, WT based techniques proliferated in medical applications ranging from the more traditional physiological signals such as ECG to the most recent imaging modalities as PET and MRI. Theoretically wavelet analysis is a reasonably complicated mathematical discipline, at least for most biomedical engineers, and consequently a detailed analysis of this technique is out of the scope of this chapter. The interested reader can find detailed references such as (Vetterli & Kovacevic, 1995) and (Mallat, 1998). The purpose of this chapter is only to emphasize the wavelet properties more related to current biomedical applications.

2.1 The wavelet transform - An overview

The wavelet transform (WT) is a signal representation in a scale-time space, where each scale represents a focus level of the signal and therefore can be seen as a result of a band-pass filtering.

Given a time-varying signal x(t), WTs are a set of coefficients that are inner products of the signal with a family of *wavelets* basis functions obtained from a standard function known as

mother wavelet. In Continuous Wavelet Transform (CWT) the wavelet corresponding to scale
s and time location τ is given by

$$\psi_{\tau,s} = \frac{1}{\sqrt{|s|}} \psi\left(\frac{t-\tau}{s}\right) \tag{1}$$

where $\psi(t)$ is the mother wavelet, which can be viewed as a band-pass function. The term
$\sqrt{|s|}$ ensures energy preservation. In the CWT the time-scale parameters vary continuously.
The wavelet transform of a continuous time varying signal $x(t)$ is given by

$$\Psi_X^{\psi}(\tau,s) = \frac{1}{\sqrt{|s|}} \int_{-\infty}^{+\infty} x(t)\psi^*\left(\frac{t-\tau}{s}\right) dt \tag{2}$$

where the asterisk stands for complex conjugate. Equation (2) shows that the WT is the
convolution between the signal and the wavelet function at scale s. For a fixed value of the
scale parameter s, the WT which is now a function of the continuous shift parameter τ, can
be written as a convolution equation where the filter corresponds to a rescaled and time-
reversed version of the wavelet as shown by equation (1) setting $t=0$. From the time scaling
property of the Fourier Transform the frequency response of the wavelet filter is given by

$$\frac{1}{\sqrt{|s|}} \psi\left(-\frac{\tau}{s}\right) \qquad \leftrightarrow \qquad \sqrt{|s|}\Psi^*(s\omega) \tag{3}$$

One important property of the wavelet filter is that for a discrete set of scales, namely the
dyadic scale $s = 2^i$ a constant-Q filterbank is obtained, where the quality factor of the filter is
defined as the central frequency to bandwidth ratio. Therefore WT provides a
decomposition of a signal into subbands with a bandwidth that increases linearly with the
frequency. Under this framework the WT can be viewed as a special kind of spectral
analyser. Energy estimates in different bands or related measures can discriminate between
various physiological states (Akay & al. 1994). Under this approach, the purpose is to
analyse turbulent hearth sounds to detect coronary artery disease. The purpose of the
approach followed by (Akay & Szeto 1994) is to characterize the states of fetal electrocortical
activity. However, this type of global feature extraction assumes stationarity, therefore
similar results can also be obtained using more conventional Fourier techniques. Wavelets
viewed as a filterbank have motivated several approaches based on reversible wavelet
decomposition such as noise reduction and image enhancement algorithms. The principle is
to handle selectively the wavelet components prior to reconstruction. (Mallat & Zhong,
1992) used such a filterbank system to obtain a multiscale edge representation of a signal
from its wavelets maxima. They proposed an iterative algorithm that reconstructs a very
close approximation of the original from this subset of features. This approach has been
adapted for noise reduction in evoked response potentials and in MR images and also in
image enhancement regarding the detection of microcalcifications in mammograms.

From the filterbank point of view the shape of the mother wavelet seems to be important in order to emphasize some signal characteristics, however this topic is not explored in the ambit of the present chapter.

Regarding implementation issues both s and τ must be discretized. The most usual way to sample the time-scale plane is on a so-called *dyadic* grid, meaning that sampled points in the time-scale plane are separated by a power of two. This procedure leads to an increase in computational efficiency for both WT and Inverse Wavelet Transform (IWT). Under this constraint the Discrete Wavelet Transform (DWT) is defined as

$$\psi_{j,k}(t) = s_0^{-j/2} \psi\left(s_0^{-j} t - k\tau_0\right) \tag{4}$$

which means that DWT coefficients are sampled from CWT coefficients. As a dyadic scale is used and therefore $s_0=2$ and $\tau_0=1$, yielding $s=2^j$ and $\tau=k2^j$ where j and k are integers.

As the scale represents the level of focus from the which the signal is viewed, which is related to the frequency range involved, the digital filter banks are appropriated to break the signal in different scales (bands). If the progression in the scale is *dyadic* the signal can be sequentially half-band high-pass and low-pass filtered.

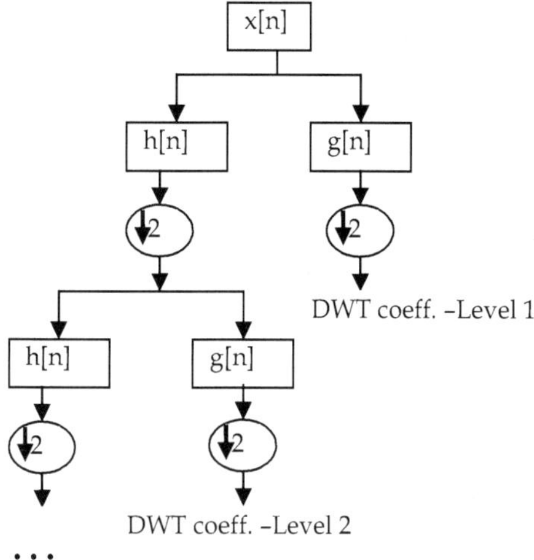

Fig. 1. Wavelet decomposition tree

The output of the high-pass filter represents the detail of the signal. The output of the low-pass filter represents the approximation of the signal for each decomposition level, and will be decomposed in its detail and approximation components at the next decomposition level. The process proceeds iteratively in a scheme known as wavelet decomposition tree, which is shown in figure 1. After filtering, half of the samples can be eliminated according to the Nyquist's rule, since the signal now has only half of the frequency.

This very practical filtering algorithm yields as Fast Wavelet Transform (FWT) and is known in the signal processing community as two-channel subband coder.

One important property of the DWT is the relationship between the impulse responses of the high-pass (g[n]) and low-pass (h[n]) filters, which are not independent of each other and are related by

$$g[L-1-n]=(-1)^n h[n]$$

(5)

where L is the filter length in number of points. Since the two filters are odd index alternated reversed versions of each other they are known as Quadrature Mirror Filters (QMF). Perfect reconstruction requires, in principle, ideal half-band filtering. Although it is not possible to realize ideal filters, under certain conditions it is possible to find filters that provide perfect reconstruction. Perhaps the most famous were developed by Ingrid Daubechies and are known as Daubechies' wavelets. This processing scheme is extended to image processing where temporal filters are changed by spatial filters and filtering is usually performed in three directions; horizontal, vertical and diagonal being the filtering in the diagonal direction obtained from high pass filters in both directions.

Wavelet properties can also be viewed as other approaches than filterbanks. As a multiscale matched filter WT have been successful applied for events detection in biomedical signal processing. The matched filter is the optimum detector of a deterministic signal in the presence of additive noise. Considering a measure model $f(t)=\psi_s(t-\Delta t)+n(t)$ where $\psi_s(t)=\psi(t/s)$ is a known deterministic signal at scale s, Δt is an unknown location parameter and $n(t)$ an additive white Gaussian noise component. The maximum likelihood solution based on classical detection theory states that the optimum procedure for estimating Δt is to perform the correlations with all possible shifts of the reference template (convolution) and to select the position that corresponds to the maximum output. Therefore, using a WT-like detector whenever the pattern that we are looking for appears at various scales makes some sense.

Under correlated situations a pre-whitening filter can be applied and the problem can be solved as in the white noise case. In some noise conditions, specifically if the noise has a fractional Brownian motion structure then the wavelet-like structure of the detector is preserved. In this condition the noise average spectrum has the form $N(w)=\sigma^2/|w|^\alpha$ with $a=2H+1$ with H as the Hurst exponent and the optimum pre-whitening matched filter at scale s as

$$(-j)^\alpha D^\alpha \psi_s(t)=C_s\psi\left(t/s\right)$$

(6)

where D^α is the αth derivative operator which corresponds to $(jw)^\alpha$ in the Fourier domain. In other words, the real valued wavelet $\psi(t)$ is proportional to the fractional derivative of the pattern ψ that must be detected. For example the optimal detector for finding a Gaussian in $O(w^{-2})$ noise is the second derivative of a Gaussian known as Mexican hat wavelet. Several biomedical signal processing tasks have been based on the detection properties of the WT such as the detection of interictal spikes in EEG recordings of epileptic patients or cardiology based applications as the detection of the QRS complex in ECG (Li & Zheng, 1993). This last application also exploits the ability of the WT to characterize singularities through the decay of the wavelet coefficients across scale. Detection of microcalcifications in mammograms is another application that successfully uses the detection properties of the WT (Strickland & Hahn, 1994).

2.2 2D Wavelet Transform

The reasoning explained in section 2.1 can be extended to the bi-dimensional space and applied to image processing. Mallat (Mallat 1989) introduced a very elegant extension of the concepts of multi-resolution decomposition to image processing. The proposed key idea is to expand the application of 1D filterbanks to the 2D in straightforward manner, applying the designed filters to the columns and to the rows separately. The orthogonal wavelet representation of an image can be described as the following recursive convolution and decimation

$$A_n(i,j) = [H_c * [H_r * A_{n-1}]_{\downarrow 2,1}]_{\downarrow 1,2} \qquad D_{n1}(i,j) = [H_c * [G_r * A_{n-1}]_{\downarrow 2,1}]_{\downarrow 1,2}$$

$$D_{n2}(i,j) = [G_c * [H_r * A_{n-1}]_{\downarrow 2,1}]_{\downarrow 1,2} \qquad D_{n3}(i,j) = [G_c * [G_r * A_{n-1}]_{\downarrow 2,1}]_{\downarrow 1,2} \tag{7}$$

where $(i,j) \in R^2$, * denotes the convolution operator, $\downarrow 2,1$ ($\downarrow 1,2$) sub-sampling along the rows (columns) and $A_0 = I(x,y)$ is the original image. H and G are low and band pass quadrature mirror filters, respectively. A_n is obtained by low pass filtering leading to a less detailed/approximation image, at scale n. The D_{ni} are obtained by band pass filtering in a specific direction, therefore encoding details in different directions. Thus these parameters contain directional detail information at scale n. This recursive filtering is no more than the extension of the scheme represented in figure 1 to a bi-dimensional space as shown in figure 2.

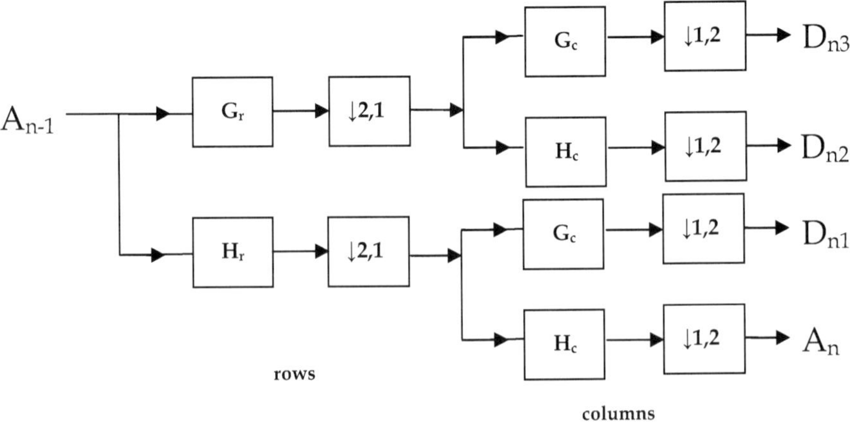

Fig. 2. Wavelet 2D decomposition tree

This 2D implementation is therefore a recursive one-dimensional convolution of the low and band pass filters with the rows and columns of the image, followed by the respective subsampling. One can note that the 2D DWT decomposition is the result at each considered scale, in subbands of different frequency content or detail, in the different orientations. A good example is illustrated in figure 3.

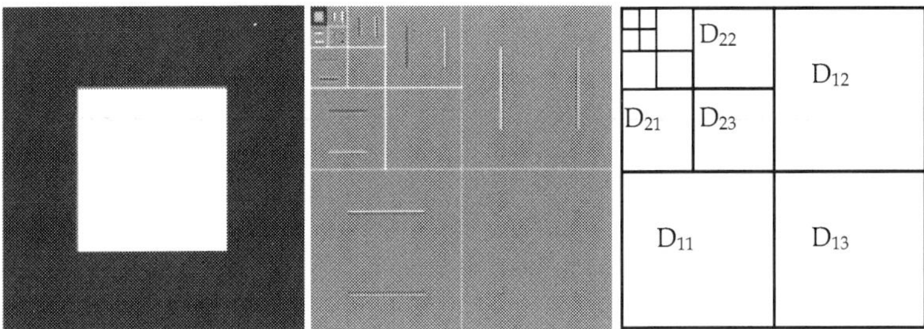

Fig. 3. Decomposition of 2D DWT in sub-bands

The application of a 2D DWT decomposition to an image of N by N pixels returns N by N wavelet coefficients, being therefore a compact representation of the original image. Furthermore, the key information will be sparsely represented, which will be the driving force for compression schemes based on DWT. The reconstruction of the image is possible through the application of the previous filterbank in the opposite direction.

2.3 Time-Frequency Localization and Wavelets

Most biomedical signals of interest include a combination of impulse-like events such as spikes and transients and also more diffuse oscillations such as murmurs and EEG waveforms which may all convey important information for the clinician and consequently regarding automatic diagnosis purposes. Classical methods based on Short Time Fourier Transform (STFT) are well adapted for the later type of events but are much less suited for the analysis of short duration pulses. Hence when both types of events are present in the data the STFT is not completely adequate to offer a reasonable compromise in terms of localization in time and frequency. The main difference of STFT and WT is that in the latter the size of the analysis window is not constant. It varies in inverse proportion of the frequency so that $s = w_0 / w$ where w_0 is the central wavelet frequency. This property enables the WT to zoom in on details, but at the expense of a corresponding loss in spectral resolution. This trade off between localization in time and localization in frequency represents the well known uncertainty principle. In this the name time-frequency analysis corresponds to the trade off between time and space to achieve a better adaptation to the characteristics of the signal.

The Morlet or Gabor wavelet given by

$$\psi(t) = e^{jw_0 t} e^{-t^2/2} \tag{8}$$

has the best time-frequency localization in the sense of the uncertainty principle since the standard deviation of its Gaussian envelope is $\sigma = s$. Its Fourier transform is also a Gaussian function with a central frequency $w = w_0/s$ and a standard deviation $\sigma_w = 1/s$. Thus each analysis template tends to be predominantly located in a certain elliptical region of the time frequency plane. The same qualitative behaviour also applies for other nongaussian wavelet functions. The area of these localization regions is the same for all templates and is constrained by the uncertainty principle as shown in figure 4.

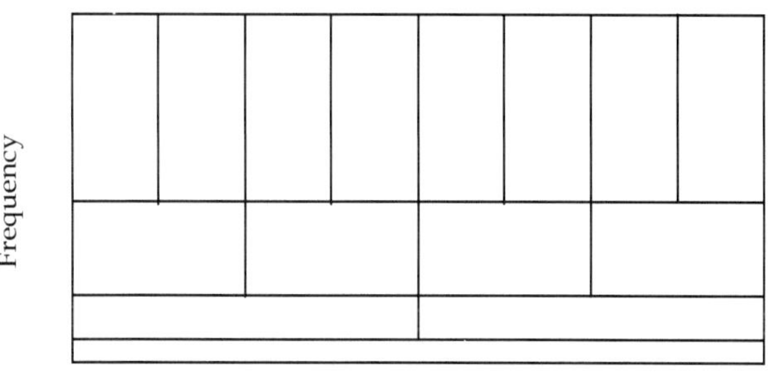

Fig. 4. Time-frequency resolution of the WT

Thus a characterization of the time frequency content of a signal can be obtained by measuring the correlation between the signal and each wavelet template. This reasoning can be extended to image processing where time is replaced by space.

Time frequency wavelet analysis have been used in the characterization of heart beat sounds (Khadra et al.1991, Obaidat 1993, Debbal & Bereksi-Reguig 2004, Debbal & Bereksi-Reguig 2007), the analysis of ECG signals including the detection of late ventricular potentials (Khadra et al. 1993, Dickhaus et al. 1994, Senhadji et al. 1995), the analysis of EEG's (Schiff et al. 1994, Kalayci & Ozdamar 1995) as well as a variety of other physiological signals (Sartene et al. 1994).

2.4 Perception and Wavelets

It is interesting to note that the WT and some of the biological information processing occurring in the first stages of the auditory and visual perception systems are quite similar. This similarity supports the use of wavelet derived methods for low-level auditory and visual sensory processing (Wang & Shamma 1995, Mallat 1989).

Regarding auditory systems, the analysis of acoustic signals in the brain involves two main functional components: 1) the early auditory system which includes the outer ear, middle ear, inner ear or the cochlea and the cochlear nucleus and 2) the central auditory system, which consists of a highly organized neural network in the cortex. Acoustic pressures impinging the outer ear are transmitted to the inner ear, transduced into neural electrical impulses, which are further transformed and processed in the central auditory system. The analysis of sounds in the early and central systems involves a series of processing stages that behave like WT's. In particular it is well known that the cochlea transforms the acoustic pressure $p(t)$ received from the middle ear into displacements $y(t,x)$ of its basilar membrane given by $y(t,x)=p(t) * h(t,x)$ where x is the curvilinear coordinate along the cochlea, $h(t,x)=h(ct/x)$ is the cochlear band-pass filter located at x and c the propagation velocity (Yang et al. 1992, Wang & Shamma 1995). Hence $y(t,x)$ is simply the CWT of $p(t)$ with the wavelet $h(t)$ at a time scale proportional to the position x/c. New Engineering applications for the detection, transmission and coding of auditory signals has been inspired in this WT property (Benedetto & Teolis 1993).

Also the visual system includes, among other complex functional units, an important population of neurons that have wavelet-like properties. These are the so-called simple cells of the occipital cortex, which receive information from the retina through the lateral geniculate nucleus and send projections to the complex and hypercomplex cells of the primary and associative visual cortices. Simple cortical cells have been characterized by their frequency response which is a directional bandpass, with a radial bandwidth almost proportional to the central frequency (constant-Q analysis) (Valois & Valois 1988). Topographically, these neurons are organized in such a way that a common preferential orientation is shared, which is not unlike wavelet channels. The receptive fields of these cells, which is the corresponding area on the retina that produces a response, consist of distinct elongated excitatory and inhibitory zones of a given size and orientation being their response approximately linear (Hubel 1982). The spatial responses of individual cells are well represented by modulated Gaussians (Marcelja 1980). Based on these properties, a variety of multichannel neural models consisting of a set of directional Gabor filters with a hierarchical wavelet based organization have been formulated (Daugman 1988, Daugman 1989, Porat & Zeevi 1989, Watson 1987). Simpler decompositions wavelet based analyses have also been considered (Gaudart et al. 1993).

2.5 Wavelets and Bioacoustics

Vibrations caused by the contractile activity of the cardiohemic system generate a sound signal if appropriate transducers are used. The phonocardiogram (PCG) represents the recording of the heart sound signal and provides an indication of the general state of the heart in terms of rhythm and contractility. Cardiovascular diseases and defects can be diagnosed from changes or additional sounds and murmurs present in the PCG. Sounds are short, impulse-like events that represent transitions between the different hemodynamic phases of the cardiac cycle. Murmurs, which are primarily caused by blood flow turbulence, are characteristic of cardiac disease such as valve defects. Given its properties the WT appears to be an appropriate tool for representing and modeling the PCG. A comparative study with other time-frequency methods (Wigner distribution and spectrogram) confirmed its adequacy for this particular application (Obaidat 1993). In particular, certain sound components such as the aortic (A2) and pulmonary (P2) valve components of the second heart sound are hardly resolved by the other methods rather than WT. More recent wavelet based approaches have considered the identification of the two major sounds and murmurs (Chebil & Al-Nabulsi 2007) and also the identification of the components of the second cardiac sound S2 (Debbal & Bereksi-Reguig 2007). Both are of utmost importance regarding diagnosis purposes. In the first case a performance of about 90% is reported which can constitute a very promising result given the difficult conditions existing in situations of severe murmurs. Particularly important in the scope of this chapter is the second situation where the objectives are to determine the order of the closure of the aortic (A2) and pulmonary (P2) valves as well as the time between these two events known as *split*. The second heart sound S2 can be used in the diagnosis of several heart diseases such as pulmonary valve stenosis and right Bundle branch block (wide split), atrial septal defect and right ventricular failure (fixed split), left bundle branch block (paradoxical or reverse split), therefore it has long been recognized, and its significance is considered by cardiologists as the "key to auscultation of the heart". However the *split* has durations from around 10 ms to 60 ms, making the classification by the human ear a very hard task (Leung et al. 1998). So, an automated method capable of measuring S2 *split* is desirable. However S2 is very hard to deal with since two very similar components (A2 and P2) must be recognized. A2 has often higher amplitude (louder) and frequency content than P2 and generally A2 precedes P2. Several approaches have been proposed to face this problem. In the ambit of this chapter we will focus on the WT since other methods can not resolve the aortic and pulmonary components as stated by (Obaidat 1993). (Debbal & Bereksi-Reguig 2007) proposed an interesting approach entirely based on WT to segment the heart sound S2. Very promising results were obtained by decomposing S2 into a number of components using the WT and chose two of the major components as A2 and P2 in order to define the *split* as the time between these components. However the method suffers from an important drawback; since the amplitudes of A2 and P2 are significantly affected by the recording locations on the chest, the two highest components obtained from WT might not always represent A2 and P2. These are strong requirements regarding diagnosis purposes that claim for high accurate measures.

Alternative methods based also on time-frequency representation by using the Wigner Ville distribution of S2 have been suggested (Xu et al. 2000, Xu et al. 2001). However the masking operation which is central to the procedure is done manually making the algorithm very sensitive to errors while performing the masking operation. This happens because A2 and P2 are reconstructed from masked time-frequency representation of the signal. Recent advances in the scope of this approach focus on the Instantaneous Frequency (IF) trajectory of S2 (Yildirim & Ansari 2007). The IF trace was analyzed by processing the data with a frequency-selective differentiator which preserves the derivative information for the spectral components of the IF data of interest. The zero crossings are identified to locate the onset of P2. While this approach appears to be robust against changes in sensor placement, since it relies only in the spectral content of the signal and not also in its magnitude, the performance of the algorithm remains to be validated. As a matter of fact murmurs change the spectral content of the signal and can compromise the algorithm performance.

Although approaches that rely on the separation of A2 and P2 are in general more susceptible to noise and sensor placement conditions robust methods based on Blind Source Separation (BSS) have also been proposed to estimate the split by separating A2 and P2 (Nigam & Priemer 2006). The main criticism of this approach is related with the independency supposition. Since A2 is generated by the closure of the valve between left ventricular and aorta and P2 by the closure of the valve between right ventricular and pulmonic artery, it is very unlikely that an abnormality in the left ventricle does not affect right ventricle too. Hence the assumption of independence between A2 and P2 needs to be validated.

High accuracy methods such as Hidden Markov Models with features extracted from WT can be more adequate than WT alone to model the phonocardiogram, especially if the wave separation is not required for training purposes. Each event (M1, T1, A2, P2 and background) is modeled by its own HMM and training can be done by HMM concatenation according to the labeling file prepared by the physician (Lima & Barbosa 2008). The order of occurrence of A2 and P2 can be obtained by the likelihood of both hypothesis (A2 preceding P2 and vice versa) and the *split* can be estimated by the backtracking procedure in the Viterbi algorithm which gives the most likely state sequence.

2.6 Wavelets and the ECG

A number of wavelet based techniques have recently been proposed to the analysis of ECG signals. Subjects as timing, morphology, distortions, noise, detection of localized abnormalities, heart rate variability, arrhythmias and data compression has been the main topics where wavelet based techniques have been experimented.

2.6.1 Wavelets for ECG delineation

The time varying morphology of the ECG is subject to physiological conditions and the presence of noise seriously compromise the delineation of the electrical activity of the heart. The potential of wavelet based feature extraction for discriminating between normal and abnormal cardiac patterns has been demonstrated (Senhadji et al., 1995). An algorithm for the detection and measurement of the onset and the offset of the QRS complex and P and T waves based on modulus maxima-based wavelet analysis employing the dyadic WT was proposed (Sahambi et al., 1997a and 1997b). This algorithm performs well in the presence of modeled baseline drift and high frequency additive noise. Improvements to the technique are described in (Sahambi et al., 1998). Launch points and wavelet extreme were both proposed to obtain reliable amplitude and duration parameters from the ECG (Sivannarayana & Reddy 1999).

QRS detection is extremely useful for both finding the fiducial points employed in ensemble averaging analysis methods and for computing the R-R time series from which a variety of heart rate variability (HRV) measures can be extracted. (Li et al., 1995) proposed a wavelet based QRS detection method based on finding the modulus maxima larger than an updated threshold obtained from the preprocessing of pre-selected initial beats. Performances of 99.90% sensitivity and 99.94% positive predictivity were reported in the MIT-BIH database. Several Algorithms based on (Li et al., 1995) have been extended to the detection of ventricular premature contractions (Shyu et al., 2004) and to the ECG robust delineation (Martinez et al., 2004) especially the detection of peaks, onsets and offsets of the QRS complexes and P and T waves.

Kadambe et al., 1999) have described an algorithm which finds the local maxima of two consecutive dyadic wavelet scales, and compared them in order to classify local maxima produced by R waves and noise. A sensitivity of 96.84% and a positive predictivity of 95.20% were reported. More recently the work of (Li et al. 1995) and (Kadambe et al. 1999) have been extended (Romero Lagarreta et al., 2005) by using the CWT, which affords high time-frequency resolution which provides a better definition of the QRS modulus maxima lines to filter out the QRS from other signal morphologies including baseline wandering and noise. A sensitivity of 99.53% and a positive predictivity of 99.73% were reported with signals acquired at the Coronary Care Unit at the Royal Infirmary of Edinburgh and a sensitivity of 99.70% and a positive predictivity of 99.68% were reported in the MIT-BIH database.

Wavelet based filters have been proposed to minimize the wandering distortions (Park et al., 1998) and to remove motion artifacts in ECG's (Park et al., 2001). Wavelet based noise reduction methods for ECG signals have also been proposed (Inoue & Miyazaki 1998, Tikkanen 1999). Other wavelet based denoising algorithms have been proposed to remove the ECG signal from the electrohysterogram (Leman & Marque 2000) or to suppress electromyogram noise from the ECG (Nikoliaev et al., 2001).

2.6.2 Wavelets and arrhythmias

In some applications the wavelet analysis has shown to be superior to other analysis methods (Yi et al. 2000). High performances have been reported (Govindan et al. 1997, Al-Fahoum & Howitt 1999) and new methods have been developed and implemented in implantable devices (Zhang et al. (1999). One approach that combines WT and radial basis functions was proposed (Al-Fahoum & Howitt 1999) for the automatic detection and classification of arrhythmias where the Daubechies D4 WT is used. High scores of 97.5% correct classification of arrhythmia with 100% correct classification for both ventricular fibrillation and ventricular tachycardia were reported. (Duverney et al. 2002) proposed a combined wavelet transform-fractal analysis method for the automatic detection of atrial fibrillation (AF) from heart rate intervals. AF is associated with the asynchronous contraction of the atrial muscle fibers is the most prevalent cardiac arrhythmia in the west world and is associated with significant morbidity. Performances of 96,1% of sensitivity and 92.6% specificity were reported.

Human Ventricular Fibrillation (VF) wavelet based studies have demonstrated that a rich underlying structure is contained in the signal, however hidden to classical Fourier techniques, contrarily to the previous thought that this pathology is characterized by a disorganized and unstructured electrical activity of the heart (Addison et al., 2000, Watson et al., 2000). Based on these results a wavelet based method for the prediction of the outcome from defibrillation shock in human VF was proposed (Watson et al., 2004). An enhanced version of this method employing entropy measures of selected modulus maxima achieves performances of over 60% specificity at 95% sensitivity for predicting a return of spontaneous circulation. The best of alternative techniques based on a variety of measures including Fourier, fractal, angular velocity, etc typically achieves 50% specificity at 95% sensitivity. This enhancement is due to the ability of the wavelet transform to isolate and extract specific spectral-temporal information. The incorporation of such outcome prediction technologies within defibrillation devices will significantly alter their function as current standard protocols, involving sequences of shocks and CPR, which can be altered according on the likelihood of success of a shock. If the likelihood of success is low an alternative therapy prior to shock will be used.

2.7 Wavelets and Medical Imaging

The impact of the Wavelet Transform in the research community is well perceived through the amount of papers and books published since the milestone works of Daubechies (Daubechies 1988) and Mallat (Mallat 1989). Accordingly with Unser (Unser 2003), more than 9000 papers and 200 books were published between the late eighties and 2003, with a significant part being focused in biomedical applications. The first paper describing a medical application of wavelet processing appeared in 1991, where was proposed a denoising algorithm based in soft-thresholding in the wavelet domain by Weaver et al. (Weaver 1991). Without the claim of being exhaustive, the main applications of wavelets in medical imaging have been:

Image denoising – The multi-scale decomposition of the DWT offers a very effective separation of the spectral components of the original image. The most tipycal denoising strategy takes advantage of this property to select the most relevant wavelet coefficients applying thresholding techniques. Some classic examples of this approach are given in (Jin 2004).

Compression of medical images – The evolution in medical imaging technology implies a fast pace increase in the amount of data generated in each exam, which generate a huge pressure in the storage and networking information systems, being therefore imperative to apply compression strategies. However the compression of medical image is a very delicate subject, since discarding small details may lead to misevaluation of exams, causing severe human and legal consequences (Schelkens 2003). Nevertheless, it should be noted that the sparse representation of the image content given by the DWT coefficients allows the implementation of different compression algorithms, that can go from a lossy compression, with very high compression ratios, to more refined, lossless compression schemes, with minimal loss of information.

Wavelet-based feature extraction and classification – The wavelet decomposition of an image allows the application of different pattern analysis techniques, since the image content is subdivided into different bands of different frequency and orientation detail. Some of the more notable applications have been the texture features extraction from the DWT coefficients, which has been successfully applied in the medical field for abnormal tissue classification (Karkanis 2003, Barbosa et al. 2008, Lima et al. 2008), given that texture can be roughly described as a spatial pattern of medium to high frequency, where the relationship of the pixels within an neighborhood presents different frequencies at different orientations, which can be modeled by the 2D DWT of the image. The use of wavelet features has also been vastly explored in the classification of mammograms, given that different wavelet approaches may be customized in order to better detect suspicious area. These are normally microcalcifications, which are believed to be cancer early indicators, and correspond to bright spots in the image, being usually detected as high frequency objects with small dimensions within the image. Some examples of this application are the works of Lemaur (Lemaur 2003) and Sung-Nien (Sung-Nien 2006).

Tomographic reconstruction – Tomography medical modalities like CT, SPECT or PET gather multiple projections of the human body that have to be reconstructed from the acquired signal, the sinogram. Therefore rely on an instable inverse problem of spatial signal reconstruction from sampled line projections, which is usually done through back projection of the sinogram signal via Radon transform and regularization for removal of noisy artifacts.

This regularization can be improved through the use of wavelet thresholding estimators (Kalifa 2003). Jin et al. (Jin 2003) proposed the noise reduction in the reconstructed through cross-regularization of wavelet coefficients.

Wavelet-encoded MRI – Wavelet basis can be used in MRI encoding schemes, taking advantage from the better spatial localization when compared with the conventional phase-encoded MRI, which uses Fourier basis. This fact allows faster acquisitions than the conventional phase encoding techniques but it is still slower than echo planar MRI (Unser 1996).

Image enhancement – Medical imaging modalities with reduced contrast may require the application of image enhancement techniques in order to improve the diagnostic potential. A typical example is the mammography, where the contrast between the target objects and the soft tissues of the breast is inherently. The easiest approach uses a philosophy similar to the image denoising techniques, where in this case instead of suppressing the unwanted wavelet coefficients one should amplify the interesting image features. Given the original data quality, redundant wavelet transforms are usually used in enhancement algorithms. Examples of enhancement algorithms using wavelets are presented in (Heinlein et al. 2003, Papadopoulos et al. 2008, Przelaskowski et al. 2007).

2.8 Breaking the limits of the DWT

The multi-resolution capability of the DWT has been vastly explored in several fields of signal and image processing, as seen in the last section. The ability of dealing with singularities is another important advantage of the DWT, since wavelets provide and optimal representation for one-dimensional piecewise smooth signal (Do 2005). However natural images are not simply stacks of 1-D piecewise smooth scan-lines, and therefore singularities points are usually located along smooth curves. The DWT inability while dealing with intermediate dimensional structures like discontinuities along curves (Candès 2000) is easily comprehensible, since its directional sensitivity is limited to three directions. Given that such discontinuity elements are vital in the analysis of any image, including the medical ones, a vigorous research effort has been exerted in order to provide better adapted alternatives by combining ideas from geometry with ideas from traditional multi-scale analysis (Candès 2005). Therefore, and as it was realized that Fourier methods were not good for all purposes, the limitations of the DWT triggered the quest for new concepts capable of overcome these limits.

Given that the focus of the present chapter is not the limits of the DWT itself, only a brief overview regarding multi-directional and multi-scale transforms will be given. The steerable pyramids, proposed in the early nineties (Simoncelli 1992, Simoncelli 1995), was one of the first approaches to this problem, being a practical, data-friendly strategy to extract information at different scales and angles. More recently, the curvelet transform (Candès 2000) and the contourlet transform (Do 2005) have been introduced, being exciting and promising new image analysis techniques whose application to medical image is starting to prove its usefulness.

Originally introduced in 2000, by Candès and Donoho, the continuous curvelet transform (CCT) is based in an anisotropic notion of scale and high directional sensitivity in multiple directions. Contrarily to the DWT bases, which are oriented only in the horizontal, vertical and diagonal directions in consequence to the previously explained filterbank applied in the 2D DWT, the elements in the curvelet transform present a high directional sensitivity, which results from the anisotropic notion of scale of this tool. The CCT is based in the tilling of the 2D Fourier space in different concentric coronae, one of each divided in a given number of angles, accordingly with a fixed relation, as can be seen in figure 5.

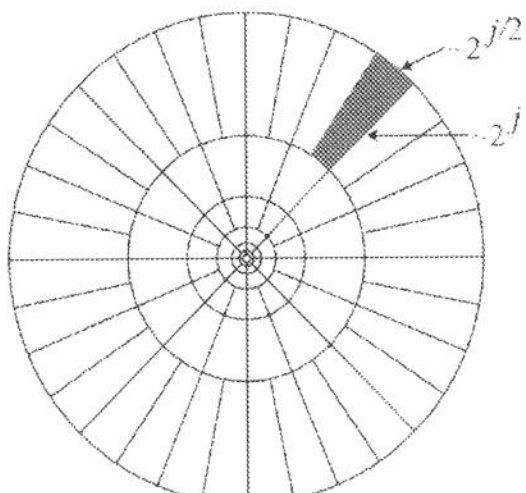

Fig. 5. Tiling of the frequency domain in the continuous curvelet transform

These polar wedges can be defined by the superposition of a radial window $W(r)$ and an angular window $V(t)$. Each of the separated polar wedges will be associated a frequency window U_j, which will correspond to the Fourier transform of a curvelet function $\varphi_j(x)$ function, which can be thought of as a "mother" curvelet, since all the curvelets at scale 2^j may be obtained by rotations and translations of $\varphi_j(x)$. The curvelets coefficients, at a given scale j and angle θ, will be then simply defined as the inner product between the image and the rotation of the mother curvelet $\varphi j(x)$.

Although a discretization scheme has been proposed with its introduction, its complexity was not very user friendly, which led to a redesign of the discretization strategy introduced in (Candès 2006). Nevertheless, the curvelet transform is a concept focused in the continuous domain and has to be discretized to be useful in image processing, given the discrete nature of the pixel grids. This fact has been the seed in (Do & Vetterli 2005), where is proposed a framework for the development of a discrete tool having the desired multi-resolution and directional sensitivity characteristics.

The contourlet tranforms is formulated as a double filter bank, where a Laplacian pyramid is first used to separate the different detail levels and to capture point discontinuities then followed by a directional filter bank to link point discontinuities into linear structures. Therefore the contourlet transform provides a multiscale and directional decomposition in the frequency domain, as can be seen in figure 6, where is clear the division of the Fourier plane by scale and angle.

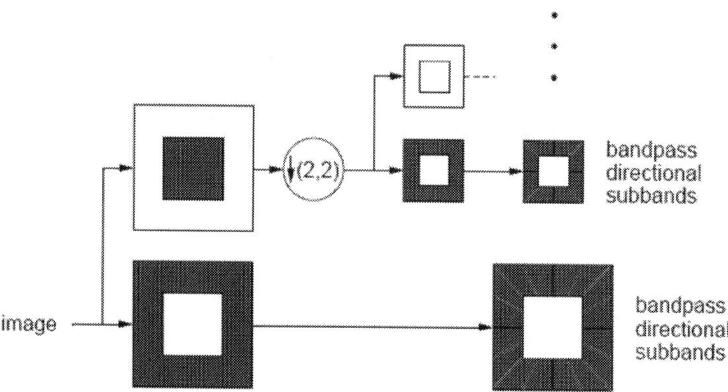

Fig. 6. The contourlet filterbank: first, a multiscale decomposition into octave bands by the Laplacian pyramid is computed, and then a directional filter bank is applied to each bandpass channel.

Although the contourlet Transform is easier to understand in the practical side, being a very elegant framework, the theoretical bases are not as robust as the ones in the curvelet Transform, in the sense that for most choices of filters in the angular filterbank, contourlets are not sharply localized in frequency, contrarily to the curvelet elements, whose location is sharply defined as the polar wedges of figure n. On the other hand, the contourlet transform is directly designed for discrete applications, whereas the discretization scheme of the curvelet transform faces some intrinsic challenges in the sampling of the Fourier plane in the outermost coronae, presenting the contourlet transform less redundancy also.

The potential of curvelet/contourlet based algorithms has been demonstrated in recent works. (Dettori & Semler 2007) compares the texture classification performance of wavelet, ridgelet and curvelet-based algorithms for CT tissue identification, where is evident that the curvelet outperforms the other methods. (Li & Meng 2009) states that the performance traditional texture extraction algorithms, in this case the local binary pattern texture operator, improves if applied in the curvelet domain. (Yang et al. 2008) proposed a contourlet-based image fusion scheme that presents better results than the ones achieved with wavelet techniques.

3. Basics on pattern recognition and hidden Markov models

3.1 Pattern recognition with HMM's

Hidden Markov Models (HMM's) make usually part of pattern recognition systems which basic principle applied to phonocardiography is shown in figure 7. An incoming pattern is classified according to a pre-trained dictionary of models. These models are in the present case HMM's, each one modeling each event in the phonocardiogram. The events are the four main waves M1, T1, A2 and P2, and the background that can accommodate systolic and diastolic murmurs. The pattern classification block evaluates the likelihood of A2 preceding P2 and vice versa and also the most likely state sequence for each hypothesis through the super HMM, which is constituted by the appropriate concatenation of the models in the dictionary. The feature extraction block takes advantage of the WT to better discriminate the wave spectral content. The signal is simultaneously viewed at three different scales each one pointing out different signal characteristics.

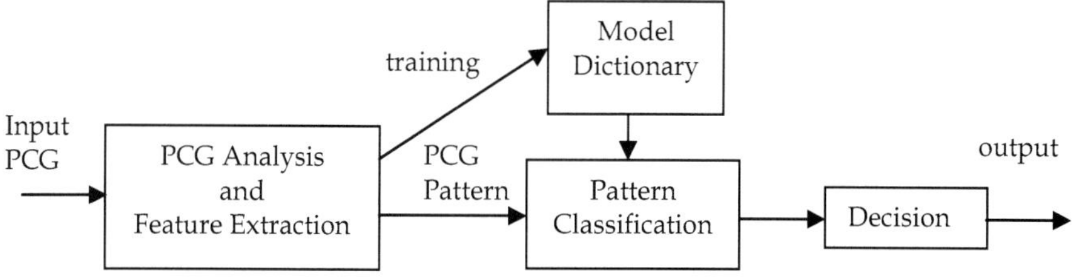

Fig. 7. Principle of a pattern recognition on PCG.

Such a system operates in two phases:

A **training phase**, during which the system learns the reference patterns representing the different PCG sounds (e.g. M1, T1, A2, P2 and background) that constitute the vocabulary of the application. Each reference is learned from labeled PCG examples and stored in the form of models that characterise the patterns properties. The learning phase necessitates efficient learning algorithms for providing the system with truly representative reference patterns.

A **recognition phase**, during which an unknown input pattern is identified by considering the set of references. The pattern classification is done computing a similarity measure between the input PCG and each reference pattern. This process necessitates defining a measure of closeness between feature vectors and a method for aligning two PCG patterns, which may differ in duration and cardiac rhythm.

By nature the PCG signal is neither deterministic nor stationary. Non-deterministic signals are frequently but not always modelled by statistical models in which one tries to characterise the statistical properties of the signal. The underlying assumption of the statistical model is that the signal can be characterised as a stochastic process, which parameters can be estimated in a precise manner. A stochastic model compatible with the non-stationary property is the Hidden Markov Model (HMM), which structure is shown in figure 4. This stochastic model consists of a set of states with transitions between them. Observation vectors are produced as the output of the Markov model according to the probabilistic transitioning from one state to another and the stationary stochastic model in each state. Therefore, the Markov model segments a non-stationary process in stationary parts providing a very rich mathematical structure for analysing non-stationary stochastic processes. So these models providing a statistical model of both the static properties of cardiac sounds and the dynamical changes that occur across them. Additionally these models, when applied properly, work very well in practice for several important applications besides the biomedical field.

3.2 Hidden Markov Models

Hidden Markov models are a doubly stochastic process in which the observed data are viewed as the result of having passed the hidden finite process (state sequence) through a function that produces the observed (second) process. The hidden process is a collection of states connected by transitions, each one described by two sets of probabilities:

A **transition probability**, which provides the probability of making a transition from one state to another.

An **output probability** density function, which defines the conditional probability of observing a set of cardiac sound features when a particular transition takes place. The continuous density function most frequently used is the multivariate Gaussian mixture.

In an HMM the goal of the decoding or recognition process is to determine a sequence of hidden (unobservables) states (or transitions) that the observed signal has gone through. The second goal is to define the likelihood of observing that particular event, given a state sequence determined in the first process. Given the Markov models definition, there are two problems of interest:

The **Evaluation Problem**: Given a model and a sequence of observations, what is the probability that the observations are generated by the model? This solution can be found using the forward-backward or Baum-Welch algorithm (Baum 1972, Rabiner 1989).

The **Learning Problem**: Given a model and a sequence of observations, what should the model's parameters be, so that it has the maximum likelihood of generating the observations? This solution can be found using the Baum-Welch or forward-backward algorithm (Baum 1972).

3.2.1 The evaluation problem

The goal of this and the next sub-section is not to broach exhaustively the HMMs theory, but only provide a basis to help in best understanding how these flexible stochastic models can be adapted to several modeling situations regarding biomedical applications. More details can be encountered in (Rabiner 1989).

When the random variables of a Markov Process take only discrete values, (frequently integers, the states are numerated by integer values) the stochastic state machine is known by Markov chain. If the state transition at each time is only dependent of the previous state, then the Markov chain is said of first order. The HMMs reviewed in this chapter are first order Markov chains.

Consider a left to right connected HMM with 6 states as illustrated in Figure 8 (for simplicity, the density probability function is not shown).

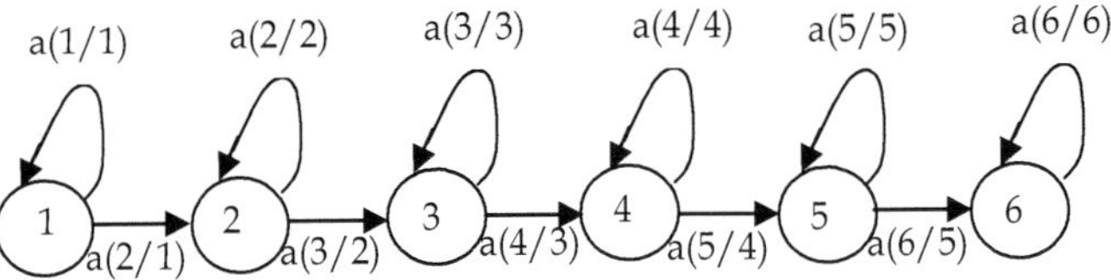

Fig. 8. A left to right HMM with 6 states

This stochastic state machine is characterised by the state transition matrix A, the probability density function in each transition B and the initial state probability vector π. The PCG signal is characterised by a time evaluating event sequence, whose properties change over time in a successive manner. Furthermore, as time increases, the state index increases or stays the same, that is, the system states proceed from left to right, and the state sequence must begin in state 1 and end in the last one for a cardiac cycle begining in an S1 sound. In this conditions a(i/j)=0, j>i and π_i have the property

$$\pi_i = \begin{cases} 0, & i \neq 1 \\ 1, & i = 1 \end{cases} \tag{9}$$

As at each time the transition comes up then a(./i)=1, where a(./i) stands for transition from state i to each other. The transition dependent probability density function is typically a finite Gaussian multivariate mixture of the form

$$f(\mathbf{y}/s_t) = \sum_{c_t=1}^{C} p_{s_t,c_t} G\left(\mathbf{y}_t, \boldsymbol{\mu}_{s_t,c_t}, \boldsymbol{\Sigma}_{s_t,c_t}\right) \qquad 1 \leq s_t \leq N \tag{10}$$

where $\mathbf{y}$ is the observation vector being modelled, p_{s_t,c_t} is the mixture coefficient for the cth mixture in state s at time t, G(.) stands for Gaussian (Normal) distribution, and N is the number of states in the model. Other types of log-concave or elliptical distributions can be used (Levinson et al. 1983).

Given a sequence of vector observations $\mathbf{Y}=\{\mathbf{y}_1, \mathbf{y}_2, \ldots \mathbf{y}_T\}$, what is the likelihood that the model generated the observations? As an example suppose T=11, and the model shown in Figure 8. One possible time indexed path through the model is 1r, 1n, 2r, 2n, 3r, 3n, 4r, 4n, 5r, 5n, 6r, when r stands for recursive transitions and n stands for next transitions. Another possible path is 1r, 1r, 1r, 1n, 2n, 3n, 4n, 5n, 6r, 6r, 6r. As the model generates observations that can arrive from any path (events mutually exclusives) then the likelihood of the sequence is the sum of the likelihood in each path. Let $\mathbf{s}=\{s_1, s_2, \ldots s_T\}$ be one considered state sequence. The likelihood of the model generates the observed vector sequence $\mathbf{Y}$ given one such fixed-state sequence $\mathbf{S}$ and the model parameters $\lambda=\{A,B,\pi\}$ is given by

$$P(\mathbf{Y}/\mathbf{S},\lambda) = f(\mathbf{y}_1/s_1,\lambda).f(\mathbf{y}_2/s_2,\lambda)...f(\mathbf{y}_T/s_T,\lambda) = \prod_{t=1}^{T} f(\mathbf{y}_t/s_t,\lambda) \tag{11}$$

The probability of such a state sequence $\mathbf{S}$ can be written as

$$P(\mathbf{S}/\lambda) = \pi_{s_1} a_{s_1 s_2} a_{s_2 s_3} ... a_{s_{T-1} s_T} \tag{12}$$

The joint probability of $\mathbf{Y}$ and $\mathbf{S}$, i.e., the probability that $\mathbf{Y}$ and $\mathbf{S}$ occur simultaneously, is simply the product of the above two terms

$$f(\mathbf{Y},\mathbf{S}/\lambda) = f(\mathbf{Y}/\mathbf{S},\lambda)P(\mathbf{S}/\lambda) \tag{13}$$

The probability of $\mathbf{Y}$ (given the model) is obtained by summing this joint probability over all possible state sequences $\mathbf{S}$ and is given by

$$f(\mathbf{Y}/\lambda) = \sum_{S} f(\mathbf{Y}/\mathbf{S},\lambda)P(\mathbf{S}/\lambda) = \sum_{s_1,s_2,...s_T} \pi_{s_1} f(\mathbf{y}_1/s_1,\lambda) a_{s_1 s_2} f(\mathbf{y}_2/s_2,\lambda)...a_{s_{T-1} s_T} f(\mathbf{y}_T/s_T,\lambda) \tag{14}$$

The interpretation of the computation in the above equation is the following. Initialy (at time t=1) the HMM is in state s_1 with probability π_{s1}=1, and generates the symbol $\mathbf{y}_1$ (in this state/transition) with probability $f(\mathbf{y}_1/s_1,\lambda)$. The clock changes from time t to $t+1$ (time=2) and the HMM make a transition to s_2 from state s_1 with probability a_{s1s2} and generates symbol $\mathbf{y}_2$ with probability $f(\mathbf{y}_{21}/s_2,\lambda)$. This process continues until the last transition (at time T) from state s_{T-1} to state s_T with probability $a_{sT-1\ sT}$ and generates symbol $\mathbf{y}_T$ with probability $f(\mathbf{y}_T/s_T,\lambda)$.

To conclude this section it is convenient rewrite the equation (14) in a more compact and useful form. Thus, substituting (10) in (14) we obtain

$$f(\mathbf{Y}/\lambda) = \sum_{S} \prod_{t=1}^{T} a_{s_{t-1}s_t} f(\mathbf{y}_t/s_t,\lambda) = \sum_{S} \prod_{t=1}^{T} a_{s_{t-1}s_t} \sum_{c_t=1}^{C} p_{s_t,c_t} G(\mathbf{y}_t,\mathbf{\mu}_{s_t,c_t},\mathbf{\Sigma}_{s_t,c_t}) \tag{15}$$

or in a more suitable and general form

$$f(\mathbf{Y}/\lambda) = \sum_{S} \sum_{C} \prod_{t=1}^{T} a_{s_{t-1}s_t} p_{s_t,c_t} f(\mathbf{y}_t/s_t,c_t,\lambda) \tag{16}$$

3.2.2 The evaluation problem

The most difficult problem of HMMs is to determine a method to adjust the model parameters (A,B,π) to satisfy a certain optimisation criterion. There is no known way to analytically solve for the model parameter set that maximises the probability of the observation sequence in a closed form. It can be, however, choose $\lambda=(A,B,\pi)$ such that its likelihood $P(\mathbf{Y}/\lambda)$, is locally maximised using an iterative procedure such as the Baum-Welch method (also known as the Expectation Maximisation (EM) method) or using gradient techniques (Levinson et al. 1983). This sub-section shows the ideas behind the EM algorithm, showing it usefulness in the resolution of problems with missing data.

Hidden Markov models are a doubly stochastic process where the first, the state sequence, is unobserved and so unknown. The observed vector sequences (observable data) are called incomplete data because they are missing the unobservable data, and data composed by observable and unobservable data are called complete data. Making use of the observed (incomplete) data and the joint probability density function of observed and unobserved data, the EM algorithm iteratively maximises the log-likelihood of observable data.

In the particular HMM case, there are a measure space $\mathbf{S}$ (state sequence) of unobservable data, corresponding to a measure space $\mathbf{Y}$ (observations) of incomplete data. Here $\mathbf{Y}$ is easy to observe and measure, while $\mathbf{S}$ contains some hidden information that is unobservable. Let $f(\mathbf{s}/\lambda)$ and $f(\mathbf{y}/\lambda)$ be members of a parametric family of probability density functions (pdf) defined on $\mathbf{S}$ and $\mathbf{Y}$ respectively for parameter λ. For a given $y\varepsilon Y$, the goal of the EM algorithm is to maximise the log-likelihood of the observable data $\mathbf{y}$, $L(\mathbf{y},\lambda)=\log f(\mathbf{y}/\lambda)$, over λ by exploiting the relationship between $f(\mathbf{y},\mathbf{s}/\lambda)$ and $f(\mathbf{s}/\mathbf{y},\lambda)$. The joint pdf $f(\mathbf{y},\mathbf{s}/\lambda)$ is given by

$$f(\mathbf{y},\mathbf{s}/\lambda) = f(\mathbf{s}/\mathbf{y},\lambda)f(\mathbf{y}/\lambda) \tag{17}$$

From the above expression the following log-likelihood can be obtained

$$\log f(\mathbf{y}/\lambda) = \log f(\mathbf{y},\mathbf{s}/\lambda) - \log f(\mathbf{s}/\mathbf{y},\lambda) \tag{18}$$

and for two parameter sets λ' and λ, the expectation of incomplete log-likelihood $L(\mathbf{y},\lambda')$ over complete data $(\mathbf{y},\mathbf{s})$ conditioned by $\mathbf{y}$ and λ is

$$E_s\left[L(\mathbf{y},\lambda')/\mathbf{y},\lambda\right] = E\left[\log f(\mathbf{y}/\lambda'/\mathbf{y},\lambda\right] = \int \log f(\mathbf{y}/\lambda')f(\mathbf{s}/\mathbf{y},\lambda)ds$$

$$= \log f(\mathbf{y}/\lambda') = L(\mathbf{y},\lambda') \tag{19}$$

where $E[./\mathbf{y},\lambda]$ is the expectation conditioned by $\mathbf{y}$ and λ over complete data $(\mathbf{y},\mathbf{s})$. Then from (18) the following expression is obtained

$$L(\mathbf{y},\lambda') = Q(\lambda,\lambda') - H(\lambda,\lambda') \tag{20}$$

where

$$Q(\lambda,\lambda') = E_s\left[\log f(\mathbf{y},\mathbf{s}/\lambda')/\mathbf{y},\lambda\right] \tag{21}$$

and

$$H(\lambda,\lambda') = E_s\left[\log f(\mathbf{s}/\mathbf{y},\lambda')/\mathbf{y},\lambda\right] \tag{22}$$

The basis of the EM algorithm lies in the fact that if $Q(\lambda,\lambda')\geq Q(\lambda,\lambda)$, then $L(\mathbf{y},\lambda')\geq L(\mathbf{y},\lambda)$, since it follows from Jensen's inequality that $H(\lambda,\lambda')\leq H(\lambda,\lambda)$ (Dempster et al. 1977). This fact implies that the incomplete log-likelihood $L(\mathbf{y},\lambda)$ increases monotonically on any iteration of parameter update from λ to λ', via maximisation of the Q function which is the expectation of log-likelihood from complete data.

From equation (15) and for the complete data we have

$$f(\mathbf{Y},\mathbf{S},\mathbf{C}/\lambda') = \prod_{t=1}^{T} a'_{s_{t-1}s_t}\, p'_{s_t,c_t}\, f(\mathbf{y}_t/s_t,c_t,\lambda') \tag{23}$$

and from equation (20) we obtain

$$Q(\lambda,\lambda') = E\big[\log P(\mathbf{Y},\mathbf{S},\mathbf{C}/\lambda')/\mathbf{Y},\lambda\big] = \sum_{S}\sum_{C} P(\mathbf{Y},\mathbf{S},\mathbf{C}/\lambda)\log f(\mathbf{Y},\mathbf{S},\mathbf{C}/\lambda') \tag{24}$$

substituting equation (23) in (24) we obtain

$$Q(\lambda,\lambda') = \sum_{S}\sum_{C} P(\mathbf{Y},\mathbf{S},\mathbf{C}/\lambda)\log \prod_{t=1}^{T} a'_{s_{t-1}s_t}\, p'_{s_t,c_t}\, f(\mathbf{y}_t/s_t,c_t,\lambda')$$

$$= \sum_{S}\sum_{C} P(\mathbf{Y},\mathbf{S},\mathbf{C}/\lambda)\sum_{t=1}^{T}\Big\{\log a'_{s_{t-1}s_t} + \log p'_{s_t,c_t} + \log f(\mathbf{y}_t/s_t,c_t,\lambda')\Big\} \tag{25}$$

At this point it is finished the expectation step of the EM algorithm. Equation (24) shows that the Q function is separately in three independent terms, one is state transition dependent, another is component mixture dependent and the last is dependent of the pdf parameters of observation incomplete data. In the second step of the EM algorithm known as the maximisation step, the Q function is maximised in order to the parameters to be estimated. For example to estimate the matrix A, the Q function must be maximised in order to the respective parameters under the constraint

$$\sum_{j=1}^{N} a'(j/i) = 1 \tag{26}$$

i.e. at each time clock the transition must occur. To estimate the mixture coefficients, the probability over all the space must be one, and express as the following constraint:

$$\sum_{c_t=1}^{C} p'_{i,c_t} = 1 \qquad 1 \le i \le N \tag{27}$$

Understanding the fundamental concepts of the EM algorithm the derivation of the reestimation formulas is straightforward. First of all we can address the most general case where the initial state is not known and must be estimated. In this situation the auxiliary Q function can be written from equations (12), (13), (14) and (25) as

$$Q(\lambda,\lambda') = \sum_{\mathbf{S}}\sum_{\mathbf{C}} P(\mathbf{Y},\mathbf{S},\mathbf{C}/\lambda)\left\{ \log \pi'_{s_1} + \sum_{t=1}^{T-1} \log a'_{s_t,s_{t+1}} + \sum_{t=1}^{T} \log p'_{s_t,c_t} + \sum_{t=1}^{T} \log f(\mathbf{y}_t / s_t, c_t, \lambda') \right\} \tag{28}$$

The auxiliary Q function can be maximized separately in order to each term, so regarding to the initial state vector the Q function can be written as

$$Q_\pi(\lambda,\pi') = \sum_{\mathbf{S}}\sum_{\mathbf{C}} f(\mathbf{Y},\mathbf{S},\mathbf{C}/\lambda)\log \pi'_{s_1} = \sum_{j}\sum_{\mathbf{C}} f(\mathbf{Y},s_1 = j,c_t / \lambda)\log \pi'_{s_j} \tag{29}$$

which results in an equation of the type

$$\sum_{j=1}^{N} w_j \log y_j \quad \text{under the constraint} \quad \sum_{j=1}^{N} y_j = 1 \tag{30}$$

Equation (29) has a global maximum at

$$y_j = \frac{w_j}{\sum_{i=1}^{N} w_i} \qquad j=1,2,...,N \tag{31}$$

Using equation (31) in the solution of equation (29) we obtain

$$\pi'_{s_j} = \frac{\sum_{\mathbf{C}} f(\mathbf{Y},s_1 = j,c_t / \lambda)}{\sum_{j}\sum_{\mathbf{C}} f(\mathbf{Y},s_1 = j,c_t / \lambda)} = \frac{f(\mathbf{Y},s_1 = j/\lambda)}{\sum_{j} f(\mathbf{Y},s_1 = j/\lambda)} = \frac{f(\mathbf{Y},s_1 = j/\lambda)}{f(\mathbf{Y}/\lambda)} \tag{32}$$

Similarly the part of the auxiliary Q function regarding to the state transition matrix can be written as

$$Q(\lambda,a'_{i,j}) = \sum_{\mathbf{S}}\sum_{\mathbf{C}} f(\mathbf{Y},\mathbf{S},\mathbf{C}/\lambda) \sum_{t=1}^{T-1} \log a'_{i,j} = \sum_{i} Q_{a_i}(\lambda,a'_{i,j}) \tag{33}$$

For a particular state i the sum in $\mathbf{S}$ in the second member of equation (32) disapears. However, as for each state i the probability of transition for any state j is the sum of the transition probabilities to all possible states j (including the state i itself) the individual Q function regarding the state transition probabilities, for a given state i can be written from equation (32) as

$$Q_{a_i}(\lambda,a'_{i,j}) = \sum_{j}\sum_{t=1}^{T-1}\sum_{\mathbf{C}} f(\mathbf{Y},s_t = i,s_{t+1} = j,c_t / \lambda)\log a'_{i,j} \tag{34}$$

From equation (31) the maximization of equation (34) can be written as

$$a'_{i,j} = \frac{\sum\limits_{t=1}^{T-1}\sum\limits_{\mathbf{C}} f(\mathbf{Y}, s_t = i, s_{t+1} = j, c_t / \lambda)}{\sum\limits_{j}\sum\limits_{t=1}^{T-1}\sum\limits_{\mathbf{C}} f(\mathbf{Y}, s_t = i, s_{t+1} = j, c_t / \lambda)} = \frac{\sum\limits_{t=1}^{T-1} f(\mathbf{Y}, s_t = i, s_{t+1} = j / \lambda)}{\sum\limits_{t=1}^{T-1} f(\mathbf{Y}, s_t = i / \lambda)} \tag{35}$$

Regarding the mixture coefficients, the individual Q function can be written from equation (28) as

$$Q(\lambda, p'_{j,c}) = \sum_{\mathbf{S}}\sum_{\mathbf{C}} f(\mathbf{Y}, \mathbf{S}, \mathbf{C} / \lambda) \sum_{t=1}^{T} \log p'_{j,c} = \sum_{j} Q_{p_j}(\lambda, p'_{j,c}) \tag{36}$$

For a particular state j equation (36) can be written as

$$Q_{p_j}(\lambda, p'_{j,c}) = \sum_{\mathbf{C}} f(\mathbf{Y}, \mathbf{S}, \mathbf{C} / \lambda) \sum_{t=1}^{T} \log p'_{j,c} = \sum_{c=1}^{C}\sum_{t=1}^{T} f(\mathbf{Y}, s_t = j, c_t = c / \lambda) \log p'_{j,c} \tag{37}$$

Which solution, obtained from equation (30) is

$$p'_{j,c} = \frac{\sum\limits_{t=1}^{T} f(\mathbf{Y}, s_t = j, c_t = c / \lambda)}{\sum\limits_{c=1}^{C}\sum\limits_{t=1}^{T} f(\mathbf{Y}, s_t = j, c_t = c / \lambda)} = \frac{\sum\limits_{t=1}^{T} f(\mathbf{Y}, s_t = j, c_t = c / \lambda)}{\sum\limits_{t=1}^{T} f(\mathbf{Y}, s_t = j / \lambda)} \tag{38}$$

Regarding the distribution parameters (excluding the mixture coefficients) the Q function is

$$Q(\lambda, f'_{s_t, c_t}) = \sum_{\mathbf{S}}\sum_{\mathbf{C}} f(\mathbf{Y}, \mathbf{S}, \mathbf{C} / \lambda) \sum_{t=1}^{T} \log f(\mathbf{y}_t / s_t, c_t, \lambda')$$

$$= \sum_{t=1}^{T}\sum_{n=1}^{N}\sum_{c=1}^{C} f(\mathbf{y}_t / s_t, c_t, \lambda) \log f(\mathbf{y}_t / s_t, c_t, \lambda') = \sum_{t=1}^{T}\sum_{n=1}^{N}\sum_{c=1}^{C} \gamma_t(n, c) \log f(\mathbf{y}_t / s_t, c_t, \lambda') \tag{39}$$

Where $\gamma_t(n,c)$ is the joint probability density function of the observation vector $\mathbf{y}_t$, the state n and the mixture component c. Assuming the observations independents and identically distributed (iid) and with Gaussian distribution, equation (39) can be written as

$$Q(\lambda, f'_{s_t,c_t}) = \sum_{t=1}^{T}\sum_{n=1}^{N}\sum_{c=1}^{C}\gamma_t(n,c)\log\prod_{i=1}^{D}G(y_{t,i},\mu'_{n,c,i},\sigma'^2_{n,c,i}) \tag{40}$$

Where $y_{t,i}$ is the ith component of the observation vector at time t, $\mu_{n,c,i}$ and $\sigma^2_{n,c,i}$ are respectively the mean and variance of the ith component of mixture c in state n and D is the dimensionality of the observation vector. Substituting the Gaussian function in equation (40) we obtain

$$Q(\lambda, f'_{s_t,c_t}) = -\sum_{t=1}^{T}\sum_{n=1}^{N}\sum_{c=1}^{C}\gamma_t(n,c)\sum_{i=1}^{D}\left[\frac{1}{2}\log\sigma'^2_{n,c,i}+\frac{(y_{t,i}-\mu'_{n,c,i})^2}{2\sigma'^2_{n,c,i}}\right] \tag{41}$$

The solution for the maximization of equation (41) is in general obtained by differentiation. For the mean we have

$$\frac{dQ(\lambda, f'_{s_t,c_t})}{d\mu'_{n,c,i}} = \sum_{t=1}^{T}\gamma_t(n,c)\frac{2}{2\sigma'^2_{n,c,i}}(y_{t,i}-\mu'_{n,c,i})=0 \tag{42}$$

Which solution is

$$\mu'_{n,c,i} = \frac{\sum_{t=1}^{T}\gamma_t(n,c)y_{t,i}}{\sum_{t=1}^{T}\gamma_t(n,c)} \tag{43}$$

Differentiating equation (41) in order to variance we obtain

$$\frac{dQ(\lambda, f'_{s_t,c_t})}{d\sigma'^2_{n,c,i}} = -\sum_{t=1}^{T}\gamma_t(n,c)\left\{\frac{1}{2\sigma'^2_{n,c,i}}-\frac{(y_{t,i}-\mu'_{n,c,i})^2}{4\sigma'^4_{n,c,i}}\right\}=0 \tag{44}$$

Which solution is given by

$$\sigma'^2_{n,c,i} = \frac{\sum_{t=1}^{T}\gamma_t(n,c)(y_{t,i}-\mu'_{n,c,i})^2}{\sum_{t=1}^{T}\gamma_t(n,c)} \tag{45}$$

The reestimation formulas given by equations (45), (43), (38), (35) and (32) can be easily calculated using the definitions of forward sequence $\alpha_t(i)=f(y_1,y_2,...y_t,s_t=i/\lambda)$ and backward sequence $\beta_t(i)=f(\mathbf{y}_{t+1},\mathbf{y}_{t+2},...\mathbf{y}_T,s_t=i/\lambda)$. This procedure is standard in the HMM implementation.

4. Wavelets, HMM's and Bioacoustics

Recently a new approach based on wavelets and HMM's was suggested for PCG segmentation purposes (Lima & Barbosa 2008). The main idea is to take advantage of the ability of HMM's to break non-stationary signals in stationary segments modelling both the static properties of cardiac sounds and the dynamical changes that occur across them. However the cardiac sound is particularly difficult to analyse since some events that must be identified are of very close characteristics, and are frequently corrupted by murmurs which are noise-like events very important concerning the diagnosis of several pathologies such as valvular stenosis and insufficiency. This approach takes also advantage of the WT to emphasize the small differences between similar events viewed at different scales, while the scales less affected by noise can be chosen for analysis purposes.

A normal cardiac cycle contains two major sounds: the first heart sound S1 and the second heart sound S2. S1 occurs at the onset of ventricular contraction and corresponds in timing to the QRS complex. S2 follows the systolic pause and is caused by the closure of the semilunar valves. The importance of S2 regarding diagnosis purposes has been recognized for a long time, and its significance is considered of utmost importance, by cardiologists, to auscultation of the heart (Leatham 1987). This approach concentrates mainly on the analysis of the second heart sound (S2) and its two major components A2 and P2. The main purposes are estimating the order of occurrence of A2 and P2 as well as the time delay between them. This delay known as *split* occurs from the fact that the aortic and pulmonary valves do not close simultaneously. Normally the aortic valves close before the pulmonary valves and exaggerated splitting of the S2 sound may occur in right ventricular outflow obstruction, such as pulmonary stenosis (PS), right bundle branch block (RBBB) and atrial and ventricular septal defect. Reverse splitting of sound S2 is due to a delay in the aortic component A2, which causes a reverse sequence of the closure sounds, with P2 preceding A2. The main causes of reverse spitting are left bundle branch block (LBBB) and premature closure of pulmonary valves. The wide *split* has duration of about 50 miliseconds compared to the normal *split* with the value of ≤ 30 ms (Leung et al. 1998). The measurement of the S2 *split*, lower or higher than 30 ms and the order of occurrence of A2 and P2 leads to a discrimination between normal and pathological cases.

4.1 Wavelet Based feature extraction

The major difficulty associated with the phonocardiogram segmentation is the similarity among its main components. For example it is well known that S1 and S2 contain very closed frequency components, however S2 have higher frequency content than S1. Another example of sounds containing very closed frequency components, which must be distinguished is the aortic and pulmonary components of S2 sound.

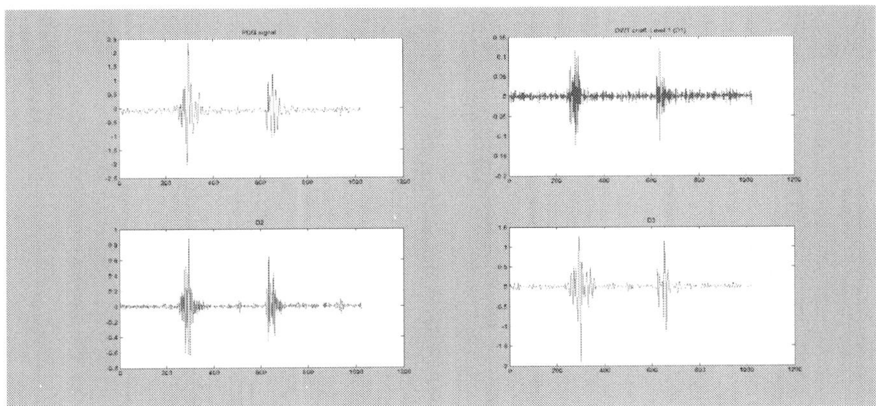

Fig. 9. Wavelet decomposition of one cycle PCG

The multiresolution analysis based on the DWT can enhance each one of these small differences if the signal is viewed at the most appropriate scale. Figure 9 shows the result of the application of the DWT one cycle of a normal PCG. From the figure we can observe that d1 level (frequency ranges of 250-500Hz) emphasize the high frequency content of S2 sound when compared with S1. D2 and d3 levels show clearly the differences in magnitude and frequency of the S2 components A2 and P2, which helps to accurately measure the *split* since A2 and P2 appear quite different. The features used in the scope of this work are simultaneous observations of d1, d3 and d4 scales, therefore the observation sequence generated after the parameter extraction is of the form $O=(o_1, o_2, \ldots o_T)$ where T is the signal length in number of samples and each observation o_t is a three-dimensional vector, i. e., the wavelet scales have the same time resolution as the original signal.

4.2 HMM segmentation of the PCG

The phonocardiogram can be seen as a sequence of elementary waves and silences containing at least five different segments; M1, T1, A2, P2 and silences. Each one of them can be modeled by a different HMM. Two different silences must be modeled since murmurs can be present and diastolic murmurs are in general different from systolic murmurs. Left to right (or Bakis) HMM's with different number of states were used, since this is the most used topology in the field of speech recognition, and the phonocardiographic signal is also a sound signal with auditory properties similar to speech signals. Each HMM models one different event and the concatenation of them models the whole PCG signal. The concatenation of these HMM's follows certain rules dependent on the sequence of events allowed. These rules define a grammar with six main symbols (four main waves and two silences of different nature) and an associated language model as shown in figure 10.

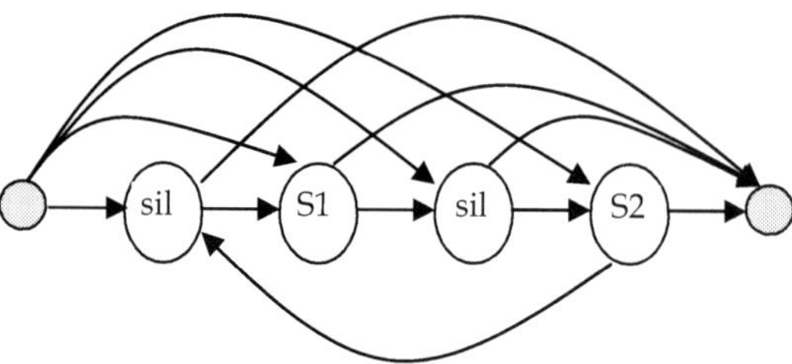

Fig. 10. Heart sound Markov Model

This HMM does not take into consideration the S3 and S4 heart sounds since these sounds are difficult to hear and record, thus they are most likely not noticeable in the records.
The acoustic HMM's are Continuous Density Hidden Markov Models (CDHMM's) and the continuous observations are frequently modeled by a Gaussian mixture. However, by observing the histograms for every state of every HMM it was observed that most of them appear to be well fitted to a single Gaussian, so a single Gaussian probability density function was used to model the continuous observations in each state/transition.
PCG elementary waves are modeled by three state HMM's and the probability density functions are simple Gaussians. The observation vector components are considered independents and identically distributed as considered in the re-estimation formulas in section 3. Silence models are one state HMM's and probabilities density functions are a mixture of three Gaussian functions.
The PCG morphologies are learned from training the HMM's. The training algorithm was the standard Baum-Welch method, also called forward-backward algorithm, which is a particular case of the expectation maximization method and is extensively explained in section 3.
The beat segmentation procedure consists on matching the HMM models to the PCG waveform patterns. This is typically performed by the Viterbi decoding algorithm, which relates each observation to an HMM state following the maximum likelihood criteria with respect to the beat model structure. Additionally the most likely state sequence is available, which allows to estimate time duration of the PCG components as the *split*. This algorithm performs well in the absence of strong murmurs. However if relatively strong murmurs are present both the silence models must be adapted for the current patient, even if murmurs exist in the training patterns. Two methods are suggested:
If the ECG is also recorded a QRS detector can be used to accurately locate diastolic murmurs that appear exactly before QRS locations. Systolic murmurs locations can also be estimated since they appear after S1 that is almost synchronous with the QRS. Having systolic and diastolic data the corresponding silence models can be updated for the current patient by using incremental training. Three cardiac cycles are enough to accurately re-estimate the silence models. Additionally using the re-estimated silence models all the other models can be updated for the current patient by using also incremental training or adaptation. Firstly the most likely wave sequence is estimated by decoding the data, then all the models except the silence models are updated on the basis of the recognition data. Two cardiac cycles are enough to adapt the wave models. This procedure incremented the system

performance of 17.25% when applied to a patient with systolic murmur, suspection of pulmonary stenosis, ventricular septal defect and pulmonary hypertension.

In the absence of ECG the most likely wave sequence can also be estimated by decoding the data and all models can be updated based on incoming data by using the formulas derived in section 3. However under severe murmur conditions the decoding can fail and the updating of the models originates model divergence. Therefore supervised adaptation is required to guarantee model convergence. Under model convergence situations and using two cardiac cycles for model adaptation purposes similar results to the previous case were obtained in the same dataset.

The performance of this algorithm is similar to the performance of (Debbal & Bereksi-Reguig 2007) algorithm in the absence of murmurs and in the most common situation where the aortic wave has higher amplitude than the pulmonary wave. However in the presence of a relatively weak systolic murmur in real data as well in noisy situations the present algorithm outperformed the (Debbal & Bereksi-Reguig 2007) algorithm.

5. Wavelets, HMM's and the ECG

Recently WT has been successfully combined with HMM's providing reliable beat segmentation results (Andreão et al., 2006). The ECG signal is decomposed in different scales by using the DWT and re-synthesized using only the most appropriate scales. Three views of the ECG at different scales were used in such a way that the re-synthesized signal has the same time resolution as the original ECG. Each wave (P, QRS, T) and segment (PQ, ST) of a heartbeat is modelled by a specific left-to-right HMM. The isolelectric line between two consecutive beats is also modelled by an HMM. The concatenation of the individual HMM's models the whole ECG signal. The continuous observations are modelled by a single Gaussian probability density function, since histograms of the observations in the various HMM's showed that the data can be well fitted to a single Gaussian. In order to improves modelling of complex patterns multiple models are created for each waveform by using the HMM likelihood clustering algorithm.

A morphological based strategy in the HMM framework have recently been proposed to take advantage of the similarities between normal and atrial fibrillation beats to improve the classifier performance by using Maximum Mutual Information (MMIE) training, in a single model/double class framework (Lima & Cardoso 2007). The approach is similar of having two different models sharing the most parameters. This approach saves computational resources at run-time decoding and improves the classification accuracy of very similar classes by using MMIE training. The idea is that if two classes have some state sequence similarities and the main morphological differences occur only in a short time slice, then setting appropriately internal state model transitions can model the differences between classes. These differences can be more efficiently emphasized by taking advantage of the well known property of MMIE training of HMM's, which typically makes more effective use of a small number of available parameters. By this reasoning the selected decoding class can be chosen on the basis of the most likely state sequence, which characterizes the most likely class.

Figure 11 shows the model structure for the atrial fibrillation and normal beats, where $a_{i,j}$ stands for transition probability from state i to state j. The behind reasoning is based on the assumption that an AF beat is similar to a normal beat without the P wave which can be modeled by a transition probability that not pass through the state which models the P wave. The recursive transition in each state can model rhythm differences by time warping capabilities. At the end of the decoding stage the recognized class can be selected by searching (backtracking) the most likely state sequence. This structure can be seen as two separate HMM's sharing the most parameters. This parameter sharing procedure is justified by the fact that ventricular conduction is normal in morphology for AF beats, and we intend to use a limited amount of parameters, just the pdf associated with the transitions from state 5 to states 6 and 7, state 6 to itself and to state 7 to reinforce the discriminative power between classes. The separation between these two classes can be increased by using an efficient discriminative training as MMIE obtained on the basis of the parameters associated with the intra-class differences, just those above mentioned. It is very important to note that this approach reinforces the HMM distance among different model structures while the distance of HMM's in the same structure (those that share parameters) are obviously decreased. However, it is believed that an appropriate discriminative training can efficiently separate the classes modeled by the same HMM. Although a recognition system fully trained by using the MMIE approach can be more effective it surely needs a much degree of computational requirements in both training and run time decoding.

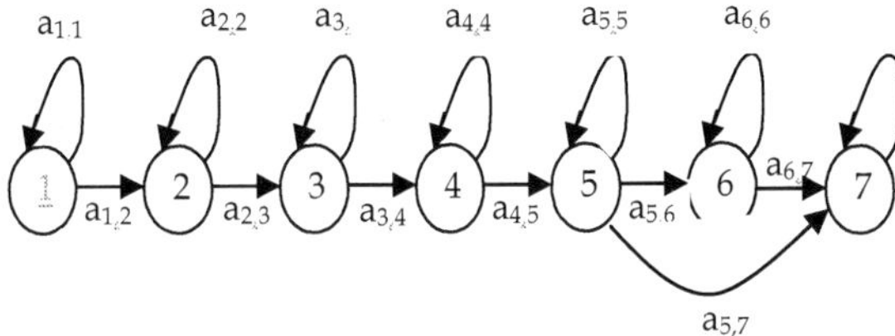

Fig. 11. HMM topology adopted for modelling normal (N) and atrial fibrillation (AF) beats.

States from 1 to 7 are concerned to the ECG events R, S, S-T, T, T-P, P, P-R.This frame state allocation concerned to the ECG events can be forced by setting (to one) the initial probability of the first state in the initial state probability vector and resetting all the other initial state probabilities, and also synchronizing the ECG feature extraction to begin in the R wave. This kind of synchronization is needed for this HMM topology where the initial state must be synchronized with the R wave, otherwise the assumption that state 6 models P-wave can not be true. We observed this evidence in our experiments. However if a back transition from the last to the initial state is added this synchronization is necessary only for the first ECG pulse decoding. The synchronization between ECG beats and the HMM model is facilitated by the intrinsic difference between the last and first state, since the last state models an isoelectric segment (weak signal) while the first state models the R wave which is a much strong signal. In other words if the HMM is in state 7 modeling an isoelectric segment the happening of a strong R wave tends to force a transition to state one which helps in model/beat synchronization. The adopted training strategy accommodate both the MMIE training and parameter sharing, or in other words an MMIE training procedure in only one HMM platform with capabilities to model two classes must be required. This compromise was obtained by estimating the shared parameters in the MLE sense. This algorithm was tested in the MIT_BIH arrhythmia database and outperforms the traditional MLE estimation algorithm.

6. Conclusion

This chapter provides a review of the WT and points out its most important properties regarding non-stationary biosignal modelling, including the extension to biomedical image processing. However practical situations often require high accurate methods capable of handling, usually by training, highly non-stationary conditions. To cope with this variability a new PCG segmentation approach was proposed relying on knowledge acquired from training examples and stored in statistical quasi-stationary models (HMM's) with features obtained from the wavelet transform. The proposed algorithm outperforms a recent wavelet only based algorithm especially under relatively light murmur situations, which are the most common in practical situations. Additionally a recent HMM algorithm based on morphological concepts concerning to arrhythmia classification was reviewed. This approach is also new and outperforms the conventional HMM training strategies.

7. References

Addison, P. S., Watson, J. N., Clegg, J. R., Holzer, M., Sterz, F. & Robertson, C. E. (2000). Evaluating arrhythmias in ECG signals using wavelet transforms. *IEEE Eng. Med. Biol.*, Vol. 19, page numbers (104-109).

Akay, Y. M., Akay, M., Welkovitz, W., & Kostis, J. (1994). Noninvasive detection of coronary artery disease. *IEEE Eng. In Med. And Biol. Mag.*, vol. 13 n°5, page numbers (761-764).

Akay, M., & Szeto, H. H., (1994). Wavelet analisis of opioid drug effects on the elctrocortical activity in fetus. *Proc. Conf. Artif. Neural Networks in Eng.*, page numbers (553-558).

Al-Fahoum, A. S. & Howitt, I. (1999). Combined wavelet transformation and radial basis neural network for classifying life-threatening cardiac arrhythmias. *Med. Biol. Eng. Comput.*, Vol. 37, page numbers (566-573).

Andreão, R. V., Dorizzi, B. & Boudy, J. (2006). ECG analysis using hidden Markov models. *IEEE Transactions on Biomedical Engineering*, Vol. 53, No. 8, page numbers (1541-1549).

Barbosa, D., Ramos, J., Tavares, A. & Lima, C. S. (2009). Detection of Small Bowel Tumors in Endoscopic Capsule Images by Modeling Non-Gaussianity of Texture Descriptors. *International Journal of Tomography & Statistics, Special Issue on Image Processing* ISSN 0972-9976. In press.

Baum, L. (1972). An inequality and associated maximisation technique in statistical estimation of probabilistic functions of Markov processes. *Inequalities,* Vol. 3, page numbers (1-8).

Benedetto, J. J., & Teolis, A. (1993). A wavelet auditory model and data compression. Appl. Computat. Harmonic. Anal., Vol. 1, page numbers (3-28).

Candès, E. & Donoho, D. (2000). Curvelets - a surprisingly effective nonadaptive representation for objects with edges. *Curves and Surfaces*, L. L. Schumaker et al., (Ed.), page numbers (105-120), Vanderbilt University Press, Nashville, TN

Candès, E.; Demanet, L.; Donoho, D. & Ying, L. (2006). Fast discrete curvelet transforms, *SIAM Multiscale Modeling Simul*, Vol. 5, No.3, September 2006, page numbers (861-899)

Chebil, J. & Al-Nabulsi, J. (2007). Classification of heart sound signals using discrete wavelet Analysis. *International Journal of Soft Compting*, Vol. 2, No. 1, page numbers (37-41).

Daugman, J. G. (1988). Complete discrete 2-D Gabor transforms by neural networks for image analysis and compression. *IEEE Trans. Acoust Speech and Signal Process.*, Vol. 36, (July. 1988) page numbers (1169-1179).

Daugman, J. G. (1989). Entropy reduction and decorrelation in visual coding by oriented neural receptive fields. *IEEE Trans. Biomed. Eng.*, Vol. 36, (Jan. 1989) page numbers (107-114).

Debbal, S. M., & Bereksi-Reguig, F. (2004). Analysis of the second heart sound using continuous wavelet transform. *J. Med. Eng. Technol.*, vol. 28, N° 4, page numbers (151-156).

Debbal, S. M., & Bereksi-Reguig, F. (2007). Automatic measure of the split in the second cardiac sound by using the wavelet transform technique, *Computers in Biology and Medicine*, vol 37, page numbers (269-276).

Dempster, A. P., Laird, N. M. & Rubin, D. B. (1977). Maximum likelihood from incomplete data via the EM algorithm. *J. Roy. Stat. Soc.*, Vol. 39, N°1, page numbers (1-38).

Dettori L. & Semler, L. (2007). A comparison of wavelet, ridgelet, and curvelet-based texture classification algorithms in computed tomography, *Computers in Biology and Medicine*, Vol. 37, No. 4, April 2007, page numbers (486-498)

Dickhaus, H., Khadra, L., & Brachmann, J., (1994). Time-frequency analysis of ventricular late potentials, *Methods of Inform. in Med.*, vol. 33 (2), page numbers (187-195).

Do, M. & Vetterli M. (2005). The Contourlet Transform: An Efficient Directional Multiresolution Image Representation, *IEEE Trans. on Image Processing*, Vol. 14, No. 12, December 2005, page numbers (2091-2106)

Donoho, D. (1995). De-noising by Soft-thresholding, *IEEE Trans. Information Theory*, Vol. 41, No. 3, May 1995, page numbers (613-617)

Duverney, D., Gaspoz, J. M., Pichot, V., Roche, F., Brion, R., Antoniadis, A. & Barthelemy, J-C. (2002). High accuracy of automatic detection of atrial fibrillation using wavelet transform of heart rate intervals. *PACE*, Vol. 25, page numbers (457-462).

Gaudart, L., Crebassa, J. & Petrakian, J. P. (1993). Wavelet transform in human visual channels. *Applied Optics*, Vol. 32, No. 22, page numbers (4119-4127).

Govindan, A., Deng, G. & Power, J. (1997). Electrogram analysis during atrial fibrillation using wavelet and neural network techniques, *Proc. SPIE 3169*, pp. 557-562.

Heinlein, P.; Drexl, J. & Schneider, W. (2003). Integrated wavelets for enhancement of microcalcifications in digital mammography, *IEEE Trans. Med. Imag.*, Vol. 22, March 2003, page numbers(402-413).

Hubel, D. H. (1982). Exploration of the primary visual cortex: 1955-1978. *Nature*, Vol. 299, page numbers (515-524).

Inoue, H. & Miyasaki, A. (1998). A noise reduction method for ECG signals using the dyadic wavelet transform. *IEICE Trans. Fundam.*, Vol. E81A, page numbers (1001-1007).

Jin, Y.; Angelini, E.; Esser, P. & Laine, A. (2003). De-noising SPECT/PET Images Using Cross-scale Regularization, *Proceedings of the Sixth International Conference on Medical Image Computing and Computer Assisted Interventions (MICCAI 2003)*, pp. 32-40, Montreal, Canada, November 2003.

Jin, Y.; Angelini, E. & Laine, A. (2004) Wavelets in Medical Image Processing: Denoising, Segmentation, and Registration, In: Handbook of Medical Image Analysis: Advanced Segmentation and Registration Models, Suri, J.; Wilson, D. & Laximinarayan, S., (Ed.), page numbers (305-358), Kluwer Academic Publishers, New York.

Kadambe, S., Murray, R. & Boudreaux-Bartels, G. F. (1999). Wavelet transform-based QRS complex detector. *IEEE Trans. Biomed. Eng.*, Vol. 46, page numbers (838-848).

Kalayci, T. & Ozdamar, O., (1995). Wavelet pre-processing for automated neural network detection of spikes. *IEEE Eng. in Med. and Biol. Mag.*, vol. 14 (2), page numbers (160-166).

Karkanis, A.; Iakovidis, D.; Maroulis, D.; Karras, D. & Tzivras, M. (2003). Computer-aided tumor detection in endoscopic video using color wavelet features, *IEEE Trans. Info. Tech. in Biomedicine*, Vol. 7, No. 3, September 2003, page numbers (142-152)

Khadra, L., Matalgah, M., El-Asir, B., & Mawagdeh, S. (1991). The wavelet transform and its applications to phonocardiogram signal analysis, In: *Med. Informat.*, vol. 16, page numbers (271-277).

Khadra, L., Dickhaus, H., & Lipp, A. (1993). Representations of ECG-late potentials in the time-frequency plane, In: J. *Med. Eng. and Technol.*, vol. 17 (6) page numbers (228-231).

Leatham, A. (1987). Auscultation and Phonocardiography: a personal view of the past 40 years. *Heart J., Vol.* 57 (B2).

Leman, H. & Marque, C. (200). Rejection of the maternal electrocardiogram in the electrohysterogram signal. *IEEE Trans. Biomed. Eng.*, Vol. 47, page numbers (1010-1017).

Lemaur, G.; Drouiche, K. & DeConinck, J. (2003). Highly regular wavelets for the detection of clustered microcalcifications in mammograms, *IEEE Trans. Med. Imag.*, Vol. 22, March 2003, page numbers (393-401)

Leung, T. S., White, P. R., Cook, J., Collis, W. B., Brown, E. & Salmon, A. P. (1998). Analysis of the second heart sound for diagnosis of paediatric heart disease. *IEE Proceedings - Science, Measurement and Technology*, Vol. 145, Issue 6, (November of 1998) page numbers (285-290).

Levinson, S. E., Rabiner, L. R. & Sondhi, M. M. (1983). An introduction to the application of the theory of probabilistic function of a Markov process to automatic speech recognition. *Bell System Tech. J.*, Vol. 62, N^a 4, page numbers (1035-1074).

Li, B. & Meng, Q. (2009). Texture analysis for ulcer detection in capsule endoscopy images, *Image and Vision Computing*, In Press

Li, C., & Zheng, C., (1993). QRS detection by wavelet transform, In: *Proc. Annu. Confl. on Eng. in Med. And Biol.*, vol. 15, page numbers (330-331).

Li, C., Zheng, C., Tai, C. (1995). Detection of ECG characteristic points using wavelet transforms. *IEEE Trans. Biomed. Eng.*, Vol. 42, page numbers (21-28).

Lima, C.S. & Cardoso, M. J. (2007). Cardiac Arrhythmia Detection by Parameters Sharing and MMI Training of Hidden Markov Models. *The 29th IEEE EMBS Annual International Conference EMBC07*, Lyon, France, 2007.

Lima, C. S. & Barbosa, D. (2008). Automatic Segmentation of the Second Cardiac Sound by Using Wavelets and Hidden Markov Models, *The 30th IEEE EMBS Annual International Conference EMBC08*, Vancouver, Canada, 2008.

Lima, C. S., Barbosa, D., Tavares, A., Ramos, J., Monteiro, L., Carvalho, L. (2008). Classification of Endoscopic Capsule Images by Using Color Wavelet Features, Higher Order Statistics and Radial Basis Functions, *The 30th IEEE EMBS Annual International Conference EMBC08*, Vancouver, Canada.

Mallat, S. G., (1989). Multifrequency channel decompositions of images and wavelet models, *IEEE Trans. Acoust., Speech and Signal Process. Patt.*, vol. 37, (December 1989) page numbers (2091-2110).

Mallat, S., & Zhong, S., (1992). Characterization of signals from multiscale edges, In: *IEEE Trans. Patt. Anal. Machine Intell.*, vol. 14, page numbers (710-732).

Mallat, S., (1998). *A wavelet tour of signal processing*, Academic Press.

Marcelja, S. (1980). Mathematical description of the responses of simple cortical cells. *J. Opt. Soc. Amer.*, Vol. 70, No. 11, page numbers (1297-1300).

Martinez, J. P., Almeida, R., Olmos, S., Rocha, A. P. & Laguna, P. (2004). A wavelet based ECG delineator: evaluation on standard data bases. *IEEE Trans. Biomed. Eng.*, Vol. 51, page numbers (570-581).

Nikoliaev, N., Gotchev, A., Egiazarian, K. & Nikolov, Z. (2001). Supression of electromyogram interference on the electrocardiogram by transform domain denoising. *Med. Biol. Eng. Comput.*, Vol. 39, page numbers (649-655).

Nigam, V. & Priemer, R. (2006). A Procedure to extract the Aortic and the Pulmonary Sounds from the Phonocardiogram, *Proceedings of the 28th Annual International Conference of the IEEE in Engineering in Medicine and Biology Society*, pp. 5715-5718, August 2006.

Obaidat, M. S., (1993). Phonocardiogram signal analysis: techniques and performance. *J. Med. Eng. and Technol.*, vol. 17, page numbers (221-227).

Papadopoulos, A.; Fotiadis, D. & Costaridou, L. (2008). Improvement of microcalcification cluster detection in mammography utilizing image enhancement techniques, *Computers in Biology and Medicine*, Vol. 38, No. 10, October 2008, page numbers (1045-1055)

Park, K. L., Lee, K. J. & Yoon H. R. (1998). Application of a wavelet adaptive filter to minimise distortion of the ST-segment. *Med. Biol. Eng. Comput.*, Vol. 36, page numbers (581-586).

Park, K. L., Khil, M. J., Lee, B. C., Jeong, K. S., Lee, K. J. & Yoon H. R. (2001). Design of a wavelet interpolation filter for enhancement of the ST-segment. *Med. Biol. Eng. Comput.*, Vol. 39, page numbers (1-6)

Porat, M. & Zeevi, Y. Y. (1989). Localised texture processing in vision: analysis and synthesis in Gaborian Space. *IEEE Trans. Biomed. Eng.*, Vol. 36, (Jan. 1989) page numbers (115-129).

Przelaskowski, A.; Sklinda, K.; Bargieł, P.; Walecki, J.; Biesiadko-Matuszewska, M. & Kazubek, M. (2007). stroke detection: Wavelet-based perception enhancement of computerized tomography exams, *Computers in Biology and Medicine*, Vol. 37, No. 4, April 2007, page numbers (524-533).

Rabiner, L. R. (1989). A tutorial on hidden Markov models and selected applications in speech recognition. *Proc. IEEE*, Vol. 77, N° 2, page numbers (257-286).

Romero Legarreta, I., Addison, P. S., Reed, M. J., Grubb, N. R., Clegg, G. R., Robertson, C. E. & Watson, J. N. (2005). Continuous wavelet transform modulus maxima analysis of the electrocardiogram: beat-to-beat characterization and beat-to-beat measurement. *Int. J. Wavelets, Multiresolution Inf. Process.* Vol. 3, page numbers (19-42).

Sahambi, J. S., Tandon, S. M. & Bhatt, R. K. P. (1997a). Using wavelet transforms for ECG characterization: an on-line digital signal processing system. *IEEE Eng. Med. Biol.*, Vol. 16, page numbers (77-83).

Sahambi, J. S., Tandon, S. M. & Bhatt, R. K. P. (1997b). Quantitative analysis of errors due to power-line interferences and base-line drift in detection of onsets and offsets in ECG using wavelets. *Med. Biol. Eng. Comput.*, Vol. 35, page numbers (747-751).

Sahambi, J. S., Tandon, S. M. & Bhatt, R. K. P. (1998). Wavelet base ST-segment analysis. *Med. Biol. Eng. Comput.*, Vol. 36, page numbers (568-572).

Sartene, R., et al., (1994). Using wavelet transform to analyse cardiorespiratory and electroencephalographic signals during sleep, In: Proc. IEEE EMBS Workshop on Wavelets in Med. and Biol., page numbers (18a-19a), Baltimore.

Schelkens, P.; Munteanu, A.; Barbarien, J.; Galca, M.; Nieto, X. & Cornelis, J. (2003). Wavelet coding of volumetric medical datasets, *IEEE Trans. Med. Imag.*, Vol. 22, March 2003, page numbers(441-458).

Schiff, S. J., Aldroubi, A., Unser, M., & Sato, S., (1994). Fast wavelet transformation of EEG, In: Electroencephalogr. Clin. Neurophysiol., vol. 91 (6), page numbers (442-455).

Senhadji, L., Carrault, G., Bellanger, J. J., & Passariello, G., (1995). Comparing wavelet transforms for recognizing cardiac patterns, In: IEEE Eng. in Med. and Biol. Mag., vol 14 (2), page numbers (167-173).

Shyu, L-Y., Wu, Y-H. & Hu, W. (2004). Using wavelet transform and fuzzy neural network for VPC detection from the Holter ECG. *IEEE Trans. Biomed. Eng.* , Vol. 51, page numbers (1269-1273).

Simoncelli, E.; Freeman, W.; Adelson, E. & Heeger, D. (1992). Shiftable multiscale transforms, *IEEE Transactions on Information Theory - Special Issue on Wavelet Transforms and Multiresolution Signal* Analysis, Vol. 38, No. 2, March 1992, page numbers (587–607).

Simoncelli, E. & Freeman, W. (1995). The Steerable Pyramid: A Flexible Architecture for Multi- Scale Derivative Computation, Proceedings of IEEE Second International Conference on Image Processing, Washington, DC, October 1995.

Sivannarayana, N. & Reddy, D. C. (1999). Biorthogonal wavelet transforms for ECG parameters estimation. *Med. Eng. Phys.*, Vol. 21, page numbers (167-174)

Strickland, R. N., & Hahn, H. I., (1994). Detection of microcalcifications in mammograms using wavelets, In: *Proc. SPIE Conf. Wavelet Applicat. in Signal and Image Process. II*, vol. 2303, page numbers (430-441), San Diego, CA.

Sung-Nien, Y.; Kuan-Yuei, L. & Huang Y. (2006). Detection of microcalcifications in digital mammograms using wavelet filter and Markov random field model, *Computerized Medical Imaging and Graphics*, Vol. 30, No. 3, April 2006, page numbers (163-173)

Tikkanen, P. E. (1999). Nonlinear wavelet and wavelet packet denoising of electrocardiogram signal. *Biol. Cybernetics*, Vol. 80, page numbers (259-267).

Valois, R. De & Valois, K. De (1988). *Spatial Vision*, Oxford Univ. Press, New York.

Vetterli, M. & Kovacevic, J. (1995). *Wavelets and Subband Coding*, Englewood Cliffs, Prentice Hall, NJ.

Wang, K., & Shamma, S. A. (1995). Auditory analysis of spectrotemporal information in acoustic signals. *IEEE Eng. in Med. and Biol. Mag.*, Vol. 14, No. 2, page numbers (186-194)

Watson, A. B. (1987). The cortex transform: rapid computation of simulated neural images. *Computer Vision Graphics Image Process.*, Vol. 39, No. 3, page numbers (311-327).

Watson, J. N., Addison, P. S., Clegg, G. R., Holzer, M., Sterz, F. & Robertson, C. E. (2000). Evaluation of arrhythmic ECG signals using a novel wavelet transform method. *Resuscitation,* Vol. 43, page numbers (121-127).

Watson, J. N., Uchaipichat, N., Addison, P. S., Clegg, G. R., Robertson, C. E., Eftestol, T., & Steen, P.A., (2008). Improved prediction of defibrillation success for out-of-hospital VF cardiac arrest using wavelet transform methods. *Resuscitation,* Vol. 63, page numbers (269-275).

Weaver, J.; Yansun, X.; Healy Jr, D. & Cromwell, L. (1991). Filtering noise from images with wavelet transforms, *Magn. Reson. Med.,* Vol. 21, October 1991, page numbers (288–295)

Xu, J., Durand, L. & Pibarot, P., (2000). Nonlinear transient chirp signal modelling of the aortic and pulmonary components of the second heart sound. *IEEE Transactions on Biomedical Engineering,* Vol. 47, Issue 10, (October 2000) page numbers (1328-1335).

Xu, J., Durand, L. & Pibarot, P., (2001). Extraction of the aortic and pulmonary components of the second heart sound using a nonlinear transient chirp signal model. *IEEE Transactions on Biomedical Engineering,* Vol. 48, Issue 3, (March 2001) page numbers (277-283).

Yang, L.; Guo, B. & Ni, W. (2008). Multimodality medical image fusion based on multiscale geometric analysis of contourlet transform, *Neurocomputing,* Vol. 72, December 2008, page numbers (203-211)

Yang, X., Wang, K., & Shamma, S. A. (1992). Auditory representations of acoustic signals. *IEEE Trans. Informat. Theory,* Vol. 38, (February 1992) page numbers (824-839).

Yi, G., Hnatkova, K., Mahon, N. G., Keeling, P. J., Reardon, M., Camm, A. J. & Malik, M. (2000). Predictive value of wavelet decomposition of the signal averaged electrocardiogram in idiopathic dilated cardiomyopathy. *Eur. Heart J.,* Vol. 21, page numbers (1015-1022).

Yildirim, I. & Ansari, R. (2007). A Robust Method to Estimate Time Split in Second Heart Sound Using Instantaneous Frequency Analysis, *Proceedings of the 29th Annual International Conference of the IEEE EMBS,* pp. 1855-1858, August 2007, Lyon, France.

Zhang, X-S., Zhu, Y-S., Thakor, N. V., Wang, Z-M. & Wang, Z. Z. (1999). Modelling the relationship between concurrent epicardial action potentials and bipolar electrograms. *IEEE Trans. Biomed. Eng.,* Vol. 46, page numbers (365-376).

4

Stochastic Differential Equations With Applications to Biomedical Signal Processing

Aleksandar Jeremic

Department of Electrical and Computer Engineering, McMaster University
Hamilton, ON, Canada

1. Introduction

Dynamic behavior of biological systems is often governed by complex physiological processes that are inherently stochastic. Therefore most physiological signals belong to the group of stochastic signals for which it is impossible to predict an exact future value even if we know its entire past history. That is there is always an aspect of a signal that is inherently random i.e. unknown. Commonly used biomedical signal processing techniques often assume that observed parameters and variables are deterministic in nature and model randomness through so called observation errors which do not influence the stochastic nature of underlying processes (e.g., metabolism, molecular kinetics, etc.). An alternative approach would be based on the assumption that the governing mechanisms are subject to instantaneous changes on a certain time scale. As an example fluctuations in the respiratory rate and/or concentration of oxygen (or equivalently partial pressures) in various compartments is strongly affected by a metabolic rate, which is inherently stochastic and therefore is not a smooth process.

As a consequence one of the mathematical techniques that is quickly assuming an important role in modeling of biological signals is stochastic differential equations (SDE) modeling. These models are natural extensions of classic deterministic models and corresponding ordinary differential equations. In this chapter we will present computational framework necessary for successful application of SDE models to actual biomedical signals. To accomplish this task we will first start with mathematical theory behind SDE models. These models are used extensively in various fields such as financial engineering, population dynamics, hydrology, etc.

Unfortunately, most of the literature about stochastic differential equations seems to place a large emphasis on rigor and completeness using strict mathematical formalism that may look intimidating to non-experts. In this chapter we will attempt to present answer to the following questions: in what situations the stochastic differential models may be applicable, what are the essential characteristics of these models, and what are some possible tools that can be used in solving them. We will first introduce mathematical theory necessary for understanding SDEs.

Next, we will discuss both univariate and multivariate SDEs and discuss the corresponding computational issues. We will start with introducing the concept of stochastic integrals and illustrate the solution process using one univariate and one multivariate example. To address the computational complexity in realistic biomedical signal models we will further discuss the aforementioned biochemical transport model and derive the stochastic integral solution for demonstration purposes. We will also present analytical solution based on Fokker-Planck equation, which establishes link between partial differential equation (PDE) and stochastic processes. Our most recent work includes results for realistic boundaries and will be presented in the context of drug delivery modeling i.e. biochemical transport and respiratory signal analysis and prediction in neonates.

Since in many clinical and academic applications researchers are interested in obtaining better estimates of physiological parameters using experimental data we will illustrate the inverse approach based on SDEs in which the unknown parameters are estimated. To address this issue we will present maximum likelihood estimator of the unknown parameters in our SDE models. Finally, in the last subsection of the chapter we will present SDE models for monitoring and predicting respiratory signals (oxygen partial pressures) using a data set of 200 patients obtained in Neonatal ICU, McMaster Hospital. We will illustrate the application of SDEs through the following steps: identification of physiological parameters, proposition of a suitable SDE model, solution of the corresponding SDE, and finally estimation of unknown parameters and respiratory signal prediction and tracking.

In many cases biomedical engineers are exposed to real-world problems while signal processors have abundance of signal processing techniques that are often not utilized in the most optimal way. In this chapter we hope to merge these two worlds and provide average reader from the biomedical engineering field with skills that will enable him to identify if the SDE models are truly applicable to real-world problems they are encountering.

2. Basic Mathematical Notions

In most cases stochastic differential equations can be viewed as a generalization of ordinary differential equations in which some coefficients of a differential equation are random in nature. Ordinary differential equations are commonly used tool for modeling biological systems as a relationship between a function of interest, say bacterial population size $N(t)$ and its derivatives and a forcing, controlling function $F(T)$ (drift, reaction, etc.). In that sense an ordinary differential equations can be viewed as model which relates the current value of $N(t)$ by adding and/or subtracting current and past values of $F(t)$ and current values of $N(t)$. In the simplest form the above statement can be represented mathematically as

$$\frac{dN(t)}{dt} \approx \frac{N(t) - N(t - \Delta t)}{\Delta t} = \alpha(t)N(t) + \beta(t)F(t) \qquad N(0) = N_0 \qquad (1)$$

where $N(t)$ is the size of population, $\alpha(t)$ is the relative rate of growth, $\beta(t)$ is the damping coefficient, and $F(t)$ is the reaction force.

In a general case it might happen that $\alpha(t)$ is not completely known but subject to some random environmental effects (as well as $\beta(t)$) in which case $\alpha(t)$ is not completely known but is given by

$$\alpha(t) = r(t) + \text{noise} \qquad (2)$$

where we do not know the exact value of the noise norm nor we can predict it using its probability distribution function (which is in general assumed to be either known or known up a to a set of unknown parameters). The main question is then how do we solve 1?

Before answering that question we first assert that the above equation can be applied in variety of applications. As an example an ordinary differential equation corresponding to RLC circuit is given by

$$L * Q''(t) + RQ'(t) + \frac{1}{C}Q(t) = U(t) \tag{3}$$

where L is the inductance, R is resistance, C is capacitance, Q is the charge on capacitor, and $U(t)$ is the voltage source connected in a circuit. In some cases the circuit elements may have both deterministic and random part, i.e., noise (.e.g. due to temperature variations).

Finally, the most famous example of a stochastic process is Brownian motion observed for the first time by Scottish botanist Robert Brown in 1828. He observed that particles of pollen grain suspend in liquid performed an irregular motion consisting of somewhat "random" jumps i.e. suddenly changing positions. This motion was later explained by the random collisions of pollen with particles of liquid. The mathematical description of such process can be derived starting from

$$\frac{dX}{dt} = b(t, X_t)dt + \sigma(t, X_t)d\Omega_t \tag{4}$$

where $X(t)$ is the stochastic process corresponding to the location of the particle, b is a drift and σ is the "variance" of the jumps. The locNote that (4) is completely equivalent to (1) except that in this case the stochastic process corresponds to the *location* and not to the population count. Based on many situations in engineering the desirable properties of random process Ω_t are

- at different times t_i and t_j the random variables Ω_i and Ω_j are independent

- Stochastic process Ω_t is stationary i.e., the joint probability density function of $(\Omega_i, \Omega_{i+1}, \dots, \Omega_{i+k})$ does not depend on t_i.

However it turns out that there does not exist reasonable stochastic process satisfying all the requirements (25). As a consequence the above model is often rewritten in a different form which allows proper construction. First we start with a finite difference version of (4) at times $t_1, \dots, t_{k_1}, t_k, t_{k+1}, \dots$ yielding

$$X_{k+1} - X_k = b_k * \Delta t + \sigma_k \Omega_k * \Delta t \tag{5}$$

where

$$\begin{aligned} b_k &= b(t_k, X_k) \\ \sigma_k &= \sigma(t_k, X_k) \end{aligned} \tag{6}$$

We replace Ω_k with $\Delta W_k = \Omega_k \Delta t_k = W_{k+1} - W_k$ where W_k is a stochastic process with stationary independent increments with zero mean. It turns out that the only such process with continuous paths is Brownian motion in which the increments at arbitrary time t are zero-mean and independent (1). Using (2) we obtain the following solution

$$X_k = X_0 + \sum_{j=0}^{k-1} b_j \Delta t_j + \sum_{j=0}^{k-1} \sigma_j \Delta W_j \tag{7}$$

When $\Delta t_j \to 0$ it can be shown (25) that the expression on the right hand side of (7) exists and thus the above equation can be written in its integral form as

$$X_t = X_0 + \int_0^t b(s, X_s)ds + \int_0^t \sigma(s, X_s)dW_s \tag{8}$$

Obviously the questionable part of such definition is existence of integral $\int_0^t \sigma(s, X_s)\,dW_s$ which involves integration of a stochastic process. If the diffusion function is continuous and non-anticipative, i.e., does not depend on future, the above integral exists in a sense that finite sums

$$\sum_{l=0}^{n-1} \sigma_i \left[W_{i+1} - W_i \right] \tag{9}$$

converge in a mean square to "some" random variable that we call the Ito integral. For more detailed analysis of the properties a reader is referred to (25).

Now let us illustrate some possible solution of the stochastic differential equations using univariate and multivariate examples.

Case 1 - Population Growth: Consider again a population growth problem in which N_0 subjects of interests are entered into an environment in which the growth of population occurs with rate $\alpha(t)$ and let us assume that the rate can be modeled as

$$\alpha(t) = r(t) + aW_t \tag{10}$$

where W_t is zero-mean white noise and a is a constant. For illustrational purposes we will assume that the deterministic part of the growth rate is fixed i.e., $r(t) = r = $ const. The stochastic differential equation than becomes

$$dN(t) = rN(t) + aN(t)dW(t) \tag{11}$$

or

$$\frac{dN(t)}{N(t)} = rdt + adW(t) \tag{12}$$

Hence

$$\int_0^t \frac{dN(s)}{N(s)} = rt + aW_t \qquad (\text{assuming } B_0 = 0) \tag{13}$$

The above integral represents an example of stochastic integral and in order to solve it we need to introduce the inverse operator i.e., stochastic (or Ito) differential. In order to do this we first assert that

$$\Delta(W_k^2) = W_k^2 + 1 - W_k^2 = (W_{k+1} - W_k)^2 + 2W_k(W_{k+1} - W_k) = (\Delta W_k)^2 + 2W_k\Delta W_k \tag{14}$$

and thus

$$\sum B_k \Delta W_k = \frac{1}{2}W_k^2 - \frac{1}{2}\sum(\Delta W_k)^2 \tag{15}$$

whici yields under regularity conditions

$$\int_0^t W_s dW_s = \frac{1}{2}W_t^2 - \frac{1}{2}t \tag{16}$$

As a consequence the stochastic integrals do not behave like ordinary integrals and thus a special care has to be taken when evaluating integrals. Using (16) it can be shown (25) for a stochastic process X_t given by

$$dX_t = udt + vdW_t \tag{17}$$

and a twice continuously differentiable function $g(t, x)$ a new process

$$Y_t = g(t, X_t) \tag{18}$$

is a stochastic process given by

$$dY_t = \frac{\partial g}{\partial t}(t, X_t)dt + \frac{\partial g}{\partial x}(t, X_t)dX_t + \frac{1}{2}\frac{\partial^2 g}{\partial x^2}(t, X_t)\cdot(dX_t)^2 \tag{19}$$

where $(dX_t)^2 = (dX_t)\cdot(dX_t)$ is computed according to the rules

$$dt\cdot dt = dt\cdot dW_t = dW_t\cdot dt = 0, \qquad dW_t\cdot dW_t = dt \tag{20}$$

The solution of our problem then simply becomes, using map $g(x, t) = \ln x$

$$\frac{dN_t}{N_t} = d\left(\ln N_t\right) + \frac{1}{2}a^2 dt \tag{21}$$

or equivalently

$$N_t = N_0\exp\left(\left(r - \frac{1}{2}a^2\right)t + aW_t\right) \tag{22}$$

Case 2 - Multivarate Case Let us consider n-dimensional problem with following stochastic processes $X_1, \ldots X_n$ given by

$$\begin{aligned}
dX_1 &= u_1 dt + v_{11}dW_1 + \ldots + v_{1m}dW_m \\
&\vdots \quad \vdots \quad \vdots \\
dX_n &= u_n dt + v_{n1}dW_1 + \ldots + v_{nm}dW_m
\end{aligned} \tag{23}$$

Following the proof for univariate case it can be shown (25) that for a n-dimensional stochastic process $\vec{X}(t)$ and mapping function $\vec{g}(t, \vec{x})$ a stochastic process $\vec{Y}(t) = \vec{g}(t, \vec{X}(t))$ such that

$$d\vec{Y}_k = \frac{\partial g_k}{\partial t}(t, \vec{X})dt + \sum_i \frac{\partial g_k}{\partial x_i}(t, \vec{X})dX_i + \frac{1}{2}\sum_{i,j}\frac{\partial^2 g_k}{\partial x_i \partial x_j}(t, \vec{X})dX_i dX_j \tag{24}$$

In order to obtain the solution for the above process we first rewrite it in a matrix form

$$d\vec{X}_t = \vec{r}_t dt + V d\vec{B}_t \tag{25}$$

Following the same approach as in Case 1 it can be shown that

$$\vec{X}_t - \vec{X}_0 = \int_0^t \vec{r}(s)ds + \int_0^t V d\vec{B}_s \tag{26}$$

Consequently the sollution is given by

$$\vec{X}(t) = \vec{X}(0) + V\vec{B}_t + \int_0^t [\vec{r}(s) + V\vec{B}(s)]ds \tag{27}$$

Case 3 - Solving SDEs Using Fokker-Planck Equation: Let $X(t)$ be an on-dimensional stochastic process and let $\ldots > t_{i-1} > t_i > t_{i+1} > \ldots$ Let $P(X_i, t_i; X_{i+1}, t_{i+1})$ denote a joint probability density function and let $P(X_i, t_i | X_{i+1}, t_{i+1})$ denote conditional (or transitional) probability density function. Furthermore for a given SDE the process $X(t)$ will be

Markov if the jumps are uncorrelated i.e., W_i and W_{i+k} are uncorrelated. In this case the transitional density function depends only on the previous value i.e.

$$P(X_i, t_i | X_{i-1}, t_{i-1}; X_{i-2}, t_{i-2}; \ldots, X_1, t_1) = P(X_i, t_i | X_{i-1}, t_{i-1}) \tag{28}$$

For a given stochastic differential equation

$$dX_t = b_t dt + \sigma_t dW_t \tag{29}$$

the transitional probabilities are given by stochastic integrals

$$P(X_{t+\Delta t}, t + \Delta t | X(t), t) = \Pr\left[\int_t^{t+\Delta t} dX_s = X(t + \Delta t) - X(t)\right] \tag{30}$$

In (3) the authors derived the Fokker-Planck equation, a partial differential equation for the time evolution of the transition probability density function and showed that the time evolution of the probability density function is given by

3. Modeling Biochemical Transport Using Stochastic Differential Equations

In this section we illustrate an SDE model that can deal with arbitrary boundaries using stochastic models for diffusion of particles. Such models are becoming subject of considerable research interest in drug delivery applications (4). As a preminalary attempt, we focus on the nature of the boundaries (i.e. their reflective and absorbing properties). The extension to realistic geometry is straight forward since it can be dealt with using Finite Element Method. Absorbing and reflecting boundaries are often encountered in realistic problems such as drug delivery where the organ surfaces represent reflecting/absorbing boundaries for the dispersion of drug particles (11).

Let us assume that at arbitrary time t_0 we introduce n_0 (or equivalently concentration c_0) particles in an open domain environment at location r_0. When the number of particles is large macroscopic approach corresponding to the Fick's law of diffusion is adequate for modeling the transport phenomena. However, to model the motion of the particles when their number is small a microscopic approach corresponding to stochastic differential equations (SDE) is required.

As before, the SDE process for the transport of particle in an open environment is given by

$$dX_t = \vec{b}(X_t, t)dt + \sigma(X_t, t)dW_t \tag{31}$$

where X_t is the location and W_t is a standard Wiener process. The function $\mu(X_t, t)$ is referred to as the drift coefficient while $\sigma()$ is called the diffusion coefficient such that in a small time interval of length dt the stochastic process X_t changes its value by an amount that is normally distributed with expectation $\mu(X_t, t)dt$ and variance $\sigma^2(X_t, t)dt$ and is independent of the past behavior of the process. In the presence of boundaries (absorbing and/or reflecting), the particle will be absorbed when hitting the absorbing boundary and its displacement remains constant (i.e. $dX_t = 0$). On the other hand, when hitting a reflecting boundary the new displacement over a small time step τ, assuming elastic collision, is given by

$$dX_t = dX_{t1} + |dX_{t2}| \cdot \hat{r}_R \tag{32}$$

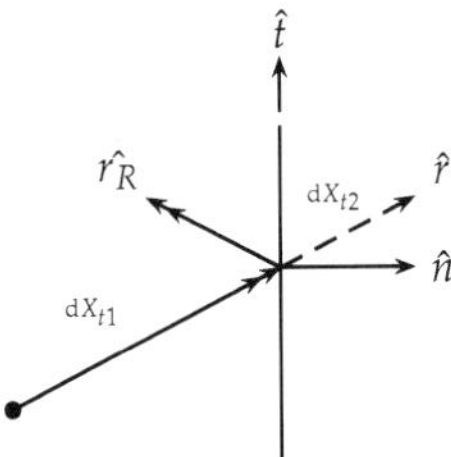

Fig. 1. Behavior of dX_t near a reflecting boundary.

where $\hat{r}_R = -(\hat{r} \cdot \hat{n})\hat{n} + (\hat{r} \cdot \hat{t})\hat{t}$, dX_{t1} and dX_{t2} are shown in Fig. (1).

Assuming three-dimensional environment $r = (x_1, x_2, x_3)$, the probability density function of one particle occupying space around r at time t is given by solution to the Fokker-Planck equation (10)

$$\frac{\partial f(r,t)}{\partial t} = \left[-\sum_{i=1}^{3} \frac{\partial}{\partial x_i} D_i^1(r) + \sum_{i=1}^{3}\sum_{j=1}^{3} \frac{\partial^2}{\partial x_i \partial x_j} D_{ij}^2(r) \right] f(r,t) \tag{33}$$

where partial derivatives apply the multiplication of D and $f(r,t)$, D^1 is the drift vector and D^2 is the diffusion tensor given by

$$\begin{aligned} D_i^1 &= \mu \\ D_{ij}^2 &= \frac{1}{2}\sum_l \sigma_{il}\sigma_{lj}^T \end{aligned} \tag{34}$$

In the case of homogeneous and isotropic infinite two-dimensional (2D) space (i.e, the domain of interest is much larger than the diffusion velocity) with the absence of the drift, the solution of Eq. (33) along with the initial condition at $t = t_0$ is given by

$$f(r, t_0) = \delta(r - r_0) \tag{35}$$

$$f(r, t) = \frac{1}{4\pi D(t - t_0)} e^{-\|r - r_0\|^2 / 4D(t - t_0)} \tag{36}$$

where D is the coefficient of diffusivity.

For the bounded domain, Eq. (33) can be easily solved numerically using a Finite Element Method with the initial condition in Eq. (35) and following boundary conditions (12)

$$f(r, t) = 0 \quad \text{for absorbing boundaries} \tag{37}$$

$$\frac{\partial f(r, t)}{\partial n} = 0 \quad \text{for reflecting boundaries} \tag{38}$$

where $\hat{n}$ is the normal vector to the boundary.

To illustrate the time evolution of $f(r,t)$ in the presence of absorbing/reflecting boundaries, we solve Eq. (33), using a FE package for a closed circular domain consists of a reflecting boundary (black segment) and an absorbing boundary (red segment of length l) as in Fig. (2). As in Figs. (3 and 4), the effect of the absorbing boundary is idle since the flux of $f(r,t)$ did not reach the boundary by then. In Fig. (5), a region of lower probability (density) appears around the absorbing boundary, since the probability of the particle to exist in this region is less than that for the other regions.

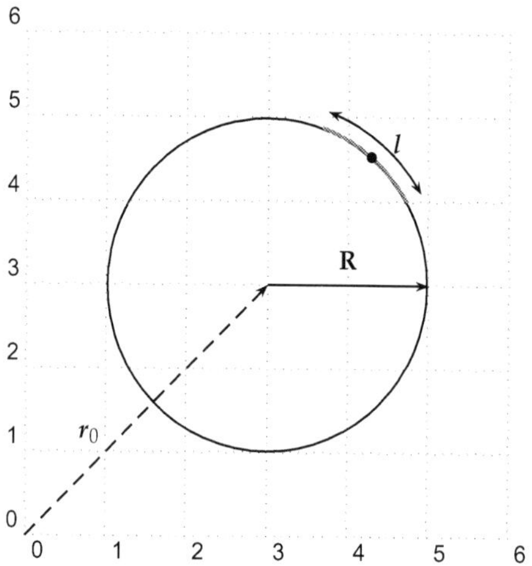

Fig. 2. Closed circular domain with reflecting and absorbing boundaries.

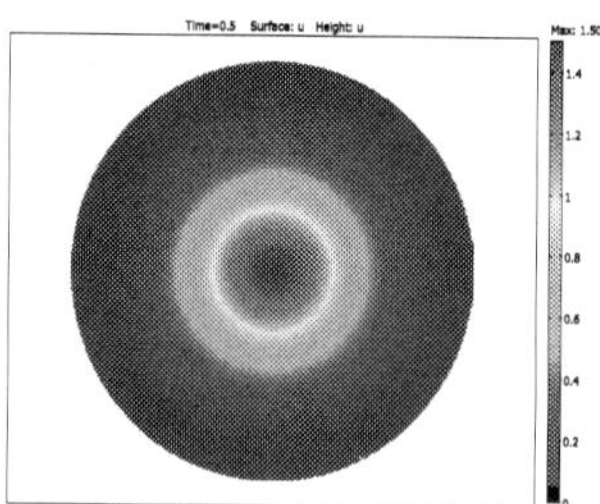

Fig. 3. Probability density function at time 5s after particle injection

Note that each of the above two solutions represents **the probability density function** of one particle occupying space around r at time t assuming it was released from location r_0 at time

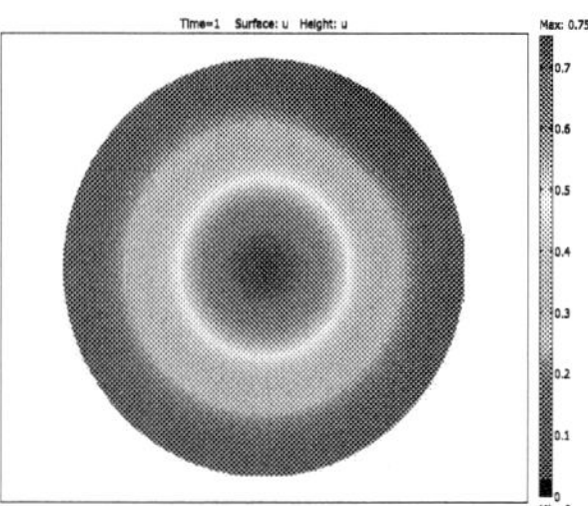

Fig. 4. Probability density function at time 10s after particle injection

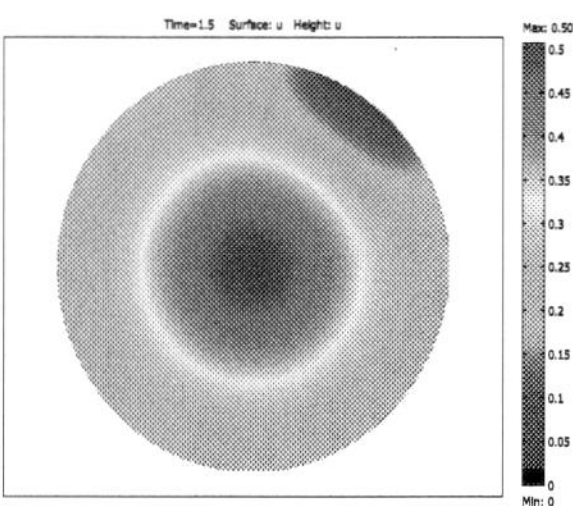

Fig. 5. Probability density function at time 15s after particle injection

t_0. These results can potentially be incorporated in variety of biomedical signal processing applications: source localization, diffusivity estimation, transport prediction, etc.

4. Estimation and prediction of respiriraty signals using stochastic differential equations

Newborn intensive care is one of the great medical success of the last 20 years. Current emphasis is upon allowing infants to survive with the expectation of normal life without handicap. Clinical data from follow up studies of infants who received neonatal intensive care show high rates of long-term respiratory and neurodevelopmental morbidity. As a consequence, current research efforts are being focused on refinement of ventilated respiratory support given to infants during intensive care. The main task of the ventilated support is to maintain the concentration level of oxygen (O_2) and carbon-dioxide (CO_2) in the blood within the physiological range until the maturation of lungs occur. Failure to meet this objective can lead to various pathophysiological conditions. Most of the previous studies concentrated on the modeling of blood gases in adults (e.g., (14)). The forward mathematical modeling of the respiratory system has been addressed in (16) and (17). In (16) the authors developed a respiratory model with large number of unknown nonlinear parameters which therefore cannot be efficiently used for inverse models and signal prediction. In (17) the authors presented a simplified forward model which accounted for circulatory delays and shunting. However, the development of an adequate signal processing respiratory model has not been addressed in these studies.

So far most of the existing research (18) focused on developing a deterministic forward mathematical model of the CO_2 partial pressure variations in the arterial blood of a ventilated neonate. We evaluated the applicability of the forward model using clinical data sets obtained from novel sensing technology, neonatal multi-parameter intra-arterial sensor which enables intra-arterial measurements of partial pressures. The respiratory physiological parameters were assumed to be known. However, to develop automated procedures for ventilator monitoring we need algorithms for estimating *unknown* respiratory parameters since infants have different respiratory parameters.

In this section we present a new stochastic differential model for the dynamics of the partial pressures of oxygen and carbon-dioxide. We focus on the stochastic differential equations (SDE) since deterministic models do not account for random variations of metabolism. In fact most deterministic models assume that the variation of partial pressures is due to measurement noise and that exchange of gasses is a smooth function. An alternative approach would result from the assumption that the underlying process is not smooth at feasible sampling rates (e.g., one minute). Physiologically, this would be equivalent to postulating, e.g., that the rate of glucose uptake by tissues varies randomly over time around some average level resulting in SDE models. Appropriate parameter values in these SDE models are crucial for description and prediction of respiratory processes. Unfortunately these parameters are often unknown and need to be estimated from resulting SDE models. In most case computationally expensive Monte-Carlo simulations are needed in order to calculate the corresponding probability density functions (pdfs) needed for parameter estimation. In Section 2 we propose two models: classical in which the gas exchange is modeled using ordinary differential equations, and stochastic in which the increments in gas numbers are modeled as stochastic processes resulting in stochastic differential equations. In Section 3 we present measurements model for both classical and stochastic techniques and discuss parameter estimation algorithms. In Section 4 we present experimental results obtained by applying our algorithms to real data set.

The schematic representation of an infant respiratory system is illustrated in Figure 1. The model consists of five compartments: the alveolar space, arterial blood, pulmonary blood, tissue, and venous blood respectively. The circulation of O_2 and CO_2 depends on two factors: diffusion of gas molecules in alveolar compartment and blood flow – arterial flow takes oxygen rich blood from pulmonary compartment to tissue and similarly, venous flow takes blood containing high levels of carbon-dioxide back to the pulmonary compartment. Furthermore, in infants there exists additional flow from right to left atria. In our model this shunting is accounted for in that a fraction α, of the venous blood is assumed to bypass the pulmonary compartment and go directly in the arteries (illustrated by two horizontal lines in Figure 1).

Classical Model

Let c_w denote the concentration of a gas (O_2 or CO_2) in a compartment w where $w \in \{p, A, a, ts, v\}$ denotes pulmonary, alveolar, arterial, tissue, and venous compartments respectively. Using the conservation of mass principle the concentrations are given by the following

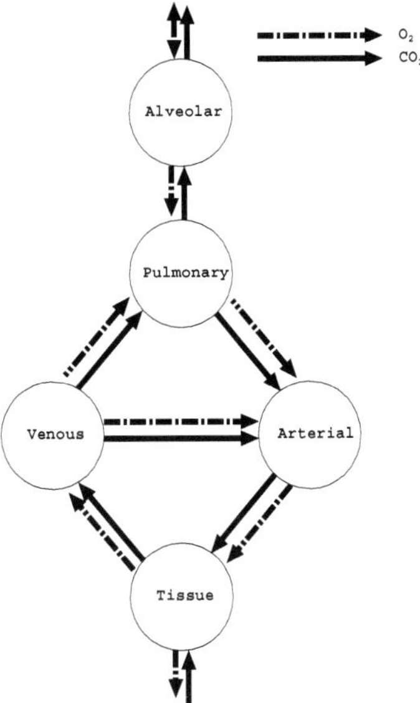

Fig. 6. Graphical layout of the model.

set of equations (18)

$$
\begin{aligned}
V_A \frac{dc_A}{dt} &= D\left(c_p - c_A\right) - e c_A \\
V_p \frac{dc_p}{dt} &= -D(c_p - c_A) + Q(1-\alpha)c_v - Q(1-\alpha)c_p \\
V_a \frac{dc_a}{dt} &= Q(1-\alpha)c_p + \alpha Q c_v - Q c_a \\
V_{ts} \frac{dc_{ts}}{dt} &= Q c_a - Q c_{ts} + r \\
V_v \frac{dc_v}{dt} &= Q c_{ts} - Q c_v
\end{aligned}
\tag{39}
$$

where e is the expiratory flow rate, D is the corresponding diffusion coefficient, Q is the blood flow rate, and r is the metabolic consumption term (determining the amount of oxygen consumed by the tissue).

Stochastic Model

In the above classical model we assumed that the metabolic rate r is known function of time. In general, the metabolic rate is unknown and time-dependent and thus needs to be estimated at *every time instance*. In order to make the parameters identifiable we propose the constrain the solution by assuming that the metabolic rate is a Gaussian random process with known mean. In that case the gas exchange can be modeled using

$$\begin{aligned}
\frac{dn_A}{dt} &= D\left(\frac{n_p}{V_p} - \frac{n_A}{V_A}\right) - e\frac{n_A}{V_A} \\
\frac{dn_p}{dt} &= -D\left(\frac{n_p}{V_p} - \frac{n_A}{V_A}\right) + Q(1-\alpha)\frac{n_v}{V_v} - Q(1-\alpha)\frac{n_p}{V_p} \\
\frac{dn_a}{dt} &= Q(1-\alpha)\frac{n_p}{V_p} + \alpha Q\frac{n_v}{V_v} - Q\frac{n_a}{V_a} \\
\frac{dn_{ts}}{dt} &= Q\frac{n_a}{V_a} - Q\frac{n_{ts}}{V_{ts}} + r \\
\frac{dn_v}{dt} &= Q\frac{n_{ts}}{V_v} - Q\frac{n_p}{V_p}
\end{aligned}$$

$$(40)$$

where we use n to denote number of molecules in a particular compartment. Note that we deliberately omit the time dependence in order to simplify notation.

Let us introduce $n = [n_A, n_p, n_a, n_{ts}, n_v]^T$ and

$$A = \begin{bmatrix}
-\frac{D+e}{V_A} & \frac{D}{V_p} & 0 & 0 & 0 \\
\frac{D}{V_A} & -\frac{D+Q(1-\alpha)}{V_p} & 0 & 0 & \frac{Q(1-\alpha)}{V_v} \\
0 & \frac{Q(1-\alpha)}{V_p} & -\frac{Q}{V_a} & 0 & \frac{\alpha Q}{V_v} \\
0 & 0 & \frac{Q}{V_a} & -\frac{Q}{V_{ts}} & 0 \\
0 & -\frac{Q}{V_p} & 0 & \frac{Q}{V_{ts}} & 0
\end{bmatrix}$$

Using the above substitutions the above the SDE model becomes

$$dn = Andt + \sigma dr \tag{41}$$

where $\sigma = [0,0,0,1,0]^T$.

In this section we derive signal processing algorithms for estimating the unknown parameters for both classical and stochastic models.

Classical Model

Using recent technology advancement we were able to obtain intra-arterial pressure measurements of partially dissolved O_2 and CO_2 in ten ventilated neonates. It has been shown (15) that intra-arterial partial pressures are linearly related to the O_2 and CO_2 concentrations in arteries i.e., can be modeled as

$$\begin{aligned}
c_a^{CO_2}(t) &= \gamma p_p^{CO_2}(t) \\
c_a^{O_2}(t) &= \gamma p_p^{O_2}(t) + c^h
\end{aligned}$$

where $\gamma = 0.016\text{mmHg}$ and c^h is the concentration of hemoglobin. Since the concentration of the hemoglobin and blood flow were measured, in the remainder of the section we will treat

c^h and Q as known constants. Let n_p be the total number of ventilated neonates and n_s the total number of samples obtained for each patient

$$
\begin{aligned}
y_{ij}^w &= [c_{A,i}^w(t_j), c_{p,i}^w, c_{a,i}^w, c_{v,i}^w, c_{t,i}^w]^T \\
y_{ij} &= [y_{CO_2}(t), y_{O_2}(t)]^T \\
i &= 1,\ldots,n_p; j = 1,\ldots,n_s; w = O_2, CO_2.
\end{aligned}
$$

Note that we use superscript ^{w} to distinguish between different vapors. Using the transient model (1) the vapor concentration can be written as

$$
y_{ij} = f_0 e^{B(\theta_i)t_j} i_a + e_i(t_j)
$$

where B is the state transition matrix obtained from model (1)

$$
B(\theta) =
\begin{bmatrix}
\frac{-D+e}{V_A} & \frac{D}{V_A} & 0 & 0 & 0 \\
\frac{D}{V_p} & -\frac{D+Q(1-\alpha)}{V_p} & 0 & 0 & \frac{Q(1-\alpha)}{V_p} \\
0 & \frac{Q(1-\alpha)}{V_a} & -Q & 0 & \frac{\alpha Q}{V_a} \\
0 & 0 & \frac{Q}{V_{ts}} & -\frac{Q}{V_{ts}} & 0 \\
0 & -\frac{Q}{V_v} & 0 & \frac{Q}{V_v} & 0
\end{bmatrix}
$$

and

$$
\theta = [V_A, V_p, V_a, V_t, V_v, r] \tag{42}
$$

is the vector of respiratory parameters for a particular neonate, and $e(t)$ is the measurement noise. Observe that we use subscript i to denote that parameters are patient dependent. We also assumed that the metabolic rate is changing slowly with time and thus can be considered as time invariant, and $i_a = [0\,0\,1\,0\,0\,0\,0\,1\,0\,0]^T$ is the index vector defined so that the intra-arterial measurements of both O_2 and CO_2 are extracted from the state vector containing all the concentrations. Note that the expiratory rate can be measured and thus will be treated as known variable.

In the case of deterministic respiratory parameters and time-independent covariance the ML estimation reduces to a problem of non-linear least squares. To simplify the notation we first rewrite the model in the following form

$$
\begin{aligned}
y_{ij} &= f_{ij} + e_{ij} \\
f_{ij} &= e^{\{A(\theta_i)t_j}
\end{aligned}
$$

The likelihood function is then given by

$$
L(y|\theta, \sigma^2) = \frac{1}{\sigma^2} \sum_{i=1}^{n} \sum_{j=1}^{n} (y_{ij} - f_{ij})^T (y_{ij} - f_{ij})
$$

The ML estimate can then be computed from the following set of nonlinear equations

$$\hat{\theta}_{ML} = \arg\min_{\theta} \sum_{i=1}^{n}\sum_{j=1}^{n}(y_{ij}-f(\theta_i))^T(y_{ij}-f(\theta_i))$$

$$\hat{\sigma}^2_{ML} = \frac{1}{n_p n_s}\sum_{i=1}^{n}\sum_{j=1}^{n}(y_{ij}-\hat{f}_{ij})^T(y_{ij}-\hat{f}_{ij})$$

$$\hat{f}_{ij} = f_0 e^{B(\hat{\theta}_i)t_j}$$

The above estimates can be computed using an iterative procedure (19). Observe that we implicitly assume that the initial model predicted measurement vector f_0 is known. In principle our estimation algorithm is applied at an arbitrary time t_0 and thus we assume $f_0 = y_{i0}$.

Stochastic Model

In their most general form SDEs need to be solved using Monte-Carlo simulations since the corresponding probability density functions (PDFs) cannot be obtained analytically. However if the corresponding generator of Ito diffusion corresponding to an SDE can be constructed then the problem can be written in a form of partial differential equation (PDE) whose solution then is the probability density function corresponding to the random process. In our case, the generator function for our model 41 is given by

$$Ap_n(n,t) = (n-\mu_r)^T \cdot \frac{\partial p_n(n,t)}{\partial n} + \frac{1}{2}\partial p_n(n,t)^T \sigma \sigma^T \partial p_n(n,t) \tag{43}$$

where

$$\mu_r = [0,0,0,\mu_r,0]^T \tag{44}$$

where μ_r is the mean of metabolic rate.

Then according to Kolmogorov forward equation (25) the PDF is given as a solution to the following PDE

$$\frac{\partial p_n(n,t)}{\partial t} = Ap_n(n,t) \tag{45}$$

In our previous work (26) we have shown that the solution to the above equation is given by

$$p_n(n,t) = \frac{1}{(2\sqrt{\pi})^5(t-t_0)^{\frac{5}{2}}} e^{-\frac{1}{2\sqrt{t-t_0}}z^T(\sigma\sigma^T)^- z}$$

$$z = n - \mu_r t - n(t_0) \tag{46}$$

where $-$ denotes Moore-Penrose matrix inverse.

Note that the above solution represents the joint probability density of number of oxygen molecules in five compartments of our compartmental model assuming that the initial number of molecules (at time t_0) is $n(t_0)$. Since in our case we can measure only intra-arterial concentration (number of particles) we need to compute the marginal density $p_{n_a}(n_a)$ given by

$$p_{n_a}(n_a,t) = \int \cdots \int p_n(n,t)dn_A dn_v dn_p dn_{ts}. \tag{47}$$

Once the marginal density is computed we can apply the maximum likelihood in order to estimate the unknown parameters

$$\hat{\theta}_i \;=\; \arg\max_{\theta} \prod_{j=1}^{m} p_{n_a}(n_a, t_j) \tag{48}$$

where we use t_j to denote time samples used for estimation and m is the number of time samples (window size). These estimates can then be used in order to construct the desired confidence intervals as will be discussed in the following section. To examine the applicability of the proposed algorithms we apply them to the data set obtained in the Neonatal Unit at St. James's University Hospital. The data set consists of intra-arterial partial pressure measurements obtained from twenty ventilated neonates. The sampling time was set to 10s and the expiratory rate was set to 1 breathe per second. In order to compare the classical and stochastic approach we first estimate the unknown parameters using both methods. In all examples we set the size of estimation window to $m = 100$ samples. Since the actual parameters are not know we evaluate the performance by calculating the 95% confidence interval for one-step prediction for both methods. In classical method, we use the parameter estimates to calculate the distribution of the measurement vector at the next time step, and in stochastic estimation we numerically evaluate the confidence intervals by substituting the parameter estimates into (36).

In Figures (7 – 11) we illustrate the confidence intervals for five randomly chosen patients. Observe that in the case of classical estimation we estimate the metabolic rate and assume that it is time-independent i.e., does not change during m samples. On the other hand for stochastic estimation, we use the estimation history to build pdf corresponding to $r(t)$ and approximate it with Gaussian distribution. Note that for the first several windows we can use density estimation obtained from the patient population which can be viewed as a training set. As expected the MLE estimates obtained using classical method provide larger confidence interval i.e., larger uncertainty mainly because the classical method assumes that the measurement noise is uncorrelated. However due to modeling error there may exist large correlation between the samples resulting in larger variance estimate.

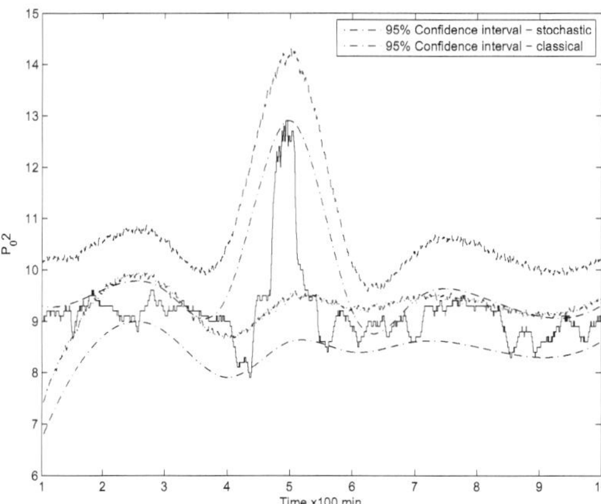

Fig. 7. Partial pressure measurements.

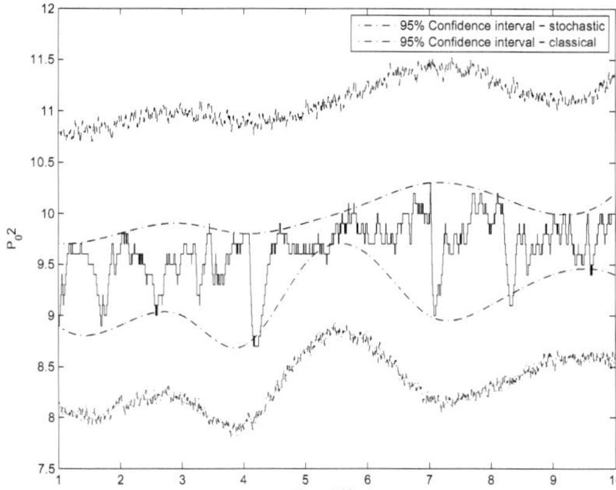

Fig. 8. Partial pressure measurements.

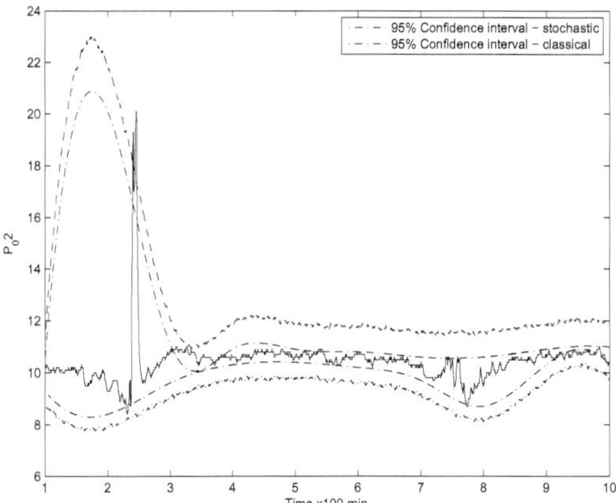

Fig. 9. Partial pressure measurements.

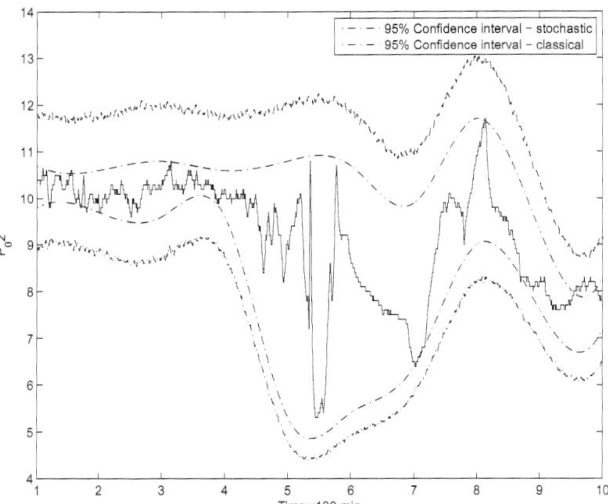

Fig. 10. Partial pressure measurements.

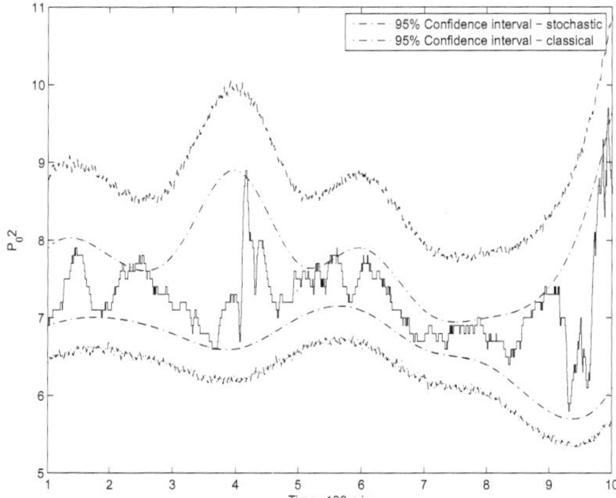

Fig. 11. Partial pressure measurements.

5. Conclusions

One of the most important tasks that affect both long- and short-term outcomes of neonatal intensive care is maintaining proper ventilation support. To this purpose in this paper we develop signal processing algorithms for estimating respiratory parameters using intra-arterial partial pressure measurements and stochastic differential equations. Stochastic differential equations are particularly amenable to biomedical signal processing due to its ability to account for internal variability. In the respiratory modeling in addition to breathing the main source of variability is randomness of the metabolic rate. As a consequence ordinary differential equations usually fail to capture dynamic nature of biomedical systems. In this paper we first model the respiratory system using five compartments and model the gas exchange between these compartments assuming that differential increments are random processes. We derive the corresponding probability density function describing the number of gas molecules in each compartment and use maximum likelihood to estimate the unknown parameters. To address the problem of prediction/tracking the respiratory signals we implement algorithms for calculating the corresponding confidence interval. Using the real data set we illustrate the applicability of our algorithms. In order to properly evaluate the performance of the proposed algorithms an effort should be made to investigate the possibility of developing real-time implementing the proposed algorithms. In addition we will investigate the effect of the window size on estimation/prediction accuracy as well.

6. References

[1] F. B. (1963). Random walks and a sojourn density process of Brownian motion. Trans. Amer. Math. Soc. 109 5686.

[2] MilshteinG. N.: Approximate Integration of Stochastic Differential Equations,Theory Prob. App. 19 (1974), 557.

[3] W. T. Coffey, Yu P. Kalmykov, and J. T. Waldron, The Langevin Equation, With Applications to Stochastic Problems in Physics, Chemistry and Electrical Engineering (Second Edition), World Scientific Series in Contemporary Chemical Physics - Vol 14.

[4] H. Terayama, K. Okumura, K. Sakai, K. Torigoe, and K. Esumi, ÒAqueous dispersion behavior of drug particles by addition of surfactant and polymer,Ó Colloids and Surfaces B: Biointerfaces, vol. 20, no. 1, pp. 73Ð77, 2001.

[5] A. Nehorai, B. Porat, and E. Paldi, "Detection and localization of vapor emitting sources," IEEE Trans. on Signal Processing, vol. SP-43, no.1, pp. 243-253, Jun 1995.

[6] B. Porat and A. Nehorai, "Localizing vapor-emitting sources by moving sensors," IEEE Trans. on Signal Processing, vol. 44, no. 4, pp. 1018-1021, Apr. 1996.

[7] A. Jeremić and A. Nehorai, "Design of chemical sensor arrays for monitoring disposal sites on the ocean floor," IEEE J. of Oceanic Engineering, vol. 23, no. 4, pp. 334-343, Oct. 1998.

[8] A. Jeremić and A. Nehorai, "Landmine detection and localization using chemical sensor array processing," IEEE Trans. on Signal Processing, vol. 48, no.5 pp. 1295-1305, May 2000.

[9] M. Ortner, A. Nehorai, and A. Jeremic, "Biochemical Transport Modeling and Bayesian Source Estimation in Realistic Environments," IEEE Trans. on Signal Processing, vol. 55, no. 6, June 2007.

[10] Hannes Risken, *The Fokker-Planck Equation: Methods of Solutions and Applications*, 2nd edition, Springer, New York, 1989.

[11] H. Terayama, K. Okumura, K. Sakai, K. Torigoe, and K. Esumi, "Aqueous Dispersion Behavior of Drug Particles by Addition of Surfactant and Polymer", Colloids and Surfaces B: Biointerfaces, Vol. 20, No. 1, pp. 73-77, January 2001.

[12] J. Reif and R. Barakat, "Numerical Solution of Fokker-Planck Equation via Chebyschev Polynomial Approximations with Reference to First Passage Time", Journal of Computational Physics, Vol. 23, No. 4, pp. 425-445, April 1977.

[13] A. Atalla and A. Jeremić, "Localization of Chemical sources Using Stochastic Differential Equations", IEEE International Conference on Acoustics, Speech and Signal Processing ICASSP 2008, pp.2573-2576, March 31 2008-April 4 2008.

[14] G. Longobardo *et al.*, "Effects of neural drives and breathing stability on breathing in the awake state in humans," *Respir. Physiol.* Vol. 129, pp 317-333, 2002.

[15] M. Revoew *et al*, "A model of the maturation of respiratory control in the newborn infant," *IEEE Trans. Biomed. Eng.*, Vol. 36, pp. 414–423, 1989.

[16] F. T. Tehrani, "Mathematical analysis and computer simulation of the respiratory system in the newborn infant," *IEEE Trans. on Biomed. Eng.*, Vol. 40, pp. 475-481, 1993.

[17] S. T. Nugent, "Respiratory modeling in infants," *Proc. IEEE Eng. Med. Soc.*, pp. 1811-1812, 1988.

[18] C. J. Evans *et al.*, "A mathematical model of CO_2 variation in the ventilated neonate," *Physi. Meas.*, Vol. 24, pp. 703–715, 2003.

[19] R. Gallant, *Nonlinear Statistical Models*, John Wiley & Sons, New York, 1987.

[20] P. Goddard *et al* "Use of continuosly recording intravascular electrode in the newborn," *Arch. Dis. Child.*, Vol. 49, pp. 853-860, 1974.

[21] E. F. Vonesh and V. M. Chinchilli, *Linear and Nonlinear Models for the Analysis of Repeated Measurements*, New York, Marcel Dekker, 1997.

[22] K. J. Friston, "Bayesian Estimation of Dynamical Systems: An Application to fMRI,", *NeuroImage*, Vol. 16, pp. 513–530, 2002.

[23] A. D. Harville, "Maximum likelihood approaches to variance component estimation and to related problems," *J. Am. Stat. Assoc.*, Vol. 72, pp. 320–338, 1977.

[24] R. M. Neal and G. E. Hinton, In *Learning in Graphical Models*, Ed: M. I. Jordan, pp. 355-368, Kluwer, Dordrecht, 1998.

[25] B. Oksendal, *Stochastic Differential Equations*, Springer, New York, 1998.

[26] A. Atalla and A. Jeremic, "Localization of Chemical Sources Using Stochastic Differential Equations," ICASSP 2008, Las Vegas, Appril 2008.

5

Spectro-Temporal Analysis of Auscultatory Sounds

Tiago H. Falk[1], Wai-Yip Chan[2], Ervin Sejdić[1] and Tom Chau[1]
[1]*Bloorview Research Institute/Bloorview Kids Rehab and the Institute of Biomaterials and Biomedical Engineering,
University of Toronto, Toronto, Canada*
[2]*Department of Electrical and Computer Engineering,
Queen's University, Kingston, Canada*

1. Introduction

Auscultation is a useful procedure for diagnostics of pulmonary or cardiovascular disorders. The effectiveness of auscultation depends on the skills and experience of the clinician. Further issues may arise due to the fact that heart sounds, for example, have dominant frequencies near the human threshold of hearing, hence can often go undetected (1). Computer-aided sound analysis, on the other hand, allows for rapid, accurate, and reproducible quantification of pathologic conditions, hence has been the focus of more recent research (e.g., (1–5)). During computer-aided auscultation, however, lung sounds are often corrupted by intrusive quasi-periodic heart sounds, which alter the temporal and spectral characteristics of the recording. Separation of heart and lung sound components is a difficult task as both signals have overlapping frequency spectra, in particular at frequencies below 100 Hz (6).

For lung sound analysis, signal processing strategies based on conventional time, frequency, or time-frequency signal representations have been proposed for heart sound cancelation. Representative strategies include entropy calculation (7) and recurrence time statistics (8) for heart sound detection-and-removal followed by lung sound prediction, adaptive filtering (e.g., (9; 10)), time-frequency spectrogram filtering (11), and time-frequency wavelet filtering (e.g., (12–14)). Subjective assessment, however, has suggested that due to the temporal and spectral overlap between heart and lung sounds, heart sound removal may result in noisy or possibly "non-recognizable" lung sounds (15). Alternately, for heart sound analysis, blind source extraction based on periodicity detection has recently been proposed for heart sound extraction from breath sound recordings (16); subjective listening tests, however, suggest that the extracted heart sounds are noisy and often unintelligible (17).

In order to benefit fully from computer-aided auscultation, both heart *and* lung sounds should be extracted or blindly separated from breath sound recordings. In order to achieve such a difficult task, a few methods have been reported in the literature, namely, wavelet filtering (18), independent component analysis (19; 20), and more recently, modulation domain filtering (21). The motivation with wavelet filtering lies in the fact that heart sounds contain large components over several wavelet scales, while coefficients associated with lung sounds quickly decrease with increasing scale. Heart and lung sounds are iteratively separated based on an adaptive hard thresholding paradigm. As such, wavelet coefficients at each scale with amplitudes above the threshold are assumed to correspond to heart sounds and the remaining coefficients are associated with lung sounds. Independent component analysis, in turn, makes use of multiple breath sound signals recorded at different locations on the chest to solve a blind deconvolution problem. Studies have shown, however, that with independent component analysis lung sounds can still be heard from the separated heart sounds and vice-versa (20). Modulation domain filtering, in turn, relies on a spectro-temporal signal representation obtained from a frequency decomposition of the temporal trajectories of short-term spectral magnitude components. The representation measures the rate at which spectral components change over time and can be viewed as a frequency-frequency signal decomposition often termed "modulation spectrum." The motivation for modulation domain filtering lies in the fact that heart and lung sounds are shown to have spectral components which change at different rates, hence increased separability can be obtained in the modulation spectral domain. In this chapter, the spectro-temporal signal representation is described in detail. Spectro-temporal signal analysis is shown to result in fast yet accurate heart and lung sound signal separation without the introduction of audible artifacts to the separated sound signals. Additionally, adventitious lung sound analysis, such as wheeze and stridor detection, is shown to benefit from modulation spectral processing.

The remainder of the chapter is organized as follows. Section 2 introduces the spectro-temporal signal representation. Blind heart and lung sound separation based on modulation domain filtering is presented in Section 3. Adventitious lung sound analysis is further discussed in Section 4.

2. Spectro-Temporal Signal Analysis

Spectro-temporal signal analysis consists of the frequency decomposition of *temporal trajectories* of short-term signal spectral components, hence can be viewed as a frequency-frequency signal representation. The signal processing steps involved are summarized in Fig. 1. First, the source signal is segmented into consecutive overlapping frames which are transformed to the frequency domain via a base transform (e.g., Fourier transform). Frequency components are aligned in time to form the conventional time-frequency representation. The magnitude of each frequency bin is then computed and a second transform, termed a modulation transform, is performed across time for each individual magnitude signal. The resulting modulation spectral axis contains information regarding the rate of change of signal spectral components. Note that if invertible transforms are used and phase components are kept unaltered, the original signal can be perfectly reconstructed (22). Furthermore, to distinguish between the two frequency axes, frequency components obtained from the base transform are termed "acoustic" frequency and components obtained from the modulation transform are termed "modulation" frequency (23).

Spectro-temporal signal analysis (also commonly termed modulation spectral analysis) has been shown useful for several applications involving speech and audio analysis. Clean speech was shown to contain modulation frequencies ranging from 2 Hz - 20 Hz (24; 25) and due to limitations of the human speech production system, modulation spectral peaks were observed at approximately 4 Hz, corresponding to the syllabic rate of spoken speech. Using such insights, robust features were developed for automatic speech recognition in noisy conditions (26), modulation domain based filtering and bandwidth extension were proposed for noise suppression (27), the detection of significant modulation frequencies above 20 Hz was proposed for objective speech quality measurement (28) and for room acoustics characterization (29), and low bitrate audio coders were developed to exploit the concentration of modulation spectral energy at low modulation frequencies (22). Alternate applications include classification of acoustic transients from sniper fire (30), dysphonia recognition (31), and rotating

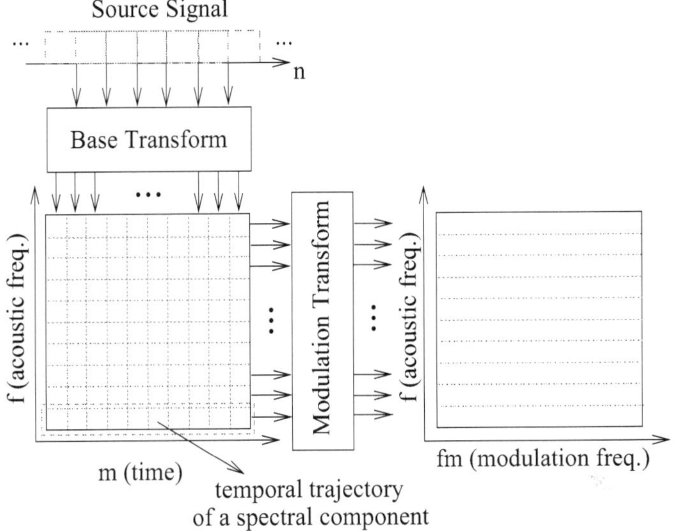

Fig. 1. Processing steps for spectro-temporal signal analysis

machine classification (32). In the sections to follow, two novel biomedical signal applications are described, namely, blind separation of heart and lung sounds from computer-based auscultation recordings and pulmonary adventitious sound analysis.

3. Blind Separation of Heart and Lung Sounds

Heart and lung sounds are known to contain significant and overlapping acoustic frequencies below 100 Hz. Due to the nature of the two signals, however, it is expected that the spectral content of the two sound signals will change at different rates, thus improved separability can be attained in the modulation spectral domain. Preliminary experiments were conducted with breath sounds recorded in the middle of the chest at a low air flow rate of 7.5 ml/s/kg to emphasize heart sounds and in the right fourth interspace at a high air flow rate 22.5 ml/s/kg to emphasize lung sounds. Lung sounds are shown to have modulation spectral content up to 30 Hz modulation frequency with more prominent modulation frequency content situated at low frequencies (< 2 Hz), as illustrated in Fig. 2 (a). This behavior is expected due to the white-noise like properties of lung sounds (33) modulated by a slow on-off (inhale-exhale) process. Heart sounds, on the other hand, can be considered quasi-periodic and exhibit prominent harmonic modulation spectral content between approximately 2-20 Hz; this is illustrated in Fig. 2 (b). As can be observed, both sound signals contain important and overlapping acoustic frequency content below 100 Hz; the modulation frequency axis, however, introduces an additional dimension over which improved separability can be attained. As a consequence, modulation filtering has been proposed for blind heart and lung sound separation (21).

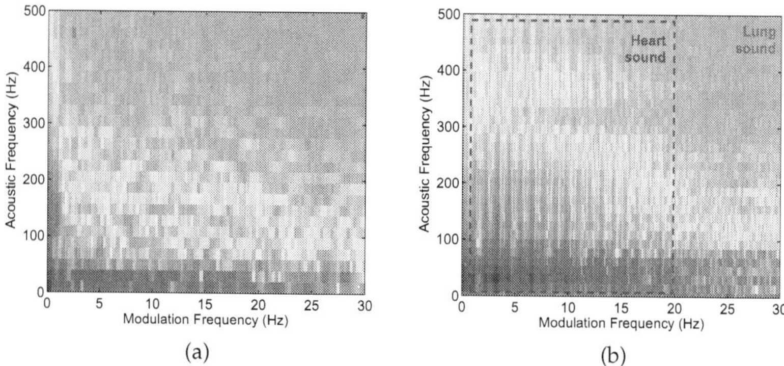

(a)   (b)

Fig. 2. Spectro-temporal representation of a breath sound recorded at (a) the right fourth interspace at a high air flow rate to emphasize lung sounds, and (b) the middle of the chest at a low air flow rate to emphasize heart sounds. Modulation spectral plots are zoomed in to depict acoustic frequencies below 500 Hz and modulation frequencies below 30 Hz.

3.1 Modulation Domain Filtering

Modulation filtering is described as filtering of the temporal trajectories of short-term spectral components. Two finite impulse response modulation filters are employed and depicted in Fig. 3. The first is a bandpass filter with cutoff modulation frequencies at 1 Hz and 20 Hz (dotted line); the second is the complementary bandstop filter (solid line). Modulation frequencies above 20 Hz are kept as they are shown to improve the naturalness of separated lung sound signals. In order to attain accurate resolution at 1 Hz modulation frequency, higher order filters are needed. Here, 151-tap linear phase filters are used; such filter lengths are equivalent to analyzing 1.5 s temporal trajectories.

For the sake of notation, let $s(f,m)$, $f = 1,\ldots,N$ and $m = 1,\ldots,T$, denote the short-term spectral component at the fth frequency bin and m^{th} time step of the short-term analysis. N and T denote total number of frequency bands and time steps, respectively. For a fixed frequency band $f = F$, $s(F,m)$, $m = 1,\ldots,T$, represents the Fth band temporal trajectory. In the experiments described herein, the Gabor transform is used for spectral analysis. The Gabor transform is a unitary transform (energy is preserved) and consists of an inner product with basis functions that are windowed complex exponentials. Doubly over-sampled Gabor transforms are used and implemented based on discrete Fourier transforms (DFT), as depicted in Fig. 4.

First, the breath sound recording is windowed by a power complementary square-root Hann window of length 20 milliseconds with 50% overlap (frame shifts of 10 milliseconds). An N-point DFT is then taken and the magnitude ($|s(f,m)|$) and phase ($\angle s(f,m)$) components of each frequency bin are input to a "modulation processing" module where modulation filtering and phase delay compensation are performed. The "per frequency bin" magnitude trajectory $|s(f,m)|, m = 1,\ldots,T$ is filtered using the bandpass and the bandstop modulation filters to generate signals $|\hat{s}(f,m)|$ and $|\check{s}(f,m)|$, respectively. The remaining modulation processing step consists of delaying the phase by 75 samples, corresponding to the group delay of the implemented linear phase filters. The outputs of the modulation processing modules are the

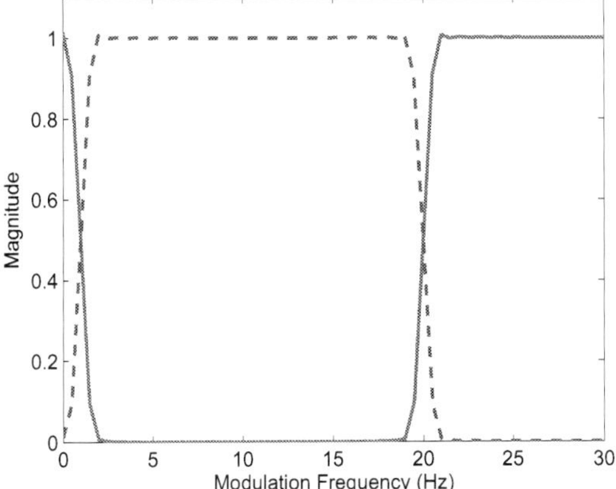

Fig. 3. Magnitude response of bandpass (dotted line) and bandstop (solid line) modulation filters.

bandpass and bandstop filtered signals and the delayed phase components $\angle\tilde{s}(f,m)$. Two N-point IDFTs are then taken. The first IDFT (namely IDFT-1) takes as input the N $|\hat{s}(f,m)|$ and $\angle\tilde{s}(f,m)$ signals to generate $\hat{s}(m)$. Similarly, IDFT-2 takes as input signals $|\tilde{s}(f,m)|$ and $\angle\tilde{s}(f,m)$ to generate $\tilde{s}(m)$. The outputs of the IDFT-1 and IDFT-2 modules are windowed by the power complementary window and overlap-and-add is used to reconstruct heart and lung sound signals, respectively. The description, as depicted in Fig. 4, is conceptual and the implementation used here exploits the conjugate symmetry properties of the DFT to reduce computational complexity by approximately 50%.

It is observed that with bandpass filtered modulation envelopes the removal of lowpass modulation spectral content may result in negative power spectral values. As with the spectral subtraction paradigm used in speech enhancement algorithms, a half-wave rectifier can be used. Rectification, however, may introduce unwanted perceptual artifacts to the separated heart sound signal. To avoid such artifacts, one can opt to filter the cubic-root compressed magnitude trajectories in lieu of the magnitude trajectories. In such instances, cubic power expansion must be performed prior to taking the IDFT. In the experiments described herein, cubic compression-expansion of bandpass filtered signals is used and negligible rectification activation rates ($<2\%$) are obtained.

3.2 Database of Breath Sound Recordings

The University of Manitoba breath sound recordings are used in the experiments; the data has been made publicly available by the Biomedical Engineering Laboratory. Data is obtained from two healthy subjects aged 25 and 30 years on three separate occasions (20). Piezoelectric contact accelerometers were used to record the respiratory sounds from the subjects in sitting position. Accelerometers were secured with double-sided adhesive tape rings at the following five locations: (1) right and (2) left midclavicular, 2nd intercostal space, (3) right and (4) left 4th intercostal space, and (5) center of chest.

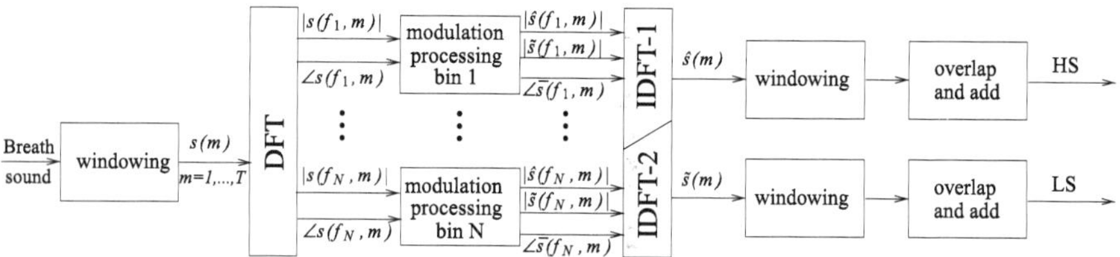

Fig. 4. Block diagram of the modulation filtering approach for blind separation of heart sounds (HS) and lung sounds (LS) from auscultation recordings.

Subjects were asked to maintain their target breathing at low (7.5 ml/s/kg), medium (15 ml/s/kg), and high (22.5 ml/s/kg) flow rates. Subjects were instructed to breathe such that one full breath occurred every two to three seconds at every flow rate and had at least five breaths at each target flow. Three recordings were made per subject and each recording consisted of approximately 20 s at each target flow and concluded with an approximate 5 s of breath hold (total of $\sim$ 65 s). During breath hold, subjects were asked to hold their breath with a closed glottis, thus allowing for a reference heartbeat signal and background noise characterization. Breath sound signals were digitized with 10240 Hz sample rate and 16-bit precision. In our experiments, data is downsampled to 5 kHz in order to reduce computational complexity.

3.3 Benchmark Separation Algorithm

For comparison purposes, a wavelet-based heart and lung sound separation algorithm is used as a benchmark (18); the reader is referred to the following references for a complete description of the algorithm: (18; 34; 35). In the experiments described herein, the threshold used was given by the standard deviation of the wavelet coefficients multiplied by a constant multiplicative factor. As suggested in a previous study (14), values used for the multiplicative factor range from $2.5 - 3.0$ (increments of 0.25) for breath sound segments of low, medium, and high air flow rates, respectively. With the wavelet filtering algorithm, heart and lung sound separation is achieved through an iterative reconstruction-decomposition process. The stopping criterion is set such that the error between two consecutive reconstruction steps drops below 10^{-5} (18).

3.4 Comparative Performance Analysis

Modulation domain and wavelet filtering algorithms are tested on breath sound signals captured at the five locations described in Section 3.2. The plots in Fig. 5 (a)-(b) illustrate short segments of separated heart and lung sounds, respectively, for both systems using signals recorded at the center of the chest during low air flow. Spectral plots of separated signals are further depicted in Fig. 6. Subplot (a) illustrates the spectra of "heart-sound-free" breath sounds and the separated lung sound signals processed by the modulation domain and wavelet filtering algorithms. Power spectra are averaged over 5 s of heart-sound-free breath sounds, which were randomly selected from segments of the breath sound recording between successive heartbeats (selected segments were within $\pm 20\%$ of the target low airflow rate). Similarly, subplot (b) depicts average power spectra of breath-hold sounds and the sep-

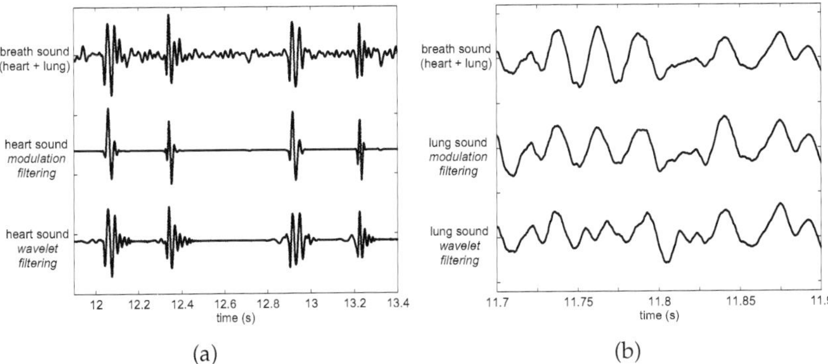

(a) (b)

Fig. 5. Breath sound signals (top) and separated (a) heart sounds and (b) lung sounds using modulation domain based filtering (center) and wavelet based filtering (bottom). Subplot (a) depicts a pair of first and second (S1-S2) heart sound tones.

arated heart sound signal. Power spectra are averaged over the approximate 5 s breath-hold duration at the end of the recording session.

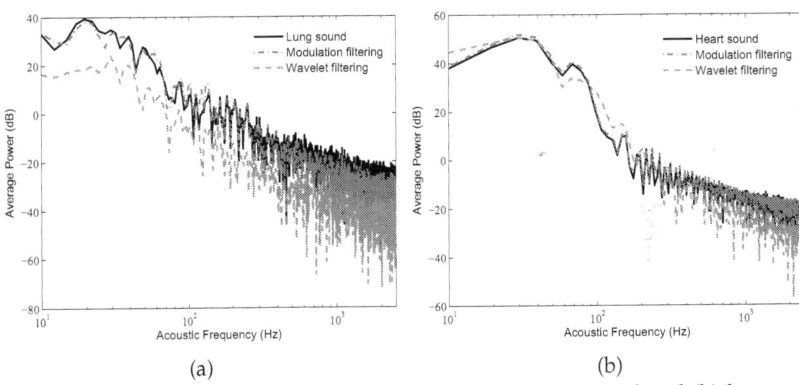

(a) (b)

Fig. 6. Spectral plots of breath sounds and (a) separated lung sound and (b) heart sound signals.

In order to quantitatively assess the performance of the blind separation methods, the average log-spectral distance (LSD) between the aforementioned breath sound spectra $P(\omega)$ and separated signal spectra $\hat{P}(\omega)$ is used. The LSD, expressed in decibel, is given by

$$LSD = \sqrt{\frac{1}{2\pi} \int_{-\omega}^{\omega} \left[10 \log_{10} \frac{P(\omega)}{\hat{P}(\omega)} \right]^2 d\omega}. \tag{1}$$

Filtering	LSD (dB)		Processing time (s)
method	Heart	Lung	
Modulation	0.61 ± 0.13	0.79 ± 0.19	2.44 ± 0.04
Wavelet	1.11 ± 0.21	1.26 ± 0.56	67.2 ± 20.86

Table 1. Log-spectral distances (LSD) and algorithm processing times for wavelet and modulation domain based filtering. Performance metrics are reported as mean $\pm$ standard deviation over the two participants and six recording sessions.

Table 1 reports LSD values obtained for wavelet and modulation domain filtering averaged over the two participants and six recording sessions. In speech coding research, two signals with $LSD < 1$ dB are considered to be perceptually indistinguishable (36). Using this same difference limen for spectral transparency, results in Table 1 suggest that audible artifacts are not introduced by modulation domain filtering; this is corroborated by subjective listening tests conducted with three listeners. For wavelet filtering, however, listeners reported that lung sounds could still be heard in heart sounds and vice versa; such finding is expected given the LSD values greater than unity reported in the table.

Execution time is also an important metric to gauge algorithm performance. Both blind separation algorithms have been implemented using Matlab version 7.6 Release 2008a and simulations were run on a PC with a 2.2 GHz Dual Core processor and 3 GB of RAM. The execution times for heart and lung sound separation, averaged over the five recorded 65 s breath sound signals, are also reported in Table 1. As observed, the computational load of the modulation filtering method is one order of magnitude lower relative to wavelet filtering (approximately 30 times lower processing time). Moreover, with modulation domain filtering, if only the bandstop filter is applied (akin to heart sound cancelation) algorithm processing time can be further decreased by a factor of 1.5. As can be seen, modulation domain filtering allows for fast, yet accurate separation of heart and lung sounds from auscultatory recordings. Separated signals are also shown to be artifact-free, an important factor for accurate clinical diagnosis. In the section to follow, an additional application is presented and shown to also benefit from spectro-temporal signal analysis.

4. Adventitious Lung Sound Analysis

Adventitious lung sounds refer to abnormal sounds present in conjunction with the normal lung sound component (37). Adventitious lung sounds often signal abnormalities in pulmonary conditions (33); representative sounds can include crackles, wheezes, and stridor. Crackles are also referred to as discontinuous sounds as they are brief (in the order of tens of milliseconds) and intermittent. Crackles are caused by fluid obstruction of the small airways often due to inflammation of the bronchi. Crackle sounds, due to their short-term characteristics, are difficult to analyze via spectro-temporal signal processing; crackles have, however, been successfully analyzed via time-frequency wavelet processing (34; 38). Wheezes and stridor, on the other hand, have longer-term behavior that can extend to more than 250 milliseconds (33), hence can be analyzed using modulation spectral analysis.

Wheezes commonly occur in patients with obstructed airways and can have acoustic frequency components ranging from 100 Hz to 1 kHz (33; 39). Wheezes are characterized by

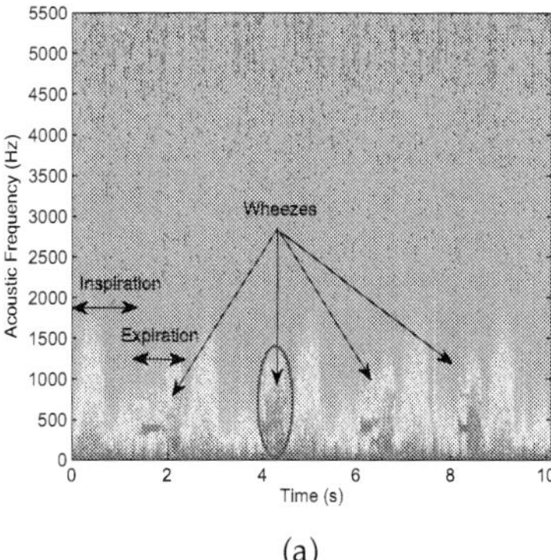

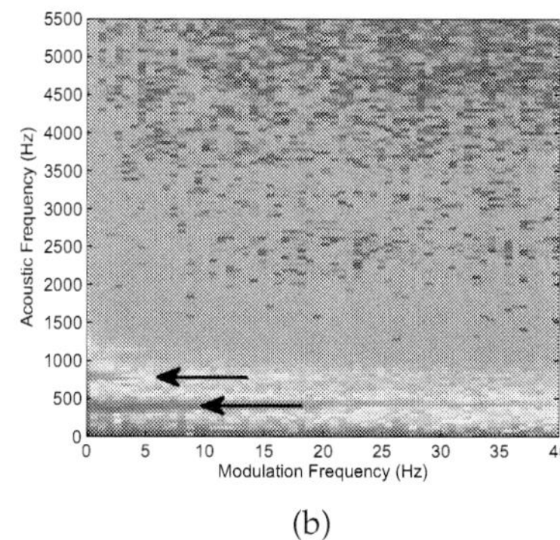

Fig. 7. Subplot (a): spectrogram of a breath sound recording with adventitious wheeze sounds indicated by arrows. Subplot (b) depicts the modulation spectrum of the approximate 0.25 s region highlighted by the ellipsoid in subplot (a).

high-pitched, musical tones manifested most prominently during expiration. Wheezes can be classified as "monophonic" or "polyphonic," if single or multiple tones are present, respectively. The perception and quantification of such properties is difficult if done subjectively via auscultation (39), hence automated methods based on spectrogram processing have been proposed (40). Figure 7 (a) depicts the spectrogram of a breath sound recording with expiratory wheezing taken from the R.A.L.E repository (41). As can be seen, tones are visible during expiration at frequencies around 400 Hz and 800 Hz and such tones are detectable with spectrogram-based methods. The two tones, however, are not easily detectable during the second respiration cycle highlighted by an ellipsoid in Fig. 7 (a). With the use of modulation spectral analysis, the two tones can be easily detected as illustrated by the arrows in Fig. 7 (b), thus can be used to assist inexperienced physicians in detecting pulmonary disorders.

Stridor, in turn, is characterized by a harsh, vibratory noise typically heard during inspiration. Stridor is caused by partial obstruction of the upper airway resulting in turbulent airflow. Figure 8 (a) depicts the spectrogram of a breath sound recording with stridor adventitious sounds taken from the R.A.L.E repository (41). Significant energy is observed at higher acoustic frequencies and tonal sounds can be seen at approximately 200 Hz and in some breath cycles at 1000 Hz. During the last breath cycle, however, the tonal components are not easily observable using spectrogram analysis. The two tonal components, however, are observable using modulation spectral analysis, as depicted by the arrows in Fig. 8 (b).

5. Conclusion

This chapter describes a spectro-temporal signal representation which is shown to be a useful tool for automatic auscultatory sound analysis. The representation, commonly termed "modulation spectrum," measures the rate at which breath sound spectral components change over time. The signal representation is successfully applied to blind heart and lung sound separation and shown to outperform state-of-the-art wavelet filtering both in terms of algorithm

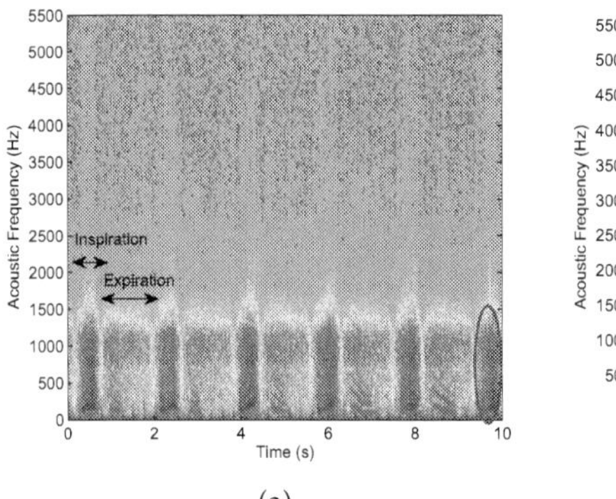
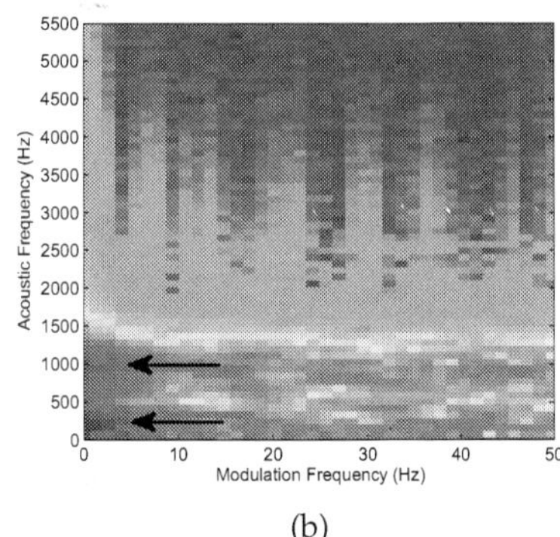

Fig. 8. Subplot (a): spectrogram of a breath sound recording with adventitious stridor sounds during inspiration. Subplot (b) depicts the modulation spectrum of the approximate 0.25 s region highlighted by the ellipsoid in subplot (a).

execution time and in separation performance. An alternate application in which the modulation spectrum can be applied, namely, adventitious lung sound detection, is also described.

6. References

[1] R. L. Watrous, "Computer-aided auscultation of the heart: From anatomy and physiology to diagnostic decision support," in *Proc. IEEE Conference of the Engineering in Medicine Biology Society*, 2006, pp. 140–143.

[2] Z. Syed, D. Leeds, D. Curtis, F. Nesta, R. A. Levine, and J. Guttag, "A framework for the analysis of acoustical cardiac signals," *IEEE Trans. on Biomedical Engineering*, vol. 54, no. 4, pp. 651–662, 2007.

[3] R. Murphy, "Computerized multichannel lung sound analysis: Development of acoustic instruments for diagnosis and management of medical conditions," *IEEE Engineering in Medicine and Biology Magazine*, vol. 26, pp. 16–19, 2007.

[4] C.-J. Hou, Y.-T. Chen, L.-C. Hu, C.-C. Chuang, Y.-H. Chiu, and M.-S. Tsai, "Computer-aided auscultation learning system for nursing technique instruction," in *Proc. IEEE Conference of the Engineering in Medicine Biology Society*, 2008, pp. 1575–1578.

[5] A. Marshall and S. Boussakta, "Signal analysis of medical acoustic sounds with applications to chest medicine," *Journal of the Franklin Institute*, vol. 344, no. 3-4, pp. 230–242, 2007.

[6] H. Pasterkamp, R. Fenton, A. Tal, and V. Chernick, "Interference of cardiovascular sounds with phonopneumography in children," *American Review of Respiratory Disease*, vol. 131, no. 1, pp. 61–64, Jan. 1985.

[7] A. Yadollahi and Z. Moussavi, "A robust method for heart sounds localization using lung sounds entropy," *IEEE Trans. on Biomedical Engineering*, vol. 53, no. 3, pp. 497–502, March 2006.

[8] C. Ahlstrom, O. Liljefeldt, P. Hult, and P. Ask, "Heart sound cancellation from lung sound recordings using recurrence time statistics and nonlinear prediction," *IEEE Signal Processing Letters*, vol. 12, no. 12, pp. 812–815, Dec. 2005.

[9] L. Hadjileontiadis and S. Panas, "Adaptive reduction of heart sounds from lung sounds using fourth-order statistics," *IEEE Trans. on Biomedical Engineering*, vol. 44, no. 7, pp. 642–648, July 1997.

[10] T. Tsalaile and S. Sanei, "Separation of heart sound signal from lung sound signal by adaptive line enhancement," in *Proc. European Signal Processing Conference*, 2007, pp. 1231–1234.

[11] M. Pourazad, Z. Moussavi, and G. Thomas, "Heart sound cancellation from lung sound recordings using time-frequency filtering," *Journal of Medical and Biological Engineering and Computing*, vol. 44, no. 3, pp. 216–225, March 2006.

[12] D. Flores-Tapia, Z. Moussavi, and G. Thomas, "Heart sound cancellation based on multi-scale products and linear prediction," *IEEE Trans. on Biomedical Engineering*, vol. 54, no. 2, pp. 234–243, Feb. 2007.

[13] S. Charleston and M. Azimi-Sadjadi, "Multi-resolution joint time delay and signal estimation for processing lung sounds," in *Proc. IEEE Conference of the Engineering in Medicine Biology Society*, 1995, pp. 985-Ǔ986.

[14] I. Hossain and Z. Moussavi, "An overview of heart-noise reduction of lung sound using wavelet transform based filter," in *Proc. IEEE Conference of the Engineering in Medicine Biology Society*, 2003, pp. 458–461.

[15] J. Gnitecki, I. Hossain, H. Pasterkamp, and Z. Moussavi, "Qualitative and quantitative evaluation of heart sound reduction from lung sound recordings," *IEEE Trans. on Biomedical Engineering*, vol. 52, no. 10, pp. 1788–1792, Oct. 2005.

[16] T. Tsalaile, S. Naqvi, K. Nazarpour, S. Sanei, and J. Chambers, "Blind source extraction of heart sound signals from lung sound recordings exploiting periodicity of the heart sound," in *Proc. International Conference on Audio, Speech, and Signal Processing*, 2008, pp. 461–464.

[17] T. Tsalaile, R. Sameni, S. Sanei, C. Jutten, and J. Chambers, "Sequential blind source extraction for quasi-periodic signals with time-varying period," *IEEE Trans. on Biomedical Engineering*, vol. 56, no. 3, pp. 646–655, 2009.

[18] L. J. Hadjileontiadis and S. M. Panas, "Separation of discontinuous adventitious sounds from vesicular sounds using a wavelet-based filter," *IEEE Trans. on Biomedical Engineering*, vol. 44, no. 12, pp. 1269–1281, 1997.

[19] J.-C. Chien, M.-C. Huang, Y.-D. Lin, and F.-C. Chong, "A study of heart sound and lung sound separation by independent component analysis technique," in *Proc. IEEE Conference of the Engineering in Medicine Biology Society*, Sept. 2006, pp. 5708–5711.

[20] M. Pourazad, Z. Moussavi, F. Farahmand, and R. Ward, "Heart sounds separation from lung sounds using independent component analysis," in *Proc. IEEE Conference of the Engineering in Medicine Biology Society*, Sept. 2005.

[21] T. Falk and W.-Y. Chan, "Modulation filtering for heart and lung sound separation from breath sound recordings," in *Proc. IEEE Conference of the Engineering in Medicine Biology Society*, Aug. 2008, pp. 1859–1862.

[22] M. Vinton and L. Atlas, "A scalable and progressive audio codec," in *Proc. International Conference on Audio, Speech, and Signal Processing*, May 2001, pp. 3277–3280.

[23] L. Atlas and S. Shamma, "Joint acoustic and modulation frequency," *EURASIP Journal on Applied Signal Processing*, vol. 7, p. 668Ǔ675, 2003.

[24] R. Drullman, J. Festen, and R. Plomp, "Effect of reducing slow temporal modulations on speech reception," *Journal of the Acoustical Society of America*, vol. 95, no. 5, pp. 2670–2680, May 1994.

[25] R. Drullman, J. Festen, and R. Plomp, "Effect of temporal envelope smearing on speech reception," *Journal of the Acoustical Society of America*, vol. 95, no. 2, pp. 1053–1064, Feb. 1994.

[26] H. Hermansky and N. Morgan, "RASTA processing of speech," *IEEE Trans. on Speech and Acoustics*, vol. 2, pp. 587–589, October 1994.

[27] T. H. Falk, S. Stadler, W. B. Kleijn, and W.-Y. Chan, "Noise suppression based on extending a speech-dominated modulation band," in *Proc. International Conference on Spoken Language Processing (Interspeech)*, 2007, pp. 970–973.

[28] D.-S. Kim, "A cue for objective speech quality estimation in temporal envelope representation," *IEEE Signal Processing Letters*, vol. 11, no. 10, pp. 849–852, Oct. 2004.

[29] T. H. Falk and W.-Y. Chan, "Temporal dynamics for blind measurement of room acoustical parameters," *IEEE Trans. on Instrumentation and Measurement*, 2009, in press, (12 pages).

[30] L. Owsley, L. Atlas, and C. Heinemann, "Use of modulation spectra for representation and classification of acoustic transients from sniper fire," in *Proc. International Conference on Audio, Speech, and Signal Processing*, 2005, pp. 1129–1133.

[31] N. Malyska, T. Quatieri, and D. Sturim, "Automatic dysphonia recognition using biologically-inspired amplitude-modulation features," in *Proc. International Conference on Audio, Speech, and Signal Processing*, 2005, pp. 873–876.

[32] S. Sukittanon, L. E. Atlas, and S. G. Dame, "Enhanced modulation spectrum using space-time averaging for in-building acoustic signature identification," in *Proc. International Conference on Audio, Speech, and Signal Processing*, 2006, pp. 153–156.

[33] H. Pasterkamp, S. Kraman, and G. Wodicka, "Respiratory sounds: Advances beyond the stethoscope," *American Journal of Respiratory and Critical Care Medicine*, vol. 156, pp. 974–987, 1997.

[34] L. Hadjileontiadis and S. Panas, "A wavelet-based reduction of heart sound noise from lung sounds," *International Journal of Medical Informatics*, vol. 52, pp. 183–190, 1998.

[35] J. Gnitecki and Z. Moussavi, "Separating heart sounds from lung sounds," *IEEE Engineering in Medicine and Biology Magazine*, vol. 26, pp. 20–29, Jan./Feb. 2007.

[36] W. B. Kleijn and K. K. Paliwal, Eds., *Speech Coding and Synthesis*. Elsevier, 1995.

[37] S. Lehrer, *Understanding lung sounds*. W.B. Saunders, 1993.

[38] S. Selloa, S. kyung Strambib, G. D. Michelea, and N. Ambrosinob, "Respiratory sound analysis in healthy and pathological subjects: A wavelet approach," *Biomedical Signal Processing and Control*, vol. 3, pp. 181–191, 2008.

[39] J. A. Fiz, R. Jane, A. Homs, J. Izquierdo, M. A. Garcia, and J. Morera, "Detection of wheezing during maximal forced exhalation in patients with obstructed airways," *Chest*, vol. 122, pp. 186–191, 2002.

[40] S. Taplidou, L. Hadjileontiadis, T. Penzel, V. Gross, and S. Panas, "WED: An efficient wheezing-episode detector based on breath sounds spectrogram analysis," in *Proc. IEEE Conference of the Engineering in Medicine Biology Society*, 2003, pp. 2531–2534.

[41] "R.A.L.E. repository." Online: http://www.rale.ca

6

Deconvolution Methods and Applications of Auditory Evoked Response Using High Rate Stimulation

Yuan-yuan Su, Zhen-ji Li and Tao Wang[*]
School of Biomedical Engineering, Southern Medical University
China

1. Introduction

An auditory-evoked potential (AEP) is electrophysiological activity within the auditory system that is stimulated by sounds. AEP components occurred at different latencies represent the regions giving rise to the responses in the auditory system. Accordingly, they are in general divided into three categories, i.e., early latency component, popularly known as auditory brainstem response (ABR), middle latency response (MLR) and later latency response (LLR). The AEP methodology has been widely used in assessing the functions of auditory system, and transmission of the electrical responses from the acoustic nerve via the brainstem to the cortex, which are associated with a series of timing different components lasting from about a few milliseconds up to several seconds. In clinic practice, AEPs, such as ABR in particular, are successfully applied to hearing screening for infants, identifying the organic or functional deafness; intraoperative monitoring for hearing preservation and restoration in acoustic surgery; intensive care unit monitoring of neurological status after severe brain injury, etc.

Due to the low-voltage nature of AEPs (microvolts level) recorded non-invasively at human scalp, distinct waveforms of AEPs have to be obtained by ensemble averaging technique, which requires hundreds or even thousands delivery of stimuli. The stimulus-intervals referred to as stimulus onset asynchrony (SOA) are inverse proportional to stimulus rates, which have to adapt to the response of interest in conjunction with the adjustment of band-pass filter settings to make sure that the duration of the transient waveform is shorter enough than that of SOA.

Many researches showed that high stimulus rates produce strong stresses on the auditory system which would benefit the diagnosis of the underlying disorders, and allow a more complete evaluation of auditory adaptation. It is reported that neuro-electrophysiological abnormalities in acoustic neuroma (Daly, 1977; Tanaka et al., 1996), multiple sclerosis (Robinson & Rudge, 1977), Bell's palsy (Uri et al., 1984) and mercury-exposed patients (Counter, 2003) are more evident and detectable under higher rate paradigms. It is also anticipated that higher rates might require less time to acquire observable responses (Bell et

---

[*] Corresponding author. Tel.: +86-20-61648276; E-mail: taowang@fimmu.com

al., 2001). However, the upper limit of the stimulus rate imposed by conventional ensemble averaging unfortunately restricts the application scopes that might be offered by the properties of rate effect. In general, one can study the responses under higher rate paradigms with uniform SOAs in terms of auditory steady state response (ASSR)—a periodic response, which can only be analyzed in frequency domain. For instance, the most investigated 40 Hz ASSRs first reported by Galambos et al. (1981), as the name indicated, are the responses to a stimulus rate at 40Hz.

One critical problem obstructs the application of high-rate stimulation is the overlapping of successive transient responses, which can be formulated mathematically as a convolution operation between the stimulus sequence and the response to individual stimulus (Jewett et al., 2004; Delgado & Ozdamar, 2004). The first technique attempted to unwrap the overlapped responses was proposed by Eyscholdt and Schreiner (1982), who employed a special family of binary impulse trains as stimuli. This method was soon widely used in the study of deriving ABRs in comparison with conventional paradigms in terms of morphology and recording efficiency (Burkard et al., 1990; Chan et al., 1992; Thornton & Slaven, 1993). In comparison with conventional ABR recording rate (maximum at 100 Hz), using MLS method, it is possible to obtain ABRs at stimulus rates up to 1000 Hz (Burkard et al., 1996a,b).

Stimulus trains of MLS must satisfy strict mathematic requirements. For example, the generation of MLS is implemented by using feedback shift registers, where the length of the binary train is solely determined by the memory number of register, moreover, the SOAs within a train must be multiples of a minimum pulse interval, which implies a wide range of jitters of SOA. Since neurosensory systems might exhibit different adaptation effects, the single derived AEP is in fact a kind of synthesis results of various responses to each stimulus. Recently, Ozdamar et al. (2004) and Jewett et al. (2004) developed similar techniques with a much lower SOA jittering to tackle this issue. These methods usually solve the convolution problem by an inverse filter in frequency domain, although it requires in practice that randomized SOAs in a stimulus sweep, the unwrapped responses, unlike in MLS paradigm, are sensitive to noise distribution along frequency bins within signal band. Wang et al. (2006) thus applied a Wiener filtering theory to attenuate amplified noise, if the power spectra of noise and signal can be estimated.

This chapter mainly focuses on introducing these techniques and applications using high stimulus rate paradigms. The rest of the chapter mainly consists of 5 Sections. Section 2 gives detailed descriptions to the theoretical framework of these techniques. Section 3 presents a simulated study on the comparison of recording efficiency using different paradigms. Section 4 proposes an iterative algorithm to the use of Wiener filter in the absence of spectral information of underlying response. Section 5 introduces applications of these techniques in clinics and practice. The conclusion with the future research directions are drawn in section 6.

2. Formulas of convolving responses and deconvolution techniques under high stimulus rates

Conventional averaging methods to obtain the transient responses assume that the response to a stimulus will be over or filtered out before next stimulus appears. Otherwise overlapped responses occur as illustrated in Fig. 1. This issue from the engineering point of view, can be described as circular convolution of transient evoked response $x(t)$ and binary stimulus sequence $h(t)$. The convolution is defined as

$$y(t) = x(t) \otimes h(t) + n(t),$$ (1)

where the symbol $\otimes$ denotes circular convolution operation. The noise $n(t)$ is assumed to be additive, which is independent with the transient evoked response $x(t)$. By the way, this model is also true for conventional case, where $x(t) \otimes h(t)$ is just a series of $x(t)$s time-locked to stimuli in $h(t)$, so that ensemble averaging is applicable as well.

The length of one period of $h(t)$ is called a sweep (see Fig.1(A)). There are usually more than eight stimuli with different SOAs in a sweep, which constitute a kind of complex stimulus presented repetitively so that conventional time-domain averaging can be carried out to obtain a noise-attenuated sweep-response as shown in Fig. 1(C). Unlike steady-state responses, the responses to all these individual stimuli appear different due to the degree of overlapping with varying SOAs. Deconvolution algorithms will thus make use of the information of such differences to estimate the underlying $x(t)$. Since additive noises may distort sweep-response, we thus conclude intuitively, that wide range SOA-jitters, such as MLS, will offer better anti-noise properties.

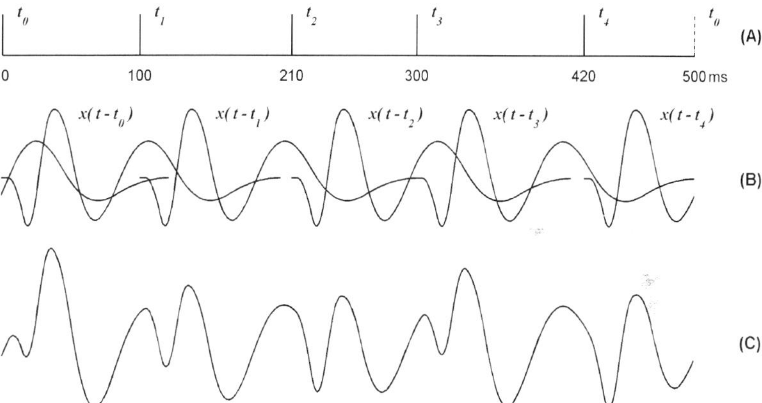

Fig. 1. Schematic illustration of deconvolution process. (A) Stimulus sequence with unequal SOAs. (B) Individual evoked response time-locked to stimuli onsets. (C) Overlapped response that is equivalent to convolution of stimulus sequence and individual evoked response.

2.1 Maximum length sequence (MLS) technique

An MLS train consists of an apparently random sequence of 0s and 1s that has a flat frequency spectrum for all frequencies. Unlike white noise, MLS trains are deterministic and therefore repeatable. It has been widely used in measuring the input impulse response of rooms for reverberation measurement.

MLS trains can be generated by a feedback shift register which is composed of binary memory elements that lined up and looped back through an operational element. The number of memory elements is referred to as the order of MLS. An example in Fig.2 illustrates the generation of three order MLS trains. The binary state of a register is denoted by $s_i(j) \in \{0, 1\}$, where $i = 1, 2, 3$, in this case designating three memory elements, and j is equivalent to a timing index control, if in electronics, by a triggering clock. An important issue of MLS generation is the feedback state $b(j)$ to the very left element which is determined by a mathematic operation on the current states of elements. This operation is directly related to a primitive polynomial defined as $f(x) = x^3 + x + 1$ used in this case, where the term with the highest power (i.e., x^3) corresponds to the feedback state to $s_2(j)$, that is determined by two other elements, $s_1(j)$ indicated by term x, and $s_0(j)$ by term 1 (i.e., x^0) in $f(x)$, respectively. Specifically,

$$b(j) = [s_1(j) + s_0(j)] \bmod(2) . \tag{2}$$

A binary value in the MLS train is thus obtained from the output state of the right memory element $s_0(j)$. As long as one specifies the initial element states, $\{s_i(0)\}$, $i = 1, 2,$ and 3, a periodic of MLS binary values, [a(0), a(1), ..., a(6)] are thus produced one by one. For instance, if the initial state of the three memory elements is [1,1,1], the MLS train would be [1, 1, 1, 0, 0, 1, 0]. Varying the initial state is equivalent to circular shift of one period of MLS.

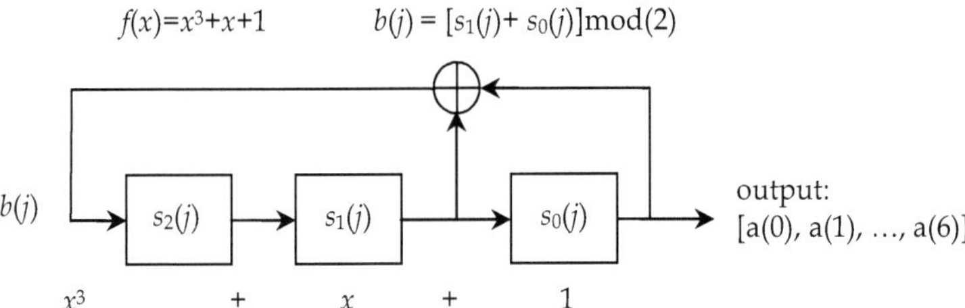

Fig. 2. Generation of three order MLS train by feedback shift register. $s_i(j)$ is the memory element of the feedback shift register, which is corresponding to the terms in primitive polynomial $f(x)$; symbol $\oplus$ stands for the calculation of feedback state $b(j)$; by specifying the initial element states, MLS binary values [a(0), a(1), ..., a(6)] are produced one by one.

Conventionally, the 1 stands for a stimulus onset and 0 for the absence of a stimulus. Thus there are 2^{m-1} 1s indicating the total number of stimuli in a m-order MLS, and the total number of 0s and 1s in a period of MLS is referred to as the sequence length $L = 2^m - 1$. Therefore one can define minimum pulse interval (MPI) as a time interval between two adjacent values (1 or 0), for instance, '1-0' or '1-1' (see Fig. 3). Consequently, the SOAs must be multiples of the MPI. The SOA-jitter measured by the ratio between maximal SOA and minimal SOA for MLS is usually in the range of 4 ~ 6.

Replacing the term 0s with -1s, gives the recovery sequence $h_r(t)$. There is a specific relationship between the MLS stimulus and recovery sequences,

$$h_s(t) \otimes h_r(-t) = \frac{L+1}{2} \delta(t) . \tag{3}$$

Eq. (3) means that the circular convolution of the stimulus sequence $h_s(t)$ and the temporal reverse of recovery sequence $h_r(-t)$ is equal to the product of a delta function $\delta(t)$ and stimuli numbers in $h_s(t)$. As the overlap procedure explained in Eq.(1), the response evoked by $h_s(t)$ is modelled as

$$y(t) = x(t) \otimes h_s(t) , \tag{4}$$

of which convolving $h_r(-t)$ with both sides, it becomes

$$y(t) \otimes h_r(-t) = x(t) \otimes h_s(t) \otimes h_r(-t) . \tag{5}$$

Substituting with Eq. (3), and knowing that $x(t) \otimes \delta(t) = x(t)$, Eq.(5) becomes

$$y(t) \otimes h_r(-t) = \frac{L+1}{2} x(t) . \tag{6}$$

According to Eq.(6), overlapped signals can be unwrapped by convolving the observed response with the temporal reverse of MLS recovery sequence. The overall process of MLS paradigm is shown in Fig.3.

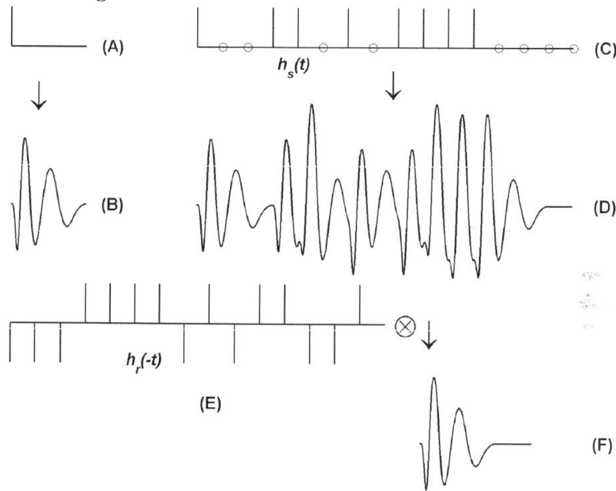

Fig. 3. Illustration of MLS paradigm. Single stimulus (A) evokes individual response (B). MLS with high stimulus rate (C) leads to overlapped sweep-response (D), which then convolves with the temporal reverse of recovery sequence (E) to retrieve the transient response (F).

2.2 Continuous loop averaging deconvolution (CLAD) technique

CLAD method was initially proposed to deconvolve the overlapped responses by matrix inverse in time domain (Delgado & Ozdamar, 2004). Similar to MLS, a sweep of stimulus $h(t)$ contains a sequence of stimuli with SOAs distributed in a random way. Mathematically, suppose $h(t)$ is binary column vector of length L, a square matrix can be constructed as

$$M = [h(t), h(t-1), h(t-2), ..., h(t-L)] , \tag{7}$$

where $h(t-j)$, represent a time-lagged version of $h(t)$. Note that $h(t)$ is treated as a periodic sequence. The overlapped response $y(t)$ is thus formulated

$$y(t) = Mx(t) . \tag{8}$$

The transient response $x(t)$ is obtained only if M is reversible.
An equivalent solution in frequency domain to this problem was also proposed later (Ozdamar et al., 2006). It is easy to derive that Eq.(8) is equivalent to a circular convolution model

$$y(t) = x(t) \otimes h(t) , \tag{9}$$

which in frequency domain is $Y(f) = X(f)H(f)$, where the capital letters denote the Fourier transforms of the counterpart signals, and f denotes frequency in Hz. Therefore,

$$X(f) = \frac{Y(f)}{H(f)} . \tag{10}$$

It is obvious that calculation in frequency domain is faster than that in time domain. However, these mathematical models must be dealt with carefully in practice since the results might be highly distorted due to the presence of noise. Incorporating the additive background noise $n(t)$ into the Eq.(9), we get the same equation as Eq.(1). If we estimate $x(t)$ in frequency domain using Eq.(10), it can be further derived

$$\hat{X}(f) = \frac{Y(f)}{H(f)} = X(f) + \frac{N(f)}{H(f)} = X(f) + \frac{H^*(f)}{|H(f)|^2} N(f) \tag{11}$$

where the symbol * denotes the complex conjugate. It is easy to find out that the inverse filtering performs poorly in case that $H(f)$ has values smaller than unity, in which condition it will amplify the noise. Moreover, zeros (very small values due to digital quantification errors) in $H(f)$ at some frequencies will lead to overflow problem. This model suggests that the frequency properties of sweep stimulus $H(f)$ substantially affect the deconvolution performance. Usually sequences with lower jitters are especially susceptive to noise. Although, one can check a sequence's quality by its spectrum behaviour, it is unfortunately inconvenient for no theoretic solution to this optimal problem.
When the noise amplification problem exists for some stimulus sequences, an optimal algorithm in terms of mean square error (MSE) was proposed by Wang et al. (2006) using Wiener filtering theory. Base on Eq.(11), if the power spectra of noise and transient response can be estimated a priori, the optimal estimate becomes

$$\hat{X}(f) = W(f)Y(f) = \frac{H^*(f)}{|H(f)|^2 + P_n(f)/P_x(f)} Y(f) \tag{12}$$

where $W(f)$ is referred to as Wiener filter, $P_n(f)$ and $P_x(f)$ are power spectra of noise $n(t)$ and transient response $x(t)$, respectively. The ratio $P_n(f)/P_x(f)$, varies across frequency that tunes the Wiener filter to suppress those frequencies dominated by noise, and less affects the inverse filter, $1/H(f)$, in signal-dominated frequencies.

2.3 Q-sequence deconvolution

As mentioned above, if the jitter-ratio of SOAs is close to 1, i.e., the stimulus sequences are quasi-periodic, it is hard to find a "good" sequence which maintains noise attenuation property. Jewett et al. (2004) investigated this issue in very details and proposed a sophisticated criterion in the selection of a good sequence to accomplish the unwrapping task which was termed as quasi-periodic sequence deconvolution (QSD). Since the underlying responses are actually confined in a range of frequency band, it is workable to allocate the frequency band as passband f^p and stopband f^s. The sequences are selected so as to in the range of $f \in f^p$, that $H(f^p)$ satisfies the requirement of noise non-amplification. While in f^s, more attenuation measures apply. Retrieving transient response $x(t)$ under this framework is also carried out by combining two estimations from passband and stopband, respectively,

$$\{\hat{X}(f)\} = \{\hat{X}(f^p)\} \cup \{\hat{X}(f^s)\} . \tag{13}$$

By setting different filters—$H(f^p)$ and $S(f^s)$ for passband and stopband respectively, impact of stopband-noise can be reduced greatly. Substitute Eq. (11) to (13), respectively

$$\hat{X}(f^p) = \frac{X(f^p)H(f^p)}{H'(f^p)} + \frac{N(f^p)}{H'(f^p)} \tag{14}$$

$$\hat{X}(f^s) = \frac{X(f^s)H(f^s)}{S(f^s)} + \frac{N(f^s)}{S(f^s)} \tag{15}$$

where $H'(f^p)$ is usually identical with $H(f^p)$. The reason for distinguishing it is to provide an alternative if the users wish to adjust it under rare circumstances that fail to obtain the desired sequence. Adjustments may include changing values of $H(f)$ at specific frequencies so as to relief the corresponding noise amplification. The adjustment will of course affect the accuracy of waveform. Thus, careful assessment should be done beforehand.

2.4 Session-jittering deconvolution technique

There is one thing in common in the aforementioned deconvolution methods. The algorithm is associated with a sweep response $y(t)$ containing overlapped $x(t)$s. Jittered SOAs must be taken within a sweep of stimuli. However, many conventional AEP devices do not provide such flexible capability of user-defined stimuli. In the study for deconvolution of 40 Hz steady-state magnetic field responses, Gutschalk et al. (1999) adopted a jittering strategy using uniform SOAs in each recording session, while only gradually changed the SOAs in different recording sessions.

Suppose there are L sessions performed. Let $y_i(t)$, where sessional index i = 1, 2,..., L, be the response to equispaced stimuli $h_i(t)$, the corresponding SOA is denoted as T_i, and $x(t)$ be the transient response to an individual stimulus assumed identical for sessions, then $y_i(t)$ = $h_i(t) \otimes x(t)$ as derived before. This model can also be expressed in matrix operation, i.e., y_i = $m_i x$, where binary matrix m_i is constructed by circular-shift versions of $h_i(t)$ in step-wise fashion. The row size of m_i is user defined which is at least larger than the length of $x(t)$. This process is the same as Eq. (7) except that $h_i(t)$ is equispaced.

Ideally, $y_i(t)$ is supposed to be a periodic steady-state response due to overlapping. By carrying out conventional ensemble averaging, gives one period of the overlapped response, $y_i(t)$, $t \in [0, T_i]$. This is equivalent to keep the column size of m_i to be T_i.

A sweep-like response $y(t)$ is formed by concatenating individual $y_i(t)$ one by one together,

$$y(t) = [y_1(t), y_2(t),..., y_i(t)] = Mx(t) , \qquad (16)$$

where $M = [m_1, m_2, ..., m_L]$. By applying the pseudo-inverse matrix M^{-1}, $x(t)$ can be retrieved. An illustration of this process is shown in Fig. 4. Note that the use of this method must be taken with care for the lack of discussions on noise effects. In fact, any matrix inverse calculation in practice might suffer the ill conditioning problem which is very sensitive to tiny disturbance.

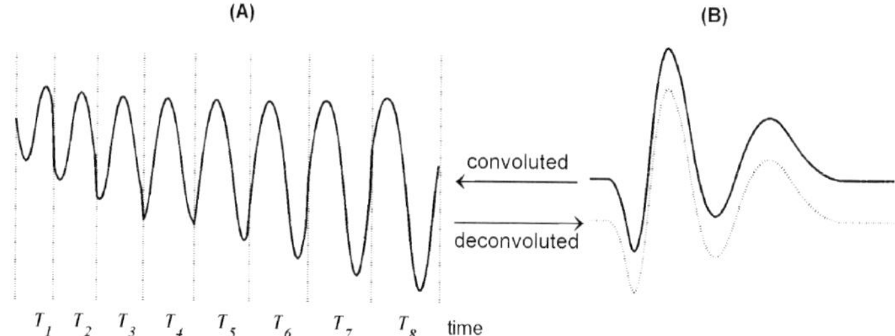

Fig. 4. The Simulation of session-jittering deconvolution. (A) Eight sessions of responses ($y_i(t)$) concatenate one by one according to a ascendant order of T_i. $T_1 \sim T_8$ corresponding to SOAs increasing with a constant step-size represent length of individual $y_i(t)$. (B) Recovered response (dotted line) obtained by deconvolution is identical with original response (solid line).

3. Recoding efficiency with high rate stimulation

Given the same number of stimulus, people expect that high rate stimulation would reduce the recording time, and the signal to noise ratio (SNR) for high rate paradigm would remain comparable with conventional counterpart. However, since the number of sweep for high rate approach is reduced by a factor of L (where L is the number of stimuli in a sweep), sweep averaged responses do not necessarily offer better SNR than conventional ones. In the processing stage of deconvolution, there are however, still chances to either improve or deteriorate SNR depending on the characteristics of sequences. Consequently, it is essential to evaluate the efficiency of these high rate paradigms in deconvolving evoked responses.

A simulated comparison among three paradigms— conventional ensemble averaging, MLS and CLAD is performed. The comparison processes are illustrated in Fig.5. First, an ideal response which convolves with a preset sequence is generated, and then both ideal and overlapped responses are added with the same level noises. The transient responses are obtained by conventional, MLS and CLAD paradigms respectively, and recording efficiencies are evaluated by measuring the correlation coefficients (CCs) and mean square errors (MSEs) of ideal and transient responses.

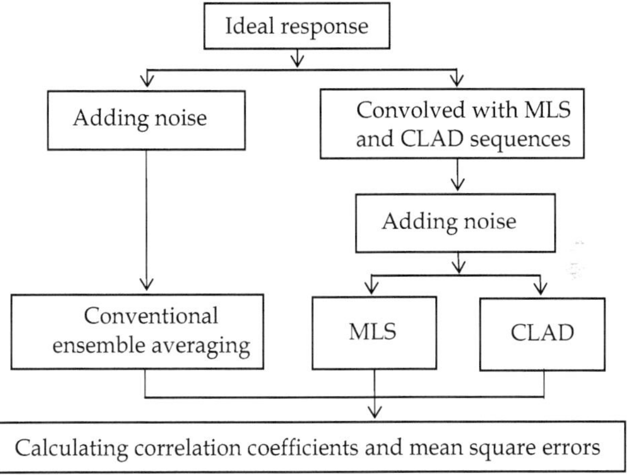

Fig. 5. The flowchart of comparison procedure of recording efficiency

For the convenience of following elaborations, we set up an artificial sampling rate of 1000 Hz. The parameters settings are as followings. The effective length of ideal response lasts 200 ms, which is composed of 5 components with different latencies, amplitudes and polarities (see Fig. 6). Background noises like EEG are modelled by pink noise—a kind of noise generally found in complex system with $1/f$ power spectra. A five order MLS sequence {1 0 0 1 0 1 1 0 0 1 1 1 1 1 0 0 0 1 1 0 1 1 1 0 1 0 1 0 0 0 0} and a lower-jittering Q-sequence (from Jewett et al., 2006) {1 5595 12228 18525 24220 29435 35394 41904 47133 53749 59088 64479 71112} are defined as fundamental sequences. These sequences are in essential dimensionless. These fundamental sequences are stretched or compressed proportionally to form 11 sequences with stimulus rates from 8 S/s (stimulus per second) to 48 S/s (i.e., step-size 4S/s), respectively. Corresponding SOAs in this range are shorter than ideal response, so that overlapping in observed signals occurs. The reason of using different rates is that the performance of deconvolution might be relevant to overlapping degrees.
The performance is evaluated by averaged CCs and MSEs over 20 runs (defined as each simulation with one mixture of noise). For different stimulus rates, the sweep numbers are adjusted to make approximately the same recording time.
As illustrated in Fig.6, the MLS response is quite similar to ideal response not only in latencies and amplitudes of their waves but in their morphology. However, there is more morphological distortion in CLAD response. Both MLS and conventional responses are

more approximate to the ideal one. The MLS method seems more efficient in higher stimulus rates, under the condition of the same recording time.

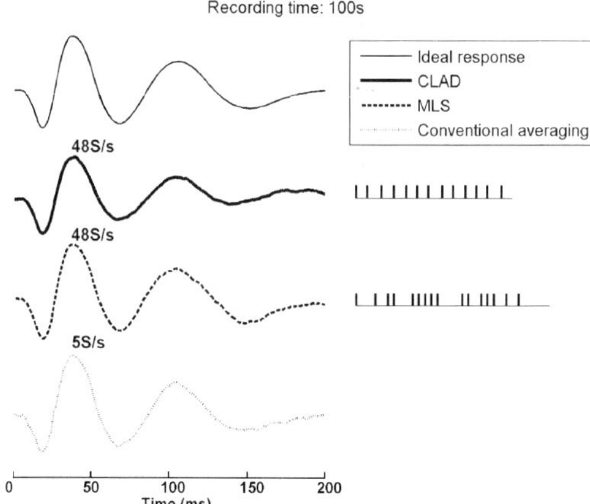

Fig. 6. Retrieved AEPs by CLAD, MLS and conventional methods indicated by legend. Stimulus sequences of CLAD and MLS are placed on the right, respectively.

Fig.7 shows the performance measured with CCs and MSEs. There is a sudden decline in correlation coefficient curve of CLAD indicating the inefficiency at some rates. The cause of this decline is not yet known. We speculated that it may be related to the different superposition enhancements at certain rates, since we observed that the amplitudes of overlapped responses were decreased at these rates.

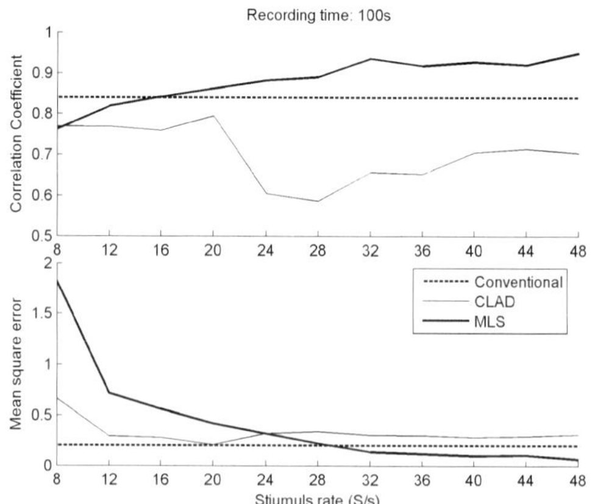

Fig. 7. CCs and MSEs at different stimulus rates, under 100 s recording time.

It is expected that MLS is better than CLAD with lower jitters under the same noise environment. The characteristic of CLAD's sweep-response is more like steady-state response than that of MLS (Fig.8), implying less recovery information available. It implies that the key in high rate paradigms lies in deconvolving the overlapped responses; merely increasing stimulus rates for lower jittered sequences may not be used as a means to improve the recording efficiency.

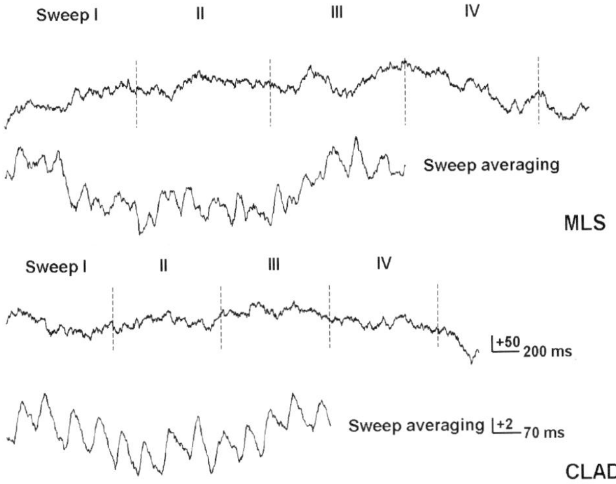

Fig. 8. Averaged sweep-responses for MLS and CLAD in the simulation. Row one and three are raw EEGs, row two and four are sweep-responses

4. Iterative Wiener filtering method

Wiener filtering has been successfully used to tackle the noise amplification problem taking place at a few frequencies bins for some lower jittered sequences (Wang et al., 2006). If the power spectra of both noise and signal are estimated correctly, the inverse filter will be able to adapt to the ratio of noise and signal in frequency domain. In general applications, estimation of signal power spectrum is not readily available in comparison with that of noise. Therefore, a method for evaluating power spectra of transient response by long term memory iterative algorithm is proposed. Fig. 9 depicts the iterative process.

First, initial value $K(f)$, say a constant unity, and adjusted factor c are preset, so the initial transient response $X_0(f)$ is recovered by Eq.(12). Assuming the power spectrum of background noise is constant, and all the estimated responses are kept and averaged to estimate power spectra of response used for next iterative calculation. If the difference of two successive estimates of $x(t)$ measured by the relative Euclidean norm is smaller than a given arbitrary minimum positive, iteration stops, otherwise repeat the iteration.

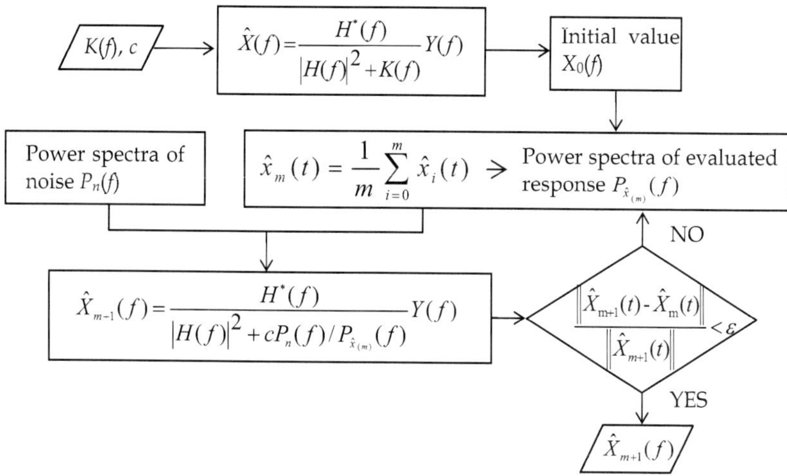

Fig. 9. Flowchart of iterative process.

In simulation data, the ideal response and additive noise are identical with that used in Section 3, and the stimulus sequence which rate is 24 S/s lasts 535 ms. The real data come from Wang's experiment (Wang et al., 2006), the rate of stimulus sequence is also 24 S/s. This sequence lasts 205ms. Both sequences have similar parameters. In order to determine the convergence of this iterative algorithm, the correlation coefficients (CCs) of present and the ideal responses are calculated. The theoretical CC in the simulation study is calculated by using the known signal power spectrum rather than the estimated ones. The parameter c (range 0~1) is introduced to weight the proportion of $K(f)$, when in the presence of strong artefacts, larger c could alleviate their effects.

The simulation results are shown in Fig. 10. The waveform obtained from the proposed algorithm (solid trace in panel D) is close to the theoretical one (doted trace). It is obvious that $K(f)$ will affect both noise and signal, the estimated responses are bias and the magnitudes tend to be suppressed.

The correlation coefficient curve also shows that the estimations (indicated by symbol $*$) are gradually approaching to the theoretical estimation (dash line).

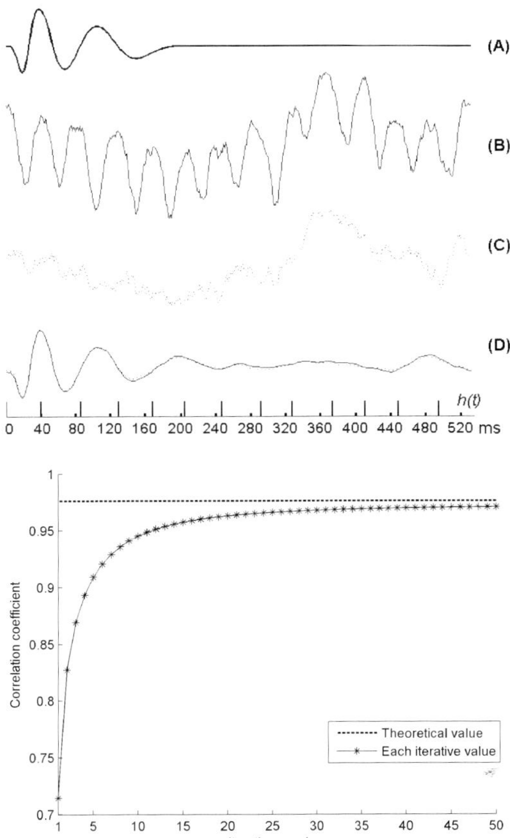

Fig. 10. Top panel shows the ideal AEP (A), sweep response (B) with the corresponding noise (C). A comparison of retrieved AEPs (D) using iterative algorithm (solid) and theoretic one (dotted). Bottom panel shows the CCs for iterative algorithm and the theoretical one.

The performance of the proposed algorithm using human recorded data as in (Wang et al., 2006) is shown in Fig.11. The very weak AEPs are buried in raw EEG and large noises, and it is hard to identify them even in the averaged sweep. However, after estimating residual noise as the background noise by $\pm$ reference method (Schimmel, 1967), the power spectra of noise are calculated and the iterative estimation can proceed. This iterative method attenuates noise greatly and highlights the feature waves $V{\sim}P_1$ out of raw EEG.

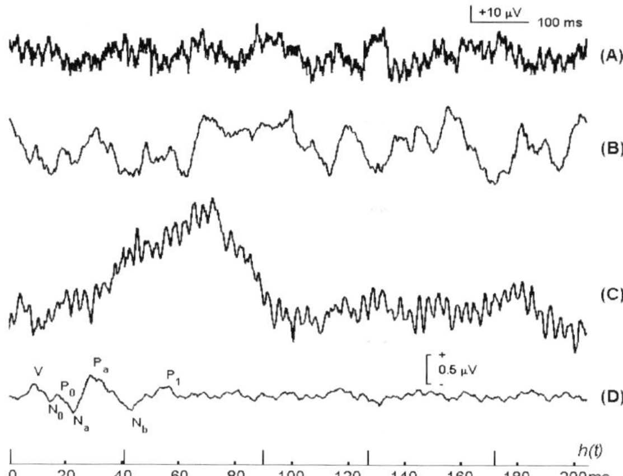

Fig. 11. Real data-processing results. (A) Raw EEG; (B) EEG processed by $\pm$ reference method; (C) Estimated residual noise; (D) Iterative recovered waveform.

The drawback of the algorithm is that there is no theoretic analysis of the convergent property. To ensure the iterative algorithm convergent in line with the correct direction, attention has to be paid to the initial states of the algorithm. If $K(f)$ is constant, signal and noise are suppressed the same over all the frequency band. The purpose of iteration is to adjust the suppression factor $K(f)$ based on the spectrum of the estimated signal. Usually at the initial stage, using a relative larger $K(f)$ will guarantee sufficient noise attenuation, although the estimated signal is also attenuated. Since the noise is more wide-band, a larger attenuation of both signal and noise is more likely to produce a better SNR signal estimation, which is able to yield a correct step-forward adjustment of $K(f)$ for next iteration.

5. Applications of high rate techniques in clinical and basic researches

Since the proposal of deconvolution techniques for high-rate stimulation, especially the early developed MLS method, researchers have been exploring the possible applications in various areas. In the study of ABR, it has been noticed that reliable ABRs were produced remarkably comparable to conventional ones in morphology (Burkard et al., 1990).

During recording ABR of premature infants by MLS, Weber and Roush (1993) found that the clarity of ABR could be well-defined under a rate as high as of about 900 S/s and the quality of MLS-ABR was even better than conventional ABR especially in large noise environment. It suggested that MLS could be applied in newborn hearing screening. This suggestion was also verified by Jiang et al. (Jiang et al., 1999). Besides, they also employed MLS in asphyxiated neonates and found that the central auditory impairment of these neonates was more detectable with this paradigm (Jiang et al, 2001).

Although MLS can raise the stimulus rate up to 1000 S/s, the rate is not the higher the better, due to adaptation effects. Thornton and Slaven (1993) found that SNR of ABR recording improved with increasing rate and came to a stop at 200 S/s, and then further increasing the rate would lead to worsening performance. Leung et al. (1998) also verified that the optimal MLS rate was in the range of 200~300 S/s during estimation of hearing threshold.

In the study of MLRs, Musiek and Lee (1997) concluded that no clear diagnostic advantage was shown for using MLS technique in patients with central nervous system lesions. While Bell et al. (2001) found that MLS could produce better wave identification and recording efficiency. Their study showed that MLS appears to produce greater improvement in recording speed for the P_a-N_b segment of the MLR than for the N_a-P_a segment, which might imply that different regions of the auditory pathway are responsible for producing the two segments of MLR. In their recently pilot study (Bell et al., 2006), MLS stimulation in conjunction with chirp stimulus sound were investigated in studying MLR variance as a potential indicator for anesthesia adequacy.

With the recently developed methods with lower-jittered sequences, CLAD or QSD paradigms are gradually applied in many studies. For instance, CLAD was implemented with other denoising techniques to assess MLRs recorded during sleep and the relation of MLRs and sleep stages was reported (Millan et al., 2006). Since the auditory MLR as well as the 40-Hz ASSR are both applicable to indicate anesthesia, the deconvolution techniques offer a way to study the relationship between the MLRs and transient ASSR during general anethesia (McNeer et al., 2009). It is found that the morphology of the transient ASSR is dependent on the stimulus rates during anesthesia. By employing CLAD to unwrap the ASSR, it was found that there was dramatic increase in amplitude of P_b component at 40 Hz and suggested that may account for the high amplitude of 40Hz-ASSR (Ozdamar et al., 2007). A further research on 40 Hz ASSR (Bohorquez & Ozdamar, 2008) also showed that the 40 Hz ASSR is a composite response mainly overlapped by ABR and MLR, and the high amplitude of ASSR at 40 Hz results from the superposition of P_b component to P_a wave.

The QSD method was also applied for investigating auditory transient ASSR which was called "G-wave" by quasi-periodic tone-pip stimulus sequences presented at 40 Hz (Larson-Priora et al., 2004). The recent finding has extended high rate techniques to other modalities, such as visual and somatosensory stimulation (Jewett et al, 2006). In this finding, they recorded a type of oscillatory waves named A-waves in the alpha rhythmic range, and found that there was a sensation-transition zone implying a range of certain stimulus rates in which the sensation of individual stimuli fuse into a continuity. Stimulus rates above and below this zone could lead to systematic differences in shape of A-wave, and the waveforms evoked above and below this zone may relate to two neuronal processing modes called "flash-memory" and "fusion-memory" respectively. They speculated that A-wave was a new evoked response phenomenon which may provide a way to reveal the mechanism of neural processing.

6. Conclusion

Despite the strong evidence of the benefits of using high-rate stimulation, technical difficulties prevent it from widespread applications in clinics. In this chapter we did an extensive literature survey on the subject of deconvolution of high rate AEPs. These techniques allow the study of more rang of rate-effects, such as ABRs up to 1000 Hz (S/s), and also allow exploring transient properties of steady-sate responses in time domain. Clinical applications are also showing a great promising in recent anesthesia investigation.

The fundamental idea behind all the techniques lies in the jittering strategy of the stimulus sequences. Unfortunately there is still no theoretical solution to the problem of finding an optimal sequence under lower jitter condition. Moreover, current methods are sill unable to deal with multivariate cases in other popular paradigms, such as oddball, where there are more than one transient response exist.

7. Acknowledgements

We would like to thank Drs. Ozdamar and Bohorque for offering valuable materials and comments. This work was supported by National Science Foundation of China (No. 60771035).

8. References

Bell, S.L.; Allen, R. & Lutman, M.E. (2001). The feasibility of maximum length sequences to reduce acquisition time of the middle latency response. *The Journal of Acoustical Society of America*, Vol. 109, No. 3, 1073-1081

Bell, S.L.; Smith, D.C.; Allen, R. & Lutman, M.E. (2006). The auditory middle latency response, evoked using maximum length sequences and chirps, as an indicator of adequacy of anesthesia. *Anesthesia and Analgesia*, Vol. 102, No. 2, 495-498

Bohorquez, J. & Ozdamar, O. (2008). Generation of the 40-Hz auditory steady-state response (ASSR) explained using convolution. *Clinical Neurophysiology*, Vol. 119, No. 11, 2598-2607

Burkard, R.; Shi, Y. & Hecox, K.E. (1990). A comparison of maximum length and Legendre sequences for the derivation of brain-stem auditory-evoked responses at rapid rates of stimulation. *The Journal of Acoustical Society of America*, Vol. 87, No. 4, 1656-1664

Burkard, R.; McGee, J. & Walsh, E. (1996a). The effects of stimulus rate on the feline BAER during development, I. Peak latencies. *The Journal of Acoustical Society of America*, Vol. 100, No. 2, 978-990

Burkard, R.; McGee, J & Walsh, E. (1996b). The effects of stimulus rate on the feline BAER during development, II. Peak amplitudes. *The Journal of Acoustical Society of America*, Vol. 100, No. 2, 991-1002

Chan, F.H.; Lam, F.K.; Poon, P.W. & Du, M.H. (1992). Measurement of human BAERs by the maximum length sequence technique. *Medical and Biological Engineering and Computing*, Vol. 30, No. 1, 32-40

Counter, S.A. (2003). Neurophysiological anomalies in brainstem responses of mercury-exposed children of Andean gold miners. *Journal of Occupational and Environmental Medicine*, Vol. 45, No. 1, 87-95

Daly, D.; Roeser, R.; Aung, M. & Daly, D.D. (1977). Early evoked potentials in patients with acoustic neuroma. *Electroencephalograph and Clinical Neurophysiology*, Vol. 43, No. 2, 151-159

Delgado, R.E. & Ozdamar, O. (2004). Deconvolution of evoked responses obtained at high stimulus rates. *The Journal of Acoustical Society of America*, Vol. 115, No. 3, 1242-1251

Eysholdt, U. & Schreiner, C. (1982). Maximum length sequences--A fast method for measuring brainstem-evoked responses. *Audiology*, Vol. 21, No. 3, 242-250

Galambos, R.; Makeig, S. & Talmachoff, P.J. (1981). A 40-Hz auditory potential recorded from the human scalp. *Proceedings of the National Academy of Sciences*, Vol. 78, No. 4, 2643-2647

Gutschalk, A.; Mase, R.; Roth, R.; Ille, N.; Rupp, A.; Hahnel, S.; Picton, T.W. & Scherg, M. (1999). Deconvolution of 40 Hz steady-state fields reveals two overlapping source activities of the human auditory cortex. *Clinical Neurophysiology*, Vol. 110, No. 5, 856-868

Jewett, D.L.; Caplovitz, G.; Baird, B.; Trumpis, M.; Olson, M.P. & Larson-Prior, L.J. (2004). The use of QSD (q-sequence deconvolution) to recover superposed, transient evoked-responses. *Clinical Neurophysiology*, Vol. 115, No. 12, 2754-2775.

Jewett, D.L.; Hart, T.; Baird, B.; Larson-Prior, L.J.; Baird, B.; Olson, M.; Trumpis, M.; Makayed, K. & Bavafa, P. (2006). Human sensory-evoked responses differ coincident with either "fusion-memory" or "flash-memory", as shown by stimulus repetition-rate effects. *BMC Neuroscience*, Vol. 7, available at http://www.biomedcentral.com /1471-2202/7/18

Jiang, Z.D.; Brosi, D.M. & Wilkinson, A.R. (1999). Brainstem auditory evoked response recorded using maximum length sequences in term neonate. *Biology of the Neonate*, Vol. 76, No. 4, 193-199

Jiang, Z.D.; Brosi, D.M. & Wilkinson, A.R. (2001). Comparison of brainstem auditory evoked responses recorded at different presentation rates of clicks in term neonates after asphyxia. *Acta Paediatrica*, Vol. 90, No. 12, 1416-1420

Larson-Prior, L.J.; Hart, M.T. & Jewett, D.L. (2004). Neural processing of high-rate auditory stimulation under conditions of various maskers. *Neurocomputing*, Vol. 58-60, 993-998

Leung, S.M.; Slaven, A.; Thornton, A.R. & Brickley, G.J. (1998). The use of high stimulus rate auditory brainstem responses in the estimation of hearing threshold. *Hearing research*, Vol. 123, No. 1-2, 201-205

McNeer, R.R.; Bohorquez, J. & Ozdamar, O. (2009). Influence of auditory stimulation rates on evoked potentials during general anesthesia: relation between the transient auditory middle-latency response and the 40-Hz auditory steady state response. Anesthesiology, Vol. 110, No. 5, 1026-1035

Millan, J.; Ozdamar O. & Bohorquez J. (2006). Acquisition and analysis of high rate deconvolved auditory evoked potentials during sleep. *Proceedings of Engineering in Medicine and Biology Society*, Vol. 1, 4987-4990

Musiek, F.E. & Lee, W.W. (1997). Conventional and maximum length sequences middle latency response in patients with central nervous system lesions. *Journal of the American Academy of Audiology*, Vol. 8, No. 3, 173-180

Ozdamar, O. & Bohorquez, J. (2006). Signal-to-noise ratio and frequency analysis of continuous loop averaging deconvolution (CLAD) of overlapping evoked potentials. *Journal of Neuroscience Methods*, Vol. 119, No. 1, 429-438

Ozdamar, O.; Bohorquez, J. & Ray, S.S. (2007). P(b)(P(1)) resonance at 40 Hz: effects of high stimulus rate on auditory middle latency responses (MLRs) explored using deconvolution. *Clinical Neurophysiology*, Vol. 118, No. 6, 1261-1273

Robinson, K. & Rudge, P. (1977). Abnormalities of the auditory evoked potentials in patients with multiple sclerosis. *Brain*, Vol. 100, 19-40

Schimmel, H. (1967). The $\pm$ reference: accuracy of estimated mean components in average response studies. *Science*, Vol. 157, No. 784, 92-94

Tanaka, H.; Komatsuzaki, A. & Hentona, H. (1996). Usefulness of auditory brainstem responses at high stimulus rates in the diagnosis of acoustic neuroma. *Journal of Oto-Rhino- Laryngology and its Related Specialties*, Vol. 58, No. 4, 224-228

Thornton, A.R. & Slaven, A. (1993). Auditory brainstem responses recorded at fast stimulation rates using maximum length sequences. *British journal of audiology*, Vol. 27, No. 3, 205-210

Wang, T.; Ozdamar, O.; Bohorquez, J.; Shen, Q. & Cheour, M. (2006). Wiener filter deconvolution of overlapping evoked potentials. *Journal of Neuroscience Methods*, Vol. 158, No. 2, 260-270

Weber, B.A. & Roush, P.A. (1993). Application of maximum length sequence analysis to auditory brainstem response testing of premature newborns. *Journal of the American Academy of Audiology*, Vol. 4, No. 3, 157-162

Uri, N.; Schuchman, G. & Pratt, H. (1984). Auditory brain-stem evoked potentials in Bell's palsy. *Archives of otolaryngology*, Vol. 100, No. 5, 301-304

7

Recent Advances in Prediction-based EEG Preprocessing for Improved Brain-Computer Interface Performance

Damien Coyle
Intelligent Systems Research Centre, University of Ulster
Northern Ireland, UK

1. Introduction

Brain-computer interface (BCI) technology is an assistive and augmentative technology that has the potential to significantly enhance the quality of the lives of those who require an alternative means of communicating and interacting with people and their environment. BCI research is growing at a significant pace (Vaughan and Wolpaw, 2006; Wolpaw et al., 2002; Mason et al., 2007; Lecuyer at al., 2008; McFarland and Wolpaw, 2008; Coyle et al., 2005a, 2006a) with many advances in signal processing and a range of BCI applications being investigated in the past few years. The depth and breadth of BCI research in progress today is indicative of its application potential – this is exemplified by the year-on-year exponential increase in peer review journal publications, regular news items in the media, formation of BCI related companies and substantial investment in BCI-specific projects. Being able to offer people with limited neuromuscular control, due to disease, spinal cord injury or brain damage (Wolpaw et al., 2002) an alternative means of communication through BCI will have an obvious impact on their quality of life. A range of studies have shown that head trauma victims diagnosed as being in a persistent vegetative state (PVS) and locked-in patients due to motor neuron disease or brainstem stroke may specifically benefit from BCI systems (Wolpaw et al., 2002; Mason et al., 2007; Owen and Coleman, 2008; Silvoni et al., 2009; Birbaumir et al., 1999; Kaiser et al., 2001) although, as BCIs improve and surpass existing assistive technologies, they will be beneficial to those with less severe disabilities (Pfurtscheller et al., 2007) and applications such as neurofeedback for stroke rehabilitation (Prasad et al., 2009), epileptic seizure prediction (Iasemidis, 2003), driver awareness/alertness detection and cognitive load monitoring. BCI is also emerging as an augmentative technology in computer games (Lecuyer at al., 2008), virtual reality (Leeb et al., 2007) and robotics (McFarland and Wolpaw, 2008).

Even though BCI technology has been under investigation concertedly for the past ten years (Vaughan and Wolpaw, 2006; Mason et al., 2007), there remain many challenges and barriers to providing this technology easily and effectively to the intended beneficiaries. These challenges include i) identification of the most appropriate mental tasks and EEG signals; ii) enhancing training through better feedback and reduced training durations; iii) developing hardware for ambulatory EEG – unobtrusive, practical, low power consumption and cost effective; iv) developing better biosignal processing algorithms (preprocessing, feature extraction/selection/translation, classification and post-processing) to improve performance (classification accuracy (CA), information transfer (IT) rates and reliability; v) enabling long-term and short-term autonomous system adaptability; vi) developing BCI-specific intelligent applications; and vii) assessing user acceptance and the service and care required at the initial stages (Wolpaw et al., 2002).

There have been significant advances in addressing these issues, but often, whilst one issue is addressed another arises. For example, it is often the case that using more electrode channels in a motor imagery based BCI provides better performance than a BCI with less channels – due to a better spatial resolution and the identification of subject-specific cortical activity topography. However increased electrodes significantly reduce the practicality of the BCI and increase the obtrusiveness of the montage. Other issues arise with large montages because the best currently available electrodes require electrolyte gels which can be messy and time consuming to apply, although dry electrodes are available but not widely used as yet (Popsecu et al., 2007). Another example of how improvements in one aspect of a BCI can have implications for other aspects is the subject-specific hyperparameter tuning problem. Almost all signal processing methods can be improved by tuning hyperparameters and tailoring signal processing methods specifically to each subject, sometimes referred to as calibrating the system. In many cases this is done offline manually or semi-automatically with heuristic approaches using data obtained via a training session. This is an effective approach and often considered essential however it does pose challenges for offering BCI widely to multiple individuals where minimal parameter tuning and operator interaction is required. BCIs require signal processing algorithm that can be applied and adapted easily and online automatically to accommodate user adaptation and drifts in attention, mood and fatigue levels. A BCI which does not require extensive parameter tuning and tightly bounded parameters but a more general set of parameters may be able to accommodate better accuracies and robustness in the face of such changes and may be more conducive to autonomous adaptation where only generalized changes to a minimal number of parameters are necessary.

A range of studies have been undertaken to address these issues but the main emphasis in BCI is on enhancing the separability of features extracted from EEG signals associated with various brain states and using advanced classification techniques to maximize the accuracy in classifying those brain states. For example, the neural-time-series-predication-preprocessing (NTSPP) framework increases data separability by predictive filtering and mapping the original EEG signals to a higher dimensional space using predictive/regression models which have been individually specialised (trained) on EEG signals associated with specific brain states (Coyle et al., 2004; 2005a; 2006a; 2006b; 2008a; 2009). Features extracted from the mapped space are more separable than those produced by the original EEG signals, in terms of increased Euclidean distance between class means and reduced inter-class correlation and intra-class variance. Preliminary results from recent work (Coyle et al., 2008a) show that NTSPP compares well to the spatial filtering approach known as common spatial patterns (CSP) (Blankertz et al., 2008; Dornhege et al., 2006; Ramouser et al., 2000) which is used extensively in BCI research. The results also indicate that CSP can complement NTSPP using a reduced electrode montage with no subject-specific parameters; producing a 3-channel BCI that achieves performance which is comparable to a 60 channel BCI in certain cases when no subject-specific parameter tuning is carried out (Coyle et al., 2008a). CSP constructs linear spatial filters that maximize the ratio of class-conditional variances of EEG sources (Ramouser et al., 2000) and can also be used to reduce the dimensionality of the feature vector by providing a surrogate data space with less data. When NTSPP is employed in a 2-class, multichannel system the data dimensionality can increase significantly whereas CSP can reduce the dimensionality of a multidimensional signal space, and both can improve separability, therefore the NTSPP-CSP combination offers significant potential for improved and stable performance in BCI systems. Additionally, it has been shown that using subject-specific discriminable frequency bands or spectral filtering (SF) improves overall BCI performance. Spectral features of the EEG are widely used in MI-based BCIs because lateralized neuronal activity in motor cortical areas is usually distinguishable in mu (8-12Hz) and central beta (18-25Hz) frequency bands (Blankertz et al., 2008; Pfurtscheller et al., 1998; Pfurtscheller, 1998; Coyle et al, 2005b; Herman et al., 2008). In addition to NTSPP and CSP, subject-specific SF can be employed, resulting in a temporal-spectral-spatio preprocessing framework (NTSPP-SF-CSP).

Developing approaches which can address all signal processing related issues is a challenge however the hypothesis of this work is that the neural-time-series-prediction-preprocessing (NTSPP) framework offers the potential of making BCI simpler (negating the need for subject-specific hyperparameters and minimizing the number of electrode channels required) whilst maintaining or enhancing performance of existing BCI methods. The aim of this chapter is to present a comprehensive analysis of NTSPP and its capacity to address a number of the issues in BCI, as outlined above, and to determine the advantages of employing multiple EEG channels in a 2 class motor imagery BCI (22 channels) compared to 2 and 3 channel montages. To achieve these aims data from twenty-three BCI subjects are used and the analysis carried out has the following objectives.

1. to compare the performance differences between BCIs employing spectral filtering (SF) only, SF and CSP combined (SF-CSP), NTSPP-SF combined, and NTSPP-SF-CSP combined.
2. to show that NTSPP can complement CSP using a reduced electrode montage with minimal subject-specific parameters.
3. to compare performances with 2 electrodes, 3 electrodes and 22 electrodes all with standard positioning.

Also, to conduct a fairer comparison[1] of all methods, a range of different classifiers have been investigated including various statistical classifiers such as Linear Discriminant Analysis (LDA), Support Vector Machines (SVM) and other distance based classifiers all of which are available in the Biosig tool box (Schlogl, 2007). A probabilistic Bayes based classification method with evidence accumulation is also tested in addition to a committee based approach involving all classifiers are also tested.

The chapter is structured as follows. Section 2 provides information on the datasets used and the data acquisition process. Section 3 describes the methods employed including NTSPP and the self-organizing fuzzy neural network (SOFNN) which is used in the NTSPP framework. CSP and feature extraction methods and a brief description of the classifier and

---

[1] Certain classifiers can work better depending on the number of dimensionality of the feature space and the number of data samples (feature vectors) available (Tebbens and Schlesinger, 2006).

analysis are presented. Section 4 contains results, including a signals and separability analysis, individual subject analysis and a statistical analysis of the methods presented. A discussion of results is presented in Section 6 which also concludes the chapter.

2. Data Acquisition and Datasets

Data from 23 subjects is used in this work. All datasets were obtained from the third and fourth international BCI competitions, BCI-III (Blankertz et al., 2005) and BCI-IV (Blankertz et al., 2008), which include datasets 2A and 2B from BCI-IV (Schlogl et al., 2008a; 2008b) and dataset IIIa from BCI-III (Schlogl et al., 2005a; 2005b). Table 1 below provides a summary of the data.

Dataset 2B - This data set consists of EEG data from 9 subjects (S1-S9). Three bipolar recordings (C3, Cz, and C4) were recorded with a sampling frequency of 250 Hz (downsampled to 125Hz in this work). The placement of the three bipolar recordings (large or small distances, more anterior or posterior) were slightly different for each subject (for more details see (Schlogl et al., 2008b; Leeb et al., 2007). The electrode position Fz served as EEG ground. The cue-based screening paradigm (cf. Fig. 1(a).1) consisted of two classes, namely the motor imagery (MI) of the left hand (class 1) and the right hand (class2). Each subject participated in two screening sessions without feedback recorded on two different days within two weeks. Each session consisted of six runs with ten trials each and two classes of imagery. This resulted in 20 trials per run and 120 trials per session. Data of 120 repetitions of each MI class were available for each person in total. Prior to the first motor imagery training the subject executed and imagined different movements for each body part and selected the one which they could imagine best (e. g., squeezing a ball or pulling a brake). For the three online feedback sessions four runs with smiley feedback were recorded whereby each run consisted of twenty trials for each type of motor imagery (cf. Fig. 1(a).2 for details of the timing paradigm for each trial). Depending on the cue, the subjects were required to move the smiley towards the left or right side by imagining left or right hand movements, respectively. During the feedback period the smiley changed to green when moved in the correct direction, otherwise it became red. The distance of the smiley from the origin was set according to the integrated classification output over the past two seconds (more details can be found in (Leeb et al., 2007)). The classifier output was also mapped to the curvature of the mouth causing the smiley to be happy (corners of the mouth upwards) or sad (corners of the mouth downwards). The subject was instructed to keep the smiley on the correct side for as long as possible and therefore to perform the MI as long as possible. A more detailed explanation of the dataset and recording paradigm is available (Schlogl et al., 2008a). In addition to the EEG channels, the electrooculogram (EOG) was recorded with three monopolar electrodes and this additional data can be used for EOG artifact removal (Schlogl et al., 2007b) but was not used in this study.

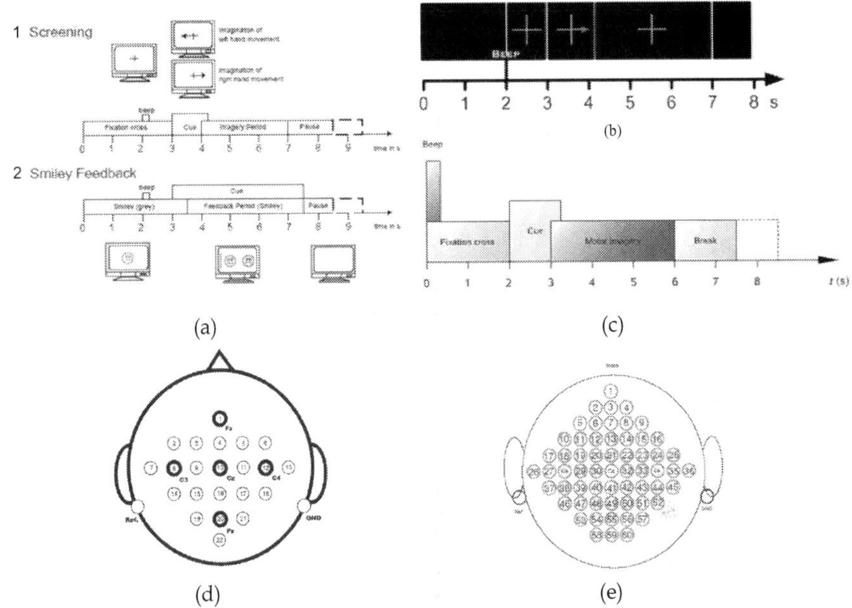

(a)   (b)   (c)

(d)   (e)

Fig. 1. (a) Timing scheme of the paradigm for recording dataset 2B; 1) the first two sessions provided training data without feedback, and 2) the last three sessions with smiley feedback. (b) Timing scheme of the paradigm for recording dataset IIIa; (c) Timing scheme of recording for dataset 2A; (d) electrode montage for recording dataset 2A; (e) electrode montage for recording dataset IIIa with the chosen subset of 22 electrodes shown (red) and electrodes used to derive bipolar channels around c3, cz and c4. For dataset 2B electrodes positions were fine tuned around positions c3, cz and c4 for each subject0 (Leeb et al., 2007)

Competition	Dataset	Subjects	Labels	Trials	Classes	Channels
BCI-IV	2B	9	S1-S9	1140	2	3
BCI-IV	2A	9	S10-S18	576	4	22
BCI-III	IIIa	3 (+2)=5	S19-S23	240-360	4	60

Table 1. Summary of datasets used from the International BCI competitions 2003 and 2008 plus additional provided datasets.

Dataset 2A - This dataset consists of EEG data from 9 subjects (S10-S18). The cue-based BCI paradigm consisted of four different motor imagery tasks, namely the imagination of movement of the left hand (class 1), right hand (class 2), both feet (class 3), and tongue (class 4) (only left and right hand trials are used in this investigation). Two sessions were recorded on different days for each subject. Each session is comprised of 6 runs separated by short breaks. One run consists of 48 trials (12 for each of the four possible classes), yielding a total of 288 trials per session. The timing scheme of one trial is illustrated in Fig. 1(c). The subjects sat in a comfortable armchair in front of a computer screen. No feedback was provided but a cue arrow indicated which motor imagery to perform. The subjects were asked to carry out the motor imagery task according to the cue and timing presented in Fig. 1(c). For each subject twenty-two Ag/AgCl electrodes (with inter-electrode distances of 3.5 cm) were used to record the EEG; the montage is shown in Fig. 1(d) left. All signals were recorded monopolarly with the left mastoid serving as reference and the right mastoid as ground. The signals were sampled with 250 Hz (downsampled to 125Hz in this work) and bandpass filtered between 0.5 Hz and 100 Hz. EOG channels were also recorded for the subsequent application of artifact processing although this data was not used in this work. A visual inspection of all data sets was carried out by an expert and trials containing artifacts were marked. For a full description of the recording procedure see (Schlogl et al., 2008b).

Dataset IIIa – This dataset was recorded from three subjects, S19-S21 using a 64-channel Neuroscan amplifier (datasets with the same recording procedure obtained from 2 additional subjects were provided by the organizers after the competition (S22-S23)). Sixty EEG channels were recorded using a 250Hz sampling rate (down-sampled to 125Hz in this work). The electrode positioning is illustrated in Fig. 1 (e). The training involved the sequential repetition of a cue based trial according to the paradigm and timing illustrated in Fig. 1(b) for each of the 5 subjects. The subjects were seated in a comfortable chair and instructed to imagine left hand, right hand, foot, or tongue movement according to the direction of the cue arrow on the screen (only left and right hand trials are used in this investigation). Each of the four motor imagery tasks was performed 10 times within each run in a randomized order. In this experiment no feedback was provided to the subject. Subjects 1 performed 360 and subjects 2-5 performed 240 trials (cf. Schlogl et al., 2005a; 2005b for further details).

To summarize, in this work only twenty of the sixty available channels for dataset IIIa are used as shown in Fig. 1(e). For all datasets 2 channel and 3 channel montages were also tested using the electrodes positioned anteriorly and posteriorly to c3, cz and c4 positions to derive 2-3 bipolar channels (i.e., the 2 channel montage involves c3 and c4, whereas the 3 channel montage also included cz). These channels are located over left, right hemisphere and central sensorimotor areas – areas which are predominantly the most active during motor imagery. As outlined all data was downsampled to 125 Hz in this work also.

3. Methods

3.1 Neural-Time-Series-Prediction-Preprocessing

NTSPP, introduced in (Coyle et al., 2005a), is a framework specifically developed for preprocessing EEG signals. NTSPP increases data separability by predictive mapping and filtering the original EEG signals to a higher dimensional space using predictive/regression models specialized (trained) on different EEG signals. The basic concept behind NTSPP is focused around exploiting the differences in prediction outputs produced by different predictor networks specialized on predicting different types of EEG signals to help improve the separability of EEG data and enhance overall BCI performance.

Consider two EEG times-series, x_i, $i \in \{1,2\}$ drawn from two different signal classes c_i, $i \in \{1,2\}$, respectively, assuming, in general, that the time series have different dynamics in terms of spectral content and signal amplitude but have some similarities. Consider also two prediction neural networks, f_1 and f_2, where f_1 is trained to predict the values of x_1 at time $t+\pi$ given values of x_1 up to time t (likewise, f_2 is trained on time series x_2), where π is the number of samples in the prediction horizon. If each network is sufficiently trained to specialize on its respective training data, either x_1 or x_2, using a standard error-based objective function and a standard training algorithm, then each network could be considered an ideal predictor for the data type on which it was trained[2] i.e., specialized on a particular data type.

In such cases the expected value of the mean error residual given predictor f_1 for signal x_1 is $E[x_1-f_1(x_1)]=0$ and the expected power of the error residual, $E[x_1-f_1(x)]^2$, would be low whereas, if x_2 is predicted by f_1 then $E[(x_2-f_1(x_2))] \neq 0$ and $E[(x_2-f_1(x_2))]^2$ would be high. The opposite would be observed when x_i, $i \in \{1,2\}$ data are predicted by predictor f_2. Based on the above assumptions, a simple set of rules could be used to determine which signal class an unknown signal type, u, belongs too. To classify u one, or both, of the following rules could be used

1. If $E[u-f_1(u)] = 0$ & $E[u-f_2(u)] \neq 0$ then $u \in C_1$, otherwise $u \in C_2$.

2. If $E[u-f_1(u)]^2 < E[u-f_2(u)]^2$ then $u \in C_1$, otherwise $u \in C_2$.

These rules are simple rules and may only work successfully in cases where the predictors are ideal. Due to the complexity of EEG data and its non-stationary characteristics, and the necessity to specify an NN architecture which approximates universally, predictors trained on EEG data will not consistently be ideal however; when trained on EEG with different dynamics e.g., left and right movement imagination (left or right motor imagery), predictor networks can introduce desirable characteristics in the predicted outputs which render them more separable than the original signals and thus aid in determining which class an unknown signal belongs to. As is shown in Section 3 this predictive filtering alters levels of variance in the predicted signals for data types and most importantly manipulates the variances differently for different classes. Instead of using only one signal channel, the hypothesis underlying the NTSPP framework is that if two or more channels are used for each signal class and more advanced feature extraction techniques and classifiers are used instead of the simple rules outlined above, additional useful information relevant to the differences introduced by the predictors for each class of signal (where the networks have been trained to specialise on particular data dynamics) can be extracted to improve overall feature separability and thus produce features that are easier classified than the original signals.

In general, the number of time-series available and the number of classes governs the number of predictor networks that must be trained and the resultant number of predicted time series from which to extract features,

$$P = M \times C \tag{1}$$

where P is the number of networks (=no. of predicted time-series), M is the no. of EEG channels and C the is number of classes. For prediction, the recorded EEG time-series data is structured so that the signal measurements from sample indices t to $t-(\Delta-1)\tau$ are used to

---

[2] Multilayered feedforward NNs and adaptive neuro fuzzy inference systems (ANFIS) are considered universal approximators due to having the capacity to approximate any function to any desired degree of accuracy with as few as one hidden layer that has sufficient neurons (Hornik et al., (1989); Jang et al., 1997).

make a prediction of the signal at sample index $t+\pi$. Parameter Δ is the embedding dimension and

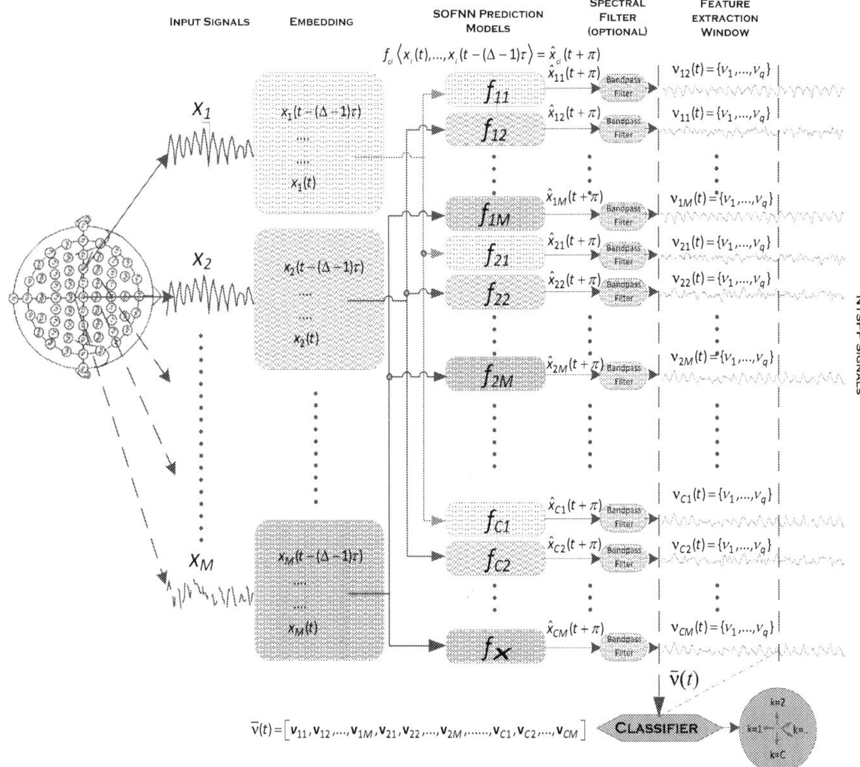

Fig. 2. Illustration of a generic multiclass or multichannel neural-time-series-prediction-preprocessing (NTSPP) framework with spectral filtering, feature extraction and classification.

$$\hat{x}_{ci}(t+\pi) = f_{ci}\left\langle x_i(t),...,x_i(t-(\Delta-1)\tau\right\rangle \tag{2}$$

where τ is the time delay, π is the prediction horizon, f_{ci} is the prediction model trained on the ith EEG channel, $i=1,..,M$, for class c, $c=1,..C$, x_i is the EEG time-series from the ith channel and $\hat{x}_{ci}$ is the predicted time series produced for the channel i by the predictor for class c, channel i. An illustration of the NTSPP framework is presented in Fig. 2.

Many different predictive approaches can be used for prediction in the NTSPP framework (Coyle, 2006). In this work the self-organizing fuzzy neural network (SOFNN) is employed (Coyle et al., 2006; 2009; Leng, 2003; Prasad et al., 2008). This is a powerful prediction algorithm capable of self-organizing its architecture, adding and pruning neurons as required. New neurons are added to cluster new data that the existing neurons are unable to cluster (cf. the following section for further details). Fine tuning parameters such as the Δ and τ may enhance the predictive performance and/or BCI performance but earlier work (Coyle et al., 2005a, Coyle 2006) has shown $\Delta=6$ and $\tau=1$ provide good performance in a two class motor imagery BCI and these values are used in this investigation. The SOFNNs are easily trained using a 3s window of event-related segments of signals drawn from between 1-10 randomly chosen, artifact free trials. Trials containing artifacts were not used to train the networks because artifact contaminated trials can prevent the networks from specializing on a particular motor imagery.

3.2 The Architecture of the SOFNN

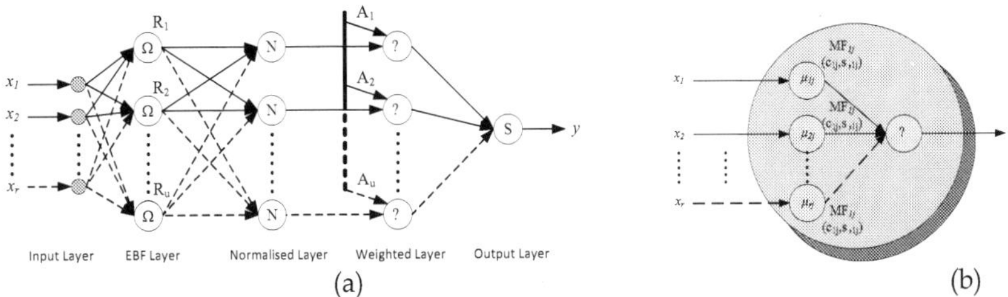

(a)   (b)

Fig. 3. (a) The architecture of the self-organising fuzzy neural network (b) Structure of the jth neuron R_j within the EBF layer

The SOFNN is a five-layer fuzzy NN and has the ability to self-organize its neurons in the learning process for implementing TS fuzzy models (Takagi and Sugeno., 1985) (cf. Fig. 3(a)). In the EBF layer, each neuron is a T-norm of Gaussian fuzzy MFs belonging to the inputs of the network. Every MF thus has a distinct centre and width, therefore every neuron has a centre and a width vector. Fig. 3(b) illustrates the internal structure of the jth neuron, where the input vector is $x = [x_1 x_2 \ldots x_r]$, $c_j = [c_{1j} c_{1j} \ldots c_{rj}]$ is the vector of centers in the jth neuron, and $\sigma_j = [\sigma_{1j} \sigma_{2j} \ldots \sigma_{rj}]$ is the vector of widths in the jth neuron. Layer 1 is the input layer with r neurons, x_i, $i=1,2,\ldots,r$. Layer 2 is the EBF layer. Each neuron in this layer represents a premise part of a fuzzy rule. The outputs of (EBF) neurons are computed by products of the grades of MFs. Each MF is in the form of a Gaussian function,

$$\mu_{ij} = \exp\left[-(x_i - c_{ij})^2 / 2\sigma_{ij}^2\right] \quad j = 1, 2, \cdots, u \tag{3}$$

where, μ_{ij} is the ith MF in the jth neuron;
           c_{ij} is the centre of the ith MF in the jth neuron;
           σ_{ij} is the width of the ith MF in the jth neuron;
           r is the number of input variables;
           u is the number of EBF neurons.

For the jth neuron, the output is

$$\phi_j = \exp\left[-\sum_{i=1}^{r}\left((x_i - c_{ij})^2 / 2\sigma_{ij}^2\right)\right] \qquad j = 1, 2, \cdots, u. \tag{4}$$

Layer 3 is the normalized layer. The number of neurons in this layer is equal to that of layer 2. The output of the jth neuron in this layer is

$$\psi_j = \phi_j \bigg/ \sum_{k=1}^{u} \phi_k \qquad j = 1, 2, \cdots, u. \tag{5}$$

Layer 4 is the weighted layer. Each neuron in this layer has two inputs and the product of these inputs as its output. One of the inputs is the output of the related neuron in layer 3 and the other is the weighted bias w_{2j}. For the TS model (Takagi and Sugeno., 1985), the bias $\mathbf{B}=[1, x_1, x_2, \ldots, x_r]^T$ and $\mathbf{A_j}=[a_{j0}, a_{j1}, a_{j2}, \ldots, a_{jr}]$ represent the set of parameters corresponding to the consequent of the fuzzy rule j which are obtained using the least square estimator or recursive LSE (RLSE). The weighted bias w_{2j} is

$$w_{2j} = \mathbf{A_j}.\mathbf{B} = a_{j0} + a_{j1}x_1 + \cdots + a_{jr}x_r \qquad j = 1, 2, \cdots, u. \tag{6}$$

This is the consequent part of the jth fuzzy rule of the fuzzy model. The output of each neuron is $f_j = w_{2j}\psi_j$. Layer 5 is the output layer where the incoming signals from layer 4 are summed, as shown in (7)

$$y(\mathbf{x}) = \sum_{j=1}^{u} f_j \tag{7}$$

where, y is the value of an output variable. If u neurons are generated from n training exemplars then the output of the network can be written as

$$\mathbf{Y} = \mathbf{W_2}\boldsymbol{\Psi}. \tag{8}$$

where for the TS model

$$\mathbf{Y} = [y_1 \quad y_2 \quad \cdots \quad y_n], \tag{9}$$

$$\boldsymbol{\Psi} = \begin{bmatrix} \psi_{11} & \cdots & \psi_{1n} \\ \psi_{11}x_{11} & \cdots & \psi_{1n}x_{1n} \\ \vdots & \vdots & \vdots \\ \psi_{11}x_{r1} & \cdots & \psi_{1n}x_{rn} \\ \vdots & \vdots & \vdots \\ \psi_{u1} & \cdots & \psi_{un} \\ \psi_{u1}x_{11} & \cdots & \psi_{un}x_{1n} \\ \vdots & \vdots & \vdots \\ \psi_{u1}x_{r1} & \cdots & \psi_{un}x_{rn} \end{bmatrix}, \tag{10}$$

and

$$\mathbf{W_2} = [a_{10} \quad a_{11} \quad \cdots \quad a_{1r} \quad \cdots \quad a_{u0} \quad a_{u1} \quad \cdots \quad a_{ur}]. \tag{11}$$

$\mathbf{W_2}$ is the parameter matrix and ψ_{jt} is the output of the jth neuron in the normalized layer for the tth training exemplar.

3.3 The SOFNN Learning Algorithm

The learning process of the SOFNN includes structure learning and parameter learning. The structure learning process attempts to achieve an economical network size by dynamically modifying, adding and/or pruning neurons. There are two criteria to judge whether or not to generate a new EBF neuron – the system *error* criterion and the *if-part* criterion. The *error* criterion considers the generalization performance of the overall network. The *if-part* criterion evaluates whether existing fuzzy rules or EBF neurons can cluster the current input vector suitably. The SOFNN pruning strategy is based on the optimal brain surgeon (OBS) approach (Hassibi and Stork, 1993). Basically, the idea is to use second derivative information to find the least important neuron. If the performance of the entire network is accepted when the least important neuron is pruned, the new structure of the network is maintained.

This section provides only a basic outline of the structure learning process, the complete structure and weight learning algorithm for the SOFNN is detailed in (Leng, 2003; Prasad et al., 2008). It must be noted that the neuron modifying, adding and pruning procedures are fully dependent upon determining the network error as the structure changes therefore a significant amount of network testing is necessary – to either update the structure based on finalized neuron changes or simply to check if a temporarily deleted neuron is significant. This can be computationally demanding and therefore an alternative approach which minimizes the computational cost of error checking during the learning process is described in (Coyle et al., 2009). A comparison of the SOFNN to the well known DENFIS is outlined in (Kasobov and Song, 2002) and it is shown that the SOFNN compares favorably to other evolving fuzzy systems in terms of structural compactness and accuracy in a range of standard benchmark tests and EEG prediction. The advantage of using the SOFNN in a BCI involving the NTSPP framework is that it has a self organizing structure and can therefore adapt autonomously to each of the time series for each class and for each subject without any parameter tuning. There are 5 standard predefined parameters of the SOFNN which govern the accuracy and complexity. The investigation presented in (Coyle et al., 2009) shows that parameters chosen via a sensitivity analysis generalize well for all subjects and all signals and these parameter values have been used in this work to apply the SOFNN autonomously.

3.4 Common Spatial Patterns(CSPs)

The CSP method, first applied for detection of abnormalities (Ramouser et al., 2000) has been used to tackle the problem of extracting the most relevant information from multiple electrode (multichannel) montages. The goal of the study in (Ramouser et al., 2000) was to design spatial filters that produce new (surrogate) time-series of which the variances are optimal for the discrimination of two classes of EEG related to left and right motor imagery.

Many advances in the CSP methods have been proposed over the past few years and this approach has shown significant potential for two-class BCIs ((Blankertz et al., 2008; Coyle et al., 2008a; Dornhege et al., 2006; Ramouser et al., 2000; Satti at al., 2008; 2009).
To utilise CSP, let Σ_1 and Σ_2 be the pooled estimates of the covariance matrices for two classes, as follows:

$$\Sigma_c = \tfrac{1}{I_c}\sum_{i=1}^{I_c} X_i X_i^t \quad (c \in \{1,2\}) \tag{12}$$

where I_c is the number of trials for class c and X_i is the $M{\times}N$ matrices containing the ith windowed segment of trial I; V is the window length and M is the number EEG channels – when CSP is used in conjunction with NTSPP, $M{=}P$ as per (1). The two covariance matrices, Σ_1 and Σ_2, are simultaneously diagonalized such that the eigenvalues sum to 1. This is achieved by calculating the generalised eigenvectors W:

$$\Sigma_1 W = (\Sigma_1 + \Sigma_2)WD \tag{13}$$

where the diagonal matrix D contains the eigenvalues of Σ_1 and the column vectors of W are the filters for the CSP projections (Blankertz et al., 2008). With this projection matrix the decomposition mapping of the windowed trials X is given as

$$E = WX \tag{14}$$

Prior to the calculation of the spatial filters, X can be processed with NTSPP and/or spectrally filtered in specific frequency bands. Many studies have shown that subject-specific frequency bands are most appropriate (Blankertz et al., 2008; Pfurtscheller et al., 1998; Pfurtscheller, 1998; Coyle et al, 2005b; Herman et al., 2008) and are normally tuned by heuristic search with a 1 Hz resolution however; in this work, to minimize the effort and time required in performing an extensive search for the best subject-specific frequency bands, only 4 bands between 8-24Hz were tested (i.e., 8-12; 8-16; 8-20, 8-24). These bands encompass the μ and β bands which are altered during sensorimotor processing (Pfurtscheller et al., 1998; Pfurtscheller, 1998). Attenuation of the spectral power in these bands indicates an event related desynchronization (ERD) whilst an increase in power indicates event-related synchronization (ERS). ERD of the mu band or ERS of the beta band is associated with activated sensorimotor areas and ERS in the mu band is associated with idle or resting sensorimotor areas. ERD/ERS has been studied widely for many cognitive studies and provides very distinctive lateralized EEG pattern differences which form the basis of left/right motor imagery based BCIs (Pfurtscheller, 1998).

3.5 Feature Extraction

Features are extracted using a 1 second window through which the data for each trial is passed either via NTSPP or the raw EEG signals and classified at rate of the sampling interval. These signals X are decomposed according to (14) and each feature vector, $\bar{v}$, is obtained using (15).

$$\bar{v} = \log(\mathrm{var}(E)) \tag{15}$$

The dimensionality of $\bar{v}$ depends on the number of surrogate signals used from E. The common practice is to use several (between 2 and 6) eigenvectors from both ends of the eigenvector spectrum, i.e., the columns of W. As can be seen from Fig. 2, if NTSPP is performed the dimensionality of X can increase as shown in (1) and becomes N×P. Depending on the number of classes and the number of signals available, the dimensionality increase can be significant. NTSPP maps the original data to a higher dimensional signal space which is more separable but also susceptible to containing redundant information in addition to increasing the dimensionality of the feature vector after features are extracted from the NTSPP (i.e., predicted) signals. Large feature vectors can result in sparse matrices for training certain classifiers when the number of exemplars is low. This can significantly impact on the performance of certain classifiers (Tebbens & Schlesinger, 2006). CSP on the other hand can be used to reduce the dimensionality of the available data and also perform a further mapping of the data to increase separability. Therefore the benefits of combining NTSPP with CSP are two fold:- 1) increasing separability and 2) maintaining a tractable dimensionality.

To quantify these benefits and the benefits of employing CSP in BCI with a low number of channels, which is not normally done in BCI, the following tests have been carried using a 2 channel montage, a 3 channel montage and a 22 channel montage as shown in Fig. 1.

- SF – spectral filtering only as a benchmark (2 and 3 channel montages only)
- SF-CSP – spectral filtering and common spatial patterns which is a normal BCI setup
- NTSPP-SF – NTSPP and spectral filtering to show the performance of NTSPP compared to CSP as a standalone preprocessing tool (2 and 3 channel montages only)
- NTSPP-SF-CSP – a combination of all preprocessing methods

Tests are not performed for the SF and NTSPP-SF tests using a 22 channel montage because without CSP the dimensionality of the feature vectors is 22 for SF (22 channels) and 44 for NTSPP-SF (22 channels x 2 classes as shown in (1)). As outlined, without employing CSP, the dimensionality of such feature vectors and the redundancy and/or noise in some channels could impact on the overall performance and therefore some method of feature selection/channel reduction is necessary. When CSP is employed tests are carried out using up to a maximum of 4 eigenvectors from either end of W. Depending on the number of EEG channels available and whether or not NTSPP is employed there are different amounts of eigenvectors to choose from and choosing the optimum number can often impact on performance therefore; when the option to have less or more eigenvectors was available, tests were performed with each number. For example, when a 2 channel montage is employed the maximum number of available eigenvectors is 1 from either end of W for SF-CSP and 2 for NTSPP-SF-CSP therefore tests are performed once with SF-CSP and 2 times with NTSPP-SF-CSP and so on.

3.6 Classification

Four different classifiers obtained from the Biosig toolbox (Schlogl, 2009) are used with all methods described. These include linear discriminant analysis (LDA), support vectors machines (SVMs), Mahalanobis distance classifier (MDA) and a generalized distance based classifier (GDBC) (cf. (Schlogl, 2009) for further details). In addition, a probabilistic Bayes based classifier involving the accumulation of evidence was employed (cf. (Duda et al., 2001;

Lemm et al., 2004) for further details). By using each of these classifiers a better general view of each methods performance was attained.

The datasets for each subject were split into two sets where half the data is used for training and validation and the other half used for testing. These tests are referred to as *5-fold* and *single trial test* sets. Using each of the 6 classification methods, a 5-fold cross-validation was carried out on the 5-fold set for each subject, where the data was partitioned into a training set (80%) and a validation set (20%). Tests were performed five times using a different validation partition each time. The mean-CA (mCA) rates on the 5-folds of validation data and 95% confidence intervals (ci) were estimated using a t-statistic. The purpose of the 5-fold cross validations was to tune any parameters and identify the point at which each subject maximized the separability between the two classes. Subsequently, all 5-fold data was utilized to train the system and the classifier was set up on the features which produced the highest mCA rate in the cross-validation on SP1. The system's generalization abilities were then tested on a one-pass single trial test on the test set – this final test corresponds to the requirement of labeling the data in online single trials test for a practically useful BCI system.

4. Results

4.1 Signals and separability analysis

To illustrate how each method enhances separability in the data for each subject a range of separability measures and visualization methods were applied to the data of each subject. Using the mean CA (mCA) on the 5-fold train and validation sets to identify the point of maximum separability, features were extracted at this time point using signals preprocessed by each of the methods from all available data (this analysis was carried out after BCI tests were performed). Using the features extracted from each signal[3] boxplots were estimated to attain a quick impression of the features' variability within and across classes, as shown in Fig. 4.

As can be seen from Fig. 4 there is substantially more interclass variability when NTSPP is employed and the NTSPP process does result in producing different median values for each of six features. The scales are different when CSP is employed so if the medians of the features obtained using the SF-CSP methods are compared with those obtained using NTSPP-SF-CSP, it can be observed that NTSPP has changed the median values of the features (i.e., features are derived using the variance calculation) and it is clear that there is more opportunity to enhance interclass variability when using NTSPP as opposed to no NTSPP. Notches display the variability of the median between samples. The width of a notch is computed so that box plots whose notches do not overlap have different medians at the 5% significance level. The significance level is based on a normal distribution assumption. Comparing box plot medians is like a visual hypothesis test, analogous to the t-test used for means and therefore it can be seen that the differences in the features produced by different NTSPP signals are significant in many cases (MATLAB®, 2009).

To quantify the separability enhancement for this subject a range of separability indices were estimated (as shown in Table 2), including the Euclidean distance (edist) between class

---

[3] Signals are c3, cz and c4 when no NTSPP is employed or signals are prefixed by the first letter of the data class that each predictor is trained on when NTSPP is employed i.e., l3, l4, and lz for the data processed by the left predictors and r3, r4, and rz for data processed by the right predictors.

means for which the objective is to maximize, the Davies-Bouldin index (dbi) which is a
cluster separability index (Davies and Bouldin, 1979) for which the objective is to minimize,
dtc is a statistical measure of the multivariate distance of each observation (feature vector).

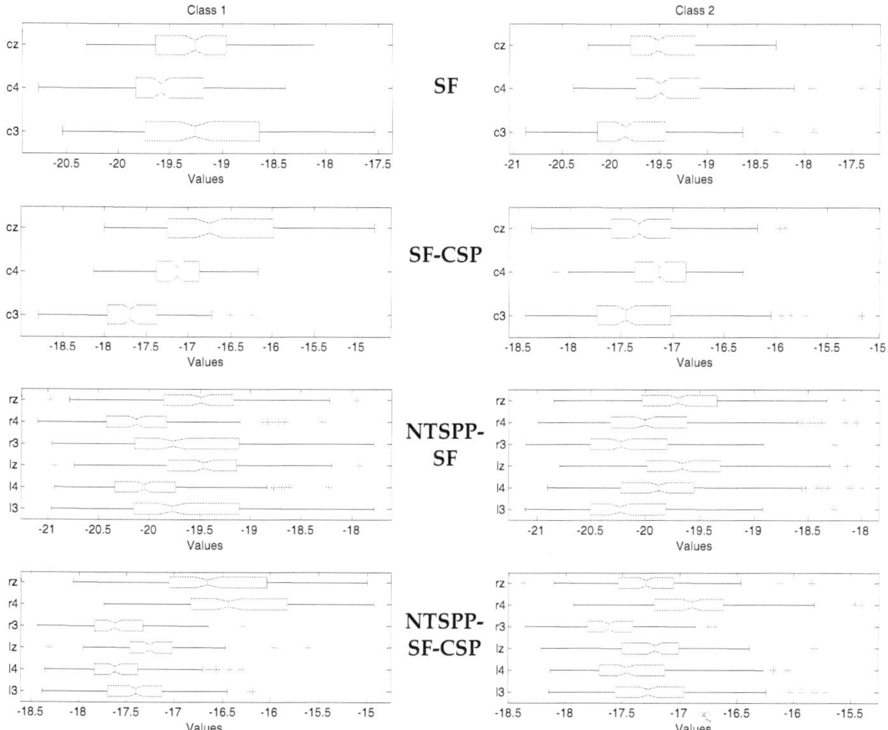

Fig. 4. Boxplots of the features extracted from each signal, for each class and for each
methodology from the center of the dataset (both classes) and the class separability index
(csi) is a measure of the average distance between each observation within class 1 to the
centre of class 2 and vice versa.

	SF	SF-CSP	NTSPP-SF	NTSPP-SF-CSP
mCA	76.43	76.43	78.57	80.00
edist	0.67	0.75	0.86	0.96
dbi	33.25	28.99	38.57	27.44
dtc	3.27	3.54	4.94	3.71
csi	1.87	2.09	2.19	2.10

Table 2. A range of separability indices for 1 subject for each of the methods (details of
separability indices are presented in the text).

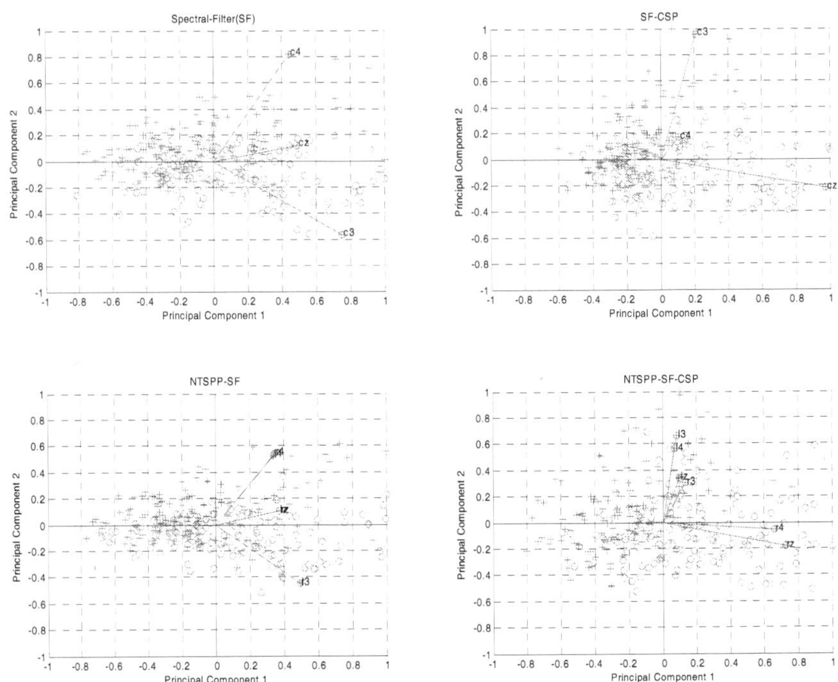

Fig. 5. Biplots showing the first 2 principle components for each of the 4 methods for 1 subject.

From Table 2 it can be seen that NTSPP produces the highest mCA on the 5 fold cross-validation. NTSPP also produces the highest separability across the data in terms of maximizing edist, minimizing dbi, and maximizing dtc and csi. It can be seen that SF alone is the worst performer on all tests, whilst SF-CSP performs better than NTSPP-SF only in dbi. Maximization of Euclidean distance with NTSPP-SF-CSP appears to be a significant benefit of employing this combination of processes which is reflected in the mCA rate which is ~4% greater than the mCA for SF-CSP with no NTSPP for this subject. With no CSP employed, NTSPP is shown to be a better preprocessor than CSP for this subject with the NTSPP-SF approach achieving higher separability than both approaches without NTSPP. The significance of the mCA results across all subjects is shown in the following section.

To aid in visualizing the multidimensional data a principle component analysis (PCA) was carried out. The two most important components for classification are shown in Fig. 5 where biplots showing the first two principle component coefficients are presented. The biplots helps visualize both the principal component coefficients for each variable and the principal component scores for each observation in a single plot.

Each of the features extracted from each signal for each method are represented in these plots by a vector, and the direction and length of the vector indicates how each variable contributes to the two principal components in the plot. The first principal component in each biplot is represented by the horizontal axis and has positive coefficients for all features for each method corresponding to the 3(6 for NTSPP) vectors directed into the right half of the plot. The second principal component, represented by the vertical axis, has positive coefficients for features obtained from c4 and cz for SF, c3 and c4 for SF-CSP, r4, l4, rz, lz for NTSPP-SF and l3, l4, lz and r3 for NTSPP-SF-CSP and has negative coefficients for the remaining five variables. This corresponds to vectors directed into the top and bottom halves of the plot, respectively. This indicates that this component distinguishes between classes that produce high values for the first set of features and low for the second, and classes that have the opposite. Overall it can be seen that the NTSPP-SF-CSP has at least 3 features which are distinguishably providing high variance for one class and two features which are providing lower variance for the other class whereas the other methods have less features that are providing this overall difference in variability, which is providing the superior separability given by NTSPP-SF-CSP in this example. This section has provided a general overview of the dynamical changes which are introduced by these NTSPP methods and the advantages produced in terms of improved separability. The following sections provide further verification of these results by providing a qualitative and statistical analysis of each of the methods when applied across the data from 23 subjects.

4.2 Classification accuracy analysis

4.2.1 Individual subject results

As per the data description in section 2 and section 3.6, results for 5-fold cross validation were obtained for all subjects. Parameter information and time point of maximum separability obtained from the cross validation were used to set up the methods for tests on the test set (single trial test), results of which provide a good indicator for online BCI performance. As outlined the objectives of the research was to compare all methods when employed with 2, 3 or 22 channels. Results for all subjects and all methods are presented in Fig. 6-Fig. 13. Multichannel datasets were not available for subjects S1-S9 therefore only results for 2 channel and 3 channel montages are presented in Fig. 6-Fig. 9. Results for subjects S10-S23 are compared for the 22 channel montages also and these results are presented Fig. 10-Fig. 13. The 22 channel results in Fig. 10 and Fig. 11 are reproduced in Fig. 12 and Fig. 13 for ease of comparison with either the 2 channel or 3 channel results respectively. Results for the Bayes based classifier and the LDA classifier provided the maximum performance in the majority of cases in the cross validation tests therefore only results for these classifiers are presented however support vectors machines (SVMs), Mahalanobis distance classifier (MDA) and a generalized distance based classifier (GDBC) did provide similar results for certain subjects (the following section provide further information on classifier performances). For SVM the regularization parameter was not tuned.

It can be seen from the results that there is quite a lot variation across subjects but in the majority of cases the accuracies for NTSPP approaches are higher than the accuracies obtained when no NTSSP is involved. The differences in accuracies are more prominent for some subjects than others and in a small number of cases the NTSPP produces lower accuracies. A statistical analysis is provided in the following section to verify the significance of the differences among each of the methods. There is a particularly noticeable increase in accuracy for the majority of subjects when 22 channels are used indicating that a 22 channel montage is much better than a 2 or 3 channel montage, however, in a number of cases 3 channel NTSPP methods produce better than or comparable performances to the 22 channel montages and in almost all cases, reduce the difference between the 3 channel results and the 22 channel results substantially more than when no NTSPP is performed using the three channel montages. These results are certainly indicative that NTSPP can improve the performance when a low number of channels are used. Again, the significance of these results is analyzed in the following section.

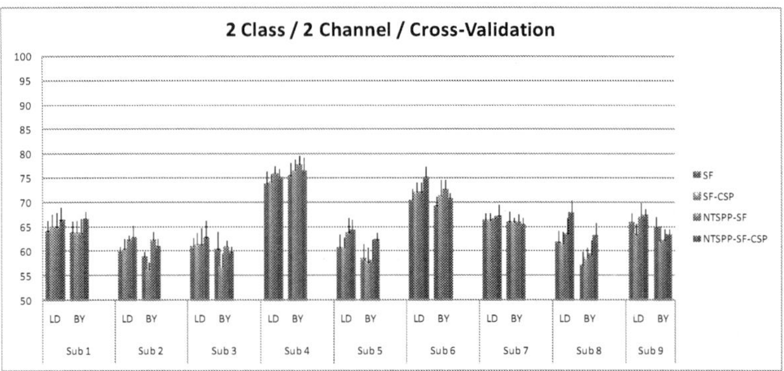

Fig. 6. mCA[%] obtained from cross validation with error bars showing the 95% confidence interval (subjects S1-S9, 2 channel).

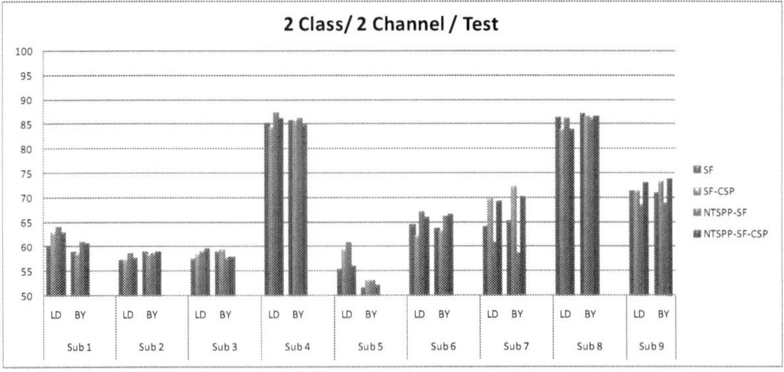

Fig. 7. CA[%] obtained from single trial tests (subjects S1-S9, 2 channel)

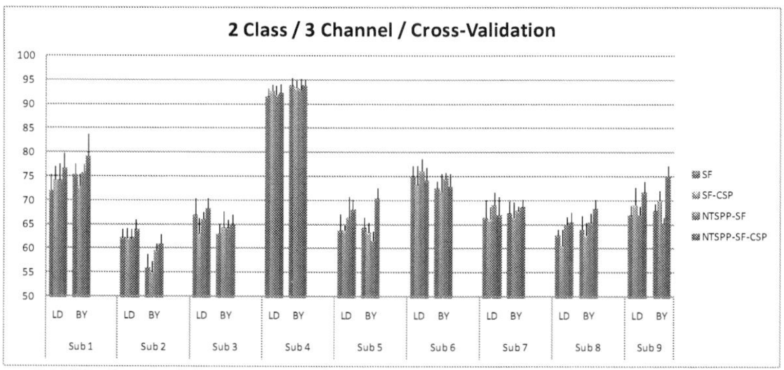

Fig. 8. mCA[%] obtained from cross validation with error bars showing the 95% confidence interval (subjects S1-S9, 3 channel)

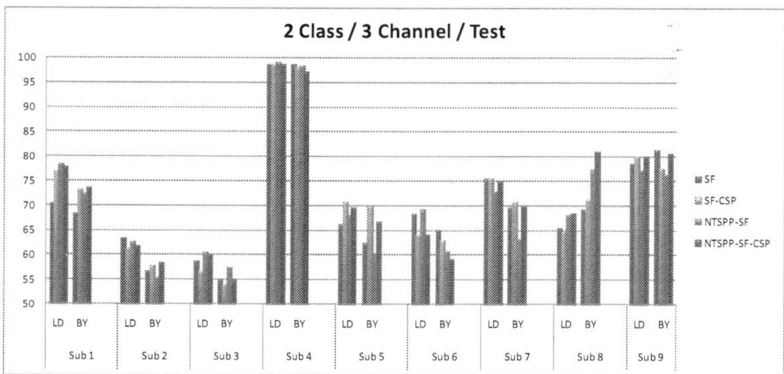

Fig. 9. CA[%] obtained from single trial tests (subjects S1-S9, 3 channel)

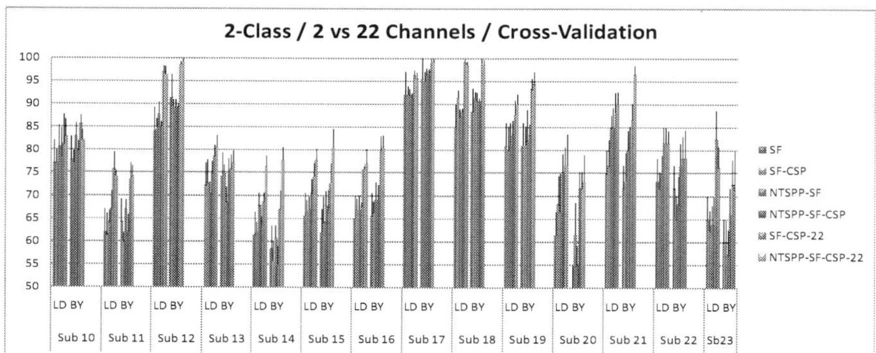

Fig. 10. mCA[%] obtained from cross validation with error bars showing the 95% confidence interval (subjects S10-S23, 2 versus 22 channel results shown)

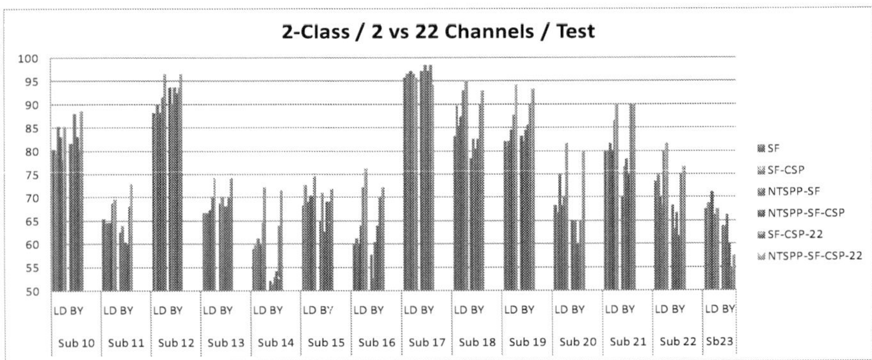

Fig. 11. CA[%] obtained from single trial tests (subjects S10-S23, 2 versus 22 channel results)

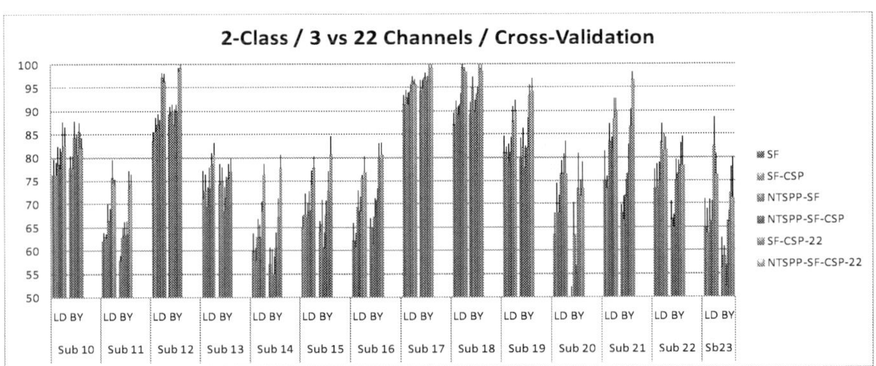

Fig. 12. mCA[%] obtained from cross validation with error bars showing the 95% confidence interval (subjects S10-S23, 3 channel versus 22 channel results shown)

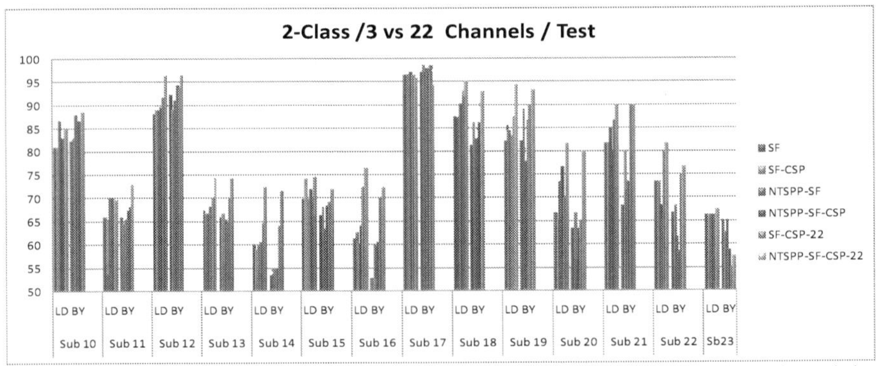

Fig. 13. CA[%] obtained from single trial tests (subjects S10-S23, 3 versus 22 channel results)

4.2.2 Statistical analysis

The results for each subject presented in the previous section show trends that NTSPP can produce better performances in many cases however there is a need to analyze all results in terms of their statistical significance, to verify whether one method is better than the other. To do this, the average accuracies for all methods across all subjects were subjected to repeated measures single factor analysis of variance (RANOVA) (Zar, 1999; Huck, 2000). This repeated measures method was preferred over standard ANOVA to account for the between subject variability which is normally substantive in BCI experiments. In this work the objective was to determine how each method compares with each other method therefore only pair-wise comparisons of means were performed which is equivalent to multiple t-tests. For a more powerful analysis RANOVA could be applied to all methods and a post hoc analysis of the ANOVA results could be performed. In this analysis it is off interest if there exists differences between one method and any of the other methods with a significance level α=0.05 however, to account for the multiple comparisons, the significance level, α, must be corrected. Based on a Bonferroni correction the corrected $\alpha = \alpha / (k.(k-1)/2)$, where k is the number of methods to be compared (i.e., k=6) therefore p<0.003 to be significant.

Table 3 and Table 4 shows the results obtained for subjects S10-S23. Only these subjects are compared as multichannel data was unavailable for Subjects S1-S9. As can be seen, average accuracies for 22 channel montages are significantly higher than those produced by the either of the 2 or 3 channel montages (p<0.003 in all cases and in some case p<0.0001).

This is evidence that there is a significant advantage in applying more channels for this two class classification problem. Although NTSPP-SF-CSP(22) is not shown to be significantly better that SF-CSP(22) for the multichannel cross-validation data, the NTSPP-SF-CSP(22) combination is significantly better than SF-CSP(22) for the single trial tests using LDA (p<0.0001) but not for Bayes. This is a strong indication that NTSPP combined with spectral filtering and CSP generalize much better to unseen data and is better for cross session single trial tests with multiple channel montages. For the 2 and 3 channel montage the results are less consistent.

For the 2 channel montage, even though NTSPP-SF-CSP produces a higher average accuracy it is not significantly better than SF-CSP for the 5-fold data and there is only a marginal difference in performance for the single trial tests using LDA. NTSPP-SF-CSP(2) has higher mean accuracy than SF alone for cross-validation tests using the LDA classifier but the results for the single trial tests have only marginal differences. There is indication from the trends in these results that NTSPP can improve performance with 2 channel systems and in many cases the difference between NTSPP methods are significantly better than the SF methods whilst the SF-CSP methods are not significantly better than SF methods. It can also be observed from Table 3 that using a 22 channel montage the difference between SF-CSP (22) and NTSPP-SF(2) or NTSPP-SF-CSP(2) is not significant using the LDA classifier on the single trial tests whereas NTSPP-SF-CSP (22 channel) produces significant differences between all the 2 channel results using LDA and the Bayes classifiers (p<0.003 in all cases). These results indicate that the 2 channel system when employed with NTSPP-SF-CSP or NTSPP-SF and LDA can produce performances which are comparable with a 22 channel system, at least in single trial tests although the 5 fold results do not show the same trends in significance levels. Overall, even though NTSPP-SF-CSP (22 channel) produce the best results, the results do confirm that NTSPP has the potential to provide better results than SF or SF-CSP using a smaller montage also.

Bayes	5-fold Mean	std	Test Mean	std	SF(2)	SF-CSP(2)	NTSPP-SF(2)	NTSPP-SF-CSP(2)	SF-CSP (22)	NTSPP-SF-CSP (22)
								Significance		
SF (2)	72.4	13.4	72.0	13.2		0.725	0.310	0.736	0.020	0.001
SF-CSP (2)	72.5	12.8	72.3	13.5	0.882		0.599	0.005	0.028	0.001
NTSPP-SF (2)	74.0	12.9	72.9	14.3	0.144	0.234		0.522	0.043	0.003
NTSPP-SF-CSP (2)	76.1	11.8	72.3	13.7	0.045	0.986	0.216		0.008	*
SF-CSP (22)	82.5	11.3	77.1	13.3	**	**	**	**		0.006
NTSPP-SF-CSP (22)	84.6	10.6	80.9	11.7	**	**	**	*	0.089	
LDA	Mean	std	Mean	std	SF(2)	SF-CSP(2)	NTSPP-SF(2)	NTSPP-SF-CSP(2)	SF-CSP (22)	NTSPP-SF-CSP (22)
SF (2)	72.9	9.9	74.1	11.0		0.185	0.065	0.093	0.002	**
SF-CSP (2)	73.9	10.3	75.0	11.2	0.191		0.620	0.009	0.006	*
NTSPP-SF (2)	75.5	9.9	75.4	11.5	0.009	0.099		0.861	0.070	*
NTSPP-SF-CSP (2)	76.9	9.3	75.3	11.3	0.003	0.625	0.154		0.031	*
SF-CSP (22)	83.1	9.4	78.3	10.9	**	**	**	*		*
NTSPP-SF-CSP (22)	83.9	8.5	82.5	10.4	**	**	**	**	0.383	

*$p < 0.001$ **$p < 0.0001$

Table 3. Results showing the average CA rates and the standard deviation across subjects S10-S23 for the cross validation (white columns) and single trial tests (grey columns) for 2 channels and 22 channels. The significance of the differences between one method and each other method is shown in white for 5-fold cross validation and in grey for single trial tests. Only results for Bayes and LDA classifiers are presented. The significance of the difference in mean for multichannel data is also presented.

Bayes	5-fold Mean	std	Test Mean	std	SF(3)	SF-CSP(3)	NTSPP-SF(3)	NTSPP-SF-CSP(3)	SF-CSP (22)	NTSPP-SF-CSP (22)
								Significance		
SF (3)	70.8	13.8	71.7	13.4		0.084	0.875	0.292	0.024	0.001
SF-CSP (3)	72.4	13.5	73.6	13.9	0.166		0.178	0.009	0.053	0.001
NTSPP-SF (3)	71.8	14.1	71.5	13.7	0.378	0.704		0.195	0.018	0.001
NTSPP-SF-CSP (3)	76.4	11.0	72.9	14.5	0.004	0.605	0.009		0.041	0.001
SF-CSP (22)	82.5	11.3	77.1	13.3	**	**	**	**		0.006
NTSPP-SF-CSP (22)	84.6	10.6	80.9	11.7	**	**	*	0.0002	0.089	
LDA	Mean	std	Mean	std	SF(3)	SF-CSP(3)	NTSPP-SF(3)	NTSPP-SF-CSP(3)	SF-CSP (22)	NTSPP-SF-CSP (22)
SF (3)	72.6	10.2	74.8	11.3		0.219	0.192	0.222	0.002	**
SF-CSP (3)	73.4	11.0	75.4	11.8	0.201		0.600	0.002	0.009	*
NTSPP-SF (3)	75.2	9.6	75.9	11.9	0.007	0.108		0.777	0.126	0.001
NTSPP-SF-CSP (3)	77.1	9.8	76.1	11.4	0.001	0.527	0.051		0.166	0.001
SF-CSP (22)	83.1	9.4	78.3	10.9	**	**	**	*		*
NTSPP-SF-CSP (22)	83.9	8.5	82.5	10.4	**	**	**	**	0.383	

*$p < 0.001$ **$p < 0.0001$

Table 4. Results showing the average CA rates and the standard deviation across subjects S10-S23 for the cross validation (white columns) and single trial tests (grey columns) for 3 channels and 22 channels. The significance of the differences between one method and each other method is shown in white for 5-fold cross validation and in grey for single trial tests. Only results for Bayes and LDA classifiers are presented. The significance of the difference in mean for multichannel data is also presented.

For the 3 channel results presented in Table 4 it can be seen that accuracies obtained using NTSPP-SF-CSP and SF-CSP are better than those produced when CSP is not employed when using the Bayes classifier in the cross validation and single trial tests. NTSPP-SF-CSP is significantly better than SF alone for cross validation but not for the single trial tests and SF-CSP is marginally better than NTSPP-SF-CSP in single trial tests using the Bayes classifier. Using the LDA classifier NTSPP-SF-CSP is marginally better than SF-CSP but not significantly better than SF alone for the single trial tests whereas NTSPP approaches are significantly better than SF alone for the cross-validation test but not better than SF-CSP. Again for the 22 channel montages, SF-CSP(22) is not significantly better than NTSPP methods using the LDA classifier but is significantly better than SF and SF-CSP (2 channels) which indicates the potential for NTSPP to produce better results than other methods on smaller montages. The NTSPP-SF-CSP(22) methods produce results which are statistically better than all 3 channel methods which indicates that NTSPP can also enhance results even with multichannel systems.

In summary, with two and three channels some results indicate that NTSPP methods can produce similar single trial performances to the 22 channel results obtained using SF-CSP, a result which indicates that NTSPP can be used to enhance the performance of BCIs with a minimal number of electrodes, reducing the burden of mounting a multiple electrodes. The results also clearly indicate that NTSPP-SF-CSP with the 22 channel montage produces significantly better single trial results than all other methods (including SF-CSP with 22 channels) for both classifiers which are considerable evidence of the NTSPP framework's capacity to stabilize cross session tests in multiple channel systems also. When all 14 subjects are taken into consideration there is substantive evidence to suggest that NTSPP significantly enhances performances when employed with SF-CSP and in many cases also when only the NTSPP-SF combination is employed. This is indicative that NTSPP can be used instead of CSP as a preprocessing methodology but, also, that combining NTSPP and CSP in addition to spectral filtering, can lead to significant performance enhancements, regardless of the number of channels or the type of classifier used therefore NTSPP and CSP are complementary approaches. It must be noted that the Bonferroni correction is conservative correction measure for significance tests. This factor, in addition to the relatively small sample size and substantive inter subjects performance variability, can have a significant impact on measuring the statistical significance of results however the results presented do prove the significance of employing NTSPP.

In term of the classifiers, in general, the Bayes classifier overall does not produce accuracies that are as high as the LDA classifier and is less stable and this may explain why SF-CSP produced marginally better single trial results than NTSPP-SF-CSP using the Bayes classifier in a small number of cases. Although the Bayes classifier may not generalize as well as other classifiers, with accumulation of evidence overtime within each trial the Bayes approach offers better within trial stability. This is achieved by using information about the classifier output from previous time points in the trial when classifying the current time point. In the majority of cases all other classifiers provide slightly lower performance than LDA. A range of RANOVA tests were carried out and it was observed that LDA outperformed all other methods in the single trial tests and that the differences in the performances were statistically significant ($p<0.05$). Different overall averages were obtained depending on the data type being classified however the results do indicate that LDA is most stable for single trial tests, although both SVM and Bayes could have been improved further by fine tuning a number of regularization parameters for each subject. In this work parameter tuning was kept to a minimum and LDA has the advantage of producing the best performance with no effort required for parameter tuning. LDA is the state-of the-art for classification in two class BCI systems and these results provide further evidence of that.

5. Discussion and Conclusions

NTSPP can act as a filter of irregular transients and noise sources, since filtering and prediction go hand in hand. However NTSPP is different to basic filtering in that different filters/predictors are developed for different data types but used to process both data types. This work has shown the value of employing NTSPP as an alternative preprocessing method to the well known CSP filtering approach. CSP has been employed in BCI systems for over ten years and is employed in a range of state-of-the-art BCI systems (Blankertz et al., 2008; Dornhege et al., 2006; Ramouser et al., 2000). It has also been shown that application of NTSPP in combination with CSP has significantly more potential than either approach employed individually. For example, as outlined, when the amount of available channels is large, CSP can be used not only to produce surrogate data which maximizes the variances for one class whilst minimizing for the other class, it can act as a signal/feature selector to reduce data dimensionality. NTSPP on the other hand also manipulates the variances of the data by predictive filtering but results in a dimensionality increase, which can be significant if the number of available EEG channels and/or classes is large. The can in some cases lead to redundancy which may have implications for classifier performance if the number of available training samples is low. By applying both approaches the manipulation of variances are complementary, in addition to CSP deriving a subset of new channels from the signals predicted by NTSPP to reduce dimensionality. The results have demonstrated the advantages in doing this for both small and multichannel montages. In (Coyle et al., 2008a) NTSPP was employed with simple features in a 4 class BCI where CSP was not employed and it was noted that there was redundancy and significant dimensionality increases and thus the results were not so consistent. An analysis is underway to show the benefits of the NTSPP-CSP combination when employed in a 4 class BCI, an approach that was employed for the multiple channel dataset in the recent International BCI competition, results of which are available online (Blankertz et al., 2008b). NTSPP has also been shown to have the capacity to reduce the latency involved in motor imagery BCIs involving continuous classification; producing higher signal separability faster (i.e., earlier in the trial) by predicting the EEG times series multiple steps ahead and subsequently features are extracted from the predicted signals. This has the potential to reduce the time required for a subject to exceed a threshold with the continuous classifier output, as NTSPP predicts characteristics of the data which are more separable multiple steps ahead in time (Coyle et al., 2004, 2009) and further work will be carried out to verify if combining CSP with the multiple step ahead prediction NTSPP framework has significant potential. In terms of improving the NTSPP framework, there is a lot that can be done. For example, a more intuitive process for selecting the embedding dimension and time lag may produce predictors which are better or more specialized and thus result in producing better variability in the outputs for different classes. However simplicity is favored over complexity in BCI development, to enable easier adaptation to each individual and continuous adaptation in the long term (Wolpaw, 2004) so the number of signals and subject specific parameters should be kept to a minimum. NTSPP increases the potentiality of using simpler feature extraction methods or reducing the necessity to fine tune parameters in more complex feature extraction methods. Also, the improved autonomy in adaptation and performance offered by the self-organizing fuzzy neural network (SOFNN) allows the NTSPP framework to be applied autonomously (no parameter tuning is necessary) (Coyle et al., 2006b; 2009).

In terms of improving all methods, the spectral filters could be tuned more precisely. In this work 4 bands were tested with a wideband 8-24 Hz being most useful in some cases whilst a narrow band (8-12Hz) being better in other cases. Fine tuning of the frequency filters in concert with the preprocessing methods, as described in (Satti et al., 2009), would undoubtedly result in better performance for some subjects if not all. Nevertheless a major objective of this work is to keep to a minimum the number of subject specific parameters and the amount of time and expert knowledge required to set up the BCI system. It is unclear whether spectral filtering prior to network training would provide better results and this will also be a topic of further investigation.

Overall this work has shown the advantages and performance gain that can be produced using NTSPP as an easily applied method for preprocessing and that NTSPP, in combination with spectral filtering and common spatial patterns, can offer superior performance than any of the approaches used independently. There is lot of potential to enhance the NTSPP framework and this is part of ongoing investigations.

6. Acknowledgment

The author would like to acknowledge and thank the organizers of the BCI Competitions III and IV, Benjamin Blankertz (Blankertz et al., 2005; 2008a), and also Gert Pfurtscheller and Alois Schlogl for providing the competition datasets IIIa, 2A and 2B and additional EEG data (Schlogl et al., 2005a; 2005b; 2008a; 2008b) and the Biosig toolbox (Schlogl et al., 2009).

7. References

Birbaumer, N.; Ghanayim, N.; Hinterberger, T.; Iversen, I.; Kotchoubey, B.; Kubler, A.; Perelmouter, J.; Taub, E.; and Flor. H. (1999). A spelling device for the paralysed. *Nature*, 398:297.298.

Blankertz et al, (2005). BCI Competition III, online: http://www.bbci.de/competition/iii/

Blankertz, B.; Tomioka, R.; Lemm, S.; Kawanabe, M.; and Müller, K-R. (2008). Optimizing spatial filters for robust EEG Analysis, *IEEE Signal Processing Magazine*, pp. 41-56.

Blankertz et al, (2008a). BCI Competition IV, online: http://www.bbci.de/competition/iv/

Blankertz et al., (2008b), BCI Competition IV Results, (submissions by Coyle et al.,), online: http://www.bbci.de/competition/iv/results/index.html

Coyle, D.; Prasad, G.; and McGinnity, T.M. (2004). Improving information transfer rates of a brain-computer interface by self-organising fuzzy neural network-based multi-step-ahead time-series prediction, *Proceedings of the 3rd IEEE Systems, Man and Cybernetics (UK&RI Chapter) conference*, pp. 230-235.

Coyle, D., Prasad, G., and McGinnity, T.M., (2005a) A time-series prediction approach for feature extraction in a brain-computer interface, *IEEE Transactions on Neural Systems and Rehabilitation Engineering*, vol. 13, no. 4, pp. 461-467.

Coyle, D.; Prasad, G.; and McGinnity (2005b). A time-frequency approach to feature extraction for a brain-computer interface with a comparative analysis of performance measures, *EURASIP JASP, Trends in Brain-Computer Interfaces (special issue)*, vol. 19, pp. 3141-3151.

Coyle, D. (2006) *Intelligent Preprocessing and Feature Extraction Techniques for a Brain Computer Interface*, PhD Thesis, Faculty of Computing and Engineering, University of Ulster, N. Ireland.

Coyle, D.; Prasad, G.; and McGinnity, T.M. (2006a). Creating a nonparametric brain-computer interface with neural time-series prediction preprocessing, *Proc. of the 28th International IEEE Engineering in Medicine and Biology Conference*, pp. 2183-2186.

Coyle, D.; Prasad, G.; and McGinnity (2006b). Enhancing autonomy and computational efficiency of the self-organizing fuzzy neural network for a brain-computer interface, *FUZZ-IEEE, World Congress on Computational Intelligence*, pp. 10485-10492.

Coyle, D.; McGinnity, T.M. and Prasad, G. (2008a) A multi-class brain-computer interface with SOFNN-based prediction preprocessing, *IEEE World Congress on Computational Intelligence*, pp. 3695-3702.

Coyle, D.; Satti, A.; Prasad, G.; and McGinnity, T.M. (2008b). Neural times-series prediction preprocessing meets common spatial patterns in a brain-computer interface, *Proceedings of the 30th International IEEE Engineering in Medicine and Biology Conference*, pp. 2626-2629.

Coyle, D.; Prasad, G.; and McGinnity, T.M. (2009). Faster self-organizing fuzzy neural network training and a hyperparameter analysis for a brain-computer interface, *IEEE Transactions on Systems, Man* and Cybernetics (Part B), vol. 39, issue 6, pp. 1458 - 1471, Dec. 2009.

Davies, D.L. and Bouldin, D.W. (1979). A cluster separation measure, *IEEE Transactions on Pattern Analysis and Machine Intelligence*. Vol. 1 No. 4, pp. 224-227.

Dornhege, G.; Blankertz, B.; Krauledat, M.; Losch, F.; Curio, G.; and Müller, K-R. (2006). Combined Optimization of Spatial and Temporal Filters for Improving Brain-Computer Interfacing, *IEEE Transactions on Biomedical Engineering*, Vol. 53, No. 11, pp. 2274-2281.

Duda, R.; Hart, P.; and Stork, D. (2001). *Pattern Classification*, 2nd ed. New York: Wiley.

Hassibi, B. and Stork, D. G. (1993). Second order derivatives for network pruning: Optimal brain surgeon, *Advances in Neural Information Processing Systems 4*, pp. 164-171.

Herman, P.; Prasad, G.; McGinnity, T.M.; and Coyle, D. (2008). Comparative analysis of spectral approaches to feature extraction for EEG-based motor imagery classification, *IEEE Transactions on Neural Systems and Rehabilitation Engineering*, Vol. 16., No. 4, pp. 317-326.

Hornik, K.; Stinchcombe, M.; and White, H. (1989). Multilayer feedforward networks are universal approximators. *Neural Networks*, Vol. 2, pp. 359–366.

Huck, S. W. (2000), *Reading Statistics and Research*. 3rd. ed. New York: Allyn&Bacon/ Longman Pub. Chapter 16.

Iasemidis, L. D. (2003). Epileptic seizure prediction and control, *IEEE Trans. on Biomedical Eng*, vol. 50, no. 5, pp. 549-558.

Jang, J.-S.R., Sun, C. -T., and Mizutani, E. (1997). *Neuro-Fuzzy & Soft Computing*, Englewood Cliffs, NJ: Prentice-Hall, 1997

Kaiser, J.; Perelmouter, J.; Iversen, I.; Neumann, N.; Ghanayim, N.; Hinterberger, T.; Kubler, A.; Kotchoubey, B.; and Birbaumer, N. (2001). Self-initiation of EEG-based communication in paralyzed patients. *Clinical Neurophysiology*, vol. 112, pp. 551–554.

Kasabov, N. K. and Song, Q. (2002). DENFIS: Dynamic evolving neural-fuzzy inference system and its application for time-series prediction, *IEEE Transactions on Fuzzy Systems,*. vol. 10, no. 2, pp. 144-154.

Kubler, A. ; Kotchoubey, B.; Hinterberger, T.; Ghanayim, N.; Perelmouter, J.; Schauer, M.; Fritsch, C.; Taub, E.; and Birbaumer, N. (1999). The thought translation device: a neurophysiological approach to communication in total motor paralysis. *Exp Brain Res.* vol. 124. pp. 223-232.

Lecuyer, A.; Lotte, F.; Reilly, R. B.; Leeb, R.; Hirose, M.; and Slater, M. (2008). Brain-computer interfaces, virtual reality and videogames, *Computer*, vol. 41, no. 10, pp. 66-71.

Leeb, R.; Lee, F.; Keinrath, C.; Scherer, R.; Bischof, H.; Pfurtscheller, G. (2007). Brain-computer communication: motivation, aim, and impact of exploring a virtual apartment. *IEEE Transactions on Neural Systems and Rehabilitation Engineering*, Vol. 15, pp. 473-482.

Leng, G. (2003). *Algorithmic Developments for Self-Organising Fuzzy Neural Networks*, PhD Thesis, University of Ulster.

Lemm, S.; Schafer, C.; and Curio, G. (2004). BCI competition—Data set III: Probabilistic modelling of sensorimotor μ rhythms for classification of imaginary hand movements, *IEEE Transaction on Biomedical Engineering*, vol. 51, no. 6, pp. 1077-1080.

Mason, S.G.; Bashashati, A.; Fatoruechi, M.; Navarro, K. F.; and Birch, G. E. (2007). A comprehensive survey of brain interface technology designs, *Annals of Biomed. Eng.*, Vol. 35, No. 2, pp. 137-169.

MATLAB® (2009) - http://www.mathworks.com/

McFarland, D. J. and Wolpaw, J. R. (2008). Brain-computer interface operation of robotic and prosthetic devices, *Computer*, vol. 41, no. 10, pp. 52-56.

Owen, A. M. and Coleman, M. R. (2008). Functional neuroimaging of the vegetative state", *Nature Reviews Neuroscience*, Vol. 9, pp. 235-243.

Pfurtscheller, G.; Guger, C.; Muller, G.; Krausz, G.; and Neuper, C. (2000). Brain oscillations control hand orthosis in a tetraplegic, *Neuroscience Letters*, vol. 292, pp. 211–214.

Pfurtscheller, G.; Neuper, C.; Schlogl, A.; and Lugger, K. (1998). Separability of EEG signals recorded during right and left motor imagery using adaptive autoregressive parameters, *IEEE Transactions on Rehabilitation Engineering*, vol.6, no.3, pp. 316-324.

Pfurtscheller, G. (1998). *Electroencephalography, Basic Principles, Clinical Application and Related Fields*, 4th Ed., E. Niedermeyer and F. L. Da Silva (Editors), Williams and Wilkins.

Popescu, F.; Fazli, S.; Badower, Y.; Müller, K-R. and Blankertz, B. (2007). Single Trial Classification of Motor Imagination Using Six Dry EEG Electrodes," *PLoS ONE*, vol. 2, 7.

Prasad, G.; McGinnity, T.M.; Leng, G.; and Coyle, D. (2008). On-line identification of self-organizing fuzzy neural networks for modelling time-varying complex systems, *In: Plamen et al. (ed.), Evolving Intelligent Systems*, John Wiley, NY, pp 302-324.

Prasad, G.; Herman, P.; Coyle, D.; McDonough, S.; and Crosbie, J. (2009). Using a motor imagery-based brain-computer interface for post-stroke rehabilitation, *Proc. of the 4th IEEE EMB Conference on Neural Engineering*, pp. 258-262.

Ramouser, H.; Muller-Gerking, J.; and Pfurtscheller, G. (2000). Optimal spatial filtering of single trial EEG during imagined hand movement, *IEEE Trans. on Rehab. Eng.*, vol. 8, no. 4, pp. 441-446.

Satti, A.; Coyle, D.; and Prasad, G. (2009). Continuous EEG Classification for a Self-paced BCI", *Proc. of the 4th IEEE EMB Conference on Neural Engineering,* pp. 315-318.

Satti, A.; Coyle, D.; and Prasad, G. (2008). Optimizing common spatial patterns for a motor imagery-based BCI by eigenvector filtration", *Biomedizinische Technik,* pp. 68-72.

Satti, A.; Coyle, D.; and Prasad, G. (2009). Spatio-spectral & temporal parameter searching using class correlation analysis and particle swarm optimization for a brain-computer interface, *Proceedings of the 2009 IEEE Systems,* Man and Cybernetics Conference, October, 2009.

Silvoni, S.; Volpato, C.; Cavinato, M.; Marchetti, M.; Priftis, K.; Merico, A.; Tonin, P.; Koutsikos, K.; Beverina, F.; and Piccione, F. (2009). P300-based brain–computer interface communication: evaluation and follow-up in amyotrophic lateral sclerosis, *Frontiers in Neuroprosthetics,* Vol. 1, pp. 1-12.

Schlogl et al, (2005a). BCI-Competition III- Dataset IIIa, online:
http://www.bbci.de/competition/iii/#data_set_iiia

Schlogl, A.; Lee, F.; Birschof, H.; and Pfurtscheller, G. (2005b) Characterization of four-class motor imagery EEG data for the BCI-competition 2005, *J. of Neural Engineering,* Vol 2, L.14-L.22.

Schlogl, A. ; Keinrath, C.; Zimmermann, D.; Scherer, R.; Leeb, R.; Pfurtscheller, G. (2007b). A fully automated correction method of EOG artifacts in EEG recordings, *Clin. Neurophys.* Vol. 118(1), pp. 98-104.

Schlogl et al, (2008a). BCI-Competition IV- Dataset 2B, online:
http://www.bbci.de/competition/iv/#dataset2b

Schlogl et al, (2008b). BCI-Competition IV- Dataset 2A, online:
http://www.bbci.de/competition/iv//#dataset2b

Schlogl, A (2009) BIOSIG – an open source software library for biomedical signal processing, online: http://biosig.sourceforge.net/

Takagi, T. and Sugeno, M. (1985). Fuzzy identification of systems and its applications to modelling and control, *IEEE Transactions on Systems, Man and Cybernetics,* vol. 15, no. 1, pp. 116-132.

Tebbens, J.D. and Schlesinger, P. (2006). "Improving Implementation of Linear Discriminant Analysis for the High Dimension/Small Sample Size Problem", *Elsevier Science.*

Wolpaw, J. R.; Birbaumer, N.; McFarland, D. J.; Pfurtscheller, G.; Vaughan, T. M. (2002). Brain-computer interfaces for communication and control, *J. Clinical Neurophysiology,* vol. 113, pp. 767-791.

Wolpaw, J. R. (2004). Brain-computer interfaces for communication and control: Current status, *Proceedings of the 2nd International Brain-Computer Interface Workshop and Training Course, Biomedizinische Technik,* pp. 43-44.

Vaughan, T.M. and Wolpaw, J. R. (2006). Guest Editorial: The Third International Meeting on Brain-Computer Interface Technology: Making a Difference, *IEEE Transactions on Neural Systems and Rehabilitation Engineering,* vol. 14, no. 2.

Zar, J. H. (1999), *Biostatistical Analysis.* 4th. ed. New-Jersey: Upper Saddle River. p. 255-259.

8

Recent Numerical Methods in Electrocardiology

Youssef Belhamadia
University of Alberta, Campus Saint-Jean
Edmonton, Alberta, Canada
email:youssef.belhamadia@ualberta.ca

1. Introduction

Heart diseases are the leading cause of death in the world. Many questions have not yet been answered regarding the electrical waves propagation in cardiac tissue, and the mechanism of ventricular fibrillation that is produced by one or many spiral propagation waves of the excitation cardiac wall. Numerical modeling can play a crucial role and provides the necessary tools to answer some of these questions. However, the mathematical models, which give the best reflection of electrophysiological waves in cardiac tissue, are extremely complicated and present a significant computational challenges.

The bidomain model is considered as the mathematical equations that have been used for simulating cardiac electrophysiological waves for many years (see Sundnes (2002), and Pierre (2006) and the reference therein). This model represents the cardiac tissue at a macroscopic scale by relating the transmembrane potential, the extracellular potential, and the ionic currents. The biodomain model consists of a system of two nonlinear partial differential equations coupled to a system of ordinary differential equations. From the numerical point of view, the model is computationally very expensive. The major difficulties are due to the computational grids size that must be very fine to get a realistic simulation of cardiac tissue. Indeed, the action potential is a wave with sharp depolarization and repolarization fronts and this wave travels across the whole computational domain calling for a very fine uniform mesh.

One popular way of reducing the computational challenges of the bidomain model is the use of the monodomain model. This model considers a single nonlinear partial differential equation coupled with the same system of ordinary differential equations for the ionic currents. Although, it has been reported that the CPU requirements are reduced when simplifying the bidomain model to a monodomain model (see Sundnes et al. (2006)), both models still encounter computational difficulties because of the need for fine meshes and small time-steps.

Many methods have been introduced in the literature to overcome these difficulties. The operator splitting is usually performed to separate the large non-linear system of ODEs and thus introduces subproblems easier to solve. A first-order (Godunov method) and a second-order (Strang method) accurate splitting technique can be employed. For more details the reader is referred to Sundnes et al. (2005), Lines, Buist, Grottum, Pullan, Sundnes & Tveito (2003); Lines, Grottum & Tveito (2003), and Weber Dos Santos et al. (2003)). To reduce the computational time at each time step, parallel computing techniques are used (see Colli Franzone & Pavarino (2004), Karpoukhin et al. (1995) and Weber dos Santos et al. (2004)). Several time-stepping strategies have also been used, fully implicit (Bourgault et al. (2003), and Murillo & Cai (2004)), and semi-implicit (Franzone & Pavarino (2004), Ethier & Bourgault (2008))

Recently, mesh adaptation methods have been introduced to reduce the size of the spatial mesh as well as the computational time. This method consists in locating finer mesh cells near the depolarisation-repolarization front position while a coarser mesh is used away from the front. In the context of isotropic unstructured meshes, the reader is referred to Cherry et al. (2003), Colli Franzone et al. (2006) and Trangenstein & Kim (2004) for more details. However, for two and three dimensional anisotropic mesh adaptation, where mesh cells are elongated along a specified direction, the reader is referred to Belhamadia (2008a;b); Belhamadia et al. (2009).

The scope of this book chapter is to present the recent adaptive technique introduced in Belhamadia (2008a;b) for simulating the two-dimensional cardiac electrical activity. The method proposed reduces greatly the size of the spatial mesh as well as the computational time. Also, an accurate prediction of the depolarization and repolarization fronts is obtained showing the advantages of the proposed method.

This work is organized as follows. Section 2 presents a brief description of the bidomain and monodomain models with Aliev-Panfilov ion kinetics. Also, the finite element discretization for these models are presented. Section 3 is devoted to a description of the time-dependent adaptive strategy while the last section presents two-dimensional numerical results representing the re-entrant waves.

2. Mathematical Models

The bidomain and modomain models will be now presented. The first model consists of a nonlinear partial differential equation for the transmembrane potential V_m coupled with an elliptic one for the extracellular potential ϕ_e, as well as an ordinary differential equation, for at least one variable, representing the ionic currents. This system of equations takes the following form:

$$
\left\{
\begin{aligned}
&\frac{\partial V_m}{\partial t} - \nabla \cdot (G_i \nabla V_m) = \nabla \cdot (G_i \nabla \phi_e) + I_{ion}(V_m, W) \\
&\qquad \nabla \cdot ((G_i + G_e) \nabla \phi_e) = -\nabla \cdot (G_i \nabla V_m) \\
&\qquad\qquad \frac{\partial W}{\partial t} = g(V_m, W),
\end{aligned}
\right.
\tag{1}
$$

where G_i and G_e are the symmetric intra- and extra-cellular conductivity tensors. The definition of the functions $I_{ion}(V_m, w)$ and $g(V_m, w)$ depends on the ionic model. Modern cardiac ionic models include generally a set of 10 to 60 ordinary differential equations. However, in this work the Aliev-Panfilov model (see Aliev & Panfilov (1996)) is presented which consists of the following equations:

$$
I_{ion} = kV_m(V_m - a)(1 - V_m) - V_m W,
$$

$$
g(V_m, W) = \left(\epsilon + \frac{\mu_1 W}{\mu_2 + V_m} \right)(-W - kV_m(V_m - a - 1)).
$$

If we assume equal anisotropy ratio of the intra- and extra-cellular media, it is well known that the bidomain equations can be reduced to the monodomain model. The resulting system consists of one nonlinear partial differential equation for the transmembrane potential

V_m coupled with an ordinary differential equation for the ionic currents. The monodomain equations using Aliev-Panfilov model take the following form:

$$\begin{cases} \dfrac{\partial V_m}{\partial t} - \nabla \cdot (G \nabla V_m) = I_{ion}(V_m, W) \\[4mm] \dfrac{\partial W}{\partial t} = g(V_m, W), \end{cases} \qquad (2)$$

Several time derivative discretization have been introduced for the bidomain model (see Ethier & Bourgault (2008), and Keener & Bogar (1998)). Also, the reader is referred to Belhamadia (2008b) for more discussion about different time schemes and their impact on two-dimensional mesh adaptation. In this work, a fully implicit backward second order scheme (Gear) is employed as time discretization. Starting from V_m^{n-1} and W^{n-1} at time t^{n-1} and from V_m^n and W^n at time t^n, Gear scheme gives:

$$\frac{\partial V_m}{\partial t}(t^{(n+1)}) \simeq \frac{3V_m^{(n+1)} - 4V_m^{(n)} + V_m^{(n-1)}}{2\Delta t},$$

and

$$\frac{\partial W}{\partial t}(t^{(n+1)}) \simeq \frac{3W^{(n+1)} - 4W^{(n)} + W^{(n-1)}}{2\Delta t}.$$

The variational formulation of the system of nonlinear equation (1) is straightforward and obtained by multiplying this system by test functions $(\psi_v, \psi_\phi, \psi_w)$ such that:

$$\begin{cases} \displaystyle\int_\Omega \frac{3V_m^{(n+1)} - 4V_m^{(n)} + V_m^{(n-1)}}{2\Delta t} \, \psi_v \, d\Omega + \int_\Omega G_i \nabla V_m^{(n+1)} \cdot \nabla \psi_v \, d\Omega \\[4mm] \displaystyle + \int_\Omega G_i \nabla \phi_e^{(n+1)} \cdot \nabla \psi_v \, d\Omega = \int_\Omega I_{ion}(V_m^{(n+1)}, W^{(n+1)}) \psi_v \, d\Omega \\[4mm] \displaystyle - \int_\Omega (G_i + G_e) \nabla \phi_e^{(n+1)} \cdot \nabla \psi_\phi \, d\Omega = \int_\Omega G_e \nabla V_m^{(n+1)} \cdot \nabla \psi_\phi \, d\Omega \\[4mm] \displaystyle \int_\Omega \frac{3W^{(n+1)} - 4W^{(n)} + W^{(n-1)}}{2\Delta t} \psi_w \, d\Omega = \int_\Omega g(V_m^{(n+1)}, W^{(n+1)}) \, \psi_w \, d\Omega. \end{cases} \qquad (3)$$

Similarly, the variational formulation of the system of nonlinear equation (2) takes the following form:

$$\begin{cases} \displaystyle\int_\Omega \frac{3V_m^{(n+1)} - 4V_m^{(n)} + V_m^{(n-1)}}{2\Delta t} \, \psi_v \, d\Omega + \int_\Omega G \nabla V_m^{(n+1)} \cdot \nabla \psi_v \, d\Omega \\[4mm] \displaystyle = \int_\Omega I_{ion}(V_m^{(n+1)}, W^{(n+1)}) \psi_v \, d\Omega \\[4mm] \displaystyle \int_\Omega \frac{3W^{(n+1)} - 4W^{(n)} + W^{(n-1)}}{2\Delta t} \psi_w \, d\Omega = \int_\Omega g(V_m^{(n+1)}, W^{(n+1)}) \, \psi_w \, d\Omega. \end{cases} \qquad (4)$$

In all numerical simulations, a quadratic (P_2) for spatial discretization and Newton's method are employed to solve the non linear system above at each time step. Linear system resulting from Newton's method is solved by iterative methods, an incomplete LU decomposition (ILU) GMRES solver Saad (1996) from the PETSc library Balay et al. (2003).

3. Adaptive Method

As already mentioned, the accurate prediction of the depolarization-repolarization fronts in cardiac tissue is crucial. It is well known that a typical simulation of time-dependent cardiac electrophysiological waves using the whole heart may require about 10^7 grid points (see Cherry et al. (2003) and Ying (2005)), which leads to numerical challenges beyond the limit of the existing computational resources. To partially avoid these challenges, the mesh has to be adapted at each time step near the depolarization-repolarization fronts while coarser mesh are sufficient away from these fronts. This can be done with appropriate mesh adaptation techniques. In the context of the electrical wave of the heart, two different methods for estimating the error, depending on the dimension of the problem, have been introduced. A hierarchical error estimator described in Belhamadia (2008b) was used for a two-dimensional case, and an error estimator based on a definition of edge length using a solution dependent metric described in Belhamadia et al. (2009) was used for a three-dimensional case.

A brief description of adaptive methods for time dependent problems will now be presented. Only the case of the monodomain model will be presented and similar strategy can be presented for the bidomain model. The objective of this method is to build at each time step t^n a fine mesh in all regions where the variables V_m and W evolve (V_m, W and ϕ_e in case of the bidomain model) and a coarse mesh in these other regions. Therefore, an accurate solution is obtained and the total number of elements is greatly reduced at each time step. The overall adaptive strategy is the following:

1. Start from the solutions $V_m^{(n-1)}$, $V_m^{(n)}$, $W^{(n-1)}$ and $W^{(n)}$ and a mesh $\mathcal{M}^{(n)}$ at time $t^{(n)}$;

2. Solve the system (2) on mesh $\mathcal{M}^{(n)}$ to obtain a first approximation of the solutions (denoted $\tilde{V}_m^{(n+1)}$ and $\tilde{W}^{(n+1)}$) at time $t^{(n+1)}$;

3. Adapt the mesh on the two expressions $\dfrac{\tilde{V}_m^{(n+1)} + V_m^{(n)} + V_m^{(n-1)}}{3}$ and $\dfrac{\tilde{W}^{(n+1)} + W^{(n)} + W^{(n-1)}}{3}$ to obtain a new mesh $\mathcal{M}^{(n+1)}$;

4. Reinterpolate $V_m^{(n-1)}$, $V_m^{(n)}$, $W^{(n-1)}$ and $W^{(n)}$ on mesh $\mathcal{M}^{(n+1)}$;

5. Solve the system (2) on mesh $\mathcal{M}^{(n+1)}$ for V_m^{n+1} and W^{n+1}.

6. Next time step: go to step 2.

4. Numerical results

The mechanism of ventricular fibrillation is believed to be produced by one or many spiral propagation waves in the myocardium. The reader is referred to Biktashev et al. (1999), Jalife (2000), and Panfilov & Kerkhof (2004) and the reference therein for a complete discussion. From the numerical point of view, there are many strategies to initiate a spiral wave (see Bourgault et al. (2003), and Ethier & Bourgault (2008)). In this section, the performance of the adaptive method will be presented. A two-dimensional problem representing the re-entrant waves will be presented using the monodomain and bidomain model.

4.1 Monodomain model

This section is devoted to a test case using the monodomain model. The computational domain is the square $[0, 100] \times [0, 100]$. Homogeneous Neumann conditions are imposed on all sides, and the following parameters values have been used:

$k = 8$	$a = 0.15$
$\epsilon = 0.002$	$\mu_1 = 0.2$
$\mu_2 = 0.3$	$G = 1$
$\Delta t = 0.5$	

Figure 1 presents the transmembrane potential V_m and the recovery variable W at the center of the computational domain as a function of time. The numerical solutions are obtained using adapted meshes with only an average of 5900 triangular elements leading to 23000 dof since we use quadratic (P_2) for spatial discretization. The total number of elements is reduced due to the use of the anisotropic adapted meshes. The reader is referred to Belhamadia (2008b) for more details about quantitative results and comparisons between structured and adapted meshes.

Figure 2 a) b) shows the solutions V_m and W at time $t = 8$ t.u. while the adapted mesh at the same time is presented in figure 2 c). A close up view of the mesh on the interface is presented in figure 2 d). It is clearly shown that the mesh is refined only in the vicinity of the front position while keeping sufficient resolution in other regions. The gain in computational time is obvious using the adaptive method since the total number of elements is greatly reduced.

4.2 Bidomain model

A test case using the bidomain model is now presented. The computational domain, the boundary conditions, and the physical parameters are the same as the previous section. However, the intra- and extra-cellular conductivity tensors are

$$G_i = \begin{pmatrix} 3 & 0 \\ 0 & 0.32 \end{pmatrix} \quad \text{and} \quad G_e = \begin{pmatrix} 2 & 0 \\ 0 & 1.37 \end{pmatrix}$$

As the previous section, the advantage of the adaptive method can be also illustrated in the case of unequal anisotropy ratios. The transmembrane potentials, and the recovery variable at the center of the computational domain as a function of time are similar to figure 1 and are not presented in this work to avoid a repetition. The numerical solutions are obtained using adapted meshes with only an average of 7100 triangular elements (29000 dof).

Figure 3 illustrates the evolution of the adapted mesh. The front position is well captured and the solution seems uniformly accurate over time steps. Finally, the numerical solutions of the transmembrane potential, the extracellular potential and the recovery variable are shown in figure 4. As could be seen, the depolarization and repolarization fronts are smooth and well captured on the adapted anisotropic meshes.

5. Conclusions

A recent numerical method for the transmembrane potential was presented. The accuracy of the method was obtained by using an anisotropic time-dependent adaptive method. A two-dimensional problem representing the re-entrant waves was shown using the monodomain and bidomain model. Although only a two dimensional case was presented, this method is general and can be extended to three dimensional case. Results using realist heart geometry and with the monodomain model are recently presented in Belhamadia et al. (2009). The method proposed in this work uses two-variable ionic model. It will be interesting to see how the method performs with more complex ionic models.

6. Acknowledgments

The authors acknowledge the financial support of NSERC.

7. References

Aliev, R. & Panfilov, A. (1996). A Simple Two-Variable Model of Cardiac Excitation, *Chaos, Solitons and Fractals* **7**(3): 293–301.

Balay, S., Buschelman, K., Eijkhout, V., Gropp, W., Kaushik, D., Knepley, M., McInnes, L. C., Smith, B. & Zhang, H. (2003). PETSc Users Manual, *Technical Report ANL-95/11-Revision 2.1.6*, Argonne National Laboratory, Argonne, Illinois. *http://www.mcs.anl.gov/petsc/*.

Belhamadia, Y. (2008a). An Efficient Computational Method for Simulation of Electrophysiological Waves, *Conf Proc IEEE Eng Med Biol Soc.* pp. 5922–5925.

Belhamadia, Y. (2008b). A Time-Dependent Adaptive Remeshing for Electrical Waves of the Heart, *IEEE Transactions on Biomedical Engineering* **55**(2, Part-1): 443–452.

Belhamadia, Y., Fortin, A. & Bourgault, Y. (2009). Towards Accurate Numerical Method for Monodomain Models Using a Realistic Heart Geometry, *Mathematical Biosciences* . 220(2): 89-10.

Biktashev, V., Holden, A., Mironov, S., Pertsov, A. & Zaitsev, A. (1999). Three Dimensional Aspects of Re-Entry in Experimental and Numerical Models of Ventricular Fibrillation, *Int. J. Bifurcation & Chaos* **9**(4): 694–704.

Bourgault, Y., Ethier, M. & LeBlanc, V. (2003). Simulation of Electrophysiological Waves With an Unstructured Finite Element Method, *Mathematical Modelling and Numerical Analysis* **37**(4): 649–662.

Cherry, E., Greenside, H. & Henriquez, C. S. (2003). Efficient Simulation of Three-dimensional Anisotropic Cardiac Tissue Using an Adaptive Mesh Refinement Method, *Chaos: An Interdisciplinary Journal of Nonlinear Science* **13**(3): 853–865.

Colli Franzone, P., Deufhard, P., Erdmann, B., Lang, J. & Pavarino, L. F. (2006). Adaptivity in Space and Time for Reaction-Diffusion Systems in Electrocardiology, *SIAM Journal on Scientific Computing* **28**(3): 942–962.

Colli Franzone, P. & Pavarino, L. F. (2004). A Parallel Solver for Reaction-Diffusion Systems in Computational Electrocardiology, *Math. Models and Methods in Applied Sciences* **14**(6): 883–911.

Ethier, M. & Bourgault, Y. (2008). Semi-implicit time-discretization schemes for the bidomain model, *SIAM Journal of Numerical Analysis* **46**(5): 2443–2468.

Franzone, P. C. & Pavarino, L. F. (2004). A parallel solver for reaction-diffusion systems in computational electrocardiology, *Mathematical Models and Methods in Applied Sciences* **14**(6): 883–912.

Jalife, J. (2000). Ventricular Fibrillation: Mechanisms of Initiation and Maintenance, *Annual Review of Physiology* **60**: 25–50.

Karpoukhin, M., Kogan, B. & Karplus, J. W. (1995). The Application of a Massively Parallel Computer to the Simulation of Electrical Wave Propagation Phenomena in the Heart Muscle Using Simplified Models, *HICSS* **5**: 112–122.

Keener, J. P. & Bogar, K. (1998). A numerical method for the solution of the bidomain equations in cardiac tissue, *Chaos* **8**: 234–241.

Lines, G., Buist, M., Grottum, P., Pullan, A., Sundnes, J. & Tveito, A. (2003). Mathematical models and numerical methods for the forward problem in cardiac electrophysiology, *Comput. Visual. Sc.* **5**: 215–239.

Lines, G., Grottum, P. & Tveito, A. (2003). Modeling the electrical activity of the heart: A bidomain model of the ventricles embedded in a torso, *Comput. Visual. Sc.* **5**: 195–213.

Murillo, M. & Cai, X. (2004). A fully implicit parallel algorithm for simulating the non-linear electrical activity of the heart, *Numerical Linear Algebra with Applications* **11**: 261–277.
URL: *http://www3.interscience.wiley.com/cgi-bin/abstract/107632540/ABSTRACT*

Panfilov, A. V. & Kerkhof, P. (2004). Quantifying Ventricular Fibrillation: in Silico Research and Clinical Implications, *IEEE Transactions on Biomedical Engineering* **51**(1): 195–196.

Pierre, C. (2006). *Modlisation et Simulation de l'Activit lectrique du Coeur dans le Thorax, Analyse Numrique et Mthodes de Volumes Finis*, PhD thesis, Universit de Nantes.

Saad, Y. (1996). *Iterative Methods for Sparse Linear Systems*, PWS Publishing Company.

Sundnes, J. (2002). *Numerical Methods for Simulating the Electrical Activity of the Heart*, PhD thesis, University of Oslo.

Sundnes, J., Lines, G. & Tveito, A. (2005). An Operator Splitting Method for Solving the Bidomain Equations Coupled to a Volume Conductor Model for the Torso, *Mathematical biosciences* **194**(2): 233–248.

Sundnes, J., Nielsen, B., Mardal, K., Cai, X., Lines, G. & A., T. (2006). On the Computational Complexity of the Bidomain and the Monodomain Models of Electrophysiology, *Ann Biomed Eng* **34**(7): 1088–1097.

Trangenstein, J. & Kim, C. (2004). Operator Splitting and Adaptive Mesh Refinement for the Luo-Rudy I Model, *Journal of Computational Physics* **196**(2): 645–679.

Weber Dos Santos, R., Plank, G., Bauer, S. & Vigmond, E. (2003). Preconditioning techniques for the bidomain equations, *Proceedings of the 15th International Conference on Domain Decomposition Methods*, Springer, Lecture Notes in Computational Science and Engineering (LNCSE)., pp. 571–580.
URL: *http://www.ddm.org/DD15/proceedings-dd15.html*

Weber dos Santos, R., Plank, G., Bauer, S. & Vigmond, E. (2004). Parallel Multigrid Preconditioner for the Cardiac Bidomain Model, *IEEE Trans. Biomed. Eng.* **51**(11): 1960–1968.

Ying, W. (2005). *A Multilevel Adaptive Approach for Computational Cardiology*, PhD thesis, Duke University, Durham, USA.

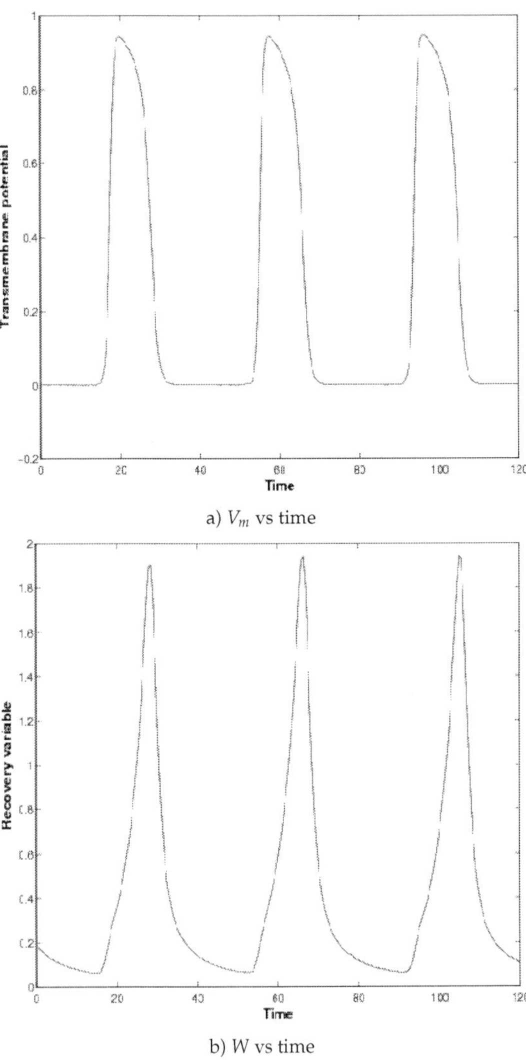

a) V_m vs time

b) W vs time

Fig. 1. Transmembrane potential and recovery variable at the point $(50,50,50)$ as a function of time using adapted meshes

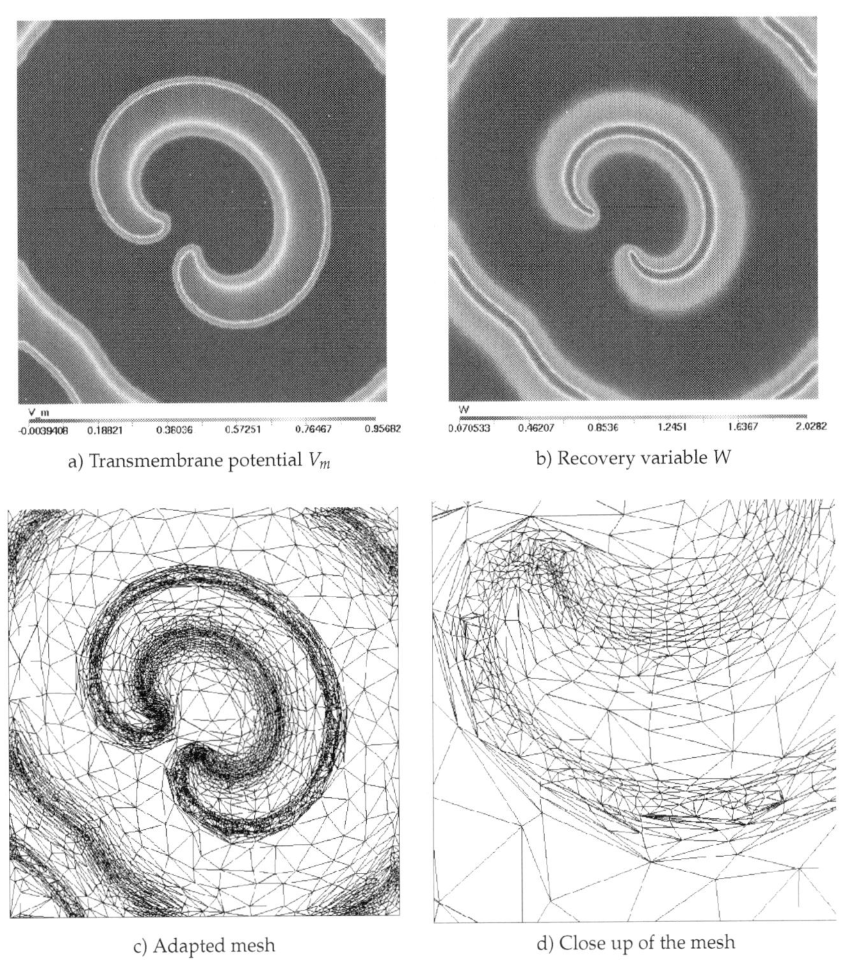

a) Transmembrane potential V_m

b) Recovery variable W

c) Adapted mesh

d) Close up of the mesh

Fig. 2. Numerical Solutions using adapted meshes: monodomain model case

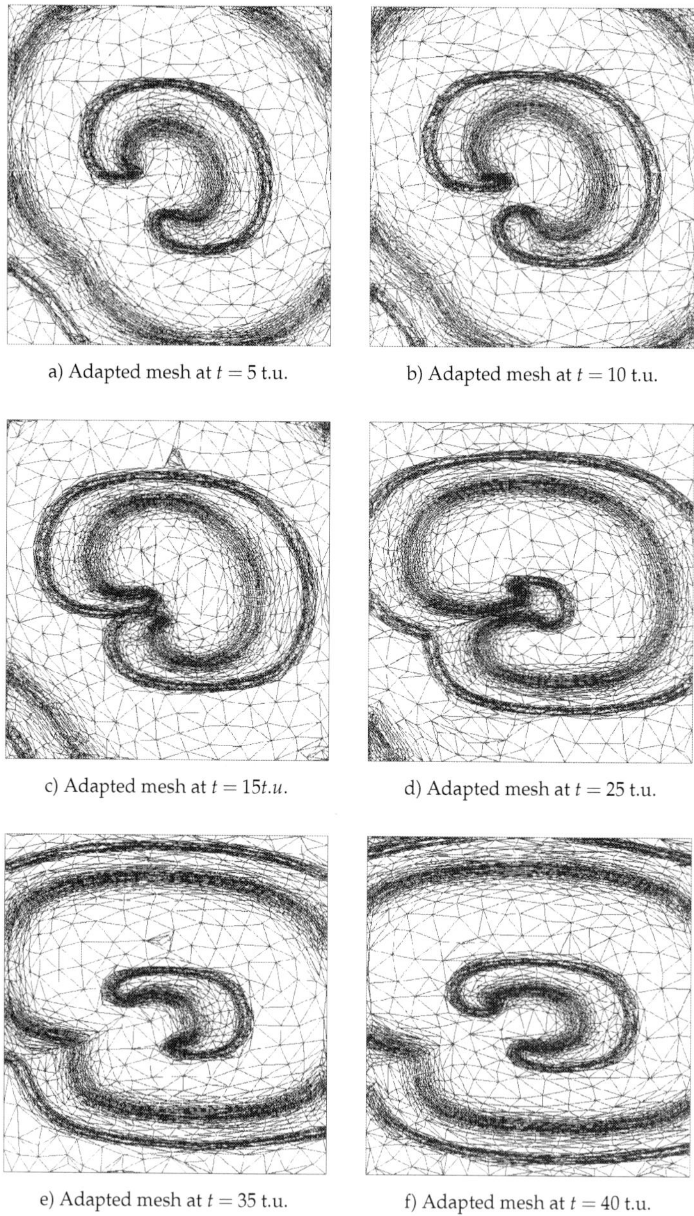

a) Adapted mesh at $t = 5$ t.u.

b) Adapted mesh at $t = 10$ t.u.

c) Adapted mesh at $t = 15t.u.$

d) Adapted mesh at $t = 25$ t.u.

e) Adapted mesh at $t = 35$ t.u.

f) Adapted mesh at $t = 40$ t.u.

Fig. 3. Mesh evolution using the bidomain model

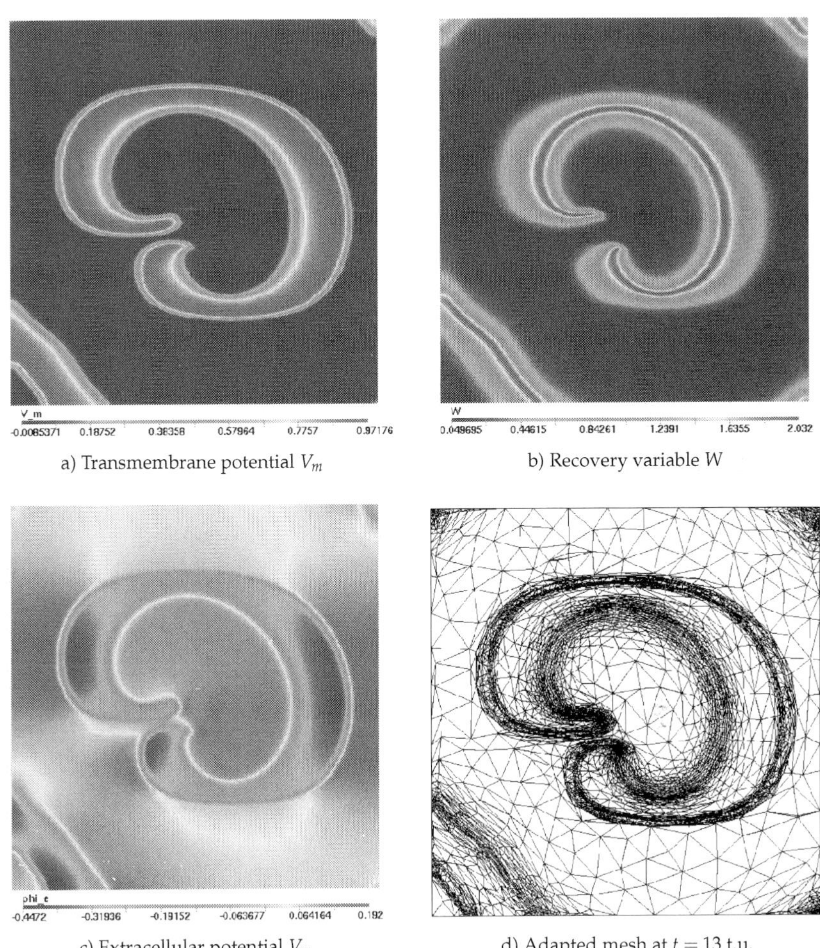

a) Transmembrane potential V_m b) Recovery variable W

c) Extracellular potential V_m d) Adapted mesh at $t = 13$ t.u.

Fig. 4. Numerical Solutions using adapted meshes: bidomain model case

9

Information Fusion in a High Dimensional Feature Space for Robust Computer Aided Diagnosis using Digital Mammograms

Saurabh Prasad, Lori M. Bruce and John E. Ball
Geosystems Research Institute
Department of Electrical and Computer Engineering
Mississippi State University
U.S.A.

1. Introduction

Most end-to-end Computer Aided Diagnosis (CAD) systems follow a three step approach – (1) Image enhancement and segmentation, (2) Feature extraction, and, (3) Classification. Although the current state-of-the-art in image enhancement and segmentation can now very accurately identify regions of interest for feature extraction, these methods typically result in very high dimensional feature spaces. Although high dimensional feature spaces can potentially provide more discrimination information for a more robust classification of images, they are typically a double-edge sword. They can adversely affect the performance of classification systems because a large feature space dimensionality necessitates a large training database to accurately model the statistics of class features (e.g. benign versus malignant classes). Further, high dimensional feature spaces affect the generalization capacity of the classification system – that is, when feature spaces are high dimensional, it is possible that the classifier can learn decision boundaries from the training data very accurately, but it's tolerance to slight variations in the statistics of test data will be poor. In other words, the system will potentially over-fit the decision boundaries to the training data. Although the extent of this reduction in generalization capacity of the classifier depends on the classification algorithm being employed, practically all classification algorithms are prone to this problem, also known as the Hughe's phenomenon in the pattern classification community.

Current state-of-the-art in mammography based CAD systems extract a wide-variety of features (for example, texture based features, shape features etc.) from the mammograms. The resulting feature spaces generated for classification are hence typically very high dimensional. To mitigate the ill-effects of high dimensionality and limited training data, most classification systems employ dimensionality reduction techniques. Algorithms such as Principal Components Analysis (PCA) and Linear Discriminant Analysis (LDA) are used in the pattern classification community for dimensionality reduction. They have their own limitations – PCA is not optimal for classification tasks [Prasad *et al*, October 2008], since it is only designed to reduce features, not optimize them for classification, and LDA requires sufficient training data to be available for learning the projections. Stepwise Linear Discriminant Analysis (S-LDA) is a more popular technique that reduces the dimensionality of the feature space by selecting a smaller subset of features from the original feature space, and then further reduces the dimensionality of this subset by an optimizing linear transformation based on the LDA algorithm. One key limitation of this approach is that it is by design sub-optimal at best, because it does not utilize all available features for estimating the final "optimizing" transformation.

In this chapter, we present a robust multi-classifier decision fusion framework that employs a divide-and-conquer approach for alleviating the affects of high dimensionality of feature vectors extracted from digital mammograms. After appropriate pre-processing of the digital mammograms (including contrast enhancement), the core region of interest is segmented, and various features are extracted from the segmented images (including morphological features, statistical features, texture features, etc.). The resulting high dimensional feature space is partitioned into multiple smaller sized subspaces, and a bank of classifiers (a multi-classifier system) is employed to perform feature optimization and classification in each partition separately. Finally, a decision fusion system merges decisions from each classifier in the bank into a single decision. Unlike previous approaches which discard potentially useful features for alleviating the over-dimensionality problem, the proposed method employs all available features for classification. The performance of the resulting CAD system is reported using overall classification accuracy, specificity and sensitivity. Results show that the proposed system results in significantly better classification performance as compared to previously employed techniques.

The outline of this chapter is as follows. In section 2, we provide an overview of mammography based CAD systems, and on common image processing methods employed in such systems. We also provide a description of the feature extraction and optimization method employed in this work, as well as conventional classification approaches and the proposed classification framework. In section 3, we present experimental results demonstrating the benefits of the proposed system, and conclude this chapter with a summary of results and future directions.

2. Computer Aided Diagnosis using Digital Mammography

Digital mammography uses x-rays to project structures in the 3D female breast onto a 2D image [Egan, 1988]. The primary use for digital mammography is for screening for breast cancer. According to the American Cancer Society (ACS), breast cancer is the leading type of cancer in women and the second most fatal type of cancer in women [ACS, 2005].

2.1 Importance of Mammography

Mammography is important for many reasons. First, early detection can increase survival rates [Rangayan, 2005] and decrease the probability that cancer cells are able to infiltrate other parts of the body [Voegeli, 1989]. The survival rate of breast-cancer patients is inversely related to the tumor size and to the number of auxiliary lymph nodes that are found with malignant cells [Lille, 1992]. Mammography can detect cancer years before physical symptoms occur [Tabar *et al*, 2001]. Often, early detection finds a minimal cancer, and the cure rate approaches 95 percent [Egan, 1991].

2.2 Challenges in Digital-Mammography Image Analysis

Digital-mammographic analysis is a very difficult problem because of the complexity of digital mammograms, poor contrast, and in many cases, a lack of a clearly defined mass border [Hughes, 1968]. First, a digital mammogram is a 2D image of a 3D and highly complex structure. Due to the complex 3D nature of breasts and the view used when taking the mammogram, some tumors may be partially obscured. Second, it is well-known that digital mammograms often have poor contrast, especially in dense breasts [Egan, 1988]. Many specialized methods have been developed to denoise and enhance digital mammographic images. Third, according to Egan, there is a wide variability in the appearance of mammograms of different patients [Egan, 1988]. Adipose tissue has a higher concentration of low-atomic-number elements, such as hydrogen and carbon, and therefore low-energy x-rays are attenuated less in adipose tissue than other tissues. The amount of adipose tissue present in the breast is important, because it provides good contrast with other structures in the breast [Egan, 1988]. Furthermore, the size of malignant lesions that can be detected depends on the adipose content of the breasts, and breasts with more fat provide the ability to detect smaller tumors than breasts with a paucity of fat [Egan, 1988]. Fourth, cancerous masses often have a similar appearance to some benign masses, or even normal fibroglandular breast tissue [Peters *et al*, 1989], and many masses have irregular or obscured borders [Egan, 1988], [Tabar *et al*, 1985]. Furthermore, most masses do not fit a distinct border type, but have mixtures of border types [Egan, 1988], [Peters *et al*, 1989]. Mass borders are a primary method radiologists use to identify benign versus malignant masses [Ball, May 2007].

2.3 Conventional Computer-Aided-Diagnosis (CAD) Systems

Many digital mammography CAD systems have been previously developed, both as experimental models in academia, and marketed and FDA-approved products for breast-cancer detection. CAD systems serve a variety of purposes, including: (1) providing a prompting system for radiologists to help them locate suspicious areas in the mammogram, (2) providing a second opinion, by analyzing the mammogram and deciding if a mass is malignant or benign, and (3) providing mammographic image enhancement, where digital mammograms can be enhanced for noise removal or to provide better contrast with the overall goal to allow better radiologist interpretation.

Qian *et al* [Qian *et al*, October 1995] and Huo *et al* [Huo *et al*, 2002] show that radiologists can benefit from the aid of CAD systems. Sahiner *et al* demonstrated that a good CAD system is comparable to expert radiologists [Sahiner *et al*, December 2001]. Burhenne *et al* show that CAD can potentially reduce radiologists' false negative rate, which is the rate at which a radiologist falsely detects a malignant mass as benign [Burhenne *et al*, 2000].

2.4 Database Description

For this study, a subset of the DDSM database consisting of 60 test cases is selected. This data subset contains 30 benign and 30 malignant cases, where 17 of the 30 malignant cases are spiculated, and none of the benign cases are spiculated. Table lists the benign and malignant cases in the study dataset.

Benign Cases	Malignant Cases
1305, 1370, 1371, 1372, 1379, 1387, 1389, 1394, 1397, 1408, 1432, 1442, 1443, 1445, 1447, 1453, 1459, 1498, 1512, 1518, 1519, 1554, 1556, 1560, 1566, 1607, 1615, 1679, 1682, 1691	1112, 1132, 1134, 1144, 1147, 1149, 1155, 1156, 1157, 1163, 1168, 1171, 1182, 1215, 1237, 1252, 1262, 1263, 1404, 1468, 1533, 1534, 1537, 1558, 1574, 1622, 1665, 1726, 1827, 1999

Table 1. Listing of case numbers for the DDSM database

Examination of figures 1 – 4 shows that the DDSM-database cases chosen comprise a relatively difficult database in terms of preprocessing, segmentation, and classification. Fig. 1 shows the ACR density-rating distribution for the test dataset. The ratings are assigned by radiologists who worked on the DDSM database [Heath *et al*, 1998]. The density rating is an integer from one to four, where a density rating of one is the least dense, and a density rating of four is the densest. In general, the higher the density rating, the more difficult segmentation may be because of increased paucity of adipose tissue, which provides mammographic contrast. Fig. 1 shows that most of the malignant tumors have density values two and three, while the benign tumors have density three and four. Also, there are mammograms for each density category, from one to four. Therefore, density is probably not a good feature for distinguishing malignant from benign cases. Fig. 2 shows the ACR Bi–RADS assessment distribution. This figure indicates that this dataset is a difficult one, since a large number of the benign cases appear in category 3. Figure 3 shows the subtlety-ratings distribution [Heath *et al*, 1998]. A subtlety rating of one indicates least subtle, while a rating of five is the most subtle. Please note that this subtlety-rating system is unique to the DDSM database, and is different from other subtlety-rating systems used in digital mammography. A case with a DDSM subtlety rating of N is N times more subtle than a case with a subtlety rating of one. There are 4 benign and 15 malignant mammograms whose subtlety is 5 (the most subtle). There are 24 out of 30 benign cases and 27 out of 30 malignant cases which have a subtlety rating from 3 to 5, as shown in Figure 3. This figure shows the database is difficult.

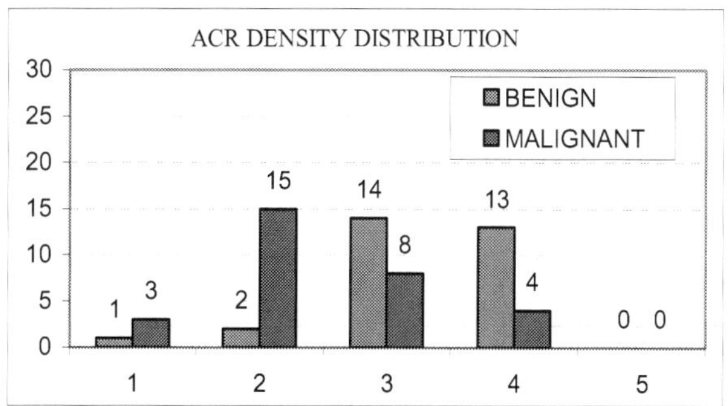

Fig. 1. Case study breast density distributions. The least dense is 1 and the most is dense is 5.

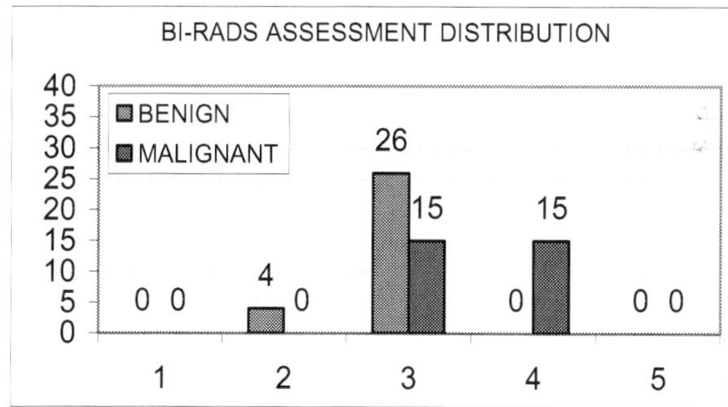

Fig. 2. Case study Bi-RADS assessment category distribution

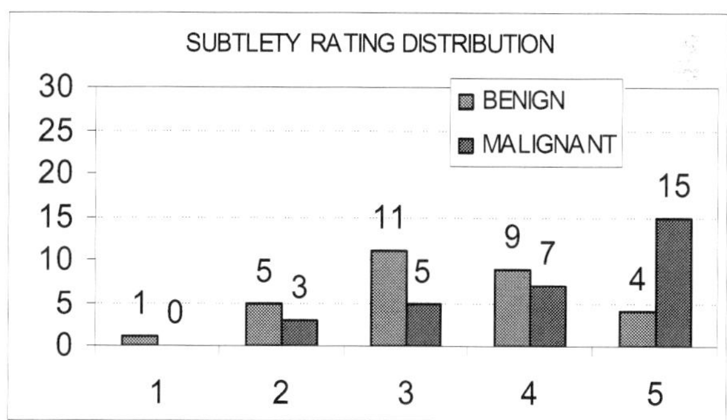

Fig. 3. Case study DDSM subtlety rating distribution. Ratings range from 1 (least subtle) to 5 (most subtle).

It is well-known that mass shape plays a very immportant factor in mammographic analysis. Fig. 4 shows the shape distribution. The shape keywords are defined in Table . The shapes are assessed by experienced radiologists. As expected, almost all irregularly shaped masses are malignant, while oval and round shapes are benign.

Keyword	Meaning	Keyword	Meaning
Oval	Shaped like an oval.	Lobulated	Shaped like breast lobes.
Irregular	Irregular shape.	Round	Circularly shaped.

Table 2. Shape keywords and their meanings

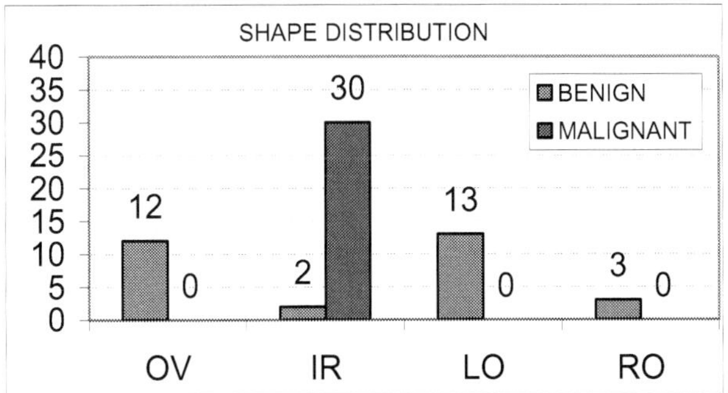

Fig. 4. Case study shape distribution. Legend: OV= Oval, IR = Irregular, LO = Lobulated, RO = Round.

2.5 Image Processing – Enhancement and Segmentation

The Catarious segmentation method (CSM) is implemented as described in [Catarious, June 2004], [Catarious, August 2004]. The original mammogram is passed through an unsharp-masking filter. The algorithm uses the DDSM supplied Region of Interest (ROI) containing a suspicious region and creates a new, square ROI sized approximately 112.6 mm^2 (245^2 pixels) centered around the seed point. The interior pixels of the square ROI are then extracted from the unsharp masked image. A circular region of radius 16 mm is selected as the initial segmentation, where interior pixels are segmented, and pixels outside of the circle are considered outside of the segmentation. Fisher's LDA (FLDA) is used to select a graylevel threshold for selection of the new boundary, which is the connected region containing the ROI centroid. Boundary constraints are applied according to the Catarious algorithm, such as interior pixels on each ray emanating from the center must not have gaps of more than d pixels, and border pixels must be within a specified city-block distance n of their immediate neighbors. This analysis is performed in the polar transform. If the stopping criterion (the boundary does not change from the previous iteration) is met, then the segmentation stops; otherwise, a new iteration is performed. It is discovered that the CSM could get in a loop wherein there will not be a state during which the segmentation does not change, and no proof of convergence is given in [Catarious, June 2004], [Catarious, August 2004]. Thus, a 40-iteration limit is added to the segmentation method. For the segmentation stage, n=2, d=3, and the unsharp-masking weighting is 0.9, which are the original parameters proposed in [Catarious, June 2004], [Catarious, August 2004]. The CSM system performed very well on Catarious' database, which is why this method was chosen as a comparison method. It provided a "successful" segmentation method against which to compare the proposed method, and also had a straightforward implementation. More details about this segmentation technique can be found in [Catarious, June 2004], [Catarious, August 2004].

2.6 Feature Extraction

This section discusses the various types of features which are typically used in mammography analysis [Ball, May 2007]. The type of features include patient information, statistical features from the pixel graylevel values, textural features, normalized radial-length (NRL) feature, based on the segmentation boundary, and morphological features based on the size and shape of the segmentation.

Patient-Information Features

It is well-known that age is the most important feature in mammographic analysis [Laws, January 1980 a], [Laws, January 1980 b]. Therefore, in this study, age will be included as a feature. The other patient information described in the previous sections will not be used in this dissertation's study.

Statistical Features

Statistical features are derived from the segmentation boundary or an extension of the segmentation boundary. The statistical features are graylevel mean value, graylevel standard deviation, and graylevel standard-deviation ratio. The standard-deviation ratio is the ratio of the graylevel standard deviation in a region from one to 200 pixels outside of the segmentation boundary to the standard deviation of pixels inside the segmentation boundary.

Textural Features

Textural features can capture important characteristics of a small area, and thus may be beneficial in image segmentation. The textural features include graylevel co-occurrence-matrix (GLCM) features derived from the RBST image, GLCM features extracted from the segmentation boundary, and Laws texture features [Ball, May 2007]. The GLCM textural features include energy, variance, correlation, inertia, inverse difference moment, and entropy [Laws, January 1980 a], [Laws, January 1980 b]. The Laws texture features include features derived from 2D Laws texture kernels. Each of these is explained in detail below.

GLCM Textural Features

In order to calculate the GLCM texture features efficiently, the image is first quantized using N bins, resulting in a quantized image whose pixel values elements are in $\{0, \cdots, N-1\}$. In this dissertation, the value for the number of quantized bins is set to N=20. Distances, d, and direction angles, θ, are selected and the associated relative-frequency matrix $P = [P_{i,j}]$ is calculated, where i and j are the pixel intensities. Following [Laws, January 1980 a], [Laws,

January 1980 b], the following equations are used to calculate the P matrix values for the distance d and the angles $\theta \in \{0°, 45°, 90°, 135°\}$:

$$P(i, j, d, 0°) = \left\{ \begin{array}{c} ((k,l),(m,n)) \in I \\ \forall \, |k - m| = 0, \; |l - n| = d \\ I(k,l) = i, \, I(m,n) = j \end{array} \right\} \tag{1}$$

$$P(i, j, d, 45°) = \left\{ \begin{array}{c} ((k,l),(m,n)) \in I \\ \forall (k - m = d, l - n = -d) \, or \, (k - m = -d, l - n = d) \\ I(k,l) = i, \, I(m,n) = j \end{array} \right\} \tag{2}$$

$$P(i, j, d, 90°) = \left\{ \begin{array}{c} ((k,l),(m,n)) \in I \\ \forall \, |k - m| = d, \; |l - n| = 0 \\ I(k,l) = i, \, I(m,n) = j \end{array} \right\} \tag{3}$$

$$P(i, j, d, 135°) = \left\{ \begin{array}{c} ((k,l),(m,n)) \in I \\ \forall (k - m = d, l - n = d) \, or \, (k - m = -d, l - n = -d) \\ I(k,l) = i, \, I(m,n) = j \end{array} \right\} \tag{4}$$

where {} denotes the number of elements that satisfy the conditions in {}, and the pixel coordinates of image I are (k,l) and (m,n).

The GLCM matrices are created from these matrices by normalizing the matrices. The matrices are normalized by dividing by R_θ for a given angle θ. That is,

$$P_{i,j} = \frac{P_{i,j}}{R_\theta}. \tag{5}$$

The values used for R_θ are given in Table 3, where n_x and n_y are the number of columns and the number of rows, respectively, in the image, and d is the user specified distance.

θ in degrees	R_θ
$0°$	$2(n_x - d)n_y$
$45°, 135°$	$2(n_x - d)(n_y - d)$
$90°$	$2n_x(n_y - d)$

Table 3. Normalizing values

Several of the GLCM features require marginal probability mass functions (PMF). The marginal PMF's, p_x and p_y, are defined by the following formulas:

$$p_x = \sum_{j=1}^{N} P(i, j)/R,$$ (6)

and

$$p_y = \sum_{i=1}^{N} P(i, j)/R,$$ (7)

where N is the number of graylevels in the quantized image, and R is the appropriate R_θ value.

The GLCM texture features are calculated as follows. The GLCM energy feature is a measure of the image uniformity. A region with little graylevel change will have a low-energy value,

$$f_{ENERGY} = \sum_i \sum_j \left[p(i, j) \right]^2.$$ (8)

The GLCM variance is a measure of the spread of the elements in the matrix. The feature is calculated from

$$f_{VARIANCE} = \sum_i \sum_j (i - \mu)^2 p(i, j),$$ (9)

where μ is the mean value of the elements in p. The GLCM correlation measure quantifies the quantized graylevel linear dependence. The GLCM correlation is calculated from

$$f_{CORRELATION} = \frac{\sum_i \sum_j (ij)p(i, j) - \mu_x \mu_y}{\sigma_x \sigma_y},$$ (10)

where μ_x, μ_y, σ_x, and σ_y are the mean values and the standard deviations of the marginal probability matrices, p_x and p_y, respectively. The entropy feature is defined as

$$f_{ENTROPY} = -\sum_i \sum_j p(i,j) \log\{p(i,j)\},\qquad(11)$$

with the convention that $\log(0) = 0$. Entropy defines a measure of randomness, and a very uniform area will have very low entropy.

Laws Textural Features
Laws [Laws, January 1980 a], [Laws, January 1980 b] developed a set of one-dimensional (1D) and 2D kernels which are designed to extract small-scale textural information from images. The 1D Laws kernels are given by

$$
\begin{aligned}
L5 &= [\ 1\ \ 4\ \ 6\ \ 4\ \ 1\ ] & E5 &= [\ \text{-}1\ \text{-}2\ \ 0\ \ 2\ \ 1\ ] \\
S5 &= [\ \text{-}1\ \ 0\ \ 2\ \ 0\ \text{-}1\ ] & W5 &= [\ \text{-}1\ \ 2\ \ 0\ \text{-}2\ \ 1\ ] \\
R5 &= [\ 1\ \text{-}4\ \ 6\ \text{-}4\ \ 1\ ]
\end{aligned}
\qquad(12)
$$

where the first letter stands for Level, Edge, Spot, Wave, and Ripple, respectively [Laws, January 1980 a], [Laws, January 1980 b]. The 2D Laws textures are sized $[5 \times 5]$, and are created by multiplying the 1D Laws kernel as a row vector by the second kernel as a column vector. Since there are five 1D Laws kernels, there will be 25 2D kernels. As an example, the L5L5 kernel is given by

$$
L5L5 = \begin{bmatrix}
1 & 4 & 6 & 4 & 1 \\
4 & 16 & 24 & 16 & 4 \\
6 & 24 & 36 & 24 & 6 \\
4 & 16 & 24 & 16 & 4 \\
1 & 4 & 6 & 4 & 1
\end{bmatrix},
\qquad(13)
$$

To create the Laws texture features, an image is convolved with each of the Laws 2D kernels. Each image is then normalized by dividing pixel-by-pixel with the $L5L5$ image, and is termed I_m for each Laws texture kernel $m \in \{1,2,\cdots,25\}$. For each Laws texture and each pixel in the convolved image, the following equation is used to calculate the texture for that pixel for the m-th texture:

$$L_m(x,y) = \sum_{j=-D}^{D} \sum_{k=-D}^{D} I_m(x+j, y+k),\qquad(14)$$

where the texture mask size is (2D+1) by (2D+1). As suggested by Laws [Laws, January 1980 a], the variable D is selected as 7, thus equation **Error! Reference source not found.** uses a $[15 \times 15]$, region centered at each pixel for analysis. Note that some applications take the absolute value before summing in this formula.

Morphological Features

Morphological features are derived from the shape characteristics of the segmented region. These features include the area, axis ratio, box ratio, circularity, convex-hull area, eccentricity, equivalent diameter, extent, extent ratio, major-axis length, minor-axis length, perimeter length, solidity, and width-to-height ratio.

The area is the number of pixels in the segmented region. The axis ratio is the ratio of the major-axis length to the minor-axis length. The box ratio is the ratio of the area to the product of the height times the width, where the height and width are defined by the bounding box of the region. Circularity is defined as the product of 4π times the region area divided by the square of the perimeter length in pixels. The convex-hull area is the size of the convex hull of the region, where the convex hull H of an arbitrary set S is the smallest convex set containing S. The equivalent diameter is defined as the diameter of a circle which has the same area as the segmented region. The extent feature is calculated as the area divided by the bounding-box area. The extent ratio is defined as max(*height, width*) / min(*height, width*). The major- and minor-axis lengths are defined as the length in pixels of the major and minor axes of the ellipse that has the same normalized second central moments as the region, respectively. The perimeter length is the number of pixels on the region perimeter. The solidity feature is defined as the region area divided by the convex-hull area. The width-to-height ratio is defined as *width* / *height*.

Normalized Radial-Length (NRL) Features

The normalized radial-length (NRL) features are derived from a normalized version of the radial-length measure [Agatheeswaran, December 2004]. First, the border pixels of the segmentation are extracted and the centroid of the segmentation region, (c_x, c_y), is calculated. Assume there are N_B border pixels and that the coordinate of the k-th border pixel is (x_k, y_k). For each border pixel, the Euclidean distance between the pixel and the centroid is calculated as $D_k = \sqrt{(x_k - c_x)^2 + (y_k - c_y)^2}$. The largest distance, D_{MAX}, is calculated, and the normalized distance is calculated by dividing the pixel Euclidean distance by the maximum distance: $NRL_k = D_k / D_{MAX}$. Table 4 summarizes the NRL features, and was adapted from [Agatheeswaran, December 2004].

Feature	Description
Entropy	A measure of the randomness of the NRL vector values. $$f_{NRL\_ENTROPY} = -\sum_{j=1}^{N_B} p_j \log_2(p_j),$$ where $\log_2(0) = 0$ and p_j is the PMF of NRL values. This PDF is estimated with a 256 bin histogram.
Length	The length of the NRL distance vector. $$f_{NRL\_LENGTH} = N_B$$
Mean	The mean value of the NRL distances. $$f_{NRL\_MEAN} = -\frac{1}{N_B}\sum_{k=1}^{N_B} NRL_k$$
Roughness	A measure of border roughness. $$f_{NRL\_MEAN} = \left[\frac{L}{N_B}\right]\sum_{j=1}^{[N_B/L]} R_j$$ where the roughness parameter R_j is given by $$R_j = \sum_{i=j}^{L+j} \left| NRL_i - NRL_{i+1} \right| \text{ with } j \in \{1, \cdots, [N_B/L]\}.$$
Standard deviation	The standard deviation of the NRL vector. $$f_{STD\_NRL} = \frac{1}{N_B-1}\sum_{j=1}^{N_B}\left[NRL_k - f_{NRL\_MEAN}\right]^2$$ Note: Some of the literature uses a biased definition for this feature, i.e. they divide by N_B and not by N_B-1. This analysis uses the unbiased estimator.
Zero crossing count	The number of times the NRL distance crosses over the NRL mean.

Table 4. NRL feature descriptions

Source: Adapted from [Agatheeswaran, December 2004].

Feature Type and source [1]	Features	Num. Features[4,5]	References
Patient age (DDSM)	Patient Age	1	[Heath *et al*, 1998]
Morphological (SB)	Area, Axis ratio, Box ratio, Circularity, Convex hull area, Eccentricity, Equivalent diameter, Extent, Extent ratio[2], Major axis length, Minor axis length, Perimeter length, Solidity, Width to height ratio	14	[Catarious, June 2004], [Catarious, August 2004]
Statistical (SB)	Graylevel mean, Graylevel std. dev, Graylevel std. dev. ratio[3]	3	[Cheng et al, August 2004]
NRL (SB)	Entropy, Length, Mean, Roughness, Std. dev., Zero crossing count	6	[Cheng et al, August 2004]
GLCM (SB)	(Note [4]) Energy, Variance, Correlation, Inertia, Inverse Difference Moment, Entropy	144	[Haralick *et al*, 1973], [Agatheeswaran, December 2004], [Cheng et al, August 2004]
GLCM (RBST)	(Note [5]) Energy, Variance, Correlation, Inertia, Inverse Difference Moment, Entropy	864	[Sahiner *et al*, April 1998], [Haralick *et al*, 1973], [Agatheeswaran, December 2004], [Cheng et al, August 2004]

Table 5. Feature list

Notes:

[1] This denotes the region from which the features were extracted. DDSM=DDSM database (there is no region, as the patient age is part of the database). SB=segmentation boundary. NRL stands for Normalized Radial Length. RBST=Rubber Band Straightening Transform. GLCM stands for gray level co-occurrence matrix. GLCM is also known as spatial gray level dependence (SGLD). [2] The extent ratio is max(length, height) / min(length, height). [3] the Gray level std. dev. ratio is the ratio of the std. dev. of the gray levels inside the segmentation to the std. dev. of gray levels outside the segmentation boundary and within 200 pixels of the segmentation boundary. [4] The GLCM SB features are calculated at distances $d=\{1,2,4,6,8,10\}$ and directions $\theta=\{0°,45°,90°,135°\}$. There will be a total of 6 GLCM features x 6 distances x 4 angles for 144 GLCM features. [5] The RBST features are the same features as the GLCM SB features. The RBST uses a parameter k to choose how many pixels before and after are used to create the normal vector to the spiculation boundary. The RBST features are calculated for distances $k=\{2,4,6,8,10,12\}$ For each value of k, there will be 144 features generated, thus there are 864 = 144 x 6 RBST features.

2.7 Feature Optimization and Statistical Pattern Classification

Conventional mammography based CAD systems employ a single classifier system to classify and label mammograms as either malignant or benign. This is typically preceeded by a feature reduction and optimization step, in an attempt to reduce the size of training data required to model the feature spaces, and to improve classification performance and generalization ability (ability to account for variability in statistics of training and testing data) of the classifier. Some common feature optimization techniques include PCA, LDA and S-LDA. These optimization techniques are at best sub-optimal. Recently, a mathematical argument was presented [Prasad *et al*, October 2008] showing that in many situations, a PCA projection can reduce the class separation in the projected space, thereby deteriorating the classification performance.

Stepwise Linear Discriminant Analysis (S-LDA)

LDA and it's variants are preferred linear feature optimization strategies, but when operating in high dimensional feature spaces, LDA can potentially fail if the amount of available training data is insufficient to estimate the within and between class scatter matrices. S-LDA employs a forward selection, backward rejection procedure to select a very small subset of features, upon which LDA is performed for feature optimization. Hence, by definition, it is sub-optimal, since it does not include a majority of the features for feature optimization. Since S-LDA will be used as a baseline feature optimization strategy, a brief description of S-LDA follows.

Stepwise linear discriminant analysis is a version of LDA which is a compromise for a full search of the feature space. In systems with a large feature vector size, an exhaustive search for the optimal solution is generally not feasible. Stepwise LDA (SLDA) with forward selection and backward rejection can be used for feature optimization. SLDA requires a discrimination metric to decide which features are better-suited to the given task, such as separating two different tumor types in medical imagery. Commonly used methods include receiver operating characteristics (ROC) area under the curve [Ball, May 2007], which is known as A_Z, Bhattacharyya Distance (BD), and Jeffries-Matusita distance (JMD).

In this work, A_Z is used as the discrimination metric, but theoretically, any appropriate metric could be used. The forward-selection procedure starts by calculating A_Z values for each feature separately, using one class as the target and all others as the non-target. The A_Z values are sorted in descending order. The feature with the highest A_Z value gets placed into a feature vector, and the ROC area, A_{Z_BEST}, is set to A_{Z1}. The second-best feature is then appended to the feature vector and A_{Z2} is computed. The second-best feature is only retained if $A_{Z2} > A_{Z\_BEST}$. In this case, A_{Z_BEST} is set to A_{Z2}. The third-best feature is then appended to the feature vector and A_{Z3} is computed. The third best feature is only retained if $A_{Z3} > A_{Z\_BEST}$. This process is continued until all the individual features are examined, or until the maximum number of features allowed is reached. The maximum number of the resulting features is determined by the minimum number of training signatures for a class. As a rule of thumb, for every five to ten training signatures, one feature can be added. Therefore, to keep five to ten features, there needs to be at least 25 to 50 training signatures for each class.

Next, backwards rejection is performed. Assume at this stage that there are b best features selected in the feature vector, and the best ROC area is A_{Z_BEST}. If $b = 1$, then no features may be removed, and the process halts. If $b > 1$, then the first feature is removed, and the ROC area A_{Z1}' is calculated. If $A_{Z1}' > A_{Z\_BEST}$, then the first feature is removed, and A_{Z_BEST} is set to A_{Z1}'. This process continues until all features have been removed and the ROC area has been recalculated. At the end of the procedure, there is a feature vector which contains the set of best features, the best A_Z value found, and the weighting coefficients.

The advantage of using SLDA is that it can produce very good results, even when individual features may not have very high A_Z values. Disadvantages of SLDA are (1) an exhaustive search is not performed, (2) a large percentage of (potentially useful) features are discarded and not considered for the classification task, and, (3) features near the end of the feature vector with tie scores to features earlier in the vector may not be chosen.

The Multi-Classifier Decision Fusion (MCDF) Framework

In recent work, Prasad *et al* [Prasad *et al*, May 2008] proposed a new divide-and-conquer paradigm for classification in high-dimensional feature spaces as pertaining to hyperspectral classification in remote sensing tasks. In this chapter, we show that this framework can be extended to other high dimensional feature spaces (features extracted from mammograms in this case), for robust classification, even when the amount of training data available is insufficient to model statistics of the classes in the high-dimensional feature space.

Figure 5 illustrates the proposed divide-and-conquer framework for mammogram classification. The algorithm is as follows. Find a suitable partition of the feature space, i.e., identify appropriate subspaces (each of a much smaller dimension). Perform "local" classification in each subspace. Finally, employ a suitable decision fusion scheme to merge the local decisions into a final malignant/benign decision per mammogram image. In our work with hyperspectral imagery, we found that the correlation structure of the feature space was approximately block-diagonal. This permitted the use of a correlation or mutual

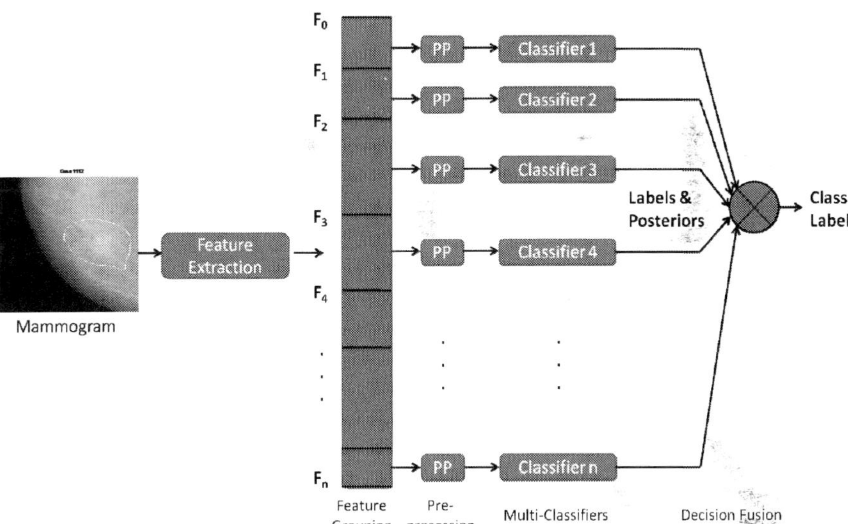

Fig. 5. The proposed MCDF framework. Training data is employed to learn an appropriate feature grouping, feature pre-processing (optimization) and class-conditional statistics. To classify mammograms as malignant/benign, the feature extraction, feature grouping and pre-processing is followed by independent classification. Each class label/posterior proabability is then combined using a decision fusion mechanism.

information based metric in the partitioning of the corresponding feature space into multiple contiguous subspaces [Prasad *et al*, May 2008]. However, unlike hyperspectral data, where the feature space comprises of reflectance values over a continuum of wavelengths, features extracted from mammogram images typically do not possess a standard correlation structure to them. This is primarily because these features are created by concatenating various different kinds of quantities, such as morphological characteristics, texture information, patient history etc. Hence, in an attempt to define a suitable partition of the feature space derived from mammogram images, we break up the feature space into small groups, each comprised of m adjacent features, where m is a small integer valued number, determined experimentally. In previous work, Ball [Ball, May 2007] found that when doing a forward selection and backward rejection of mammography features, patient age was always selected as an important feature in the final feature selection. Hence, in this work, patient age was injected into each partition/subspace generated above to strengthen each local classifier.

Since each subspace is of a much smaller dimensionality than the dimension of the original feature space, a suitable preprocessing (such as LDA) may prove beneficial before making the local classification decisions. After creating multiple subspaces as described above, an LDA based pre-processing is performed in each subspace. The benefits of LDA based pre-processing are well known and documented in the pattern classification literature [Fukunaga, 1990]. Employing LDA in the proposed setup indeed further strengthens each classifier by improving class separation in the LDA projected space. Since the dimension of each subspace is small as compared to that of the original feature space, LDA based dimensionality reduction at the local subspace level is going to be well conditioned, even when a single LDA projection over the original feature space is ill conditioned. After LDA based pre-processing, a classifier is allocated to each subspace. The multi-classifier system is hence essentially a bank of classifiers that make "local" decisions in the partitioned subspaces. These can be parametric classifiers such as maximum likelihood classifiers, or non parametric classifiers such as k nearest neighbors classifiers, neural network based classifiers etc. In this work, we use quadratic maximum likelihood classifiers [Fukunaga, 1990]. These classifiers assume Gaussian class distributions for the i'th class, $p(x/w_i) \sim N(\mu_i, \Sigma_i)$. Assuming equal priors, the class membership function for such a classifier is given by

$$p(w_i \mid x) = -\frac{1}{2}(x - \mu_i)^T \Sigma_i^{-1}(x - \mu_i) - \frac{1}{2}\ln|\Sigma_i|. \qquad (15)$$

Here, w_i is the class label, x is the feature vector in the subspace, μ_i and Σ_i are the mean vector and covariance matrix of the i'th class respectively. Local classification decisions from each subspace are finally merged (fused) into a single class label (malignant or benign) per mammogram using an appropriate decision fusion rule. Decision fusion can occur either at the class label level (hard fusion), or at the posterior probability level (soft fusion). We test our system with decision fusion at both of these levels.

In hard decision fusion, we arrive at a final classification decision based on a vote over individual class labels (hard decisions) from each subspace. Unlike soft fusion based techniques, the overall classification of majority voting (MV) based fusion is not very sensitive to inaccurate estimates of posterior probabilities. However, in situations where posterior probabilities can be accurately estimated, soft fusion methods are likely to provide stable and accurate classification. A form of majority voting that incorporates a non uniform weight assignment [Prasad *et al*, May 2008] is given by:

$$w = \arg\max_{i \in \{1,2...C\}} N(i)$$

$$\text{where, } N(i) = \sum_{j=1}^{n} \alpha_j I(w_j = i) \tag{16}$$

where α_j is the confidence score / weight (e.g., training accuracies) for the j'th classifier, I is the indicator function, w is the class label from one of the C possible classes for the test pixel, j is the classifier index, n is the number of subspaces / classifiers, and $N(i)$ is the number of times class i was detected in the bank of classifiers. A popular soft decision fusion strategy – the Linear Opinion Pool (LOP) uses the individual posterior probabilities of each classifier (j = 1, 2,... n), $p_j(w_i/x)$ to estimate a global class membership function:

$$C(w_i \mid x) = \sum_{j=1}^{n} \alpha_j p_j(w_i \mid x)$$

$$w = \arg\max_{i \in \{1,2...C\}} C(w_i \mid x) \tag{17}$$

This is essentially a weighted average of posteriors across the classifier bank. In this work, uniform weights are assigned to decisions from the bank of classifiers, although, theoretically, non-uniform weight assignments can be made using "training accuracy assessment" [Prasad *et al*, May 2008].

In addition to resolving the over-dimensionality and small-sample-size problems, the MCDF framework provides another advantage – Irrespective of whether we use hard or soft decision fusion, it provides a natural framework to fuse information from different modalities (in this case, different types of physical features extracted from mammograms), and hence allows simultaneous exploitation of a diverse variety of information.

3. Experimental Setup and Classification Performance

Classification experiments were conducted in the proposed framework using the database described in section 2.4, using a leave-one-out (i.e. N-fold cross validation) testing methodology [Fukunaga, 1990] for unbiased accuracy estimates. Under this scheme, a mammogram is sequestered for testing, while the system (all sub-components, i.e., Multi-classifier system, LDA etc.) is trained on the features extracted from the remaining mammograms. This is repeated in a round-robin fashion until all mammograms have been employed for testing. After segmenting the region of interest, features were extracted for each mammogram. After this stage, the multi-classifier decision fusion framework takes over. This was repeated per iteration of the leave-one-out scheme.

Table 6 depicts the results from the experimental setup described above. Results from a conventional stepwise LDA, single classifier system are also included as baseline (for comparison). Performance of a binary classification in CAD applications is typically quantified by: (1) Overall accuracy - proportion of correctly identified malignant and benign cases, (2) Sensitivity -proportion of true positives (true malignant cases) identified correctly, and, (3) Specificity - proportion of true negatives (true benign cases) identified correctly. These numbers, expressed in percentage are provided in Table 6. The 95% Confidence interval in estimation of the overall accuracy is also reported, in order to account for the

Table 6. Classification performance of the proposed system with the DDSM dataset. OA: Overall Accuracy; CI: 95% Confidence Interval; SE: Sensitivity; SP: Specificity (all expressed in percentage); m: partition size

Stepwise LDA (Baseline)					MV based fusion (Proposed)				LOP based Fusion (Proposed)			
OA	CI	SE	SP	(m)	OA	CI	SE	SP	OA	CI	SE	SP
				2	85	3.8	87	83	85	3.8	87	83
				3	90	3.2	90	90	88	3.4	90	87
				4	85	3.8	83	87	85	3.8	83	87
82	4	80	83	5	80	4.2	77	83	82	4.1	80	83
				6	85	3.8	83	87	83	3.9	83	83
				7	82	4.1	80	83	82	4.1	80	83
				8	82	4.1	80	83	82	4.1	80	83
				15	78	4.4	73	83	78	4.4	73	83

finite sample size. Classification performance is studied over a range of values of m, the size of each partition in the multi-classifier framework.

For the baseline Stepwise LDA, single-classifier system, the overall accuracy, sensitivity, and specificity were 82%, 80%, and 83%, respectively. These values are all higher for the proposed multi-classifier, decision fusion system for small window sizes (e.g., feature subsets have dimensionality of 2,3,4), regardless of whether MV and LOP based decision fusion is utilized. This improvement is highest for $m = 3$, where the overall accuracy, sensitivity, and specificity were each 90% when MV based fusion is used. If m is increased, these performance metrics start to drop for the proposed system, and as m is increased to 15, the classification accuracy and sensitivity of the system eventually fall below that of the baseline system.

4. Conclusion

To conclude, the proposed multi-classifier, decision fusion system significantly outperforms the baseline single-classifier based system for small partition sizes (m). By employing the proposed system, the overall accuracy, sensitivity and specificity of the binary classification task improve by as much as 10%. Hence, the multi-classifier, decision fusion framework promises robust classification of mammographic masses even though the dimensionality of feature vectors extracted from these mammograms is very high. In this study, the multi-classifier decision fusion approach proves to be very promising and certainly warrants future study. The proposed information fusion based approach also provides a natural framework for integrating different physical characteristics derived from the mammogram images (e.g., combining morphological, textural and statistical information). Additional patient information, if available, can also be added to the feature stream without over-burdening the classification system. In future work, we will explore the benefits of a nonlinear pre-processing of the feature space and an adaptive weight assignment based decision fusion system within the proposed framework.

5. References

Agatheeswaran, A., *"Analysis of the effects of JPEG2000 compression on texture features extracted from digital mammograms"*. Masters Thesis in Electrical and Computer Engineering. Starkville, MS: Mississippi State University, pp. 20-37, 42-43, Dec. 2004.

Andolina, V.F., Lillé, S.L., and Willison, K.M., *Mammographic Imaging: A Practical Guide*. New York, NY: Lippincott Williams & Wilkins, 1992.

American Cancer Society, *"American Cancer Society: Breast Cancer Facts & Figures 2005-2006,"* pp. 1-28, 2006. Available: http://www.cancer.org/downloads/STT/CAFF2005BrF.pdf.

Ball, J. *Three Stage level Set Segmentation of Mass Core, Periphery, and Spiculations for Automated Image Analysis of Digital Mammograms*, Ph.D. in Electrical Engineering. Starkville, Mississippi: Mississippi State University, May 2007.

Burhenne, L. J. W., et. al., "Potential Contribution of 164 Computer-aided Detection to the Sensitivity of Screening Mammography," *Radiology*, vol. 215, no. 2, pp. 554-562, 2000.

Catarious, D. M., *"A Computer-Aided Detection System for Mammographic Masses."* Ph.D. Dissertation in Biomedical Engineering. Durham, NC: Duke University, Aug. 2004.

Catarious, D.M., Baydush, A.H., and Floyd, C.E., Jr., "Incorporation of an iterative, linear segmentation routine into a mammographic mass CAD system," *Medical Physics*, vol. 31, no. 6, pp. 1512-1520, Jun. 2004.

Cheng, H.D., et. al., "Approaches for automated detection and classification of masses in mammograms," *Pattern Recognition*, vol. 39, no. 4, pp. 646-668, Apr. 2006.

Egan, R.L., *Breast Imaging: Diagnosis and Morphology of Breast Diseases*. Philadelphia, PA: W. B. Saunders Co., 1988.

Egan, R., *"The new age of breast care,"* Administrative Radiology, p. 9, Sept. 1989.

Fukunaga, K., *Introduction to Statistical Pattern Recognition*, Academic Press, 1990.

Haralick, R. M., Dinstein, I., and Shanmugam, K., "Textural features for image classification," *IEEE Transactions on Systems, Man, and Cybernetics*, vol. SMC-3, pp. 610-621, Nov. 1973.

Heath, M., et. al., "Current status of the Digital Database for Screening Mammography," in *Digital Mammography*, N. Karssemeijer, M. Thijssen, J. Hendriks, and L. van Erning, Eds. Boston, MA: Kluwer Academic Publishers, pp. 457-460, 1998.

Hughes, G. *"On the mean accuracy of statistical pattern recognizers,"* IEEE Trans. on Information Theory, vol. 14, no. 1, pp. 55-63, 1968.

Huo, Z., Giger, M.L, Vyborny, C.J., and Metz, C.E., *"Breast Cancer: Effectiveness of Computer-aided Diagnosis – Observer Study with Independent Database of Mammograms,"* Radiology, vol. 224, no. 2, pp. 560-568, 2002.

Kundel H. L. and Dean, P.B., "Tumor Imaging," in *Image Processing Techniques for Tumor Detection*, R. N. Strickland, Ed. New York, NY: Marcel Dekker, Inc., pp. 1-18, 2002.

Laws, K., *"Textured Image Segmentation."* Ph.D. in Electrical Engineering. Los Angeles, CA: Image Processing Institute, University of Southern California, Jan. 1980 a.

Laws, K., "Rapid Texture Identification," *Proc. of the Image processing for missile guidance seminar*, San Diego, CA, pp. 376-380, Jan. 1980 b.

Lillé, S. L., "Background information and the need for screening," *in Mammographic Imaging: A Practical Guide*. New York, NY: Lippincott Williams & Wilkins, pp. 7-17, 1992.

Peters, M.E., Voegeli, D.R., and Scanlan, K.A., *Breast Imaging*. New York, NY: Churchhill Livingstone, 1989.

Prasad, S., Bruce, L. M., "Limitations of Principal Components Analysis for Hyperspectral Target Recognition," in *IEEE Geoscience and Remote Sensing Letters*, Vol. 5, Issue 4, pp 625-629, October 2008.

Prasad, S., Bruce, L. M., "Decision Fusion with Confidence based Weight Assignment for Hyperspectral Target Recognition," in *IEEE Transactions on Geoscience and Remote Sensing*, Vol. 46, No. 5, May 2008.

Qian, W., Clarke, L.P, Baoyu, Z., Kallergi, M. and Clark, R., "Computer assisted diagnosis for digital mammography," *IEEE Engineering in Medicine and Biology Magazine*, vol. 14, no. 5, pp. 561-569, Sep.-Oct. 1995.

Rangayyan, R. M., "The Nature of Biomedical Images," in *Biomedical Image Analysis*, M. R. Neuman, Ed. Boca Raton, FL: CRC Press, pp. 22-27, 2005.

Sahiner, B., Petrick, N., Heang-Ping, C., Hadjiiski, L.M., Paramagul, C., Helvie, M.A., and Gurcan, M.N., "Computer-aided characterization of mammographic masses: accuracy of mass segmentation and its effects on characterization," *IEEE Trans. on Medical Imaging*, vol. 20, no. 12, pp. 1275-1284, Dec. 2001.

Sahiner, B., Chan, H.-P., Petrick, N., Helvie, M.A., and Goodsitt, MM., "Computerized characterization of masses on mammograms: The rubber band straightening transform and texture analysis," *Medical Physics*, vol. 25, no. 4, pp. 516-526, Apr. 1998.

Tabár, L. and Dean, P.B., *Teaching Atlas of Mammography*, vol. 2nd revised ed. New York, NY: Georg Thieme Verlag, 1985.

Tabár, L., Vitak, B., Chen, H.-H.T., Yen, M.-F. , Duffy, S. W., and Smith, R.A., "*Beyond randomized controlled trials*," Cancer, vol. 91, no. 9, pp. 1724-1731, 2001.

Voegeli, D. R., "Mammographic Signs of Malignancy," in *Breast Imaging*, R. L. Eisenberg, Ed. New York, NY: Churchhill Livingstone, pp. 183-217, 1989.

Willison, K. M. "Breast anatomy and physiology," in *Mammographic Imaging: A Practical Guide New York*, NY: Lippincott Williams & Wilkins, pp. 119-161, 1992.

10

Computer-based diagnosis of pigmented skin lesions

Hitoshi Iyatomi
Hosei University, Faculty of Science and Engineering
Japan

1. Introduction – Malignant melanoma and dermoscopy

The incidence of malignant melanoma has increased gradually in most parts of the world. There is a report that the incidence of melanoma is now approaching 50 cases per 100,000 population in Australia (Stolz et al., 2002) and another report describes that a total of 62,480 incidence and 8,420 deaths are estimated in United States in 2008 (Jemal et al., 2008). Although advanced malignant melanoma is often incurable, early-stage melanoma can be cured in many cases, particularly before the metastasis phase. For example, patients with a melanoma less than or equal to 0.75 mm in thickness have a good prognosis and their five-year survival rate is greater than 93% (Meyskens et al., 1998). Therefore, early detection is crucial for the reduction of melanoma-related deaths. On the other hand, however, it is often difficult to distinguish between early-stage melanoma and Clark nevus, one of melanocytic pigmented skin lesion, with the naked eye, especially when small lesions are involved.
Dermoscopy, a non-invasive skin imaging technique, was introduced to improve accuracy in the diagnosis of melanoma (Soyer et al., 1987). It uses optical magnification and either liquid immersion and low angle-of-incidence lighting or cross-polarized lighting to make the contact area translucent, making subsurface structures more easily visible when compared to conventional macroscopic (clinical) images (Tanaka, 2006). Fig 1 shows examples of (a) a clinical image of early stage of melanoma and (b) a dermoscopy image of the same lesion. The dermoscopy image has no defused reflection on the skin surface and shows the internal structures clearly. In this case, an experienced dermatologist found regression structures (tint color areas) in the dermoscopy image and concluded that this lesion should be malignant.
Several diagnostic schemes based on dermoscopy have been proposed and tested in clinical practice including the ABCD rule (Stolz et al., 1994), Menzies' scoring method (Menzies et al., 1996), the 7-point checklist (Argenziano et al., 1998), the modified ABC-point list (Blum et al., 2003), and the 3-point checklist (Soyer et al., 2004). A systematic review covering Medline entries from 1983 to 1997 revealed that dermoscopy had 10-27% higher sensitivity (Mayer et al., 1997). However, dermoscopic diagnosis is often subjective and is therefore associated with poor reproducibility and low accuracy especially in the hands of inexperienced dermatologists. Despite the use of dermoscopy, the accuracy of expert dermatologists in diagnosing melanoma is estimated to be about 75-84% (Argenziano et al., 2003).

In order to overcome the above problems, automated and semi-automated procedures for classification of dermoscopy images and related techniques have been investigated since the late 1990s. This chapter introduces the recent advancement of those investigations with Internet based melanoma screening system developed by authors.

The following of the chapter is organized as follows: section 2 describes the diagnostic scheme of melanomas and outlines computer-based melanoma diagnosis in methodology and past studies; section 3 introduces an outline of our web-based melanoma screening system and its architectonics; section 4 explains Asian specific melanomas found in acral volar regions and their automated method for diagnosis; section 5 describes the remaining issues needing to be addressed in this field and the conclusion is given in section 6.

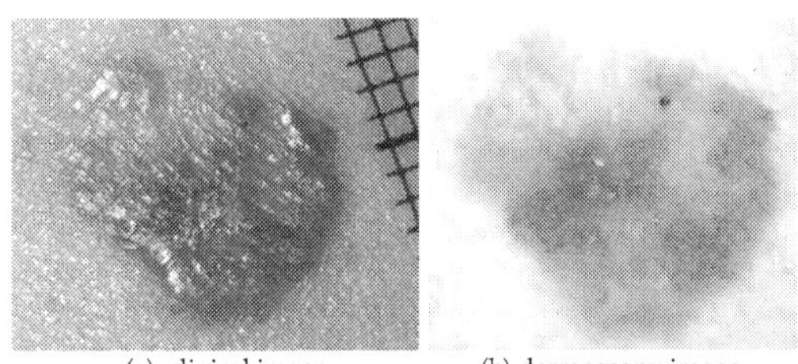

(a) clinical image   (b) dermoscopy image

Fig. 1. Sample of (a) clinical image and (b) dermoscopy image of same lesion (malignant melanoma)

2. Diagnosis of melanoma

This section firstly introduces the diagnosis scheme for melanomas, namely how dermatologists diagnose melanomas, and then introduces the computer-based diagnosis in terms of methodological outline and past studies.

2.1 Diagnosis scheme for melanomas

This subsection introduces well-known and commonly-used diagnosis scheme for dermoscopy images, the ABCD rule (Stolz et al., 1994) and the 7-point checklist (Argenziano et al., 1998) for further understanding.

2.1.1 ABCD rule

This is one of the most well-known semi-quantitative diagnosis schemes. It quantifies the asymmetry (A), border sharpness (B), color variation (C) and the number of differential structures (D) present in a lesion. Table 1 summarizes these definitions and their relative weights. A describes the degree of asymmetry of the tumor. Assuming a pair of orthogonal symmetry axes intersecting at the centroid of the tumor, A can be 0 (symmetry along both axes), 1 (symmetry along one axis), or 2 (no symmetry). B represents the number of border octants with sharp transitions. C indicates the number of significant colors present in the tumor, of which six are considered to be significant: white, red, light-brown, dark-brown, blue-gray, and black. Finally, D represents the number of differential structures (pigment network, structureless or homogeneous areas, streaks, dots, and globules) present in the tumor. Using the ABCD rule, the total dermoscopy score (TDS) is calculated as follows:

$$TDS = (A \times 1.3) + (B \times 0.1) + (C \times 0.5) + (D \times 0.5). \tag{1}$$

TDS below 4.75 indicates benignity, whereas TDS above 5.45 indicates malignancy. A score between these limits corresponds to a suspicious case that requires clinical follow-up.

Fig.2 shows the sample dermoscopy image. Dermatologists will find no symmetry border (A=2), more than half of the tumor border has sharp color transition (B=5), four colors (white, light-brown, dark-brown, blue-gray) in the tumor area (C=4) and five defined structures (pigment network, structureless or homogeneous areas, streaks, dots, and globules) (D=5).With these criteria, TDS becomes 7.6 (>5.45) and they can conclude this tumor is malignant.

Criterion	Description	score	weight
Asymmetry	Number of asymmetry axes	0-2	× 1.3
Border	Number of border octants with sharp transition	0-8	× 0.1
Color	Number of significant colors from: white, red, light-brown, dark-brown, bule-gray, and black	1-6	× 0.5
Differential structures	Number of differential structures from: pigment network, structureless, streaks, dots, and globules	0-5	× 0.5

Table 1. Brief summary of ABCD rule (Stolz et al., 1994)

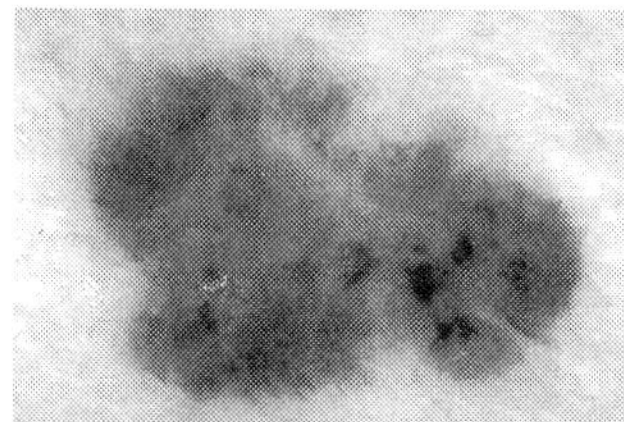

Fig. 2. Sample of dermoscopy image (malignant melanoma)

2.1.2 7-point checklist

This is another well-known diagnostic method that requires the identification of seven dermoscopic structures that are shown in Table 2. The score for a lesion is determined as the weighted sum of the structures present in it. Using the 7-point checklist, the total score (TS) is calculated as follows:

$$TS = (\#_{major} \times 2) + (\#_{minor}). \tag{2}$$

Here $\#_{major}$ and $\#_{minor}$ are the number of dermoscopic structures (see Table 2) present in the image. If TS is greater than or equal to 3, then the lesion is considered to be malignant.

In Fig. 2, dermatologists will find "blue-whitish veil", "irregular streaks", "irregular pigmentation", "irregular dots/globules", and "regression structures". Accordingly, TS becomes 6 (≥3) and they consider this tumor to be malignant. Note again that the scores in the above examples may vary among physicians. See (Argenziano et al., 2003) in detail.

Major criterion	weight
1. Atypical pigment network	× 2
2. Blue-whitish veil	× 2
3. Atypical vascular pattern	× 2
Minor criterion	weight
4. Irregular streaks	× 1
5. Irregular pigmentation	× 1
6. Irregular dots / globules	× 1
7. Regression structures	× 1

Table 2. Brief summary of 7-point checklist (Argenziano et al., 1998)

2.2 Computer-based diagnosis of melanomas

Several groups have developed automated analysis procedures to overcome the above mentioned problems – difficulty, subjectivity and low reproducibility of diagnosis, and reported high levels of diagnostic accuracy. The pioneering study of fully automated diagnosis of melanoma was conducted by Green et al. (Green et al., 1991). In their study tumor images were captured using a CCD color video camera.

Table 3 shows the list of recent studies in this topic. The diagnosis process of most automated diagnosis methods can be divided into three steps:

(1) Determination of tumor area from dermoscopy image,

(2) Extraction of image features from image,

(3) Building of the classification model and evaluation.

In the following section, outline of these steps is described with our Internet-based system as an example.

Reference	Classifier	#Images	SE(%)	SP(%)	comments
Gunster et al., 2001	k-NN	5363	73.0	89.0	(not dermoscopy images)
Elbaum et al., 2001	Linear	246	100	85.0	
Rubegni et al., 2002	ANN	550	94.3	93.8	
Hoffmann et al.,2003	Logistic	2218	-	-	AUC*=0.844
Blum et al., 2003	ANN	837	82.3	86.9	
Oka et al., 2004	Linear	247	87.0	93.1	**Internet-based**
Burroni et al., 2004	Linear	174	71.1	72.1	Only melanoma in situ
Seidenari et al., 2005	Linear	459	87.5	85.7	AUC*=0.933
Menzies et al., 2005	Logistic	2420	91.0	65.0	
Celebi et al., 2007b	SVM	564	93.3	92.3	
Iyatomi et al., 2008b	ANN	1258	85.9	86.0	**Internet-based** AUC=0.928

* area under the ROC (receiver operating characteristics) curve

Table 3. Recent studies in automated diagnosis for melanomas

3. Internet-based melanoma screening system

The software-based approaches introduced in the section 2, however, have several problems or limitations for practical use. For example, results of these studies are not comparable because of the different image sets used in each one. In addition, these studies were designed to develop a screening system for new patients using standalone systems and therefore they have not been opened to the public.

In 2004, authors developed the first Internet-based melanoma screening system and opened it for public use with the intention to solve abovementioned issues (Oka et al., 2004). The URL of the site has changed and it is now http://dermoscopy.k.hosei.ac.jp. Here we show the current top page of the site in Fig.3(a). When one uploads a dermoscopy image, inputs photographed body region of the tumor and the associated clinical data (Fig. 3(b)), the system extracts the tumor area, calculates the tumor characteristics and reports a diagnosis based on the output of built linear or artificial neural network classifier (Fig. 3(c)). Collecting many dermoscopy images for building a classifier is the most important issue to ensure system accuracy and generality. However, this is not a trivial task because obtaining the diagnosis information, dermatologists usually need histopathological tests or long term clinical follow-up. To address this issue, our system is designed to store the uploaded dermoscopy images into our database and waiting a final diagnosis by pathological examination etc. as a feedback from the users, if available.

Since we made this system open to the public, we have identified several issues that would make the system more practical. We have thus focused on the following topics: (1) expansion of the image database for building a classifier, (2) development of a more accurate tumor area extraction algorithm, (3) extraction of more discriminative diagnostic features, (4) development of an effective classification model, and (5) reduction of the system response time.

The latest version of our system (Iyatomi et al., 2008b) features a sophisticated tumor-area extraction algorithm that attains superior extraction performance to conventional methods (Iyatomi et al., 2006) and linear and back-propagation artificial neural network classifiers. The system has a capability to accept the usual melanocytic pigmented lesions (e.g. Clark nevi, Spitz nevi, dermal nevi, blue nevi, melanomas etc. - research target of most conventional studies as listed in Table 1) and it can also accept acral volar skin lesions that are found specifically in palm and sole area of non-white people. Acral lesions have completely different appearances and therefore a specific classification model is required to analyze these lesions (details are described in section 4). Our system automatically selects the appropriate diagnostic classifier based on the location of lesions provided by the user and yields the final diagnosis results in the form of a malignancy score between 0 and 100 within 3-10 seconds (see Fig.3(c)).

For non-acral lesions, the system achieved 85.9 % SE, 86.0% SP and 0.928 area under the receiver operating characteristics (ROC) curve (AUC) using a leave-one-out cross-validation test on a set of 1258 dermoscopy images (1060 nevi and 198 melanomas) and for acral volar lesions, 93.3% SE, 91.1% SP and 0.991 AUC on a set of 199 dermoscopy images (169 nevi and 30 melanomas). Fig. 4 shows the ROC curve for our latest screening system for (1) non-acral and (2) acral lesions.

In this section, key components of our web-based system, namely determination of tumor area, extraction and selection of important image features, building classifiers, and their performances are described. In the following section (section 4), introduction of acral volar skin lesions and their automated diagnosis is explained.

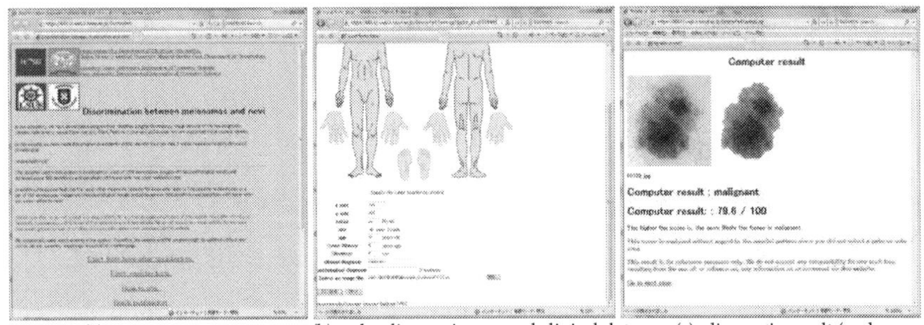

| (a) top page | (b) uploading an image and clinical data | (c) diagnosis result (melanoma) |

Fig. 3. (a) Top page, (b) uploading an image and corresponding clinical data, (c) sample of result page

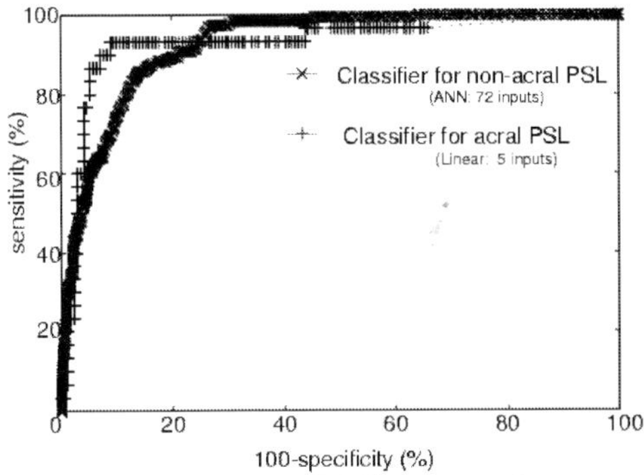

Fig. 4. Receiver operating characteristics (ROC) curves for our latest Internet-based melanoma screening system (classifier for non-acral lesions and acral lesions)

3.1 Tumor area extraction from surrounding skin

Diagnostic accuracy highly depends on the accurate extraction of the tumor area. Since the late 90s, numerous solutions that address this issue have been reported (Celebi et al., 2009). A notable problem with these studies is that the computer-extracted regions were often smaller than the dermatologist-drawn ones resulting in the area immediately surrounding the tumor, an important feature in the diagnosis of melanoma, being excluded from the subsequent analysis (Grana et al., 2003). Therefore, there is need for developing a more accurate tumor area extraction algorithm that produces results similar to those determined by the dermatologists.

We developed "dermatologist-like" tumor area extraction algorithm (Iyatomi et al., 2006) introduces a region-growing approach that aims to bring the automatic extraction results closer to those determined by expert dermatologists. To the best of author's knowldge, this algorithm was developed based on the largest number of manual extraction results by expert dermatologists at present and quantitatively evaluated performance showed that is had almost equivalent extraction performance to that by expert dermatologists. With those reasons, this algorithm is now used on our web-based screening system.

In this section, a brief summary of our method is introduced and explained. For more detailed information on this topic, please see survey paper (Celebi et al., 2009).

The "dermatologist-like" tumor area extraction algorithm is developed based on a total of 319 dermoscopy images from EDRA-CDROM (Argenziano et al., 2000) (244 melanocytic nevi and 75 melanomas) and their manual extraction results of tumor area by five expert dermatologists. The algorithm consists of four phases:

(1) initial tumor area decision,
(2) regionalization,
(3) tumor area selection, and
(4) region-growing.

In the following subsections, we introduce the method briefly and show some examples. For more details, please refer to the original article (Iyatomi et al., 2006).

3.1.1 Initial tumor area decision phase

This method uses two filtering operations before the selection of a threshold. First, the image was processed with a Gaussian filter to eliminate the sensor noise. Then, the Laplacian filter was applied to the image and the pixels in the top 20% of the Laplacian value were selected. Only these selected pixels were used to calculate a threshold. The threshold was determined by maximizing the inter-group variance (Otsu, 1988) with blue channel of image and the darker area was taken as a tentative tumor area.

3.1.2 Regionalization phase

Because many isolated small regions were created in the previous phase, these needed to be merged in order to obtain a continuous or a small set of tumor areas. First, a unique region number was assigned to each connected region. Second, a region smaller than predefined certain size (ratio to the image size) was combined with the adjacent larger region that shares the longest boundary. This phase makes it possible to manipulate the image as an assembly of regions.

3.1.3 Tumor area selection phase

Tumor areas were experimentally determined by selecting appropriate areas from the segmented regions using experimentally decided rules. The main objective of this phase is to eliminate undesired surrounding shadow areas that are sometimes produced by narrow shooting area of the dermoscopy. The regions that fulfilled these specific conditions were selected as the tumor region.

3.1.4 Region-growing phase

The extracted tumor area was expanded along the pre-defined border by a region-growing algorithm in order to bring it closer to the area selected by dermatologists. This method traverses the border of the initial tumor using a window of S×S pixels. When the color properties of the inner V_{in} and outer V_{out} regions of the tumor are similar, all of the neighborhood pixels are considered as part of the tumor area. This procedure is performed on each and every border pixel. This modification makes the tumor size larger and the border of the tumor is redefined. This procedure is repeated iteratively until the size of tumor becomes stable.

3.1.5 Evaluation of tumor area extraction

We used a total of 319 dermoscopy images and evaluated the algorithm from a clinical perspective using manually determined borders from five expert dermatologists. Five dermatologists, with an average of 11 years of experience manually determined the borders of all tumors using a tablet computer. Even though these were expert dermatologist, their manual extraction results of the tumor area showed more than minor differences from each other (standard deviation of the extracted area is 8.9% of the tumor size in average) and therefore the determination of the standard tumor area (STA) for each image was necessary to be done in advance. We compared the extraction results from 5/5 medical doctor (5/5 MD) area (the region that is selected by all five dermatologists) to 1/5 MD area (the region that is selected by at least one dermatologist) and evaluated the standard deviation (SD) of the selected area. We concluded that the area extracted by two or more dermatologists (2/5 MD area) could be taken as the standard tumor area (STA).

Fig. 5 shows examples of tumor extraction results. From left to right: (a) dermoscopy image, (b) extraction result by conventional thresholding method, (c) extraction result by our "dermatologist-like" method, and (d) manual extraction result by five expert dermatologists. In manual the extraction results, the black area represents the area selected by all five dermatologists and the gray one is that selected by at least one dermatologist.

We used *precision* and *recall* criteria for performance evaluation. Their definitions are as follows:

$$precision = \frac{correctly\ extracted\ area}{extracted\ area}. \qquad recall = \frac{correctly\ extracted\ area}{STA}. \qquad (3)$$

Note that "correctly extracted area" is the intersectional parts of the STA and the extracted area. The *precision* indicates "How accurate the extracted area was" and *recall* indicates "How well the tumor area was extracted". Those are ambivalent criteria and good extraction requires both precision and recall in high levels.

The summary of evaluation results for tumor area extraction is shown in Table 4. The conventional thresholding method showed excellent precision (99.5%) but low recall (87.6%), because this method tended to extract the inner area of the STA. This score indicated that the extracted area was smaller and almost all of the extracted area was in the tumor area. The characteristics of peripheral part of tumors are important for diagnosing melanoma so that inadequate extraction could have lost important information. Other computer-based methods using the clustering technique showed a similar trend; they had high precision but low recall when compared with the results of dermatologists. Given that the SD of the tumor areas manually extracted by five dermatologists was 8.9%, the precision of the proposed algorithm can be considered to be high enough and the extracted areas were almost equivalent to those determined by dermatologists. In addition, this algorithm provided better performance compared with that by non-medical individuals. With this result, we can consider we don't have to prepare manual interface for tumor area extraction when we widen the target audience of the system for non medically-trained individuals.

Celebi *et al.* compared recent seven tumor area extraction algorithms using a total of 90 dermoscopy images with manual extraction results by three expert dermatologists as a gold standard (Celebi et al., 2007a). In their evaluation, our dermatologist-like tumor area extraction algorithm achieved the lowest error in the benign category (mean $\pm$ SD = 10.66$\pm$5.13%) and the second lowest in the overall image set (11.44$\pm$6.40%).

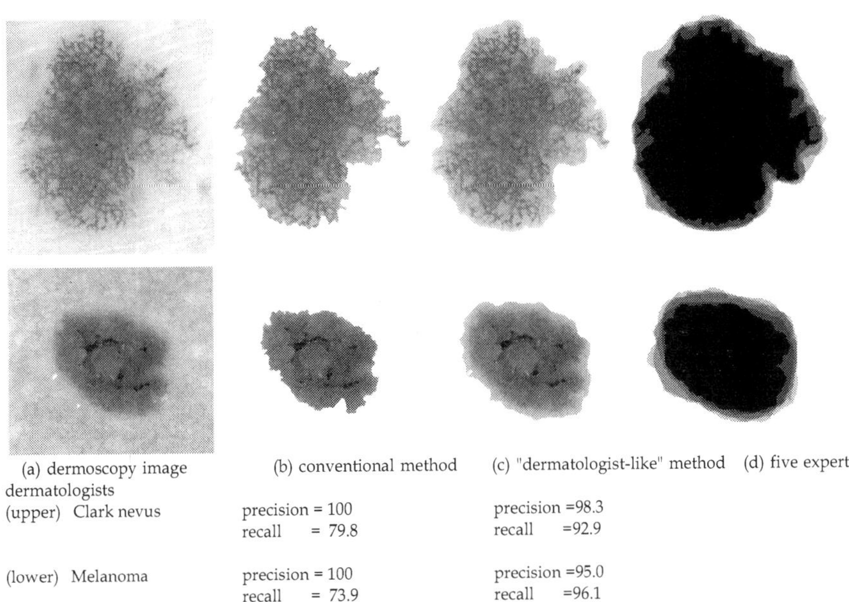

(a) dermoscopy image	(b) conventional method	(c) "dermatologist-like" method	(d) five expert

dermatologists
(upper) Clark nevus   precision = 100   precision =98.3
                              recall   = 79.8   recall   =92.9

(lower) Melanoma   precision = 100   precision =95.0
                              recall   = 73.9   recall   =96.1

Fig. 5 Comparison of tumor area extraction results: From left to right: dermoscopy image, extraction result by conventional thresholding method, extraction result by our "dermatologist-like" method, and manual extraction result by five expert dermatologists.

Methods	precision	recall
Conventional thresholding	99.5	87.6
Average of 10 non-medical individuals	97.0	90.2
Dermatologist-like	94.1	95.3

Table 4. Summary of tumor extraction performance

3.1.6 Importance of tumor area extraction from diagnostic performance

The effectiveness of our extraction method for the diagnostic accuracy was evaluated using a total of 319 dermoscopy images (same dataset). We extracted a tumor area by conventional and dermatologist-like methods, calculated a total of 64 image features (Oka et al., 2004) from each image, and then built a linear classifier using a incremental stepwise input selection method. The final diagnostic accuracy was evaluated by drawing the ROC curve of each classifier and the area under the each ROC curve (AUC) was evaluated. Our dermatologist like tumor extraction algorithm had improved diagnostic accuracy over the other conventional methods. AUC increased from 0.795 to 0.875 with improvement of tumor extraction algorithm. When the diagnostic threshold was defined at a sensitivity of 80%, our extraction method showed approximately 20% better accuracy in specificity.

3.2 Feature extraction from the image

After the extraction of the tumor area, the tumor object is rotated to align its major axis with the Cartesian x-axis. We extract a total of 428 image related objective features (Iyatomi et al., 2008b). The extracted features can be roughly categorized into asymmetry, border, color and texture properties. In this section, a brief summary is described, please refer the original article for more details.

(a) Asymmetry features (80 features): We use 10 intensity thresholds values from 5 to 230 with a stepsize of 25. In the extracted tumor area, thresholding is performed and the areas whose intensity is lower than the threshold are determined. From each such area, we calculate 8 features: area ratio to original tumor size, circularity, differences of the center of gravity between original tumor, standard deviation of the distribution and skewness of the distribution.

(b) Border features (32 features): We divide the tumor area into eight equi-angle regions and in each region, we define an $S_B \times S_B$ window centered on the tumor border. In each window, a ratio of color intensity between inside and outside of the tumor and the gradient of color intensity is calculated on the blue and luminance channels, respectively. These are averaged over the 8 equi-angle regions. We calculate four features for eight different window sizes; $1/5, 1/10, 1/15, 1/20, 1/25, 1/30, 1/35$ and $1/40$ of the length of the major axis of the tumor object L.

(c) Color features (140 features): We calculated minimum, average, maximum, standard deviation and skewness value in the RGB and HSV color spaces, respectively (subtotal 30) for the whole tumor area, perimeter of the tumor area, differences between the tumor area and the surrounding normal skin, and that between peripheral and normal-skin ($30 \times 4 = 120$). In addition, a total of 20 color related features are calculated; the number of colors in the tumor area and peripheral tumor area in the RGB and HSV color spaces quantized to 8^3 and 16^3 colors, respectively (subtotal 8), the average color of normal skin (R, G, B, H, S, V: subtotal 6), and average color differences between the peripheral tumor area and inside of the tumor area (R, G, B, H, S, V subtotal 6). Note that peripheral part of the tumor is defined as the region inside the border that has an area equal to 30% of the tumor area based on a consensus by several dermatologists.

(d) Texture features (176 features): We calculate 11 different sized co-occurrence matrices with distance value δ ranging from $L/2$ to $L/64$. Based on each co-occurrence matrix, energy, moment, entropy and correlation were calculated in four directions (0, 45, 90 and 135 degrees).

3.3 Feature selection and build a classifier

Feature selection is one of the most important steps for developing a robust classifier in any case. It is also well known that building a classifier with highly correlated parameters was adversely affected by so called "multi collinearity" and in such a case the system loses accuracy and generality.

In our research, we usually prepare two types of feature sets, (1) original image feature set and (2) orthogonal feature set. Using the original image feature set, the extracted image features are used directly as input candidates in the classifier and therefore we can clearly observe the relationship between image features and the target (e.g. diagnosis). However, using the original image features has the above mentioned potential risk. Note that the risk of multi collinearity is greatly reduced by appropriate input selection. On the other hand using the orthogonal feature set, finding the relationship between the image features and the target (e.g. diagnosis) becomes complicated, but this can show us the global trends with further investigation. To calculate the orthogonal image features, we extracted a total of 428 features per image and transformed them into the [0, 1] range using z-score normalization and then orthogonalized them using the principal component analysis (PCA).

The parameters used in melanoma classifiers are selected by an incremental stepwise method which determines the statistically most significant input parameters in a sequential manner. This method searches appropriate input parameters one after the other according to the statistical rule. This input selection method rejects statistically ignorable features during incremental selection and therefore, these highly correlated features were automatically excluded from the model. Note that using orthogonal feature sets frees from this problem.

The details of the feature selection is as follows:

(Step 0) Set the base parameter BP=null and number of the base parameter $\#_{BP}=0$.

(Step 1) Search one input parameter x^* from all parameters x where regression model with x^* yields best performance (lowest residual) among all. Set BP to x^* and $\#_{BP}=1$.

(Step 2) Build linear regression models whose input elements are BP and x' without redundancy $\forall x' \in x$, number of input is $\#_{BP}+1$ and select one input candidate $x^\wedge$ which has the highest partial correlation coefficient among x'.

(Step 3) Calculate the variance ratio (F-value) between the regression sum of squares and the residual sum of squares of the built regression model.

(Step 4) Perform statistical F-test (calculate p value) in order to verify that the model is reliable.

If $p<0.05$: BP $\leftarrow$ BP $+ x^\wedge$, $\#_{BP} \leftarrow \#_{BP}+1$ and return to (step 2). Else if $0.05 \leq p < 0.10$: discard $x^\wedge$ and return to (step 2) and find the next best candidate.Else if the developed model has a statistically negligible parameter $x^\wedge$ ($0.10 \leq p$) among currently selected input, exclude $x^\wedge$ from BP, $\#_{BP} \leftarrow \#_{BP}-1$ and return to (step 2). Otherwise terminate the feature selection process.

Based on selected image features by above mentioned method, we built a back propagation artificial neural network (ANN) to classify dermoscopy images into benign or malignant.

Although ANNs have excellent learning and function approximation abilities, it is desirable to restrict the number of hidden-neurons and input nodes to a minimum in order to obtain a general classification model that performs well on future data (Reed et al., 1993).

In our network design, we had only one output node. This is because our aim was to classify the input as malignant or benign. All nevi such as Clark nevi, Reed nevi, blue nevi, and dermal nevi are equally considered as benign. Note that we assigned a training signal of 0.9 and 0.1 to melanoma and benign classes, respectively. If the output of the ANN exceeded the diagnostic threshold θ, we judged the input tumor as being malignant.

On a separate note, our system provides the screening results not only in the form of ``benign'' or ``malignant'', but also as a malignancy score between 0 and 100 based on the output of the ANN classifier. We assigned a malignancy score of 50 to the case where the output of the ANN was θ. For other values, we adjust this score of 0, 20, 80, and 100 according to the output of the ANN of 0, 0.2, 0.8 and 1.0, respectively using linear interpolation. This conversion is based on the assumption that the larger score of the classifier is, the more malignancy is. Although this assignment procedure is arbitrary, we believe the malignancy score can be useful in understanding the severity of the case.

We also built a linear classifier using the same method as a baseline for the classification performance comparison.

3.4 Performance evaluation

We used a total 1258 dermoscopy images with diagnosis (1060 cases of melanocytic nevi and 198 melanomas) from three European university hospitals (University of Naples, Graz, and Vienna) and one Japanese university hospital (Keio University). The diagnostic performance was evaluated by leave-one-out cross-validation test.

The incremental stepwise method selected 72 orthogonalized features from 428 principal components and all selected features were statistically significant (p<0.05). In this experiment, the basic back-propagation algorithm with constant training coefficients achieved the best classification performance among the tested training algorithms. The ANN classifier with 72 inputs - 6 hidden neurons achieved the best performance of 85.9% in SE, 86.0% in SP, and an AUC value of 0.928. Introducing a momentum term boosted the convergence rate at the expense of reduced diagnostic accuracy (Note that linear model with same inputs achieved 0.914 in AUC).

The classification performance is quite good considering that the diagnostic accuracy of expert dermatologists was 75-84% and that of histological tissue examination on difficult case sets was as low as 90% (Argenziano et al., 2003). In this study, we used ANN and linear models for classification. Using other models such as support vector machine classifier may improve performance, however importance of model selection is less than selecting efficient features in this task.

On the other hand, despite the good classification performance obtained, our system has several limitations regarding the acceptable tumor classes and the condition of the input images. At the present, the diagnostic capability of our system does not match that of expert dermatologists.The primary reason for this is the lack of a large and diverse dermoscopy image set.

4. Diagnosis of Asian specific melanomas

In non-white populations, almost half of the melanomas are found in acral volar areas and nearly 30% of melanomas affect the sole of the foot (Saida et al., 2004). Saida *et al.* also reported that melanocytic nevi are also frequently found in their acral skin and approximately 8% of Japanese have melanocytic nevi on their soles. They reported that about 90% of melanomas in this area have the parallel ridge pattern (ridge areas are pigmented) and 70% of melanocytic nevi have the parallel furrow pattern (furrow areas are pigmented). In fact, the appearance of these acral volar lesions is largely different from pigmented skin lesions found in other body areas and accordingly the development of a specially designed classifier is required for these lesions.

Fig. 6 shows sample dermoscopy images from acral volar areas. Expert dermatologists focus on parallel patterns and diagnose this lesion. However, automatic detection of the parallel ridge or parallel furrow patterns is often difficult to achieve due to the wide variety of dermoscopy images (e.g. fibrillar pattern, sometimes looks similar to parallel ridge pattern) and there has been no published methods on computerized classification of this diagnostic category. Recently authors found key features to recognize parallel patterns and developed a classification model for these lesions (Iyatomi et al., 2008a).

In this chapter, we introduce the methodology and results briefly and then discuss them.

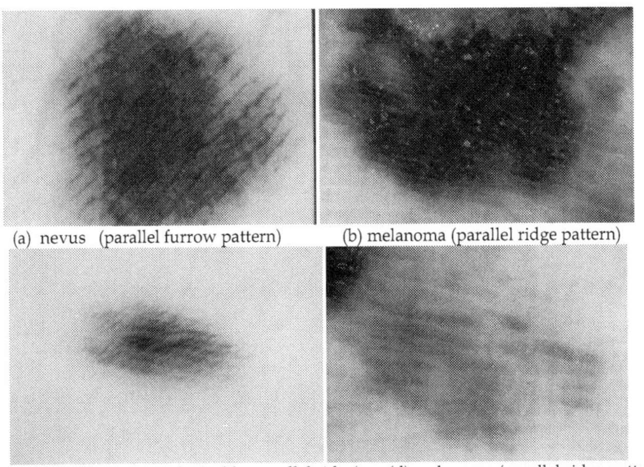

(a) nevus (parallel furrow pattern)   (b) melanoma (parallel ridge pattern)

(c) nevus (fibrillar pattern – looks like parallel ridge) (d) melanoma (parallel ridge pattern)

Fig. 6. Sample of acral volar pigmented skin lesions.

4.1 Strategy for diagnosis of acral volar lesions

A total of 213 acral volar dermoscopy images; 176 clinically equivocal nevi and 37 melanomas from four Japanese hospitals (Keio University, Toranomon, Shinshu University, and Inagi Hospitals) and two European university hospitals (University of Naples, Italy, University of Graz, Austria) as part of the EDRA-CDROM (Argenziano et al., 2000) were used in our study.

Identification of parallel ridge or parallel furrow patterns is an efficient clue for the diagnosis of acral volar lesions, however as described before, automatic detection of these patterns from dermoscopy image are often difficult. Therefore we did not extract these patterns (structures) directly but instead we constructed a parametric approach as we searched for non-acral lesions, namely by determining the tumor area extracting image features and classifying the image.

In our study,we developed an acral melanoma-nevus classifier and three detectors for typical patterns of acral volar lesions: parallel ridge pattern, parallel furrow pattern and fibrillar pattern. For melanoma-nevus classifier, the training signal of 1 or -1 was assigned to each melanoma and nevus case, respectively. Similarly, a training signal of 1 (positive) or -1 (negative) was assigned to each dermoscopic pattern. The dermoscopic patterns were identified by three experienced dermatologists and only those patterns of which at least two dermatologists agreed were considered. Note here that dermoscopic patterns were assessed independently of each other and therefore some cases received multiple or no assignments. As for a classification model, we used a linear model with the confirmation of whose enough performance for separating malignant tumors from others. The classification performance was evaluated by leave-one-out cross-validation.

4.2 Computer-based diagnosis of acral volar lesions

4.2.1 Determination of tumor area and details of material

The dermatologist-like tumor area extraction algorithm successfully extracted tumor area in 199 cases out of 213 cases ($\approx$ 93.4%). In 14 cases (7 nevi and 7 melanomas), tumor area extraction process failed. This was due to the size of the tumor being larger than about 70% of the dermoscope field. Our algorithm is mainly for early melanomas which usually fit in the frame. Note that most of automated tumor area extraction algorithms meet this difficulty. Tumors in dermoscopy images have a wide variety of colors, shapes and sizes, and accordingly the pre-definition of the characteristics of tumor areas is difficult. Automated algorithms are designed to extract intended areas from the image for most cases with cost of mis-extraction of irregular cases.

Since larger lesions are relatively easy to diagnose, we deem that computer-based screening is not necessary. Also note that the false-extraction rate for melanomas was higher (19%) than that of nevi (4%) and therefore if extraction fails we can consider the lesion as potentially malignant in the first screening step.

Out of 169 nevi, parallel ridge, parallel furrow and fibrillar patterns were found in 5, 133 and 49 cases, respectively. A total of 11 cases of nevi had no specific patterns and, 28 nevi had both parallel furrow pattern and fibrillar pattern. One nevus had both a parallel ridge and a fibrillar pattern. In 30 melanomas, parallel ridge, parallel furrow and fibrillar patterns were found in 24, 2 and 1 cases, respectively. Five of the melanomas had no specific patterns and one of the melanomas had all three patterns.

4.2.2 Developed model

A total of 428 image features were transformed into orthogonal 198 principal components (PCs). From these PCs, we selected the effective ones for each classifier. Table 5 summarizes the number of selected PCs for each classification model (#PC), determination coefficient with adjustment of the degree of freedom R^2, standard deviation of mean estimated error E, the order number of the first 10 PCs lined by the selected sequence by stepwise input-selection method, and the classification performance in terms of SE, SP and AUC under leave-one-out cross-validation test. The SE and SP values shown are those that have the maximum product. The numbers in parentheses represent the performance when 14 unsuccessful extraction cases are considered as false-classification. Even though the number of the test images was limited, good recognition and classification performance was achieved as well for acral volar pigmented skin lesions.

Classifier type	#PC	R^2	E	Selected PCs (first 10)	SE(%)	SP(%)	AUC
Melanoma	45	.807	.315	**2,9,6,1,3**,15,91,40,20,98	100 (81.1†)	95.9 (92.1†)	0.993
Parallel ridge	40	.736	.363	**2,9,1,6,3**,59,20,88,77,33	93.1	97.7	0.985
Parallel furrow	35	.571	.614	**6,2**,145,15,**3**,98,70,24,59,179	90.4	85.9	0.931
Fibrillar	24	.434	.654	106,66,56,145,137,94,111,169,131,5	88.0	77.9	0.890

† When 14 unsuccessful extraction cases are treated as false-classification.

Table 5. Modeling result and classification performance for acral volar lesions

4.2.3 Important features for recognition of acral lesions

Since we used an orthogonalized image feature set in our analysis, we reached interesting results that compares to the clinical findings of a dermatologist.

For the melanoma-nevus classifier, many significant (small numbered) PCs were found in the first 10 selected features. The parallel ridge and parallel furrow detector were also composed of significant PCs, on the other hand, fibrillar pattern detector showed a different trend. The melanoma classifier and the parallel ridge detector have many common PCs. Particularly, the top five PCs for the two (2nd, 9th, 6th, 1st and 3rd PCs) were completely the same. Note that parameters chosen early in the stepwise feature selection were thought to be more important for the classification because the most significant parameters were statistically selected in each step. The common PCs are mainly related to asymmetry and structural properties rather than color. (See details in original manuscript (Iyatomi et al., 2008a)) The linear classifier using only these five components achieved 0.933 AUC, 93.3% SE, and 91.1% SP using a leave-one out cross validation test. Since the system with a smaller number of the inputs should have high generality in general and a linear model is the most simple architecture, we integrated this 5-input linear classifier on our server.

Dermatologists evaluate parallel patterns using the intensity distribution of the images and they consider the peripheral area of the lesion as important. We confirmed that our computer-based results also focus on similar characteristics as the dermatologists.

5. Open issues in this field

In order to improve system accuracy and generality, there is no doubt that the system should be developed with many samples as much as possible. The number of cases used in any of conventional studies is not enough for practical use at present. On the other hand, even if we can collect a large enough number of images and succeed at finding robust features for diagnosis, the accuracy of the diagnosis cannot reach 100%. In the current format, most of the conventional studies provide only the final diagnosis or diagnosis with limited information. It is desirable that the system provides the grounds for diagnostic results in accordance with quantitatively scored common clinical structures, such as those defined in the ABCD rule, the 7-point checklist, or others. However, since these dermoscopic structures are defined subjectively, their automated quantification is still difficult.

Recent studies on high-level dermoscopic feature extraction include (i) two studies on pigment network (Fleming et al.,1998) and globules (Caputo et al.,2002), (ii) four systematic studies on dots (Yoshino et al., 2004), blotches (Stoecker et al., 2005)(Pellacani et al.,2004), and blue-white areas (Celebi et al.,2008), and (iii) a recent study on parallel-ridge and parallel-furrow patterns (Iyatomi et al.,2008a). Although several researchers attempted to extract these features using image processing techniques, to the best of authors' knowledge, no general solution has been proposed, especially the evaluation of structural features such as pigment networks and streaks have remained an open issue.

We also find that when we widen the target user of an automated diagnostic or screening system from "dermatologist only" to physicians with other expertise or not-medically trained people, the system should have pre-processing schemes to exclude non melanocytic lesions such as basel cell carcinoma (BCC), seborrheic keratosis, and hemangioma. Identification of melanomas from those lesions is in not small cases easier than that from melanocytic lesion (e.g. Clark nevi) by expert dermatologists, but this is also important issue and almost no published results examine this topic.

6. Conclusion

In this chapter, recent investigations in computer-based diagnosis for melanoma are introduced with authors' Internet-based system as an example. Even though recent studies shows good classification accuracy, these systems still have several limitations regarding the acceptable tumor classes, the condition of the input images, etc. Note here again that the diagnostic capability of the present automated systems does not match that of an expert dermatologist. On the other hand, they would be efficient as a diagnosis support system with further improvements and they have the capability to find early stage hidden patients.

7. References

Argenziano, G.; Fabbrocini G, Carli P et al. (1998) Epiluminescence microscopy for the diagnosis of ABCD rule of dermatoscopy and a new 7-point checklist based on pattern analysis, *Archives of Dermatology*, No. 134, pp. 1536-1570.

Argenziano, G.; Soyer HP, De Giorgi V et al. (2000). *Interactive atlas of dermoscopy CD*: EDRA Medical Publishing and New Media, Milan.

Argenziano, G.; Soyer HP, Chimenti S et al. (2003) Dermoscopy of pigmented skin lesions: Results of a consensus meeting via the Internet, *Journal of American Academy of Dermatology* , Vol. 48, No.5, pp. 679-693.

Blum, A.; Rassner G & Garbe C. (2003) Modified ABC-point list of dermoscopy: A simplified and highly accurate dermoscopic algorithm for the diagnosis of cutaneous melanocytic lesions, *Journal of the Americal Academy of Dermatology*, Vol. 48, No. 5, pp. 672-678.

Blum, A.; Luedtke H, Ellwanger U et al. (2004) Digital image analysis for diagnosis of cutaneous melanoma. Development of a highly effective computer algorithm based on analysis of 837 melanocytic lesions, *British Journal of Dermatology*, Vol. 151, pp. 1029-1038.

Burroni, M.; Sbano P, Cevenini G et al. (2005) Dysplastic naevus vs. in situ melanoma: digital dermoscopy analysis, *British Journal of Dermatology*, Vol. 152, pp. 679-684.

Caputo, B.; Panichelli V, Gigante GE. (2002) Toward a quantitative analysis of skin lesion images, *Studies in Health Technology and Informatics*, Vol. 90, pp. 509-513.

Celebi, ME.; Aslandogan YA, Stoecker WV et al. (2007a) Unsupervised border detection in dermoscopy images, *Skin Research and Technology*, Vol. 13, pp. 1-9.

Celebi, ME.; Kingravi HA, Uddin B et al. (2007b) A methodological approach to the classification of dermoscopy images, *Computerized Medical Imaging & Graphics*, Vol. 31, No. 6, pp. 362-373.

Celebi, ME.; Iyatomi H, Stoecker WV et al. (2008) Automatic Detection of Blue-White Veil and Related Structures in Dermoscopy Images, *Computerized Medical Imaging and Graphics*, Vol. 32, No. 8, pp. 670-677.

Celebi, ME.; Iyatomi H & Gerald S. (2009) Lesion border detection in dermoscopy images, *Computerized Medical Imaging and Graphics*, Vol. 33, No. 2, pp. 148-153.

Elbaum, M.; Kopf AW, Rabinovitz HS et al. (2001) Automatic differentiation of melanoma from melanocytic nevi with multispectral digital dermoscopy: a feasibility study, *Journal of American Academy of Dermatology* , Vol. 44, pp. 207-218.

Fleming, MG.; Steger C, Zhang J et al. (1998) Techniques for a structural analysis of dermatoscopic imagery, *Computerized Medical Imaging and Graphics*, Vol. 22, No. 5, pp. 375-389.

Ganster, H.; Pinz A, Rohrer R et al. (2001) Automated melanoma recognition, *IEEE Trans. on Medical Imaging*, Vol. 20, No. 3, pp. 233-239.

Grana, C.; Pellacani G, Cucchiara R et al. (2003) A new algorithm for border description of polarized light surface micriscopic images of pigmented skin lesions, *IEEE Trans. on Medical Imaging*, Vol 22, No. 8, pp. 959-964.

Green, A.; Martin N, McKenzle G et al. (1991) Computer image analysis of pigmented skin lesions, Melanoma Research, Vol. 1, pp. 231- 236.

Hoffmann, K.; Gambichler T, Rick A et al. (2003) Diagnostic and neural analysis of skin cancer (DANAOS). A multicentre stidy for collection and computer-aided analysis of data from pigmented skin lesions using digital dermoscopy. *British Journal of Dermatology*, Vol. 149, pp. 801-809.

Iyatomi, H.; Oka H, Saito M et al. (2006) Quantitative assessment of tumour area extraction from dermoscopy images and evaluation of the computer-based methods for automatic melanoma diagnostic system, *Melanoma Research*, Vol. 16, No. 2, pp. 183-190.

Iyatomi, H.; Oka H, Celebi ME et al. (2008a) Computer-Based Classification of Dermoscopy Images of Melanocytic Lesions on Acral Volar Skin, *Journal of Investigative Dermatology*, Vol. 128, pp. 2049-2054.

Iyatomi, H.; Oka H, Celebi ME et al.(2008b) An improved Internet-based melanoma screening system with dermatologist-like tumor area extraction algorithm, *Computerized Medical Imaging and Graphics*, Vol. 32, No. 7, pp. 566-579.

Jemal, A.; Siegel R, Ward E et al. (2008) Cancer Statistics, *A Cancer Journal for Clinicians*, Vol. 58, No. 2, pp. 71-96.

Mayer, J.; (1997) Systematic review of the diagnostic accuracy of dermoscopy in detecting malignant melanoma, *Med. Journal of Australia*, Vol. 167, No. 4, pp. 206-210.

Menzies, SW.; Bischof L, Talbot H, et al. (2005) The performance of SolarScan - An automated dermoscopy image analysis instrument for the diagnosis of primary melanoma, *Archives of Dermatology*, Vol. 141, No. 11, pp. 1388-1396.

Meyskens, FL Jr.; Berdeaux DH, Parks B et al. (1998). Natural history and prognostic factors incluencing survival in patients with stage I disease, *Cancer*, Vol. 62, No. 6, pp. 1207-1214.

Oka, H.; Hashimoto M, Iyatomi H et al. (2004) Internet-based program for automatic discrimination of dermoscopic images between melanoma and Clark nevi, *British Journal of Dermatology*, Vol. 150, No. 5, p. 1041.

Otsu, N. (1998) An automatic threshold selection method based on discriminant and least square criteria, *Trans. of IEICE*, Vol. 63, pp. 349-356.

Pellacani, G.; Grana C, Cucchiara R et al. (2004) Automated extraction and description of dark areas in surface microscopy melanocytic lesion images, *Dermatology*, Vol. 208, No. 1, pp. 21-26.

Reed, R. (1993) Pruning algorithms - a survey, *IEEE Trans. on Neural Networks*, Vol. 4, No. 5, pp. 740-747.

Rubegn ,P.; Cevenini G, Burroni M et al. (2002) Automated diagnosis of pigmented skin lesions, *International Journal of Cancer* , Vol. 101, pp. 576-580.

Saida, T.; Miyazaki A, Oguchi S et al. (2004) Significance of dermoscopic patterns in detecting malignant melanoma on acral volar skin, Arch Dermatol, Vol. 140, pp. 1233-1238.

Seidenari, S; Pellacani G & Grana C. (2005) Pigment distribution in melanocytic lesion images: a digital parameter to be employed for computer-aided diagnosis, *Skin Research and Technology*, Vol. 11, pp. 236-241.

Stoecker, WV.; Gupta K, Stanley RJ et al. (2005) Detection of asymmetric blotches (asymmetric structureless areas) in dermoscopy images of malignant melanoma using relative color, *Skin Research and Technology*, Vol. 11, No. 3, pp. 179-184.

Stolz, W.; Riemann A, Cognetta AB et al. (1994) ABCD rule of dermatoscopy: a new practical method for early recognition of malignant melanoma, *European Journal of Dermatology*, Vol. 4, No. 7, pp. 521-527.

Stolz W.; Falco OB., Bliek P et al. (2002). *Color Atlas of Dermatoscopy -- 2nd enlarged and completely revised edition*, Berlin: Blackwell publishing, ISBN: 978-1-4051-0098-4, Berlin.

Soyer, HP.; Smolle J, Kerl H et al. (1987) Early diagnosis of malignant melanoma by surface microscopy, *Lancet*, No. 2, p. 803.

Soyer, HP.; Argenziano G, Zalaudek I et al. (2004) Three-Point Checklist of Dermoscopy: A New Screening Method for Early Detection of Melanoma, *Dermatology*, Vol. 208, pp. 27-31.

Tanaka M. (2006) Dermoscopy, *Journal of Dermatology*, Vol. 3, pp. 513-517.

Yoshino, S.; Tanaka T, Tanaka M et al. (2004) Application of morphology for detection of dots in tumor, *Procs. SICE Annual Conference*, Vol. 1, pp. 591-594.

11

Quality Assessment of Retinal Fundus Images using Elliptical Local Vessel Density

Luca Giancardo[1,2], Fabrice Meriaudeau[1], Thomas P Karnowski[2],
Dr Edward Chaum[3] and Kenneth Tobin[2]

[1]*Université de Bourgogne*
France
[2]*Oak Ridge National Laboratory*
USA
[3]*University of Tennessee - Hamilton Eye Institute*
USA

1. Introduction

Diabetic retinopathy is the leading cause of blindness in the Western world. The World Health Organisation estimates that 135 million people have diabetes mellitus worldwide and that the number of people with diabetes will increase to 300 million by the year 2025 (Amos et al., 1997). Timely detection and treatment for DR prevents severe visual loss in more than 50% of the patients (ETDRS, 1991). Through computer simulations is possible to demonstrate that prevention and treatment are relatively inexpensive if compared to the health care and rehabilitation costs incurred by visual loss or blindness (Javitt et al., 1994).

The shortage of ophthalmologists and the continuous increase of the diabetic population limits the screening capability for effective timing of sight-saving treatment of typical manual methods. Therefore, an automatic or semi-automatic system able to detect various type of retinopathy is a vital necessity to save many sight-years in the population. According to Luzio et al. (2004) the preferred way to detect diseases such as diabetic retinopathy is digital fundus camera imaging. This allows the image to be enhanced, stored and retrieved more easily than film. In addition, images may be transferred electronically to other sites where a retinal specialist or an automated system can detect or diagnose disease while the patient remains at a remote location.

Various systems for automatic or semi-automatic detection of retinopathy with fundus images have been developed. The results obtained are promising but the initial image quality is a limiting factor (Patton et al., 2006); this is especially true if the machine operator is not a trained photographer. Algorithms to correct the illumination or increase the vessel contrast exist (Chen & Tian, 2008; Foracchia et al., 2005; Grisan et al., 2006; Wang et al., 2001), however they cannot restore an image beyond a certain level of quality degradation. On the other hand, an accurate quality assessment algorithm can allow operators to avoid poor images by simply re-taking the fundus image, eliminating the need for correction algorithms. In addition, a quality metric would permit the automatic submission of only the best images if many are available.

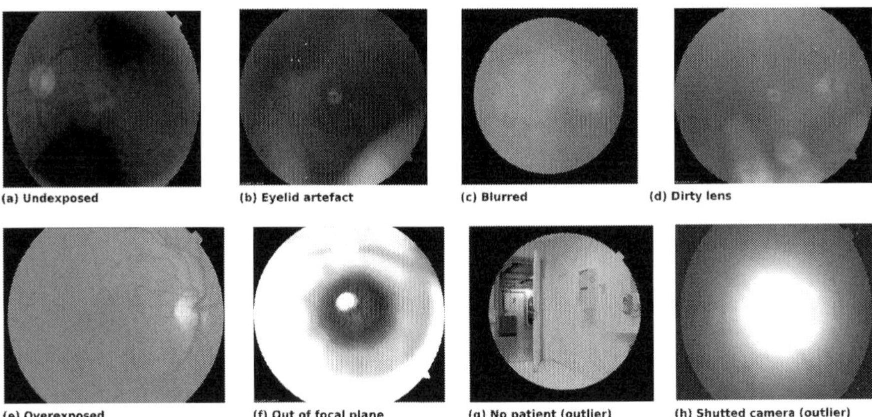

(a) Undexposed   (b) Eyelid artefact   (c) Blurred   (d) Dirty lens

(e) Overexposed   (f) Out of focal plane   (g) No patient (outlier)   (h) Shutted camera (outlier)

Fig. 1. Examples of Poor Quality Fundus Images (images extracted from datasets used in this study, see Section 4.1).

The measurement of a precise image quality index is not a straightforward task, mainly because quality is a subjective concept which varies even between experts, especially for images that are in the middle of the quality scale. In addition, image quality is dependent upon the type of diagnosis being made. For example, an image with dark regions might be considered of good quality for detecting glaucoma but of bad quality for detecting diabetic retinopathy. For this reason, we decided to define quality as the *"characteristics of an image that allow the retinopathy diagnosis by a human or software expert"*.

Fig. 1 shows some examples of macula centred fundus images whose quality is very likely to be judged as poor by many ophthalmologists. The reasons for this vary. They can be related to the camera settings like exposure or focal plane error (Fig. 1.(a,e,f)), the camera condition like a dirty or shuttered lens (Fig. 1.(d,h)), the movements of the patient which might blur the image (Fig. 1.(c)) or if the patient is not in the field of view of the camera (Fig. 1.(g)). We define an outlier as any image that is not a retina image which could be submitted to the screening system by mistake.

Existing algorithms to estimate the image quality are based on the length of visible vessels in the macula region (Fleming et al., 2006), or edges and luminosity with respect to a reference image (Lalonde et al., 2001; Lee & Wang, 1999). Another method uses an unsupervised classifier that employs multi-scale filterbanks responses (Niemeijer et al., 2006). The shortcomings of these methods are either the fact that they do not take into account the natural variance encountered in retinal images or that they require a considerable time to produce a result.

Additionally, none of the algorithms in the literature that we surveyed generate a "quality measure". Authors tend to split the quality levels into distinct classes and to classify images in particular ones. This approach is not really flexible and is error prone. In fact human experts are likely to disagree if many categories of image quality are used. Therefore, we think that a normalised "quality measure" from 0 to 1 is the ideal way to approach the classification problem.

Processing speed is another aspect to be taken into consideration. While algorithms to assess the disease state of the retina do not need to be particularly fast (within reason), the time

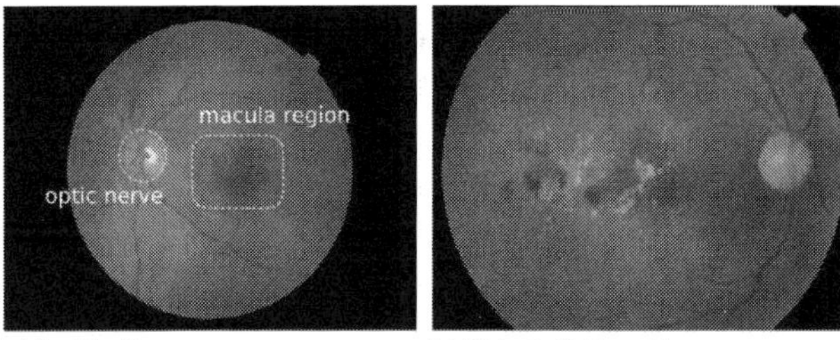

(a) Healthy Eye   (b) Diabetic Retinopathy

Fig. 2. Comparison of fundus images of an healthy and an unhealthy patient (images extracted from our datasets, see Section 4.1).

response of the quality evaluation method is key towards the development of an automatic retinopathy screening system.

This chapter is structured as follows. The rest of the introduction gives an brief overview of the anatomy of the retina and about diabetic retinopathy, which is useful to fully comprehend the algorithms that will be presented. Section 2 is a survey of existing techniques to evaluate the quality of retina fundus images. In Section 3 we introduce a quality assessment technique based on a new set of features called ELVD. Section 4 describes the tests and results obtained. Section 5 concludes the chapter.

1.1 Anatomy of the Retina

The retina is a multi-layered sensory tissue that lies on the back of the eye. It contains millions of photoreceptors that capture light rays and convert them into electrical impulses. These impulses travel along the optic nerve to the brain where they are converted into images. Many retinal blood vessels supply oxygen and nutrients to the inner and outer layers of the retina. The former are visible, the latter are not since they are situated in the choroid (the back layer of the retina) (Cassin & Solomon, 1990).

There are two types of photoreceptors in the retina: rods and cones, named after their shape. Rod cells are very sensitive to changes in contrast even at low light levels, hence able to detect movement, but they are imprecise and insensitive to colour. They are generally located in the periphery of the retina and used for scotopic vision (night vision). Cones, on the other hand, are high precision cells capable of detecting colours. They are mainly concentrated in the macula, the area responsible for photopic vision (day vision). The very central portion of the macula is called the fovea, which is where the human eye is able to distinguish visual details at its best. While loss of peripheral vision may go unnoticed for some time, damage to the macula will result in loss of central vision, which has serious effects on the visual perception of the external world (Wyszecki & Stiles, 2000).

All the photoreceptors are connected to the brain through a dense network of roughly 1.2 million of nerves (Jonas et al., 1992). These leave the eye in a unique bundle, the optic nerve. Fig. 2.(a) shows where the macula and fovea areas are located.

1.2 Diabetic Retinopathy

Diabetes mellitus (DM) is a chronic, systemic, life-threatening disease characterised by disordered metabolism and abnormally high blood sugar (hyperglycaemia) resulting from low levels of the hormone insulin with or without abnormal resistance to insulin's effects (Tierney et al., 2002). DM has many complications that can affect the eyes and nervous system, as well as the heart, kidneys and other organs. Diabetic retinopathy (DR) is a vascular complication of DM which causes damages to the retina which leads to serious vision loss if not treated promptly. People with diabetes are 25 times more likely to develop blindness than individuals without diabetes. For any type of diabetes, the prevalence of diabetic retinopathy in people more than 40 years of age was reported to be 40.3% (Baker et al., 2008).

The National Eye Institute divides diabetic retinopathy in four subsequent stages:

- *Mild Nonproliferative Retinopathy:* At this earliest stage, microaneurysms occur. They are small areas of balloon-like swelling in the retina's tiny blood vessels.

- *Moderate Nonproliferative Retinopathy:* As the disease progresses, some blood vessels that nourish the retina are blocked. Lesions like exudates (fat deposits) and haemorrhages start to appear.

- *Severe Nonproliferative Retinopathy:* Many more blood vessels are blocked, depriving several areas of the retina with their blood supply. These areas of the retina send signals to the body to grow new blood vessels for nourishment.

- *Proliferative Retinopathy (PDR):* At this advanced stage, the signals sent by the retina for nourishment trigger the growth of new blood vessels. These new blood vessels are abnormal and fragile. They grow along the retina and along the surface of the clear, vitreous gel that fills the inside of the eye. By themselves, these blood vessels do not cause symptoms or vision loss. However, they have thin, fragile walls. If they leak blood, vision loss and even blindness can result.

2. State of the Art of Fundus Images Quality Assessment

Computerised evaluation of image quality is a problem not only in the field of medical imaging but in many other image processing systems, such as image acquisition, compression, restoration and enhancement. Over the years, a number of researchers have developed general purpose algorithms to objectively assess the image quality with a good consistency with human judgements, regardless the type, scale or distortion of the image (Sheikh et al., 2006). In this section we present only techniques that are designed specifically for retinal fundus images. These methods attempt to simulate the judgement of an expert ophthalmologist rather than a generic human vision system. The methods are grouped in three different categories depending on the technique used: Histogram Based Methods, Retina Morphology Methods and "Bag-of-Words" Methods.

2.1 Histogram Based Methods

Besides some reference to Quality Assessment (QA) in research reports in the OPHTEL EU project (Mann, 1997), the first authors that have explicitly addressed the problem of automatic detection of fundus image quality are Lee and Wang (Lee & Wang, 1999). Their approach starts from a pure signal processing perspective with the aim of providing a quantitative measure to compare and evaluate retinal images enhancement methods in further studies. They used 20 images with excellent quality extracted from a set of 360. These reference images are used to compute an ideal template intensity histogram discarding any information about the colour. The template histogram is adjusted in order to approximate a Gaussian distribution as follows:

$$f(i) = A \cdot \exp\left(\frac{-(i - M)^2}{2\sigma^2}\right) \qquad (1)$$

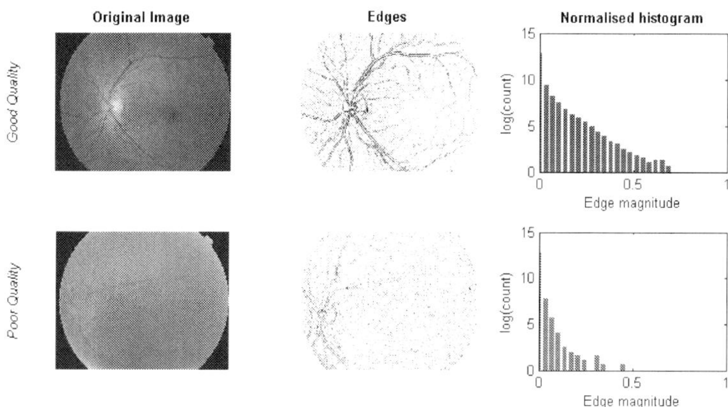

Fig. 3. Comparison of edges between a good and poor quality image

where i (from 0 to 255) is the pixel intensity, A is the peak value of the Gaussian curve, M and σ are respectively the mean and standard deviation of all the training histograms. In their tests, the authors estimated that $\sigma = R/6$ where R is the histogram spread. The quality of a target image is assessed by convolving its histogram with the template histogram and by computing a quality index Q. The index Q is normalised between 0 and 1 by employing the self correlation of the template histogram as the maximum value possible.

The key discriminating features in this method are the image contrast (i.e. the histogram spread), brightness and signal-to-noise ratio (SNR). New subsequent publications challenged the idea that pure histogram similarity is correlated with image quality. For example, Lalonde et al. (2001) found poor quality images whose histogram resembled the template histogram and also good quality images with markedly different histograms. Therefore, they tried to extend the approach of Lee and Wang maintaining the idea that a model of a good image is defined using a set of images of excellent quality but using two different sets of features: the distribution of the edge magnitudes in the image and the local distribution of the pixel intensity, as opposed to the global histogram of Lee and Wang. Their notion of quality differs from the one of Lee and Wang. Rather than viewing it from a pure signal processing perspective where quality is correlated with noise, they are closer to the medical field needs, whose concept of quality depends on the experts' ability to diagnose retinopathy.

Lalonde et al. notice that the edge magnitude histogram in a ophthalmic image has a shape that is similar to a Rayleigh distribution. In Fig. 3 the edge distributions are compared. The authors found that the edge distribution of poor images fall more rapidly than good images (notice that in the figure the histogram is plotted on a logarithmic scale). They evaluate the difference between two edges magnitude histogram using an equation similar to the χ^2 statistic:

$$d_{edge}(T, R) = \sum_i \frac{(R_i - T_i)^2}{R_i + T_i}, \quad \forall i | R_i + T_i \neq 0 \tag{2}$$

where R is the reference histogram and T is the edge histogram of the target image.

The second set of features used is a localised version of the global histogram of Lee and Wang. They retrieve the global histogram and segment it into uniform region by the standard histogram-splitting algorithm from Ohlander et al. (1978). Regions below a certain threshold are discarded. The dissimilarity W between reference and target image is calculated as follows:

$$W(h_1, h_2) = \left[\frac{\mu_{h_1} - \mu_{h_2}}{min(\mu_{h_1} \mu_{h_2})} \right] \tag{3}$$

It should be noticed that only the mean of the histogram is used in the equation; all the other information is discarded.

Finally, they classified the target images into three classes by using on the similarity measures given from Eq. 2 and 3. Using a dataset of 40 images they obtained 77% images classified correctly.

2.2 Retina Morphology Methods

Usher et al. (2003) were the first authors to consider features unique to retina images for QA. They noticed a correlation between image blurring and visibility of the vessels. By running a vessel segmentation algorithm and measuring the area of detected vessels over the entire image, the authors estimated if the quality of the image was sufficient for screening since images that are out of focus or blurred will not have visible smaller vessels. The classification between good and poor is performed by means of a threshold value. The authors employed a dataset of 1746 images taken from a retinopathy screening program obtaining a sensitivity of 84.3% and a specificity of 95.0%.

Fleming et al. (2006) found a problem in the previous approach: even if some vessels are undetectable in cases of image distortions, large vessels can remain visible, especially in the main arcades coming out from the optic nerve. These vessels have a substantial area which can easily be greater than the classifier threshold.

Consequently, they developed a method based on the image grading system used in the Grampian Diabetes Retinal Screening Programme in Aberdeen, Scotland. The QA score is divided into two aspects: image clarity and field definition. Image clarity is graded as follows:

- *Excellent:* Small vessels are clearly visible and sharp within one optic disc diameter around the macula. The nerve fibre layer is visible.

- *Good:* Either small vessels are clearly visible but not sharp within one optic disc diameter around the macula or the nerve fibre layer is not visible.

- *Fair:* Small vessels are not clearly visible within one optic disc diameter around the macula but are of sufficient clarity to identify third-generation branches within one optic disc diameter around the macula.

- *Inadequate:* Third-generation branches within one optic disc diameter around the macula cannot be identified.

Field definition is graded as follows:

- *Excellent:* The entire macula and optic disc are visible. The macula is centred horizontally and vertically in the image.

- *Good:* The entire macula and optic disc are visible. The macula is not centred horizontally and vertically in the image, but both main temporal arcades are completely visible and the macula is complete.

- *Inadequate:* Either a small-pupil artefact is present, or at least one of the macula, optic disc, superior temporal arcade, or inferior temporal arcade is incomplete.

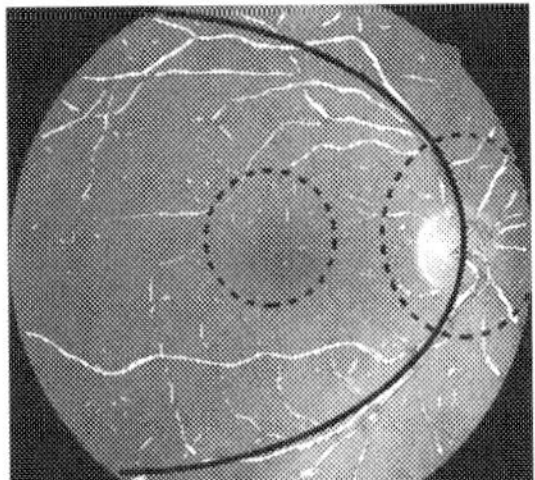

Fig. 4. Detected vessels (white) with the semiellipse fitted to the temporal arcades and the search regions for fovea and optic disk with the method described by Fleming et al. (2006).

First, a search is made for the arcade vessels. The generalised Hough transform (Ballard, 1981) is used to identify large-scale vessels between 10 and 30 pixels by employing semielliptical templates with different sizes, orientations and eccentricities. The process is quite computationally expensive. Hence, the image is subsampled by a factor of 32.
The authors estimate the average optic nerve diameter (OND) to be 246 pixels, based on a manual estimation of its the mean size in the dataset. The rightmost (or leftmost depending on the arcade template detected) point of the semiellipse fitted to the temporal arcades is used as a search centre for the optic disk. The search space is restricted to a region with height 2.4 x 2.0 times OND. Within this region a Hough transform is applied to detect the optic disk with a circular template.
The search area for the fovea is restricted to a circular region with diameter 1.6 OND centred on a point that is 2.4 OND from the optic disk and on a line between the detected optic disk and the centre of the temporal arcades. The fovea is actually found by identifying the maximum cross-correlation between the image and a predefined foveal model in the search area. Figure 4 shows the search region for the optic disk and fovea.
The image clarity was assessed taking into consideration the vessel area. However, instead of measuring it globally like Usher et al. (2003), only the area in the foveal region is used. The size of measured area is again relative to OND: a square of 3.5 OND if the foveal cross-correlation coefficient is large enough, otherwise a square sized 4.5 OND. The rationale for the choice of such area is the fact that in the foveal region there are the thinnest vessels, the ones that are more likely to disappear when the image is degraded.
The second aspect considered is the field definition. A fundus image with an adequate field definition has to satisfy the following constraints[1]:

- Distance between optic disk and the edge of the image < 0.5 OND
- Distance from the fovea to the edge of the image > 2 OND
- Angle between the fovea and the optic disk between 24.7° and -5.7°
- Length of the vessel arcades > 2.1 OND

The final classification of the overall quality is obtained by combining the two measures of image clarity and field definition. The authors reported a sensitivity and specificity respectively of 99.1% and 89.4% on a dataset of 1039 images. In this context, the sensitivity represents the "good quality" images correctly classified, while the specificity represents the correct classification on "poor quality" images.

---

[1] The measurement of all these constraints are possible thanks to the initial segmentation step.

2.3 "Bag of Words" Methods

Niemeijer et al. (2006) found various deficiencies in previous QA methods. They highlight that it is not possible to consider the natural variance encountered in retinal images by taking into account only a mean histogram of a limited set of features like Lalonde et al. (2001); Lee & Wang (1999). Niemeijer et al. acknowledge the good results of Fleming et al. (2006) but having to segment many retinal structures is seen as a shortcoming. In fact, detecting the segmentation failure in case of low quality is not trivial. Finally, they proposed a method that is comparable to the well known "Bag-of-Words" classification technique, used extensively in pattern recognition tasks in fields like image processing or text analysis (Fei-Fei & Perona, 2005; Sivic et al., 2005).

"Bag-of-Words" methods work as follows. First, a feature detector of some sort is employed to extract all the features from the complete training set. Because the raw features are too numerous to be used directly in the classification process, a clustering algorithm is run to express the features in a compact way. Each cluster is analogue to a "word" in a dictionary. In the dictionary, words do not have any relative information about the class they belong to or their relative location respect others. Instead, they are simply image characteristics that are often repeated throughout the classes, therefore they are likely to be good representatives in the classification process. Once the dictionary is built, the features of each sample are mapped to words and a histogram of word frequencies for each image is created. Then, these histograms are used to build a classifier and the learning phase ends. When a new image is presented to this type of system, its raw features are extracted and their word representation is searched in the dictionary. Then, the word frequency histogram is built and presented to the trained classifier which makes a decision on the nature of the image.

Niemeijer et al. employ two sets of feature to represent image quality: colour and second order image structure invariants (ISI). Colour is measured through the normalised histograms of the RGB planes, with 5 bins per plane. ISI are proposed by Romeny (ter Haar Romeny, 2003) who employed filterbanks to generate features invariant to rotation, position or scale. These filters are based on the gauge coordinate system, which is defined in each point of the image L by its derivative. Each pixel has a local coordinate system $(\vec{v}, \vec{w})$ where $\vec{w}$ points in the direction of the gradient vector $\left(\frac{\delta L}{\delta x}, \frac{\delta L}{\delta y}\right)$, and $\vec{v}$ is perpendicular to it. Because the gradient is independent of rotation, any derivative expressed in gauge coordinates is rotation independent too. Table 1 shows the equations to derive the gauge coordinates from the (x,y) coordinate system up to the second order. Notice that L is the luminosity of the image, L_x is the first derivative in the x direction, L_{xx} is the second derivative on the x direction, etc.

The ISI are made scale invariant by calculating the derivatives using Gaussian filters at 5 different scales, i.e. Gaussian with standard deviation $\sigma = 1, 2, 4, 8, 16$. Therefore the total number of filters employed is 5 x 5 = 25.

In Niemeijer et al. (2006), the authors derived the "visual words" from the feature by randomly sampling 150 response vector from the ISI features of 500 images. All vectors are scaled to zero mean and unit variance, and k-means clustering is applied. The frequency of the words is used to compute a histogram of the ISI "visual words" which, in conjunction with the RGB histogram is presented to the classifier.

Niemeijer et al. tested various classifiers on a dataset of 1000 images: Support Vector Machine with radial basis kernel (SVM), a Quadratic Discriminant Classifier (QDC), a Linear Discriminant Classifier (LDC) and a k-Nearest Neighbour Classifier (kNNC). The best accuracy is 0.974 obtained through SVM classifier.

Feature	Expression
L	L
L_w	$\sqrt{L_x^2 + L_y^2}$
L_{vv}	$\dfrac{-2L_x L_{xy} L_y + Lxx L_y^2 + L_x^2 L_{yy}}{L_x^2 + L_y^2}$
L_{vw}	$\dfrac{-L_x^2 L_{xy} + L_y^2 L_{xy} + L_x L_y (Lxx - L_{yy})}{L_x^2 + L_y^2}$
L_{ww}	$\dfrac{L_x^2 L_{xx} + 2L_x L_{xy} L_y + L_y^2 L_{yy}}{L_x^2 + L_y^2}$

Table 1. Derivation of the irreducible set of second order image structure invariants (Niemeijer et al., 2006).

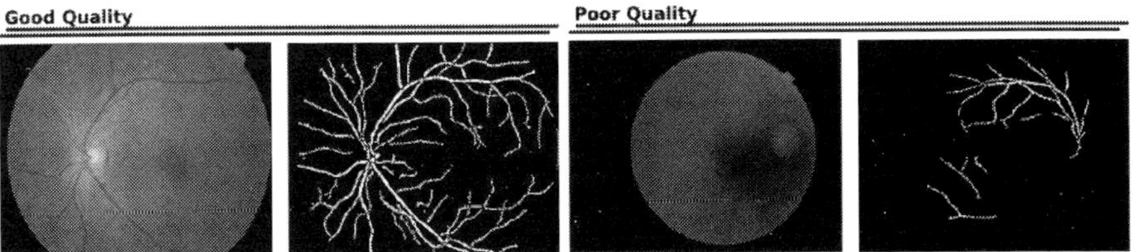

Fig. 5. Comparison of the vessel segmentation by our implementation of Zana & Klein (2001) in a good and a poor quality fundus image.

The whole QA process is called "image structure clustering" (ISC). They estimated a time of around 30 seconds to QA a new image[2].

3. Methodology

The QA proposed aims to be: *accurate* in its QA of patients of different ethnicities, *robust* enough to be able to deal with the vast majority of the images that a fundus camera can produce (outliers included), *independent* of the camera used, *computationally inexpensive* so that it can produce a QA in a reasonable time and, finally it should produce a *quality index* from 0 to 1 which can be used as input for further processing.

Our approach is based on the hypothesis that a vessel segmentation algorithm's ability to detect the eye vasculature correctly is partly related to the overall quality of an image. Fig. 5 shows the output of the vessel segmentation algorithm in images with different quality. It is immediately evident that the low vessel density in the bottom part of the right image is due to an uneven illumination and possibly to some blurring. However, a global measure of the vessel area (or vessel density) is not enough to discriminate good from bad quality images. One reason is that a considerable quantity of vessels area is taken by the two arcades which are likely to be detected even in a poor quality image as in Usher et al. (2003). Another problem is that the illumination or blurring might be uneven, making only part of the vessels undetectable. The visible vessels area can be enough to trick the QA into a wrong decision. Finally, this type of measure does not take into account outliers, artefacts caused by smudges on the lens or different Field of View (FOV) of the camera.

---

[2] Niemeijer et al. did not reported the hardware configuration for their tests, however in our implementation we obtained similar results (see Section 4.4)

The algorithm presented is divided in three stages: Preprocessing, Features Extraction and Classification. An in depth illustration of the full technique follows in the next sections.

3.1 Preprocessing
Mask Segmentation

The mask is defined as "a binary image of the same resolution of the fundus image whose positive pixels correspond to the foreground area". Depending on the settings, each fundus camera has a mask of different shape and size. Knowing which pixels belongs to the retina is a step that helps subsequent analysis as it gives various information about the effective size and shape of the image analysed.

Some fundus cameras (like the Zeiss Visucam PRO NM^{TM}) already provide the mask information. However, having the ability to automatically detect the mask has some benefits. It improves the compatibility across fundus cameras because it does not need to be interfaced with any sort of proprietary format to access the mask information. Also, if the QA is performed remotely, it reduces the quantity of information to be transmitted over the network. Finally, some image archives use a variety of fundus cameras and the mask is not known for each image.

The mask segmentation is based on region growing (Gonzales & Woods, 2002). It starts by extracting the green channel of the RGB fundus image, which contains the most contrast between the physiological features in the retina (Teng et al., 2002), hence this channel best describes the boundary between background and foreground. It is also the channel that is typically used for vessel segmentation. Then, the image is scaled down to 160x120, an empirically derived resolution which keeps the computational complexity as low as possible. Four seeds are placed on the four corners of the image with an offset equals to 4% of the width or height:

$$offset_w \leftarrow round(imageWidth \cdot 0.04)$$
$$offset_h \leftarrow round(imageHeight \cdot 0.04)$$
$$seed_{tl} = [offset_w; offset_h]$$
$$seed_{tr} = [imageWidth - offset_w; offset_h]$$
$$seed_{bl} = [offset_w; imageHeight - offset_h]$$
$$seed_{br} = [imageWidth - offset_w; imageHeight - offset_h]$$

where $seed_{xy}$ is the location of a seed. The reason for the offsets is to avoid regions getting "trapped" by watermarks, ids, dates or other labels that generally appear on one of the corners of the image.

The region growing algorithm is started from the 4 seeds with the following criteria:

1. The absolute grey-level difference between any pixel to be connected and the mean value of the entire region must be lower than 10. This number is based on the results of various experiments.

2. To be included in one of the regions, the pixel must be 4-connected to at least one pixel in that region.

3. When no pixel satisfies the second criterion, the region growing process is stopped.

When four regions are segmented, the mask is filled with negative pixels when it belongs to a region and positive otherwise. The process is completed scaling back the image to its original size by using bilinear interpolation. Even if this final step leads to a slight quality loss, the advantages in terms of computational time are worth the small imperfections at the edges of the mask.

"Virtual" FOV Identification

During the acquisition of a macula centred image, the patient is asked to look at fixed point visible at the back of the camera lens. In this way the macula is roughly located at the centre of the image Field of View (FOV). Even if the area viewed by different cameras is standardised, various vendors crop some part of the fundus images that do not contain useful information for diagnosis purposes.

In order to develop an algorithm that runs independently from the lost information, the "Virtual" FOV (VFOV) is extracted. The VFOV consists of an ellipse that represents the contour of the fundus image as if it was not cropped. This measure allows a simplification of the algorithm at further stages and it is the key component that makes the method independent of the camera FOV and resolution.

The classical technique to fit a geometric primitive such as an ellipse to a set of points is the use of iterative methods like the Hough transform (Leavers, 1992) or RANSAC (Rosin, 1993). Iterative methods, however, require an unpredictable amount of computational time because the size of the image mask could vary. Instead, we employ the non-iterative least squares based algorithm presented by Halir & Flusser (2000) which is extremely computationally efficient and predictable.

The points to be fitted by the ellipse are calculated using simple morphological operations on the mask. The complete procedure follows:

$\alpha \leftarrow$ erode($maskImage$)
$\gamma \leftarrow maskImage - \alpha$
fitEllipse(γ)

The erosion is computed with a square structuring element of 5 pixels. The binary nature of the image in this step (Fig. 6.b) makes the erosion very computationally efficient.

Vessel Segmentation

The ability to discern vessels from other structure is a preprocessing step of great importance in many medical imaging applications. For this reason many vessel segmentation algorithms

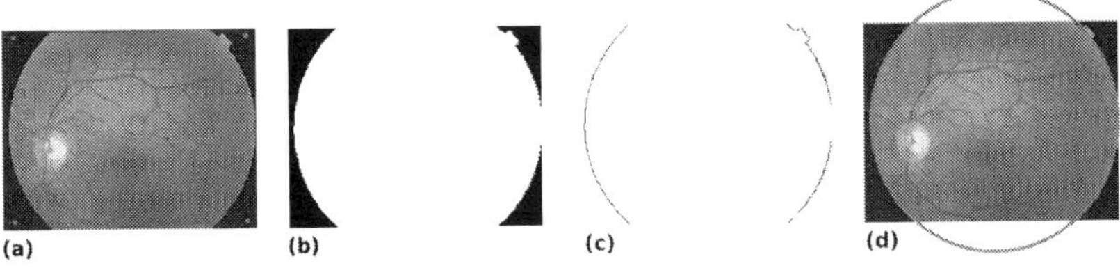

(a)　　　　　(b)　　　　　(c)　　　　　(d)

Fig. 6. (a) Original image with the 4 seeds (in red) placed. (b) Mask segmentation results. (c) Points used for VFOV detection. (d) VFOV detected.

have been presented in the literature (such as Lam & Hong, 2008; Patton et al., 2006; Ricci & Perfetti, 2007).

The technique chosen to segment veins and arteries visible in fundus images is based on the mathematical morphology method introduced by Zana and Klein (Zana & Klein, 2001). This algorithm proved to be effective in the telemedicine automatic retinopathy screening system currently developed in the Oak Ridge National Laboratory and the University of Tennessee at Memphis (Tobin et al., 2006). Having multiple modules that share the same vessel segmentation algorithm is a benefit for the system as a whole to prevent redundant processing.

Although there are more recently developed algorithms with somewhat improved performance relative to human observers, the Zana & Klein algorithm is useful because it does not require any training and its sensitivity to the quality of the image actually benefits the global QA.

This algorithm makes extensive use of morphological operations; for simplicity's sake the following abbreviations are used:

erosion: $\epsilon_B(S)$

dilation: $\delta_B(S)$

opening: $\gamma_B(S) = \delta_B(\epsilon_B(S))$

closing: $\phi_B(S) = \epsilon_B(\delta_B(S))$

geodesic reconstruction (or opening): $\gamma^{rec}_{S_{marker}}(S_{mask})$

geodesic closing: $\phi^{rec}_{S_{marker}}(S_{mask}) = N_{max} - \gamma^{rec}_{N_{max}-S_{marker}}(N_{max} - S_{mask})$

where B is the structuring element and S is the image to which it is applied, S_{marker} is the marker, S_{mask} is the mask and S_{max} is the maximum possible value of the pixel. A presentation of these morphological operators can be found in Vincent (1993).

The vessel segmentation starts using the inverted green channel image already extracted by the mask segmentation. In fact, the blue channel appears to be very weak without many information about vessels. On the other hand, the red band is usually too saturated since vessels and other retinal features emit most of their signal in the red wavelength.

The initial noise is removed while preserving most of the capillaries on the original image S_0 as follows:

$$S_{op} = \gamma^{rec}_{S_0}(Max_{i=1\ldots12}\{\gamma_{L_i}(S_0)\}) \tag{4}$$

where L_i is a linear structuring element 13 pixels long and 1 wide for a fundus image. For each i, the element is rotated of $15°$. The authors specify that the original method is not robust for changes of scale. However, since we have an estimation of the VFOV, we are in a position

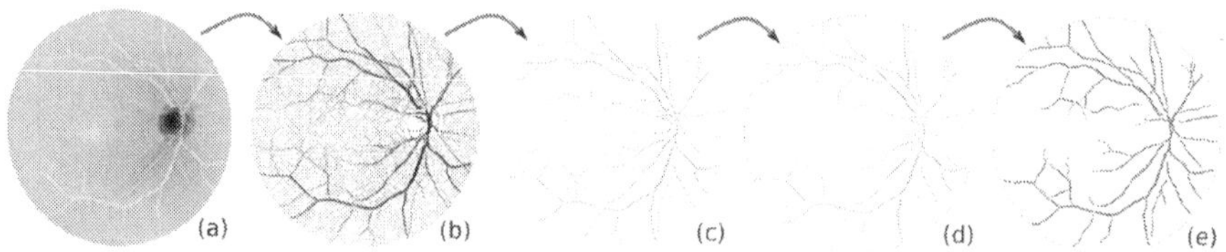

Fig. 7. Vessel segmentation summary. (a) Initial image (green channel). (b) Image after Eq. 5. (c) Image after Gaussian and Laplacian filter. (d) Image after Eq. 8. (e) Final segmentation after binarisation and removal of small connected components. All images, apart from the first one, have been inverted to improve the visualisation.

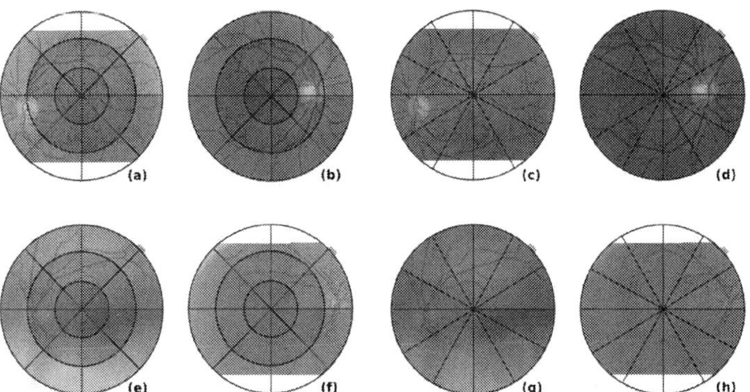

Fig. 8. Elliptical local vessel density examples. Even and odd columns respectively contain left and right retina images. In top row good quality images are shown, in the bottom row bad quality ones. The 4 images on the left use ELVD with $\theta = 8$ and $r = 3$; the 4 images on the right are the same ones but the parameters for ELVD are $\theta = 12$ and $r = 1$.

to improve it by dynamically changing the size elements depending on the length of the axes in the VFOV.

Vessels can be considered as linear bright shapes identifiable as follows:

$$S_{sum} = \sum_{i=1}^{1} 2(S_{op} - \gamma_{L_i}(S_0))\tag{5}$$

The previous operation (a sum of top hats) improves the contrast of the vessels but at the same time various unwanted structures will be highlighted as well. The authors evaluate the vessel curvature with a Gaussian filter (width=7px; $\sigma = 7/4$) and a Laplacian (size=3x3) obtaining the image S_{lap}. Then alternating the following operation the final result is obtained and the remaining noise patterns eliminated:

$$S_1 = \gamma_{S_{lap}}^{rec}(Max_{i=1...12}\{\gamma_{L_i}(S_lap)\})\tag{6}$$

$$S_2 = \phi_{S_1}^{rec}(Min_{i=1...12}\{\phi_{L_i}(S_1)\})\tag{7}$$

$$S_{res} = (Max_{i=1...12}\{\gamma_{L_i}^2(S_2)\} \geq 1)\tag{8}$$

As the last step of our implementation, we binarise the image and remove all the connected components that have an area smaller than 250 pixels. Once again this value is scaled depending on the VFOV detected. Fig. 7 shows a visual summary of the whole algorithm.

3.2 Feature Extraction
Elliptical Local Vessel Density (ELVD)
By employing all information gathered in the preprocessing phase, we are able to extract a local measure of the vessel density which is camera independent and scale invariant. Other authors either measure a similar feature globally like Usher et al. (2003), or they use a computationally expensive method like Fleming et al. (2006) whose approach requires a vessel segmentation, a template cross correlation and two different Hough transforms. Instead, we

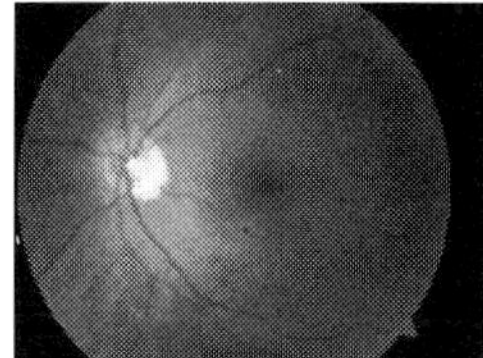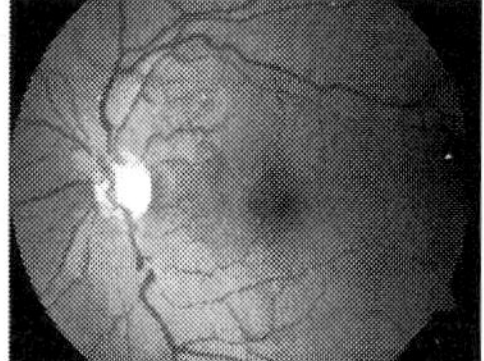

Fig. 9. Pigmentation difference between Caucasian (on the left) and African American (on the right) retinas. Images extracted from the datasets used in our tests (see section 4.1).

employ an "adaptable" polar coordinate system (θ, r) with the origin coincident with the origin of the VFOV. It is adaptable in the sense that its radius is not constant but it changes according to the shape of the ellipse. This allows to deal with changes of scale not proportional between height and width.

The Elliptical Local Vessel Density (ELVD) is calculated by measuring the vessel area under each local window, then normalised with zero mean and unit variance[3]. The local windows are obtained sampling r and θ. Different values of r and θ will tolerate or emphasize different problems with the image quality. In Fig. 8 for example, the 4 images on the left ($\theta = 8$ and $r = 3$) have 8 windows each on the centre of VFOV where the macula is located. In this fashion, ELVD features can detected a misaligned fundus image. On the other hand, the ELVD in the 4 images on the right ($\theta = 12$ and $r = 1$) will be more robust to macula misalignment, but more sensitive to vessel detection on both vascular arcades.

The idea behind ELVD is to create local windows that are roughly placed in consistent positions throughout different images. In the even or odd columns of Fig. 8, note that vessels close to the ON are in the same or nearby local windows, even if images have different FOVs. The power of this new style of windowing is its capability of capturing morphological information about fundus images without directly computing the position of ON, macula or arcade vessels, since these operations are computational expensive and prone to errors if the image has a very poor quality.

Luminosity/Colour Information

The analysis of the global colour information of the fundus image can contain useful information for the quality of the image. The method of Lee & Wang (1999) employed the histogram of the grey-level obtained from the RGB image as the only means to describe the image quality. The much more refined method of Niemeijer et al. (2006) uses 5 bins of each channel of the RGB histogram as additional features as input to the classifier. The authors presented results demonstrating that this piece of RGB information improved their classification respect to pure ISI features, even if ISI is representative of most of the retinal structures.

Inspired by Niemejer et al. we use colour information to represent aspects of quality that cannot be entirely measured with ELVD such as over/underexposed images in which the vasculature is visible or outliers with many features that are recognised as vessels.

All RGB channels are evaluated by computing the histogram for each plane. The histogram is normalised by the size of the mask in order to make this measure scale independent. It is noticed that people from different ethnic origin have a different pigmentation on the retina; this aspect is particularly noticeable in the blue and red channel. For example while Caucasians

---

[3] The zero mean and unit variance is calculated for each feature across all the training images.

have a fundus with a very strong red component people of African descent have a darker pigmentation with a much stronger blue component (see figure 9). In our case this is not an issue because we ensure we have adequate examples of different ethnic groups in our training library.

Also, the HSV colour space is employed as a feature. Only the saturation channel is used which seems to play an important role in the detection of the over/under exposition of the images. The reason is the channel relative independence from pigment and luminosity. Once again, the global histogram is extracted and normalised with the image mask.

Other Features

In addition to ELVD and colour information two other sets of features are considered as candidates to represent quality:

- *Vessel Luminosity:* Wang et al. (2001) noted that the grey level values of corresponding to the vessels can be used as a good approximation of the background luminosity. They proposed an algorithm that exploits this information to normalise the luminosity of the fundus images. If the vessel luminosity with the same elliptical windows used for the ELVD, we can measure the luminosity spread in the image. This can be particularly useful because poor quality images have often an uneven illumination.

- *Local Binary Patterns (LBP):* Texture descriptors are numerical measures of texture patterns in an image. LBP are capable of describing a texture in a compact manner independently from rotation and luminosity (Ojala & Pietikainen, 1996). The LBP processing creates binary codes depending on the relation between grey levels in a local neighbourhood. In the QA context this type of descriptor can be useful to check if the particular patterns found in a good quality retina are present in the image. This is accomplished by generating an histogram of the LBP structures found.

3.3 Classification

The majority of the authors who developed a QA metric for retinal images approached the classification in a similar way (Lalonde et al., 2001; Lee & Wang, 1999; Usher et al., 2003). The training phase consists of creating models of good and poor quality images (in some cases more intermediate models are employed) by calculating the mean of the features of the training sets. When a new retinal image is retrieved, its features are computed and the it is classified based on the shortest distance[4] to one of the models. This type of approach works reasonably well if the image to be classified is similar enough to one of the models. Also, it simplifies the calculation of a QA metric between 0 and 1 because distances can be easily normalised. However, this approach has a major drawback: the lack of generalisation on images with a large distance from the both models. This problem limits the method applicability in a real world environment.

Niemejer et al. (Niemeijer et al., 2006) are the only authors to our knowledge that approach the QA as a classic pattern classification problem. During the training phase they do not try to build a model or to make any assumption about the distribution of the data. Instead, they label each samples in one of the two classes and train one of the following classifiers: Support Vector Machines (SVM), Quadratic Discriminant Classifier (QDC), Linear Discriminant Classifier (LDC) and k-Nearest Neighbour Classifier (KNNC). Finally, they selected the classifier

---

[4] Distances calculations vary; some use Euclidean distance, others are based on correlation measures.

with the best performance (in their case a SVM with radial basis kernel) by testing it with a separate dataset.

Our classification technique is similar to the one of Niemeijer et al., but with two major differences. The first one is that the feature vector is created directly from the raw features without any need of pre-clustering, which can be computationally expensive, especially if a large number of features are used in a high dimensional space. The second difference is the fact that the classifier needs to output a posterior probability rather than a clear cut classification of a particular class. This probability will allow the correct classification of fair quality images even if the training is performed on two classes only.

4. Tests and Results

In this section, a summary of the most significant experiments performed during the development of the ELVD quality estimator are presented. The first section contains an overview of the datasets used. We then show the tests used for an initial evaluation of the QA proposed, the comparison with existing techniques and the choice of the classifier. Then, an analysis on possible optimisations of the feature set is performed. Finally the final QA system is tested on all the datasets and its computational performance is evaluated.

4.1 Data Sets

Various datasets are employed in the following tests. Each of them has peculiar characteristics that make it useful to test particular aspects of the QA classifier. The list follows:

- *"Abramoff"*: dataset composed of 10862 retinal images compiled by M. Abramoff as part of a study in the Netherlands. They were obtained using with different settings (FOV, exposure, etc.) on healthy and ill patients (Niemeijer et al., 2007). Three different cameras were used: Topcon NW 100, Topcon NW 200 and the Canon CR5-45NM. Unfortunately their quality was not labelled by the physicians.

- *"Aspen"*: dataset composed of 98 images that targets mainly patients with retinopathy conditions. This images were captured as part of a non-research teleophtalmology program to identify diabetic retinopathy in people leaving in the Aspen Health Region of Alberta, Canada (Rudnisky et al., 2007). Once again the quality was not labelled by the physicians.

- *"Chaum"*: this set is composed of 42 images extracted from the Abramoff dataset labelled as good and poor quality. They are good representatives of various aspects of the quality aspects of fundus images. These images were labelled by an expert in the field (Dr. E. Chaum) in order to facilitate the development of the QA system.

- *"ORNL"*: it is composed of 75 images extracted from the Abramoff dataset and labelled as good, fair and poor quality. These images were compiled at the Oak Ridge National Laboratory for the analysis of various aspects of the automatic diagnosis of diabetic retinopathy.

- *"African American"*: it contains 18 retina images of African American patients. All these images were labelled as good quality by Dr. E. Chaum. This dataset is of particular importance because it is very likely that most of the patients in Netherlands are Caucasian[5], but our system deployment is targeted toward the deep-to-mid South region of the United States of America where there is a large population of African Americans.

- *"Outliers"*: it is composed of 24 images containing various types of image outliers, all captured with a fundus camera.

4.2 Classifier Selection

In order to select the most appropriate classifier, a series of comparative tests is run on the "ORNL" and "Outliers" dataset. The results are compared with our implementation of the QA by Niemeijer et al. (2006), the most recent method found in the literature. The feature vector used by our classifiers is composed of ELVD with 3 slices and 8 wedges (ELVD 3x8) and the RGB colour histogram with 5 bins per channel. These tests were presented in the EMBC conference of 2008 and led to encouraging results (Giancardo et al., 2008).

The testing method used a randomised 2-fold validation, which works as follows. The samples are split in two sets A and B. In the first phase A is used for training and B for testing, then roles are inverted and B is used for training and A for testing. The performance of a classifier are evaluated using the Area Under the ROC curve (AUR) for $\frac{TruePositiveRate}{FalsePositiveRate}$ (TPR/FPR) and $\frac{TrueNegativeRate}{FalseNegativeRate}$ (TNR/FNR). See (Fawcett, 2004) for more details.

	ORNL set		ORNL + Outliers dataset	
Classifier	TPR/FPR	TNR/FNR	TPR/FPR	TNR/FNR
Nearest Neighbour	1	1	1	1
KNN (K=5)	1	1	0.99	0.98
SVM (Linear)	1	1	0.92	0.79
SVM (Radial)	1	1	1	1
ISC by Niemeijer et al.	1	0.88	1	0.88

Table 2. Good/Poor classifier test on "ORNL" and "Outliers" dataset. For the first four classifiers the feature vector used is ELVD 3x8 + RGB histogram with 5 bins.

In the two columns on left, table 2 shows the Good/Poor classification results for the "ORNL" dataset. All the classifiers using our feature vector have perfect or near-perfect performance in the selection between good and poor class, which is not the case for the Niemeijer et al. method (note that only the good and poor classes are used).

In the two columns on the right, all the Outliers dataset were added as test samples. An outlier image can have an enormous variability, therefore we feel that the training on this type of images might bias the classifier. Ideally, a classifier should be able to classify them as poor even if they are not fundus images as such. In this test, the classifiers performed differently, the best results are given by Nearest Neighbour classifier and SVM with a radial kernel.

Recall that the aim of this system is to generate a quality score from 0 to 1 to judge the image quality. In order to analyse this aspect, means and standard deviations of the scores obtained are displayed in Fig. 10. The classifiers are again trained on Good and Poor class (with 2-fold validation) but the Fair class is added to the testing samples without any explicit training on it. This allows to test the generalisation of the system. The most striking result of this test is the fact that the classifier with the poorest average AUR (SVM with a linear kernel) is also the one that achieves the best class separation, with an average score separation between Good and Poor classes of more than 0.8. The Fair class in this test has a mean score located at the middle of the scale.

---

[5] For privacy reasons the ethnicity of the subjects in the Abramoff dataset was not known.

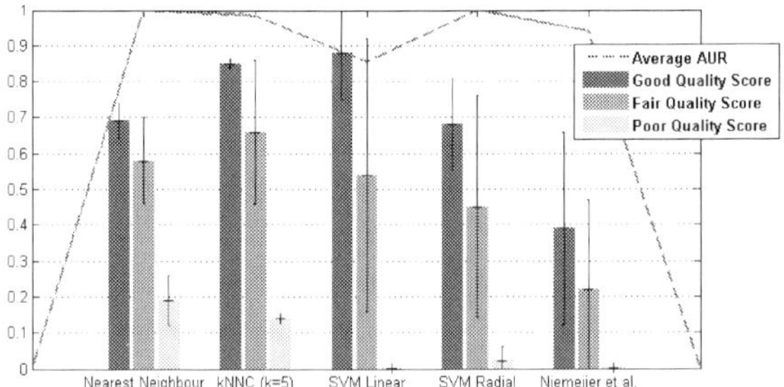

Fig. 10. Classifier scores test on "ORNL" dataset. For the first four classifiers the feature vector used is ELVD 3x8 + RGB histogram with 5 bins.

This apparent contradiction makes the selection of the classifier difficult. Therefore another series of tests was run on the more challenging "Chaum" dataset. In this case a leave-one-out strategy is used, i.e. the classifier is trained multiple times removing a different sample from the training set and using it as test target each time. This technique allows us to run complete tests using a relative small dataset.

Table 3 shows the results obtained employing the same classifiers and feature vector as before. While no classifier obtained ideal performance, the SVM with a linear kernel seems to have a good compromise between AUR and score separation. The small AUR advantages of KNN and Nearest Neighbour do not justify the computational performance issues that these type of classifiers have when many training samples in a high dimensional space are used, and also these classifiers have relatively low score difference between Good and Poor class.

Classifier	AUR TPR/FPR	AUR TNR/FNR	Average Good/Poor score difference
Nearest Neighbour	0.97	0.97	0.51
KNN (K=5)	0.97	0.97	0.51
SVM (Linear)	0.97	0.94	0.76
SVM (Radial)	0.94	0.91	0.54

Table 3. Good/Poor classifier test on "Chaum" dataset. The feature vector used is ELVD 3x8 + RGB histogram with 5 bins (the error bars show the average standard deviation).

The main problem of SVM with a linear kernel is its poor performance on the outliers, especially when compared with the results obtained by the other classifiers tested. For a better understanding of this behaviour part of the sample vectors are projected on a hyperplane which allows their representation in 2 dimensions. The hyperplane is calculated using the Linear Discriminant Analysis (Duda et al., 2001) on the Good and Poor samples, allowing a visualization of the space from the "point of view of the classifier".

Fig. 11 shows the result of the LDA calculation. While the distribution of Good and Poor class are well defined, the Outliers are spread throughout the LDA space. Nonlinear classifiers like Nearest Neighbour, KNN or SVM (Radial) can easily isolate the cluster of Good samples from the rest, but this is not a problem solvable by a linear function like the one employed by SVM (Linear).

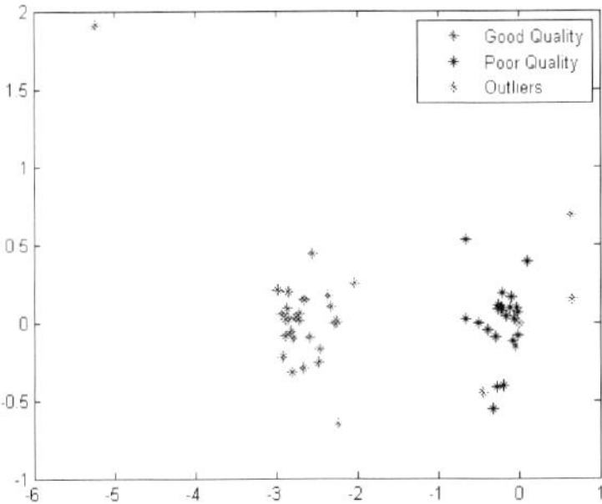

Fig. 11. 2D LDA Space Projection for ELVD features (Outliers not included in the LDA calculation).

4.3 Features Selection

It would be desirable to use the SVM (Linear) given its good score separation properties. One solution to this problem is the selection of new feature capable of linearising the space. However, the selection of adequate features allowing the SVM hyperplane to split the good quality samples from all the rest is not a straightforward task. Testing all the possible combination of the feature sets mentioned is impractical. Each feature set has many parameters: ELVD 36 (3 sets of radial section and 12 sets of wedges), Vessel Luminosity 36 (same as previously), RGB histogram 80 (all the channel combinations which can be normalised or not and 5 sets of histogram bins), HSV histogram 80 (same as previously) and LBP 4 (2 sets of radii length and 2 sets of LBP codes), for a total of 33 177 600 possible combinations.

Therefore an empirical approach was adopted. Firstly, it is assumed that all feature sets represent independent aspects of the fundus image quality. While this assumption is rather far-fetched, it does allow us to run only 324 tests to check all the possible permutation in each feature set, and also gives a feeling for what features are worth testing. Table 4 shows which are the parameters that achieved the best results for each feature set on the "Chaum" dataset. This dataset was chosen because is the most authoritative representation of good and poor quality image in most of the different aspects.

If feature sets were actually independent, the ideal feature vector would be composed by all of them with the parameters shown in Table 4. However, because there is almost certainly some degree of correlation, various parameters of the feature sets are selected based on their relative AUR and Good/Poor score difference and they are combined together for a total of 16 800 tests.

Surprisingly optimal results (Avg AUR of 1) and excellent good/poor score separability (0.91) are obtained with a relatively simple feature vector composed of:

- ELVD with 6 wedges and a single radial section

- The mask normalised histogram of the saturation with 2 bins

Feature Set	Parameters	Avg AUR	Average Good/Poor score difference
ELVD	16 rad. sec. & 6 wedges	0.98	0.74
RGB Hist	4 bins per ch. & mask norm.	0.81	0.51
HSV Hist	5 bins of Sat. & mask norm.	0.85	0.59
Vessel Luminosity	16 rad. sec. & 6 wedges	0.98	0.74
LBP	8 px radius & 8 codes	0.85	0.59

Table 4. Best results of each independent feature set on the "Chaum" dataset. The test is a leave-one-out with a SVM Linear classifier.

As it was suspected, the parameters that lead to the best results in this test are not the combination of the parameters found in each independent feature set test (table 4). However, they allowed to reduce the parameters search space and obtain excellent results with a relative simple combination.

4.4 Computational Performance

The performance of the C++ implementation of the ELVD QA is evaluated with a standard benchmarking technique. The complete ELVD QA system is run on 25 images randomly chosen from the "Chaum" dataset, during each iteration the time required to run the total system and each separate algorithm is recorded and averaged. All the images are scaled to the common resolution of 756x576 in order to have fairly consistent measurements. All the test were run on a 3.4 GHz Intel Pentium 4 machine with 2 GB of RAM.

Stage	Time (in milliseconds)
Mask Detection	116
VFOV	16
Vessel Segmentation	1920
ELVD	15
Saturation Histogram	25
Classification + Memory Allocation	38
Total	2130

Table 5. Relative performance of the different components in the ELVD QA C++ implementation.

The total time required to obtain a quality score for a single image is 2130 milliseconds. Table 5 shows how each system component contributes to the global computational time. The vessels segmentation is by far the main contributor having more the 10 times the computational cost of all the other algorithms summed together. The mask detection and the classification, two possibly expensive operations, are actually quite efficient considering the needs of this system. For comparison, a global benchmark was run on our implementation of the Niemeijer et al. QA classification (Niemeijer et al., 2006). The result obtained is well over 30 seconds, a time one order of magnitude greater than our approach. This is due to the many filterbanks that must be executed to calculate the raw features and the nearest neighbour operations to obtain the "words". However, the comparison between the two techniques should be taken with a bit of perspective because of the different implementation platforms. In fact the Niemeijer et al. algorithm is implemented in Matlab, a slower language than C++ because of its interpreted language nature. Nevertheless, we should point out that in our tests Matlab uses fast native code thanks to the Intel IPP libraries (Intel, 2007) for all the filtering operations, and these are very computationally efficient regardless of programming language choice.

5. Conclusion

At the beginning of the chapter, the quality assessment for fundus images was defined as "the characteristics of an image that allow the retinopathy diagnosis by a human or software expert". The literature was surveyed to find techniques which could help to achieve this goal. General image QA does not seem well suited for our purposes, as they are mainly dedicated to the detection of artefacts due to compression and they often require the original non-degraded image, something that does not make much sense in the context of QA for retinal images.

Our survey found five publications which tackled a problem comparable to the one of this project. They were divided into 3 categories: "Histogram Based", "Retina Morphology" and "Bag-of-Words". The authors of the first category approached the problem by computing relatively simple features and comparing them to a model of a good quality image. Although this approach might have advantages like speed and ease of training, it does not generalise well on the natural variability of fundus images as highlighted by Niemeijer et al. (2006) and Fleming et al. (2006). "Retina Morphology" methods started to take into account features unique to the retina, such as vessels, optic nerve or temporal arcades. This type approach considerably increased the QA accuracy. Remarkably, Fleming et al. developed a very precise way to judge the quality of image clarity and field definition which closely resembled what an ophthalmologist would do. The main drawbacks are time required to locate the various structures and the fact that if the image quality is too poor, some of the processing steps might fail, giving unpredictable results. This is unlikely to happen in the problem domain of Fleming et al. because they worked with images taken by trained ophthalmologists, but this is not the case with systems that can be used by personnel with basic training. The only method of the "Bag-of-Words" category is the one developed by Niemeijer et al. Their technique is based on pattern recognition algorithms which gave high accuracy and specificity. The main drawback is again speed of execution.

The new approach described in this chapter was partially inspired by all these techniques: colour was used as features as in the "Histogram Based" technique, the vessels were segmented as a preprocessing step like in the "Retina Morphology" techniques and the QA was computed by a classifier similar to the one used in the "Bag-of-Words" techniques. New features were developed and used such as ELVD, VFOV and the use of the HSV colour space, which was not evaluated by any of the previous authors for QA of fundus images. This made possible the creation of a method capable of classifying the quality of an image with a score from 0 to 1 in a period of time much shorter than "Retina Morphology" and "Bag-of-Words" techniques.

Features, classifier types and other parameters were selected based on the results of empirical tests. Four different types of datasets were used. Although none are very large (none contained more than 100 images) they were fairly good representative of the variation of fundus images in terms of quality, camera used and patient's ethnicity. In the literature, the method which seemed to perform best and which had the best generalisation was the one of Niemeijer et al. It was implemented and compared to our algorithm. Our results are in favour of the method presented in this chapter in terms of classification performance and speed. However, while our method has a clear advantage in terms of speed (it runs one order of magnitude faster because of the lower computational complexity), the comparison in terms of classification should be taken with care. In fact, Niemeijer et al. employed a dataset larger than ours to train the system.

The final algorithm was implemented in C++. Tests showed that it was able to produce a QA score in 2 seconds, also considering the vessel segmentation which can later be used by other modules of the global diabetic retinopathy diagnosis system.

In February 2009, the first clinic in a telemedicine network performing teleophthalmology went on-line in Memphis, Tennessee under the direction of Dr. E. Chaum. This network addresses an under served population and represents a valuable asset to broad-based screening of diabetic retinopathy and other diseases of the retina. A secure web-based protocol for submission of images and a database archiving system has been developed with a physician reviewing tool. All images are acquired from non-dilated retinal images obtained in primary care clinics and are manually reviewed by an ophthalmologist. As part of the submission process, all images undergo an automatic quality estimation using our C++ implementation of the ELVD QA.

6. References

Amos, A. F., McCarty, D. J. & Zimmet, P. (1997). The rising global burden of diabetes and its complications: estimates and projections to the year 2010., *Diabetic Medicine* **14 Suppl 5**: S1–85.

Baker, M. L., Hand, P. J., Wang, J. J. & Wong, T. Y. (2008). Retinal signs and stroke: revisiting the link between the eye and brain., *Stroke* **39**(4): 1371–1379.

Ballard, D. (1981). Generalizing the hough transform to detect arbitrary shapes, *Pattern Recognition* **13**: 111–122.

Cassin, B. & Solomon, S. (1990). *Dictionary of Eye Terminology*, Gainsville, Florida: Triad Publishing Company.

Chen, J. & Tian, J. (2008). Retinal vessel enhancement based on directional field, *Proceedings of SPIE*, Vol. 6914.

Duda, R. O., Hart, P. E. & Stork, D. G. (2001). *Pattern Classification*, Wiley-Interscience.

ETDRS (1991). Early photocoagulation fior diabetic retinopathy. early treatment diabetic retinopathy study report number 9, *Ophthalmology* **98**: 766–785.

Fawcett, T. (2004). Roc graphs : Notes and practical considerations for researchers, *Technical report*, HP Laboratories, 1501 Page Mill Road, Palo Alto, CA 94304, USA.

Fei-Fei, L. & Perona, P. (2005). A bayesian heirarcical model for learning natural scene categories, *Proceedings of CVPR*.

Fleming, A. D., Philip, S., Goatman, K. A., Olson, J. A. & Sharp, P. F. (2006). Automated assessment of diabetic retinal image quality based on clarity and field definition., *Investigative Ophthalmology and Visual Science* **47**(3): 1120–1125.

Foracchia, M., Grisan, E. & Ruggeri, A. (2005). Luminosity and contrast normalization in retinal images., *Medical Image Analysis* **9**(3): 179–190.

Giancardo, L., Abramoff, M. D., Chaum, E., Karnowski, T. P., Meriaudeau, F. & Tobin, K. W. (2008). Elliptical local vessel density: a fast and robust quality metric for retinal images, *Proceedings of IEEE EMBS*.

Gonzales, R. C. & Woods, R. E. (2002). *Digital Image Processing*, Prentice-Hall.

Grisan, E., Grisan, E., Giani, A., Ceseracciu, E. & Ruggeri, A. (2006). Model-based illumination correction in retinal images, *in* A. Giani (ed.), *Proceedings of 3rd IEEE International Symposium on Biomedical Imaging: Nano to Macro*, pp. 984–987.

Halir, R. & Flusser, J. (2000). Numerically stable direct least squares fitting of ellipses, *Department of Software Engineering, Charles University, Czech Republic* .

Intel (2007). *Intel Integrated Performance Primitives for the Windows OS on the IA-32 Architecture*, 318254-001us edn.
    URL: *http://developer.intel.com*

Javitt, J., Aiello, L., Chiang, Y., Ferris, F., Canner, J. & Greenfield, S. (1994). Preventive eye care in people with diabetes is cost-saving to the federal government, *Diabetes Care* **17**: 909–917.

Jonas, J. B., Schneider, U. & Naumann, G. O. H. (1992). Count and density of human retinal photoreceptors, *Graefe's Archive for Clinical and Experimental Ophthalmology* **230**: 505–510.

Lalonde, M., Gagnon, L. & Boucher, M. C. (2001). Automatic visual quality assessment in optical fundus images, *Proceedings of Vision Interface*, pp. 259–264.

Lam, B. S. Y. & Hong, Y. (2008). A novel vessel segmentation algorithm for pathological retina images based on the divergence of vector fields, *IEEE Transaction on Medical Imaging* **27**(2): 237–246.

Leavers, V. F. (1992). *Shape Detection in Computer Vision Using the Hough Transform*, Springer-Verlag New York, Inc. Secaucus, NJ, USA.

Lee, S. & Wang, Y. (1999). Automatic retinal image quality assessment and enhancement., *Proceedings of SPIE Image Processing*, pp. 1581–1590.

Luzio, S., Hatcher, S., Zahlmann, G., Mazik, L., Morgan, M. & Liesenfeld, B. (2004). Feasibility of using the tosca telescreening procedures for diabetic retinopathy, *Diabetic Medicine* **21**: 1121.

Mann, G. (1997). Ophtel project, *Technical report*, European Union.

Niemeijer, M., Abramoff, M. D. & van Ginneken, B. (2006). Image structure clustering for image quality verification of color retina images in diabetic retinopathy screening., *Medical Image Analysis* **10**(6): 888–898.

Niemeijer, M., Abramoff, M. D. & van Ginneken, B. (2007). Segmentation of the optic disc, macula and vascular arch in fundus photographs, *IEEE Trans Med Imag* **26**(1): 116–127.

Ohlander, R., Price, K. & Reddy, D. R. (1978). Picture segmentation using a recursive region splitting methods, *Computer Graphic and Image Processing* **8**: 313–333.

Ojala, T. & Pietikainen, M. (1996). A comparative study of texture measures with classification based on feature distribution, *Pattern Recognition* **29**: 51–59.

Patton, N., Aslam, T. M., MacGillivray, T., Deary, I. J., Dhillon, B., Eikelboom, R. H., Yogesan, K. & Constable, I. J. (2006). Retinal image analysis: concepts, applications and potential, *Progress in retinal and eye research* **25**(1): 99–127.

Ricci, E. & Perfetti, R. (2007). Retinal blood vessel segmentation using line operators and support vector classification, *IEEE Transaction on Medical Imaging* **26**(10): 1357–1365.

Rosin, P. L. (1993). Ellipse fitting by accumulating five-point fits, *Pattern Recognition Letters*, Vol. 14, pp. 661–699.

Rudnisky, C. J., Tennant, M. T. S., Weis, E., Ting, A., Hinz, B. J. & Greve, M. D. J. (2007). Web-based grading of compressed stereoscopic digital photography versus standard slide film photography for the diagnosis of diabetic retinopathy, *Ophthalmology* **114**(9): 1748–1754.

Sheikh, H. R., Sabir, M. F., Bovik, A. C., Sheikh, H., Sabir, M. & Bovik, A. (2006). A statistical evaluation of recent full reference image quality assessment algorithms, *IEEE Transactions on image processing* **15**(11): 3440–3451.

Sivic, J., Russell, B., Efros, A., Zisserman, A. & Freeman, W. (2005). Discovering object categories in image collections, *Proceedings of International Conference Computer Vision, Beijing*.

Teng, T., Lefley, M. & Claremont, D. (2002). Progress towards automated diabetic ocular screening: a review of image analysis and intelligent systems for diabetic retinopathy, *Medical and Biological Engineering and Computing* **40**(1): 2–13.

ter Haar Romeny, B. M. (2003). *Front-End Vision and Multi-Scale Image Analysis*, 1st edn, Springer.

Tierney, L. M., McPhee, S. J. & Papadakis, M. A. (2002). *Current medical Diagnosis & Treatment. International edition.*, New York: Lange Medical Books/McGraw-Hill.

Tobin, K. W., Chaum, E., Govindasamy, V. P., Karnowski, T. P. & Sezer, O. (2006). Characterization of the optic disc in retinal imagery using a probabilistic approach, *Proceedings of SPIE*, Vol. 6144.

Usher, D., Himaga, M. & Dumskyj, M. (2003). Automated assessment of digital fundus image quality using detected vessel area, *Proceedings of Medical Image Understanding and Analysis*, British Machine Vision Association (BMVA), pp. 81–84.

Vincent, L. (1993). Morphological grayscale reconstruction in image analysis: applications and efficient algorithms, *IEEE Journal of Image Processing* **2**(2): 176–201.

Wang, Y., Tan, W. & S C Lee, S. (2001). Illumination normalization of retinal images using sampling and interpolation, *Proceedings of SPIE*, Vol. 4322.

Wyszecki, G. & Stiles, W. S. (2000). *Color science: Concepts and methods, quantitative data and formulae.*, 2nd edn, New York, NY: John Wiley & Sons.

Zana, F. & Klein, J. C. (2001). Segmentation of vessel-like patterns using mathematical morphology and curvature evaluation, *IEEE Transaction on Image Processing* **10**(7): 1010–1019.

12

3D-3D Tubular Organ Registration and Bifurcation Detection from CT Images

Jinghao Zhou[1], Sukmoon Chang[2], Dimitris Metaxas[3] and Gig Mageras[4]

[1]*Department of Radiation Oncology*
The Cancer Institute of New Jersey
Robert Wood Johnson Medical School
University of Medicine and Dentistry of New Jersey
USA
[2]*Computer Science, Capital College, Pennsylvania State University*
USA
[3]*CBIM, Rutgers University*
USA
[4]*Department of Medical Physics*
Memorial Sloan-Kettering Cancer Center
USA

1. Introduction

The registration of tubular organs (pulmonary tracheobronchial tree or vasculature) of 3D medical images is critical in various clinical applications such as surgical planning and radiotherapy. For example, the pulmonary tracheobronchial tree or vascular structures can be used as the landmarks in lung tumor resection planning; the quantifying treatment effectiveness of the radiotherapy on lung nodules is based on the registration of the pulmonary tracheobronchial tree or vessels; the planning inter-patients partial liver transplants use registered contrast injection angiography (CTA) to create digital-subtraction contrast injection angiography (CTA) of liver vessels. The bifurcation of the tubular organs plays a critical role in clinical practices as well. Inflammation caused by bronchitis alters the airway branching configuration which causes various breathing problems (Luo et al., 2007). Atherosclerotic disease at the bifurcation has been widely known as a risk factor for cerebral ischemic episodes and infarction (Binaghi et al., 2001). The bifurcation points (or the branching points) have been chosen to build the validation protocol of the registration methods (Gee et al., 2002).

Many researchers have developed various methods for registration of tubular organs from medical images. Baert et al. (2004) used an intensity based 2D-3D registration algorithm to register the pre-operative 3D Magnetic Resonance Angiogram (MRA) data to the interventional digital subtraction angiography (DSA) images. Chan et al. (2004) proposed a 2D-3D vascular registration algorithm based on minimizing the sum of squared differences between the projected image and the reference DSA image. However, these registration methods are all developed for applications with 2D-3D registration. Chan & Chung (2003) solves a 3D-3D registration problem by transform the problem into 2D-3D registration problem. Aylward et al. (2003) presented a registration method by registering a model of the tubes in the source image directly with the target images. This method extracted an accurate model of the tubes in the source image and multiple target images without extractions could be registered with that model. However, this method does not utilize the information in the bifurcation points of the tubular organs.

In this chapter, we present a rigid registration method of the tubular organs based on the automatically detected bifurcation points of the tubular organs. There are two steps in our approach. We first perform a 3D tubular organ segmentation method to extract the centerlines of tubular organs and radius estimation in both planning and respiration-correlated CT images. This segmentation method automatically detects the bifurcation points by applying Adaboost algorithm with specially designed filters. We then apply a rigid registration method which minimizes the least square error of the corresponding bifurcation points between the planning CT images and the respiration-correlated CT (RCCT) images.

2. Method

Our method consists of two steps: the first step is the 3D tubular organ segmentation method to extract the centerlines of tubular organs in both planning and respiration-correlated CT images with the analysis of the Hessian matrix and bifurcation detection using Adaboost with specially designed filters (Zhou et al., 2007); in the second step, we apply a rigid registration method which minimizes the least square error of the corresponding bifurcation points between the planning and respiration-correlated CT images. Without loss of generality, we assume that the tubular organs appear brighter than the background and their centerlines coincide with the ridges in the intensity profile. When the vessel tree is segmented, the original CT images will be used. When the pulmonary tracheobronchial tree is segmented, the inverted CT images will be used.

2.1 Tubular organ segmentation and bifurcation detection
2.1.1 Tubular organ direction estimation and normal plane extraction

The eigenanalysis of the Hessian matrix is a widely used method for tubular organs detection (Danielsson & Lin, 2001; Lorenz et al., 1997; Zhou et al., 2006). The signs and ratios of the eigenvalues provide the indications of various shapes of interest, as summarized in Table 1. Also, the eigenvector corresponding to the largest eigenvalue can be used as an indicator of the elongated direction of tubular organs.

Given an image $I(x)$, the local intensity variations in the neighborhood of a point x_0 can be expressed with its Taylor expansion:

$$I(x_0 + h) \approx I(x_0) + h^T \nabla I(x_0) + h^T H(x_0)h$$

Eigenvalues	Shape
$\lambda_1 \leq 0, \lambda_2 \leq 0, \lambda_3 \leq 0$	blob
$\lambda_1 \leq 0, \lambda_2 \leq 0, \lambda_3 \approx 0$	tube
$\lambda_1 \leq 0, \lambda_2 \approx 0, \lambda_3 \approx 0$	plane
$\lambda_1 \leq 0, \lambda_2 \leq 0, \lambda_3 \geq 0$	double cone

Table 1. Criteria for eigenvalues and corresponding shapes.

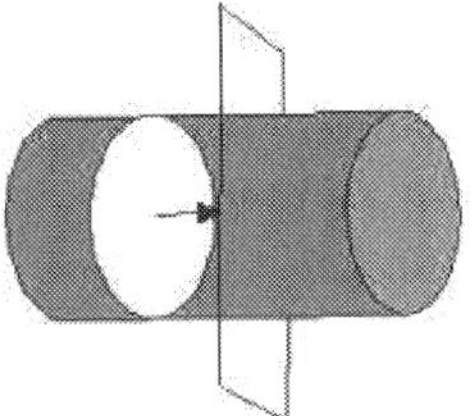

Fig. 1. Tracing along the direction of the tubular organs. Figure shows $\vec{e_3}$ and the normal plane defined by $\vec{e_1}$ and $\vec{e_2}$.

where, $\nabla I(x_0)$ and $H(x_0)$ denote the gradient and the Hessian matrix of I at x_0, respectively. Let $\lambda_1, \lambda_2, \lambda_3$ and $\vec{e_1}, \vec{e_2}, \vec{e_3}$ be the eigenvalues and eigenvectors of H such that $\lambda_1 \leq \lambda_2 \leq \lambda_3$ and $|\vec{e_i}| = 1$.

Tracing the centerlines of tubular organs by integrating along the elongated direction of tubular organs may be less sensitive to image noise (Aylward & Bullitt, 2002). Our method for tracing the centerlines of tubular organs starts from a preselected point (and, thereafter, from the point selected in the previous step) and follows the estimated direction of tubular organs to extract intensity ridges. The intensity ridges in 3D must meet the following constraints:

$$\lambda_1 \ll 0, \quad \lambda_2 \ll 0$$
$$\vec{e_1} \cdot \nabla I(x) \approx 0 \quad \text{and} \quad \vec{e_2} \cdot \nabla I(x) \approx 0$$

Note that the intensity reduces away from the ridge: $\lambda_1/\lambda_2 \approx 0$. Also note that the ridge point must be a local maximum of the plane defined by $\vec{e_1}$ and $\vec{e_2}$, while $\vec{e_3}$ is normal to the plane. Thus, $\vec{e_1}$ and $\vec{e_2}$ define the cross-sectional plane orthogonal to the tubular organs, while $\vec{e_3}$ provides the estimate of the tubular organs direction. Therefore, to trace tubular organs centerlines, the cross-sectional plane defined by $\vec{e_1}$ and $\vec{e_2}$ is shifting a small step along the direction of the tubular organs given by $\vec{e_3}$ (Fig. 1).

2.1.2 Bifurcation detection using AdaBoost

Boosting is a method for improving the performance of any weak learning algorithm which, in theory, only needs to perform slightly better than random guessing. A boosting algorithm called AdaBoost improves the performance of a given weak learning algorithm by repeatedly running the algorithm on the training data with various distributions and then combining the classifiers generated by the weak learning algorithm into a single final classifier (Freund & Schapire, 1996; Schapire, 2002). The proposed method uses AdaBoost with specially designed filters for fully automatic detection of bifurcation points.

We design three types of linear filters to capture the local appearance characteristics: 2D Gaussian filters to capture low frequency information; the first order derivatives of 2D Gaussian filters to capture high frequency information, i.e., edges; the second order derivatives of 2D Gaussian filters to capture local maxima, i.e., ridges (Lindeberg, 1999). These filters function as weak classifiers for AdaBoost.

We design three types of linear filters to capture the local appearance characteristics: 2D Gaussian filters to capture low frequency information; the first order derivatives of 2D Gaussian filters to capture high frequency information, i.e., edges; the second order derivatives of 2D

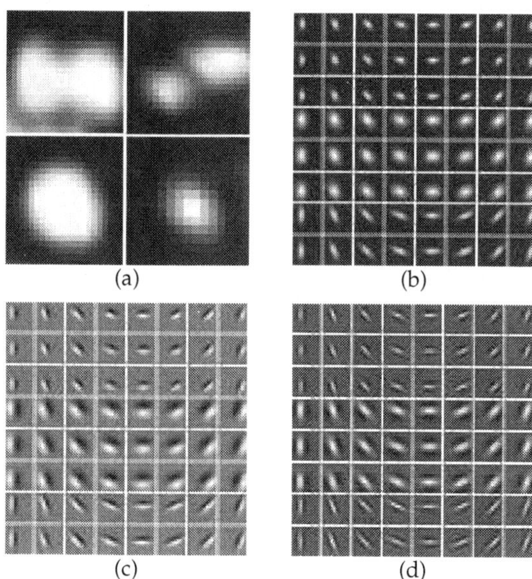

Fig. 2. (a) The cross-sectional planes of the pulmonary tracheobronchial tree with bifurcation (top row) and without bifurcation (bottom row), (b) 2D Gaussian used for low frequency information detection, (c) the first derivatives of Gaussian used for edge detection, and (d) the second derivatives of Gaussian used for ridge detection.

Gaussian filters to capture local maxima, i.e., ridges (Lindeberg, 1999). These filters function as weak classifiers for AdaBoost.

Let $G = G(\mu_x, \mu_y, \sigma_x, \sigma_y, \theta)$ be an asymmetric 2D Gaussian, where

$$\begin{pmatrix} \mu_x \\ \mu_y \end{pmatrix} = R \times \begin{pmatrix} x - x_0 \\ y - y_0 \end{pmatrix}, \quad R = \begin{pmatrix} \cos\theta & -\sin\theta \\ \sin\theta & \cos\theta \end{pmatrix}$$

and, (σ_x, σ_y), (x_0, y_0), and θ are the standard deviation, translation, and rotational parameters of G, respectively. We set the derivatives of G to have the same orientation as G:

$$G' = G_x \cos(\theta) + G_y \sin(\theta)$$
$$G'' = G_{xx} \cos^2(\theta) + 2\cos(\theta)\sin(\theta)G_{xy} + G_{yy}\sin^2(\theta)$$

From the above equations, we tune x_0, y_0, σ_x, σ_y, and θ to generate the desired filters. For a 15×15 sized window, we designed the total of $16,200$ filters—$x_0 \times y_0 \times (\sigma_x, \sigma_y) \times \theta = 10 \times 10 \times 3 \times 18 = 5,400$ filters for each of G, G', and G''. Some of the filter are shown in Fig. 2.

We then normalized the cross-sectional planes obtained from the previous step to the size of the filters and collected an example set containing both positive (i.e., samples with bifurcation) and negative (i.e., samples without bifurcation) examples from the normalized planes. The AdaBoost method is used to classify positive training examples from negative examples by selecting a small number of critical features from a huge feature set previously designed and creating a weighted combination of them to use as a strong classifier. Even when the strong classifier consists of a large number of individual features, AdaBoost encounters relatively few overfitting problems (Viola & Jones, 2001).

During the boosting process, every iteration selects one feature from the entire feature set and combines it with the existing classifier obtained from previous iterations. After a sufficient number of iterations, the weighted combination of the selected features become a strong classifier with high accuracy. That is, the output of the strong classifier is the weighted sum of the outputs of the selected features (i.e., weak classifiers): $F = \sum_t \alpha_t h_t(x)$, where α_t and h_t are weights and outputs of weak classifiers, respectively. We call F the bifurcation criterion. AdaBoost classifies an example plane as a sample with bifurcation when $F > 0$ and as a sample without bifurcation when $F < 0$.

To estimate the generalization error of AdaBoost in classification, we applied bootstrapping (Efron, 1983). We trained and tested the method on a bootstrap sample, i.e., a sample of size m chosen uniformly at random with replacement from the original example set of size m. the test error continues improving even after the training error has already become zero and converges to error rate of 3.9% after about 20 iterations of boosting steps, i.e., 95% confidence interval of 3.1~4.6%.

2.1.3 Tubular organs radius estimation for 3D reconstruction

We use a deformable sphere model to estimate the radii of the tubular organs for 3D tubular organs reconstruction (Zhou et al., 2007). At each of the detected center points as well as the detected branching points, a deformable sphere is initialized. The position of points on the model are given by a vector-valued, time varying function of the model's intrinsic coordinates $\vec{u}$:

$$\vec{x}(\vec{u},t) = (x_1(\vec{u},t), x_2(\vec{u},t), x_3(\vec{u},t))^T = \vec{c}(t) + \vec{R}(t)\vec{s}(\vec{u},t)$$

where, $\vec{c}(t)$ is the origin of a noninertial, model-centered reference frame Φ, $\vec{R}(t)$ is the rotation matrix for the orientation of Φ, and $\vec{s}(\vec{u},t)$ denotes the positions of points on the reference shape relative to the model frame Metaxas (1997). The reference shape of a sphere is generated in spherical coordinate system with fixed intervals along longitude and latitude directions in the parametric (u,v) domain:

$$\vec{e}(u,v) = \begin{pmatrix} x \\ y \\ z \end{pmatrix} = a_0 \cdot \begin{pmatrix} a_1 \cdot \cos u \cdot \cos v \\ a_2 \cdot \cos u \cdot \sin v \\ a_3 \cdot \sin u \end{pmatrix}$$

where, $a_0 \geq 0$ is a scale parameter and $0 \leq a_1, a_2, a_3 \leq 1$ are deformation parameters that control the aspect ratio of the cross section of the sphere. We collected the parameters in $\vec{e}(u,v)$ into the parameter vector

$$\vec{q}_s = (a_0, a_1, a_2, a_3)^T$$

The velocity of a point on the model is

$$\dot{\vec{x}} = \dot{\vec{c}} + \dot{\vec{R}}\vec{s} + \vec{R}\dot{\vec{s}} = \dot{\vec{c}} + \vec{B}\dot{\vec{\theta}} + \vec{R}\dot{\vec{s}} = \begin{bmatrix} I & B & RJ \end{bmatrix} \dot{\vec{q}} = L\dot{\vec{q}}$$

where, $\vec{\theta}$ is the vector of rotational coordinates of the model, $\vec{B} = \left[\partial(\vec{R}\vec{s})/\partial\vec{\theta} \right]$, $\vec{J} = [\partial\vec{s}/\partial\vec{q}_s]$, $\vec{q} = (\vec{q}_c^T, \vec{q}_\theta^T, \vec{q}_s^T)^T$, $\vec{q}_c = \vec{c}$, $\vec{q}_\theta = \vec{\theta}$, and $\vec{L}$ is the model's Jacobian matrix that maps generalized coordinates $\vec{q}$ into 3D vectors. When initialized near a vessel, the model deforms to fit to the vessel due to the overall forces exerted from the edge of the vessel and comes to rest when $\vec{q}$ is found that minimizes the simplified Lagrangian equation of motion:

$$\dot{q} = \vec{f}_{\vec{q}} = \int \vec{L}^T \vec{f} du$$

where, $\vec{f}_{\vec{q}}$ is the generalized external forces associated with the degrees of freedom $\vec{q}$ of the model and $\vec{f}$ is the external force exerted from the images. In this paper, we use Gradient Vector Flow (GVF) field computed from the images as the external force (Xu & Prince, 1998).

2.2 Tubular organs registration

The registration is formulated as a rigid global deformation. We denote the bifurcation points in the planning CT images as the source points and the corresponding bifurcation points in the respiration-correlated CT images as the target points. Since our tubular organs tracing starts from preselected points, the correspondence between the source points and the target points can be easily determined. The global deformation is a transformation of a point $\vec{x}$ in the planning CT image coordinate system into a point $\vec{x}'$ in the respiration-correlated CT image coordinate system, that is, $\vec{x}' = \vec{M} \cdot \vec{x}$, where $\vec{M}$ is the transformation matrix. Let $\vec{X}^P$ and $\vec{X}^B$ be the bifurcation points for the planning CT images and respiration-correlated CT images, respectively. The global deformation of $\vec{X}^P$ onto $\vec{X}^B$ is achieved by finding the parameters of a 3D transformation that minimizes the least square error:

$$\varepsilon = \sum_{i=1}^{n} \left\| \vec{x}_i^B - \vec{M} \cdot \vec{x}_i^P \right\|^2$$

where, $\vec{x}_i$ is the i-th point of a deformable model in the homogeneous coordinate system. We use Levenberg-Marquardt optimization method with the following Jacobian of the transformation as the metric to provide transformation parameter gradients:

$$\frac{\partial \varepsilon}{\partial \vec{M}} = -\sum_{i=1}^{n} 2(\vec{x}_i^B - \vec{M} \cdot \vec{x}_i^P)(\vec{x}_i^P)^T$$

3. Results

We applied our method on clinical lung CT data from six different patients. Each patient has one planning CT data set and ten respiration-correlated CT (RCCT) data sets taken in one complete respiratory cycle. They represent CT images at ten different points in the patient's breathing cycle. The number of slices in each CT scan ranged from 83 to 103 with 2.5mm slice thickness(and also digitally resliced to obtain cubic voxels, resulting in 206 to 256 slices), each of which are of size 512×512 pixels, with in-plane resolution of 0.9mm. All experiments were performed on a PC with 2.0GHz processor and 2.0GB of memory. We first extracted 507 cross-sectional planes from the VOIs using cross-sectional plane extraction method. The extracted planes were originally of size 30*30 pixels and were normalized to be the same size as the filter, i.e., 15*15 pixels. The smallest diameter of bronchi in our samples was 3 pixels. These example planes contained 250 positive (i.e., with bifurcation) and 257 negative (i.e., without bifurcation) examples. Our method was trained with 150 positive and 150 negative examples and tested on 100 positive and 107 negative examples. We performed bootstrapping

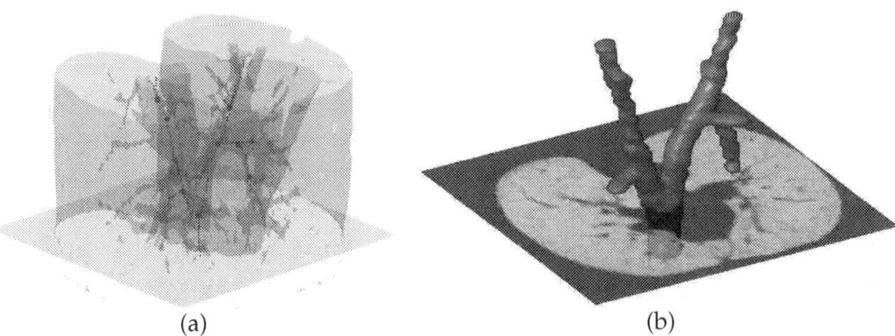

(a)   (b)

Fig. 3. Pulmonary tracheobronchial tree segmentation and bifurcation detection. (a) center-lines superimposed on an isosurface of the initial image, (b) 3D reconstruction of pulmonary tracheobronchial tree from the graph representation in (a). Blue points in (a) shows the bifurcation points detected by our method.

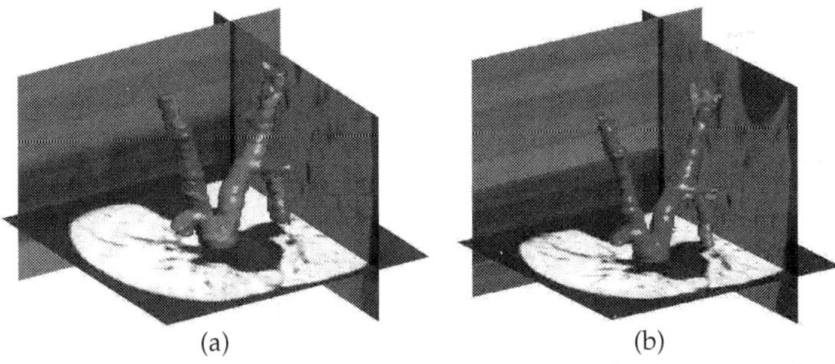

(a)   (b)

Fig. 4. Registration results. Blue shows the 3D reconstruction of pulmonary tracheobronchial tree in the registered planning images and red shows 3D reconstruction of pulmonary tracheobronchial tree in the respiration-correlated images.

to estimate the generalization error of our method, obtaining the mean error rate of 3.1~4.6%, which is 95% confidence interval, as described in previous section.

Fig. 3 illustrates further visual validation of our segmentation method applied to the pulmonary tracheobronchial structures. In Fig. 3(a), the extracted centerlines are superimposed on the isosurface of the original CT images along with the detected bifurcation points by the Adaboost learning method (shown in blue). Fig. 3(b) shows the 3D reconstruction of the pulmonary tracheobronchial tree from the centerlines and bifurcation points in Fig. 3(a). Fig. 4 shows the registration results. The results are also summarized in Table 2. It shows that, on average, the mean distance and the root-mean-square error (RMSE) of the corresponding bifurcation points between the respiration-correlated images and the registered planning images are less than 2.7 mm. There are breathing-induced deformations in the tracheobronchial tree, owing to the different amount of lung inflation in the different RCCT data sets. These may partly explain the mean distance and the root-mean-square error (RMSE) in Table 2.

Dataset	Mean distance (mm)	Root mean square error (mm)
Best	1.51	1.63
Worst	3.08	3.38
Average	2.17	2.63

Table 2. Results of the registration method on clinical datasets.

4. Conclusion

In this chapter, we present a novel method for tubular organs registration based on the automatically detected bifurcation points of the tubular organs. We first perform a 3D tubular organ segmentation method to extract the centerlines of tubular organs and radius estimation in both planning and respiration-correlated CT images. This segmentation method automatically detects the bifurcation points by applying Adaboost algorithm with specially designed filters. We then apply a rigid registration method which minimizes the least square error of the corresponding bifurcation points between the planning CT images and the respiration-correlated CT images. Our method has over 96% success rate for detecting bifurcation points. We present bery promising results of our method applied to the registration of the planning and respiration-correlated CT images. On average, the mean distance and the root-mean-square error (RMSE) of the corresponding bifurcation points between the respiration-correlated images and the registered planning images are less than 2.7 mm.

5. References

Aylward, S. & Bullitt, E. (2002). Initialization, noise, singularities, and scale in height ridge traversal for tubular object centerline extraction, *IEEE Transactions on Medical Imaging* **21**(2): 61–75.

Aylward, S., Jomier, J., Weeks, S. & Bullitt, E. (2003). Registration and analysis of vascular images, *International Journal of Computer Vision* **55**: 123–138.

Baert, S., Penney, G., van Walsum, T. & Niessen, W. (2004). Precalibration versus 2d-3d registration for 3d guide wire display in endovascular interventions, *MICCAI* **3217**: 577–584.

Binaghi, S., Maeder, P., Uské, A., Meuwly, J.-Y., Devuyst, G. & Meuli, R. (2001). Three-dimensional computed tomography angiography and magnetic resonance angiography of carotid bifurcation stenosis, *European Neurology* **46**: 25–34.

Chan, H. & Chung, A. (2003). Efficient 3d-3d vascular registration based on multiple orthogonal 2d projections, *Biomedical Image Registration* **2717**: 301–310.

Chan, H., Chung, A., Yu, S. & Wells, W. (2004). 2d-3d vascular registration between digital subtraction angiographic (dsa) and magnetic resonance angiographic (mra) images, *IEEE International Symposium on Biomedical Imaging* pp. 708–711.

Danielsson, P.-E. & Lin, Q. (2001). Efficient detection of second-degree variations in 2d and 3d images, *Journal of Visual Communication and Image Representation* **12**: 255–305.

Efron, B. (1983). Estimating the error rate of a prediction rule: Improvement on cross-validation, *Journal of the American Statistical Association* **78**: 316–331.

Freund, Y. & Schapire, R. (1996). Experiments with a new boosting algorithm, *the 13th International Conference on Machine Learning*, pp. 148–156.

Gee, J., Sundaram, T., Hasegawa, I., Uematsu, H. & Hatabu, H. (2002). Characterization of regional pulmonary mechanics from serial mri data, *MICCAI* pp. 762–769.

Lindeberg, T. (1999). Principles for automatic scale selection, *in* B. J. et al. (ed.), *Handbook on Computer Vision and Applications*, Academic Press, Boston, USA, pp. 239–274.

Lorenz, C., Carlsen, I.-C., Buzug, T. M., Fassnacht, C. & Weese, J. (1997). Multi-scale line segmentation with automatic estimation of width, contrast and tangential direction in 2d and 3d medical images, *CVPRMed-MRCAS*, pp. 233–242.

Luo, H., Liu, Y. & Yang, X. (2007). Particle deposition in obstructed airways, *Journal of Biomechanics* **40**: 3096–3104.

Metaxas, D. N. (1997). *Physics-Based Deformable Models: Applications to Computer Vision, Graphics and Medical Imaging*, Kluwer Academic Publishers.

Schapire, R. (2002). The boosting approach to machine learning: An overview, *MSRI Workshop on Nonlinear Estimation and Classification*.

Viola, P. & Jones, M. (2001). Robust real-time object detection, *Second International Workshop on Statistical and Computational Theories of Vision—Modeling, Learning, and Sampling*.

Xu, C. & Prince, J. (1998). Snakes, shapes, and gradient vector flow, *IEEE Transactions on Image Processing* **7**(3): 359–369.

Zhou, J., Chang, S., Metaxas, D. & Axel, L. (2006). Vessel boundary extraction using ridge scan-conversion and deformable model, *IEEE International Symposium on Biomedical Imaging* pp. 189–192.

Zhou, J., Chang, S., Metaxas, D. & Axel, L. (2007). Vascular structure segmentation and bifurcation detection, *IEEE International Symposium on Biomedical Imaging* pp. 872–875.

13

On breathing motion compensation in myocardial perfusion imaging

Gert Wollny[1,2], María J. Ledesma-Carbayo[1,2],
Peter Kellman[3] and Andrés Santos[1,2]
[1]*Biomedical Image Technologies, Department of Electronic Engineering, ETSIT,
Universidad Politécnica de Madrid, Spain*
[2]*Ciber BNN, Spain,*
[3]*Laboratory of Cardiac Energetics, National Heart, Lung and Blood Institute, NIH, DHHS,
Bethesda, MD
USA*

1. Introduction

First-pass gadolinium enhanced, myocardial perfusion *magnetic resonance imaging* (MRI) can be used to observe and quantify blood flow to the different regions of the myocardium. Ultimately such observation can lead to diagnosis of coronary artery disease that causes narrowing of these arteries leading to reduced blood flow to the heart muscle.

A typical imaging sequence includes a pre-contrast baseline image, the full cycle of contrast agent first entering the right heart ventricle (RV), then the left ventricle (LV), and finally, the agent perfusing into the LV myocardium (Fig. 1). Images are acquired to cover the full first pass (typically 60 heartbeats) which is too long for the patient to hold their breath. Therefore, a non-rigid respiratory motion is introduced into the image sequence which results in a misalignment of the sequence of images through the whole acquisition. For the automatic analysis of the sequence, a proper alignment of the heart structures over the whole sequence is desired.

1.1 State of the art

The mayor challenge in the motion compensation of the contrast enhanced perfusion imaging is that the contrast and intensity of the images change locally over time, especially in the region of interest, the left ventricular myocardium. In addition, although the triggered imaging of the heart results in a more-or-less rigid representation of the heart, the breathing movement occurs locally with respect to the imaged area, yielding non-rigid deformations within the image series. Various registration methods have been proposed to achieve an alignment of the myocardium. For example, Delzescaux et al. (Delzescaux et al., 2003) proposed a semi-automated approach to eliminate the motion and avoid the problems of intensity change and non-rigid motion: An operator selects manually the image with the highest gradient magnitude, from which several models of heart structures were created as a reference. By using potential maps and gradients they eliminated the influence of the intensity change and restricted the processing to the heart region. Registration was then achieved through translation only.

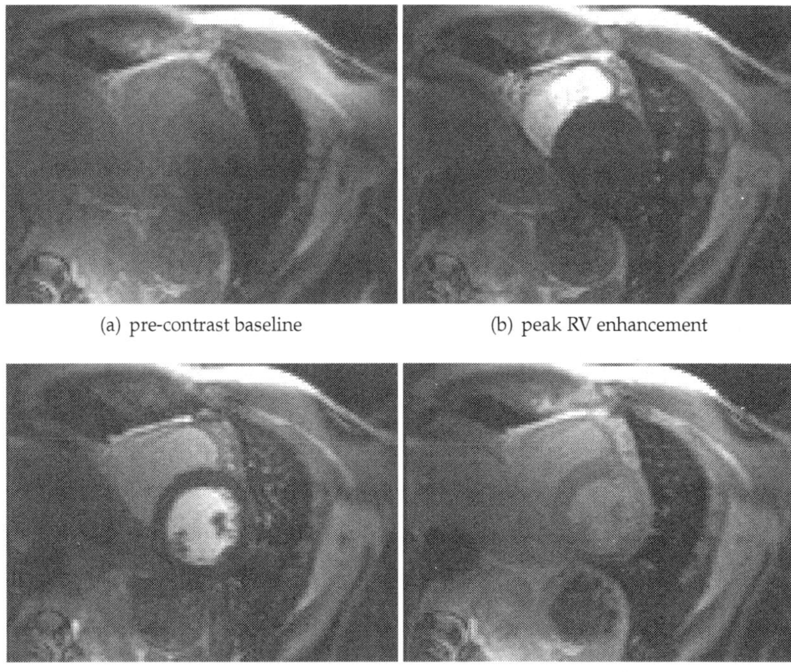

(a) pre-contrast baseline   (b) peak RV enhancement

(c) peak LV enhancement   (d) peak myocardial enhancement

Fig. 1. Images from a first-pass gadolinium enhanced, myocardial perfusion MRI of a patient
with chronic myocardial infarction (MI).

In (Dornier et al., 2003) two methods where described that would either use simple rectangular masks around the myocardium or an optimal masks, where the area with the high intensity change where eliminated as well. Rigid registration was then achieved by employing a
spline-based multi-resolution scheme and optimizing the sum of squared differences. They reported, that using an optimal mask yields results that are comparable to gold standard data set
measurements, whereas using the rectangular mask did not show improvements over values
obtained from the raw images. A two step registration approach was introduced by (Gupta
et al., 2003), the first step comprising the creation of a binary mask of the target area in all
images obtaining an initial registration by aligning their centers of mass. Then, in the second step, they restricted the evaluation of the registration criterion to a region around the
center of mass, and thereby, to the rigidly represented LV myocardium. By optimizing the
cross-correlation of the intensities, complications due to the intensity change were avoided
and rigid registration achieved.
Others measures that are robust regarding differences in the intensity distribution can be
drawn from Information Theory. One such measure is, e.g. *Normalized Mutual Information*(NMI) (Studholme et al., 1999). Wong et al. (Wong et al., 2008) reported its successful
use to achieve rigid motion compensation if the evaluation of the registration criterion was

restricted to the LV by a rectangular mask. One more sophisticated approach to overcome the problems with the local intensity change was presented by Milles et al. (Milles et al., 2007). They proposed to identify three images (base-line, peak RV enhancement, peak LV enhancement) by using Independent Component Analysis (ICA) of the intensity curve within the left and the right ventricle. These three images then form a vector base that is used to create a reference image for each time step by a weighted linear combination, hopefully exhibiting a similar intensity distribution like the according original image to be registered. Image registration of the original image to the composed reference image is then achieved by a rigid transformation minimizing the Sum of Squared Differences (SSD). Since the motion may also affect the ICA base images, this approach was later extended to run the registration in two passes (Milles et al., 2008).

Since rigid registration requires the use of some kind of mask or feature extraction to restrict the alignment process to the near-rigid part of the movement, and, since non-rigid deformations are not taken into account by these movements other authors target for non-rigid registration. One such example was presented in (Ólafsdóttir, 2005): All images were registered to the last image in the series were the intensities have settled after the contrast agent passed through the ventricles and the myocardium, and non-rigid registration was done by using a B-spline based transformation model and optimizing NMI. However, the evaluation of NMI is quite expensive in computational terms, and, as NMI is a global measure, it might not properly account for the local intensity changes.

Some other methods for motion compensation in cardiac imaging have been reported in the reviews in (Makela et al., 2002) and (Milles et al., 2008).

1.2 Our contribution

In order to compensate for the breathing movements, we use non-rigid registration, and to avoid the difficulties in registration induced by the local contrast change, we follow Haber and Modersitzki (Haber & Modersitzki, 2005) using a modified version of their proposed image similarity measure that is based on *Normalized Gradient Fields* (NGF). Since this cost function does not induce any forces in homogeneous regions of the chosen reference image, we combine the NGF based measure with SSD. In addition, we use a serial registration procedure, where only images are registered that follow in temporal succession, reducing the influence of the local contrast change further. The remainder of this chapter first discusses non-rigid registration, then, we focus on the NGF based cost measure and our modifications to it as well as combining the new measure with the well known SSD measure. We give some pointers about the validation of the registration, and finally, we present and discuss the results and their validation.

2. Methods

2.1 Image registration

Image registration can be defined as follows: consider an image domain $\Omega \subset \mathbb{R}^d$ in the d-dimensional Euclidean space and an intensity range $\mathbb{V} \subset \mathbb{R}$, a moving image $M : \Omega \to \mathbb{V}$, a reference image $R : \Omega \to \mathbb{V}$, a domain of transformations $\Theta := \{T : \Omega \to \Omega\}$, and the notation $M_T(\mathbf{x}) := M(T(\mathbf{x}))$, or short $M_T := M(T)$. Then, the registration of M to R aims at finding a transformation $T_{\text{reg}} \in \Theta$ according to

$$T_{\text{reg}} := \min_{T \in \Theta} \left(F(M_T, R) + \kappa E(T) \right). \tag{1}$$

F measures the similarity between the (transformed) moving image M_T and the reference, E ensures a steady and smooth transformation T, and κ is a weighting factor between smoothness and similarity. With non-rigid registration, the domain of possible transformations Θ is only restricted to be neighborhood-preserving. In our application, the F is derived from a so called voxel-similarity measure that takes into account the intensities of the whole image domain. In consequence, the driving force of the registration will be calculated directly from the given image data.

2.1.1 Image similarity measures

Due to the contrast agent, the images of a perfusion study exhibit a strong local change of intensity. A similarity measure used to register these images should, therefore, be of a local nature. One example of such measure are Normalized Gradient Fields (NGF) as proposed in (Haber & Modersitzki, 2005).

Given an image $I(\mathbf{x}) : \Omega \to \mathbb{V}$ and its noise level η, a measure ϵ for boundary "jumps" (locations with a high gradient) can be defined as

$$\epsilon := \eta \frac{\int_\Omega |\nabla I(\mathbf{x})| d\mathbf{x}}{\int_\Omega d\mathbf{x}}, \tag{2}$$

and with

$$\|\nabla I(\mathbf{x})\|_\epsilon := \sqrt{\sum_{i=1}^{d} (\nabla I(\mathbf{x}))_i^2 + \epsilon^2}, \tag{3}$$

the NGF of an image I is defined as follows:

$$\mathbf{n}_\epsilon(I, \mathbf{x}) := \frac{\nabla I(\mathbf{x})}{\|\nabla I(\mathbf{x})\|_\epsilon}. \tag{4}$$

In (Haber & Modersitzki, 2005), two NGF based similarity measures where defined,

$$F_{\text{NGF}}^{(\cdot)}(M, R) := -\frac{1}{2} \int_\Omega \|\mathbf{n}_\epsilon(R, \mathbf{x}) \cdot \mathbf{n}_\epsilon(M, \mathbf{x})\|^2 d\mathbf{x} \tag{5}$$

$$F_{\text{NGF}}^{(\times)}(M, R) := \frac{1}{2} \int_\Omega \|\mathbf{n}_\epsilon(R, \mathbf{x}) \times \mathbf{n}_\epsilon(M, \mathbf{x})\|^2 d\mathbf{x} \tag{6}$$

and successfully used for rigid registration. However, as discussed in (Wollny et al., 2008) for non-rigid registration, these measures resulted in poor registration: (5) proved to be numerically unstable resulting in a non-zero gradient even in the optimal case $M = R$, and (6) is also minimized, when the gradients in both images do not overlap at all. Therefore, we define another NGF based similarity measure:

$$F_{\text{NGF}}(M, R) := \frac{1}{2} \int_\Omega \|(\mathbf{n}_\epsilon(M) - \mathbf{n}_\epsilon(R)) \cdot \mathbf{n}_\epsilon(R)\|^2 d\mathbf{x}. \tag{7}$$

This cost function needs to be minimized, is always differentiable and its evaluation as well as the evaluation of its derivatives are straightforward, making it easy to use it for non-rigid registration. In the optimal case, $M = R$ the cost function and its first order derivatives are zero and the evaluation is numerically stable. $F_{\text{NGF}}(\mathbf{x})$ is minimized when $\mathbf{n}_\epsilon(R, \mathbf{x})$ and $\mathbf{n}_\epsilon(M, \mathbf{x})$ are parallel and point in the same direction and even zero when $\mathbf{n}_\epsilon(R, \mathbf{x})(\mathbf{x})$ and $\mathbf{n}_\epsilon(M, \mathbf{x})(\mathbf{x})$ have the same norm. However, the measure is also zero when $\mathbf{n}_\epsilon(R, \mathbf{x})$ has zero norm, i.e.

in homogeneous areas of the reference image. This requires some additional thoughts when good non-rigid registration is to be achieved. For that reason we also considered to use a combination of this NGF based measure (7) with the Sum of Squared Differences (SSD)

$$F_{SSD}(M, R) := \frac{1}{2} \int_{\Omega} (M(\mathbf{x}) - R(\mathbf{x})^2 \, d\mathbf{x} \tag{8}$$

as registration criterion. This combined cost function will be defined as

$$F_{Sum} := \alpha F_{NGF} + \beta F_{SSD} \tag{9}$$

with α and β weighting between the two parts of the cost functions.

2.1.2 Regularization, transformation space and optimization

Two measures are taken to ensure a smooth transformation: On one hand, the transformation is formulated in terms of uniform B-splines (Kybic & Unser, 2003),

$$T(x) := \sum_{i=0}^{(m-D)} P_i \beta_{i,D}(x - x_i) \tag{10}$$

with the control points P_i, the spline basis functions $\beta_{i,D}$ of dimension D, knots x_i, and a uniform knots spacing $h := x_i - x_{i-1} \forall i$. The smoothness of the transformation can be adjusted by the knot spacing h.
On the other hand, our registration method uses a Laplacian regularization (Sánchez Sorzano et al., 2005),

$$E_L(T) := \int_{\Omega} \sum_i^d \sum_j^d \left\| \frac{\partial^2}{\partial x_i \partial x_j} T(\mathbf{x}) \right\|^2 d\mathbf{x}. \tag{11}$$

As given in eq. (1) the latter constraint will be weighted against the similarity measure by a factor κ. To solve the registration problem by optimizing (1), generally every gradient based optimizer could be used. We employed a variant of the Levenberg-Marquardt optimizer (Marquardt, 1963) that will optimize a predefined number of parameters during each iteration which are selected based on the magnitude of the cost function gradient.

2.2 Serial registration

As the result of the myocardic perfusion imaging over N time steps $\mathfrak{S} := \{1, 2, ..., N\}$, a series of N images $\mathfrak{J} := \{I_i : \Omega \to \mathbb{V} | i \in \mathfrak{S}\}$ is obtained. In order to reduce the influence of the changing intensities, a registration of all frames to one reference frame has been rules out and replaced by a serial registration. In order to be able to choose a reference frame easily, the following procedure is applied: For each pair of subsequent images (I_i, I_{i+1}) registration is done twice, one selecting the earlier image of the series as a reference (backward registration), and the second by using the later image as the reference (forward registration). Therefore, for each pair of subsequent images I_i and I_{i+1}, a forward transformation $T^{i,i+1}$ and a backward transformation $T^{i+1,i}$ is obtained. Now, consider the concatenation of two transformations

$$T_a(T_b(\mathbf{x})) := (T_b \oplus T_a)(\mathbf{x}); \tag{12}$$

in order to align all image of the series, a reference frame i_ref is chosen, and all other images I_i are deformed to obtain the corresponding aligned image $I_i^{(\text{align})}$ by applying the subsequent forward or backward transformations

$$
I_i^{(\text{align})} := \begin{cases} I_i\left(\bigoplus_{k=i_\text{ref}}^{i+1} T^{k,k-1}(\mathbf{x}) \right) & \text{if } i < i_\text{ref}, \\ I_i\left(\bigoplus_{k=i_\text{ref}}^{i-1} T^{k,k+1}(\mathbf{x}) \right) & \text{if } i > i_\text{ref}, \\ I_{i_\text{ref}} & \text{otherwise.} \end{cases} \tag{13}
$$

In order to minimize the accumulation of errors for a series of n images one would usually choose $i_\text{ref} = \lfloor \frac{n}{2} \rfloor$ as the reference frame. Nevertheless, with the full set of forward and backward transformations at hand, any reference frame can be chosen.

2.3 Towards validation

In our validation, we focus on comparing perfusion profiles obtained from the registered image series to manually obtained perfusion profiles, because these profiles are the final result of the perfusion analysis and their accuracy is of most interest. To do so, in all images the myocardium of the left ventricle was segmented manually into six segments $S = \{S_1, S_2, ..., S_6\}$ (Fig. 2).

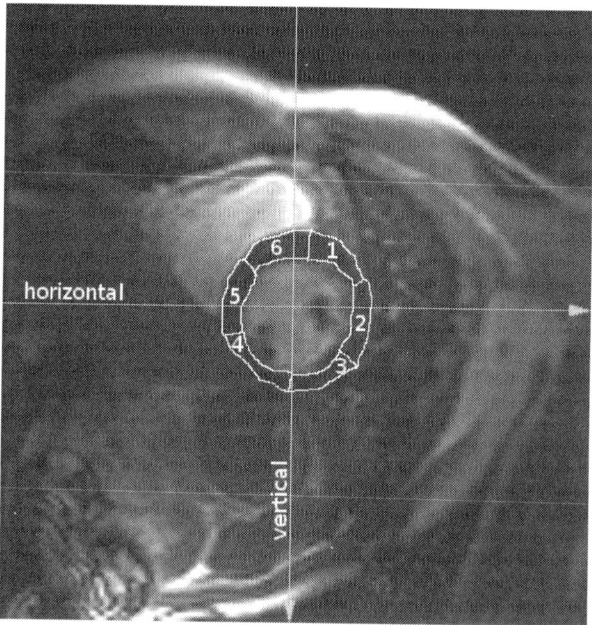

Fig. 2. Segmentation of the LV myocardium into six regions and horizontal as well as vertical profiles of the original image series.

The hand segmented reference intensity profiles $P_\text{hand}^{(s)}$ of the sections $s \in S$ over the image series were obtained by evaluating the average intensities in these regions and plotting those over the time of the sequence (e.g. Fig. 4). By using only the segmentation of the reference image I_{ref} as a mask to evaluate the intensities in all registered images, the registered intensity profiles $P_{\text{reg}}^{(s)}$ were obtained. Likewise, the intensity profiles $P_{\text{org}}^{(s)}$ for the unregistered, original series were evaluated based on the unregistered images.

In order to make it possible to average the sequences of different image series for a statistical analysis, the intensity curves K were normalized based on the reference intensity range $[v_{\min}, v_{\max}]$, with $v_{\min} := \min_{s \in S, t \in G} P_{\text{hand}}^{(s)}(t)$ and $v_{\max} := \max_{s \in S, t \in G} P_{\text{hand}}^{(s)}(t)$ by using

$$\hat{P} := \left\{ \left. \frac{v - v_{\min}}{v_{\max} - v_{\min}} \right| v \in P \right\}. \tag{14}$$

To quantify the effect of the motion compensation, the quotient of the sum of the distance between registered and reference curve as well as the sum of the distance between unregistered and reference curve are evaluated, resulting in the value Q_s as quality measure for the registration of section s:

$$Q_S := \frac{\sum_{t \in G} |\hat{P}_{\text{reg}}^{(s)}(t) - \hat{P}_{\text{hand}}^{(s)}(t)|}{\sum_{t \in G} |\hat{P}_{\text{org}}^{(s)}(t) - \hat{P}_{\text{hand}}^{(s)}(t)|} \tag{15}$$

As a result $Q_s > 0$ and smaller values of Q_s will express better registration.

As a second measure, we also evaluated the squared Pearson correlation coefficient R^2 of the manually estimated profiles and the unregistered respective the registration profiles. The range of this coefficient is $R^2 \in [0, 1]$ with higher values indicating a better correlation between the data sets. Since the correlation describes the quality of linear dependencies, it doesn't account for an error in scaling or an intensity shift. Finally, we consider the standard deviation of the intensity in the six sections S_i of the myocardium $\sigma_{s_i, t}$ for each time step $t \in G$. Since the intensity in these regions is relatively homogeneous, only noise and the intensity differences due to disease should influence this value. Especially, in the first part of the perfusion image series, when the contrast agent passes through the right and left ventricle, this approach makes it possible to assess the registration quality without comparing it to a manual segmentation: Any mis-alignment between the section mask of the reference image and the corresponding section of the analyzed series frame will add pixels of the interior of the ventricles to one or more of the sections, increasing the intensity range, and hence its standard deviation. With proper alignment, on the other hand, this value will decrease.

3. Experiments and results

3.1 Experiments

First pass contrast enhanced myocardial perfusion imaging data was acquired during free-breathing using 2 distinct pulse sequences: a hybrid GRE-EPI sequence and a trueFISP sequence. Both sequences were ECG triggered and used 90 degree saturation recovery imaging of several slices per R-R interval acquired for 60 heartbeats. The pulse sequence parameters for the true-FISP sequence were 50 degree readout flip angle, 975 Hz/pixel bandwidth, TE/TR/TI= 1.3/2.8/90 ms, 128x88 matrix, 6mm slice thickness; the GRE-EPI sequence parameters were: 25 degree readout flip angle, echo train length = 4, 1500 Hz/pixel bandwidth, TE/TR/TI=1.1/6.5/70 ms, 128x96 matrix, 8 mm slice thickness. The spatial resolution was approximately 2.8mm x 3.5mm. Parallel imaging using the TSENSE method with acceleration factor = 2 was used to improve temporal resolution and spatial coverage. A single dose of contrast agent (Gd-DTPA, 0.1 mmol/kg) was administered at 5 ml/s, followed by saline flush. Motion compensation was performed for seven distinct slices of two patient data sets covering different levels of the LV-myocardium. All in all we analyzed 17 slices from six different patients, three breathing freely, one holding his breath during the first half of the sequence, and breathing with two deep gasps in the second half, and two breathing shallow.

The registration software was implemented in C++, the registration procedure used B-Splines of degree 2 and varying parameters for the number $l \in \{1, 2, 3\}$ of multi-resolution levels, the knot spacing $h \in \{14, 16, 20\}$ pixels for the B-Spline coefficients, and the weight $\kappa \in \{0.8, 1.0, 2.0, 3.0\}$ of the Laplacian regularization term. Estimating the noise level of images is a difficult problem, we approximated η by $\sigma(\nabla I)$ standard deviation of the intensity gradient.

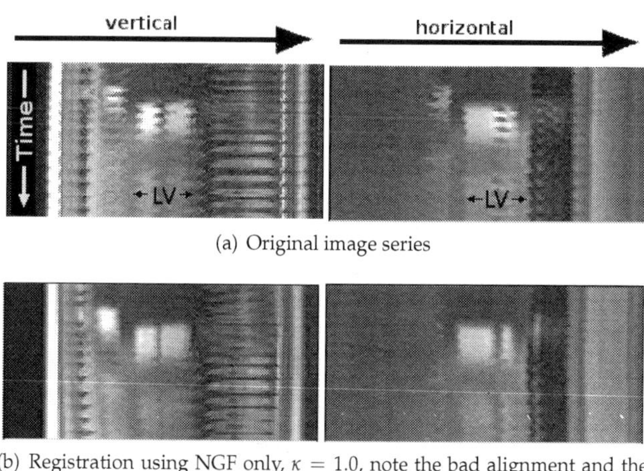

(a) Original image series

(b) Registration using NGF only, $\kappa = 1.0$, note the bad alignment and the drift in the second (lower) half of the series

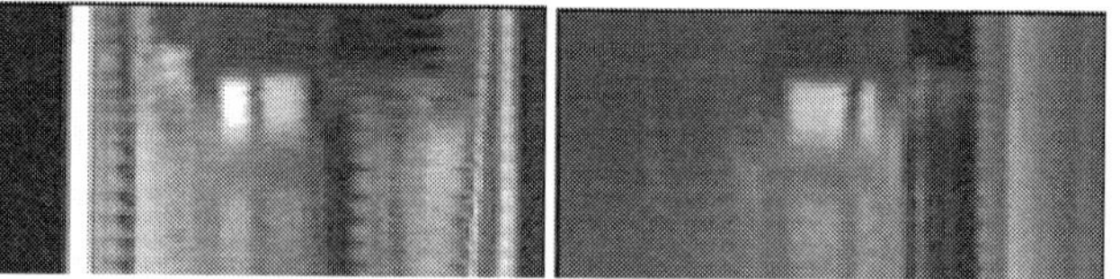

(c) Registration using NGF + 0.1 SSD, $\kappa = 2.0$, the drift vanished and alignment is in general better then with NGF only

Fig. 3.   Registration result by using $l = 3$ multi-resolution levels, and a knot spacing $h = 16mm$. Left: vertical cut, right: horizontal cut.

To ensure registration driving forces exist over the whole image domain, we also run experiments with the combined cost function (9), setting $\alpha = 1.0$ and $\beta \in 0.1, 0.5, 1.0$. Since all images are of the same modality, we expect that combining the two measures will yield the same or better results. Tests showed that applying F_{SSD} as only registration criterion doesn't yield usable results.

3.2 Registration results

Fully automatic alignment of a series of 60 images, including 118 image-to-image registrations at the full resolution of size 196x256 pixels and the transformation of the images to the reference frame 30, was achieved in approximately 5 minutes running the software on a Linux workstation (Intel(R) Core(TM)2 CPU 6600). This time could be further reduced if a bounding box were to be applied and by exploiting the multi-core architecture of the processing and running the registrations in parallel.

First, the quality of the registration was assessed visually observing videos as well as horizontal and vertical profiles through the time-series stack. An example of the profiles location is given in Fig. 2.

In terms of the validation measure, we obtained the best results using $l = 3$ multi-resolution levels and a knot-spacing of $h = 16$ pixels in each spacial direction. For the registration using NGF, a regularizer weight $\kappa = 1.0$ yielded best results, whereas for the combination of NGF and SSD $\kappa = 2.0$ was best. The registration by using F_{NGF} yields good results for the first half of the sequence, where the intensity contrast is higher, and the gradients are, therefore, stronger. In the second half, the sequential registration resulted in a bad alignment and a certain drift of the left ventricle (Fig. 3 (b)).

Combining F_{NGF} and F_{SSD} results in a significant improvement of the alignment for the second part of the sequence (Fig. 3 (c)) and provided similar results for the first half. Best results where obtained for $\beta = 0.5$. Following this scheme, a good reduction of the breathing motion was achieved in all of the analyzed slices.

The registration procedure performed equally well for all types of patient data - freely breathing, shallow breathing, and partial breath holding. It has to be noted though, that for some slices the registration didn't perform very well, resulting in errors that are then propagated through the far part of the series as seen from the reference point.

For the validation, the intensity curves before and after registration were obtained and compared to manually segmented ones (Fig. 4). In most cases, the intensity curves after registration resemble manual obtained ones very well, correlation between the two curves increased considerably 1.

		Mean	SD	Median	Min	Max
Q_s smaller is better		0.68	0.42	0.55	0.16	2.72
R^2 larger is better	unregistered	0.87	0.16	0.93	0.02	1.00
	registered	0.97	0.05	0.99	0.61	1.00
$\sigma_{*,*}$ smaller is better	unregistered	0.63	0.54	0.51	0.05	8.99
	registered	0.50	0.33	0.44	0.03	4.01
	segmented	0.46	0.22	0.41	0.04	1.30

Table 1. The registration quality Q_s, correlation R^2, and section intensity variation σ for the optimal parameters as given in the text.

The average and median of the quality measure Q_s support the findings of a generally good motion compensation, as do the improved correlation R^2 between the intensity profiles and the reduced intensity variations in the myocardium sections $\sigma_{*,*}$.

However, the maxima of Q_s above 1.0 indicate that in some cases motion compensation is not, or only partially achieved. For our experiments, which included 17 distinct slices and, hence, 102 myocardium sections, registration failed partially for 16 sections. This is mostly due to

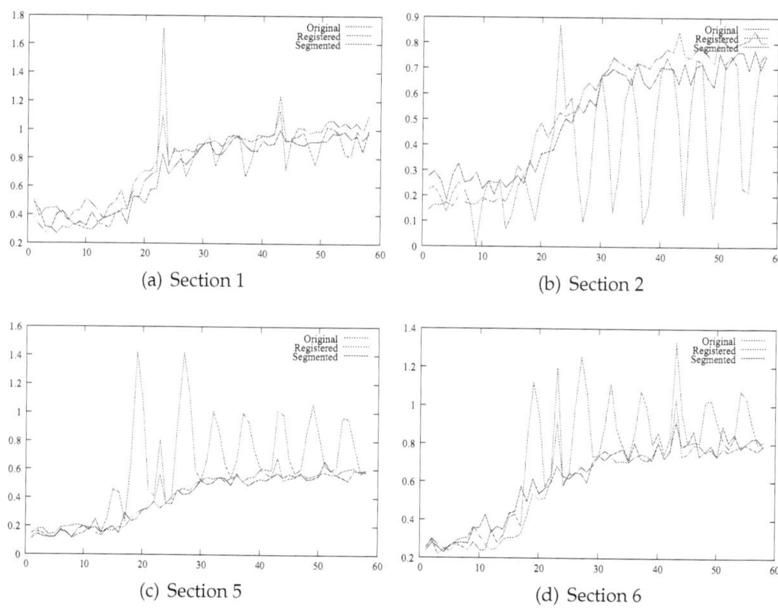

(a) Section 1

(b) Section 2

(c) Section 5

(d) Section 6

Fig. 4. Intensity curves before and after registration compared to the manually obtained ones. The alignment was evaluated by using frame 30 as reference. Note the periodic intensity change in the unregistered series that results from the breathing movement, and how well the registered series resembles the manually obtained intensity curve.

the serial registration procedure, where one failed registration of an image pair will propagate and small registration errors might accumulate when the final deformation is evaluated according to (13) and with respect to a certain reference image $I_{i_{ref}}$. In Fig. 5, these problems are illustrated: The registration of two frames, namely 13 and 14 in one of the analyzed series failed, resulting in partial misalignment of all images on the far side of this image pair with respect to the reference frame. For one section of the myocardium, this resulted in large errors for most of the first 13 frames in its intensity profile (Fig. 5(a)) which is also reflected by an increase of the standard deviation (Fig. 5(b)). In the second half of the series, registration errors accumulate, resulting in an ever increasing deviation of the intensity profile obtained by hand segmentation.

Note however, if only a part of the intensity profile is of interest, it is possible to minimize this accumulation of errors by selecting a proper reference frame and reducing the analysis to the part of the intensity profile. In the above example (Fig. 5), by restricting evaluation to the frames 15-35, and thereby, focusing on the upslope, it is shown that the registration quality is sufficient to analyze this part of the perfusion process, although a complete registration could not be achieved. This can be expressed in terms of the registration quality Q_s, which is greater than 1.0 in section 3 for two distinct reference frames when analyzing the full series, but smaller in the sub-range (Table 2).

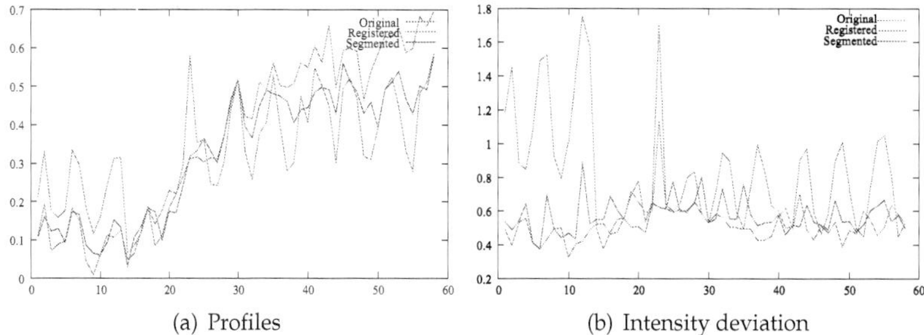

(a) Profiles (b) Intensity deviation

Fig. 5. In this intensity profile (a) the accumulation of registration errors is apparent which are in part reflected by the increased standard deviation (b).

Q_s	Sections of the myocardium					
(smaller is better)	1	2	3	4	5	6
full series, reference 30	0.88	0.42	1.52	0.31	0.17	0.29
full series, reference 25	0.77	0.35	1.07	0.38	0.18	0.36
frames 15-35, reference 30	0.80	0.31	0.56	0.22	0.12	0.23
frames 15-35, reference 25	0.48	0.24	0.29	0.26	0.12	0.34

Table 2. The registration quality Q, of a whole example series versus a part of it. Note, the dependence of the quality from the reference frame and the significantly better registration quality of the subset compared to the whole series.

4. Conclusion

In this work, we proposed a new scheme for breathing motion compensation in MRI perfusion studies based on non-rigid registration. In order to reduce the influence of the change of intensity, which is induced by the contrast agent as it passes through the both heart ventricles and the myocardium, we used a serial registration scheme where only subsequent images of the series are registered. In addition, we have introduced a new image similarity measure that is based on normalized gradient fields and was improved over the previous proposal in (Haber & Modersitzki, 2005). This measure is of a very local nature, and therefore, well suited to obtain non-rigid registration for images with local contrast change, as it is the case in myocardial perfusion MRI. Our experiments show that using this measure alone yields a good registration only for the images of the series that exhibit a high contrast and, hence, strong gradients in the regions of interest. When the intensity contrast is low, small registration errors may occur and, because of the serial registration scheme, these errors accumulate resulting an increasing misalignment over the series time course.

We were able to improve these results by combining the normalized gradient field based cost function with the sum of squared differences, so that the first would take precedence in regions with high contrast and, hence, strong gradients, while the latter ensures a steady registration in areas with low contrast and, therefore, small gradients.

The serial registration approach results in a high dependency on a good registration of all neighboring image pairs, if one is to obtain a good registration of the whole image series.

In addition, all over registration quality may vary depending on the reference frame chosen. However, for an analysis of only a part of the series, it is possible to reduce the influence of accumulating errors by selecting a reference close or within the time frame of interest resulting in sufficiently good registration.

5. ACKNOWLEDGMENTS

This study was partially supported by research projects TIN2007-68048-C02-01, CDTI-CDTEAM and SINBAD (PS-010000-2008-1) from SpainŠs Ministry of Science and Innovation.

6. References

Delzescaux, T., Frouin, F., Cesare, A. D., Philipp-Foliguet, S., Todd-Pokropek, A., Herment, A. & Janier, M. (2003). Using an adaptive semiautomated self-evaluated registration technique to analyze mri data for myocardial perfusion assessment, *J. Magn. Reson. Imaging* **18**: 681âŞ 690.

Dornier, C., Ivancevic, M., Thevenaz, P. & Vallee, J.-P. (2003). Improvement in the quantification of myocardial perfusion using an automatic spline-based registration algorithm, *J. Magn. Reson. Imaging* **18**: 160–168.

Gupta, S., Solaiyappan, M., Beache, G., Arai, A. E. & Foo, T. K. (2003). Fast method for correcting image misregistration due to organ motion in time-series mri data, *Magnetic Resonance in Medicine* **49**: 506 âŞ514.

Haber, E. & Modersitzki, J. (2005). Beyond mutual information: A simple and robust alternative, *in* A. H. Hans-Peter Meinzer, Heinz Handels & T. Tolxdorff (eds), *Bildverarbeitung für die Medizin 2005*, Informatik Aktuell, Springer Berlin Heidelberg, pp. 350–354.

Kybic, J. & Unser, M. (2003). Fast parametric elastic image registration, *IEEE Transactions on Image Processing* **12**(11): 1427–1442.

Makela, T., Clarysse, P., Sipila, O., Pauna, N., Pham, Q., Katila, T. & Magnin, I. (2002). A review of cardiac image registration methods, *IEEE Transactions on Medical Imaging* **21**(9): 1011–1021.

Marquardt, D. (1963). An Algorithm for Least-Squares Estimation of Nonlinear Parameters, *SIAM J. Appl. Math.* **11**: 431–441.

Milles, J., van der Geest, R. J., Jerosch-Herold, M., Reiber, J. H. & Lelieveldt, B. P. (2007). Fully automated registration of first-pass myocardial perfusion MRI using independent component analysis., *Inf Process Med Imaging* **20**: 544–55.

Milles, J., van der Geest, R., Jerosch-Herold, M., Reiber, J. & Lelieveldt, B. (2008). Fully automated motion correction in first-pass myocardial perfusion mr image sequences, *Medical Imaging, IEEE Transactions on* **27**(11): 1611–1621.

Ólafsdóttir, H. (2005). Nonrigid registration of myocardial perfusion MRI, *Proc. Svenska Symposium i Bildanalys, SSBA 2005, Malmø, Sweden,* SSBA. http://www2.imm.dtu.dk/pubdb/p.php?3599.

Sánchez Sorzano, C., Thévenaz, P. & Unser, M. (2005). Elastic registration of biological images using vector-spline regularization, *IEEE Transactions on Biomedical Engineering* **52**(4): 652–663.

Studholme, C., Hawkes, D. J. & Hill, D. L. G. (1999). An overlap invariant entropy measure of 3d medical image alignment, *Pattern Recognition* **32**(1): 71–86.

Wollny, G., Ledesma-Carbayo, M. J., Kellman, P. & Santos, A. (2008). A New Similarity Measure for Non-Rigid Breathing Motion Compensation of Myocardial Perfusion MRI, *Proc. of the 30th Int. Conf. of the IEEE Eng. in Medicine and Biology Society*, Vancouver, BC, Canada, pp. 3389–3392.

Wong, K., Yang, E., Wu, E., Tse, H.-F. & Wong, S. T. (2008). First-pass myocardial perfusion image registration by maximization of normalized mutual information, *J. Magn. Reson. Imaging* **27**: 529–537.

Silhouette-based Human Activity Recognition Using Independent Component Analysis, Linear Discriminant Analysis and Hidden Markov Model

Tae-Seong Kim and Md. Zia Uddin
Kyung Hee University, Department of Biomedical Engineering
Republic of Korea

1. Introduction

In recent years, Human Activity Recognition (HAR) has evoked considerable interest in various research areas due to its potential use in proactive computing (Robertson & Reid, 2006; Niu & Abdel-Mottaleb, 2004; Niu & Abdel-Mottaleb, 2006). Proactive computing is a technology that proactively anticipates peoples' necessity in situations such as health-care or life-care and takes appropriate actions on their behalf. A system capable of recognizing various human activities has many important applications such as automated surveillance systems, human computer interaction, and smart home healthcare systems. The most common method for activity recognition so far is based on video images from which features are extracted and compare with the pre-defined activity features. Hence, effective feature extraction, modeling, learning, and recognition technology play vital roles in a HAR system.

In general, binary silhouettes (i.e., binary shapes or contours) of various human activities are commonly employed to represent different human activities (Niu & Abdel-Mottaleb, 2004; Niu & Abdel-Mottaleb, 2006; Yamato et al., 1992). In (Niu & Abdel-Mottaleb, 2004) and (Niu & Abdel-Mottaleb, 2006), Principal Component (PC) of binary silhouette features were applied for view invariant human activity recognition. In (Yamato et al., 1992), 2-D mesh features of binary silhouettes extracted from video frames were used to recognize several tennis activities in time sequential images. In (Cohen & Lim, 2003), the authors used a view independent approach utilizing 2-D silhouettes captured by multiple cameras and 3-D silhouette descriptions with Support Vector Machine (SVM) for recognition. In (Carlsson & Sullivan, 2002), a silhouette matching key frame based approach was proposed to recognize forehand and backhand strokes from tennis video clips. In addition to the binary silhouette features, motion features have also been used in HAR (Ben-Arie et al., 2002; Nakata, 2006; Niu & Abdel-Mottaleb, 2004; Niu & Abdel-Mottaleb, 2006; Robertson & Reid, 2006; Sun et al., 2002). In (Ben-Arie et al., 2002), the authors proposed multi-dimensional indexing to recognize different actions represented by velocity vectors of major body parts. In (Nakata, 2006), the authors applied the Burt-Anderson pyramid to extract useful features consisting of multi-resolutional optical flows to recognize human activities. In (Niu & Abdel-Mottaleb, 2004) and (Niu & Abdel-Mottaleb, 2006), the authors augmented the optical flow motion features with the PC-based binary silhouette features to recognize different activities. In (Robertson & Reid, 2006), the authors described human action with trajectory information (i.e., position and velocity) and a set of local motion descriptors. In (Sun et al., 2002), the authors used affine motion parameters and optical flow for activity recognition.

Regarding fore-mentioned features so far, the most common feature extraction technique applied in video-based human activity recognition is Principal Component Analysis (PCA) (Niu & Abdel-Mottaleb, 2004; Niu & Abdel-Mottaleb, 2006). PCA is an unsupervised second order statistical approach to find useful basis for data representation. It finds PCs at the optimally reduced dimension of the input. For human activity recognition, it focuses on the global information of the binary silhouettes, which has been actively applied. However, PCA is only limited to second order statistical analysis, allowing upto decorrelation of data. Lately, a higher order statistical method called Independent Component Analysis (ICA) is being actively exploited in the face recognition area (Bartlett et al., 2002; Kwak & Pedrycz, 2007; Yang et al., 2005) and has shown superior performance over PCA. It has also been utilized successfully in other fields such as speech recognition (Kwon & Lee, 2004) and functional magnetic resonance imaging signals (Mckeown et al., 1998) but rarely on HAR.

Various pattern classification techniques are applied on the features in the reduced dimensional space for recognition from the time sequential events. Among them, Hidden Markov Models (HMM) have been used effectively in many works (Nakata, 2006; Niu & Abdel-Mottaleb, 2006; Niu & Abdel-Mottaleb, 2004; Sun et al., 2002; Yamato et al., 1992). In (Nakata, 2006) and (Sun et al., 2002), the authors utilized optical flows to build HMMs for recognition. In (Niu & Abdel-Mottaleb, 2004) and (Niu & Abdel-Mottaleb, 2006), the authors applied binary silhouette and optical flow motion features in combination with HMM. In (Yamato et al., 1992), the binary silhouettes were employed to develop distinct HMMs for different activities.

In this chapter, we present a novel approach utilizing independent binary silhouette-component and HMM for HAR (Uddin et al., 2008a; Uddin et al., 2008b). ICA is used for the first time on the activity silhouettes obtained from the activity video to extract the local features rather than global features produced by PCA. With the extracted features, HMM, a strong probabilistic tool to encode the time sequential information is employed to train and recognize different human activities from video. The IC-feature based approach shows better performance in recognition over PC features. In addition, the IC-features are further enhanced by Linear Discriminant Analysis (LDA) by finding out the underlying space that better discriminates the features of different activities, which leads further improvement in the recognition rate of HAR.

2. Methodology of the HMM-based Recognition System

Our recognition system consists of binary silhouette extraction, feature extraction, vector quantization, modeling, and recognition via HMM. The feature extraction is done over the extracted silhouettes from the activity video frames. The extracted features are then vector quantized by means of vector quantization to generate discrete symbol sequences for HMM for training and recognition. Fig. 1 shows the basic procedures of the silhouette feature-based activity recognition system using HMM.

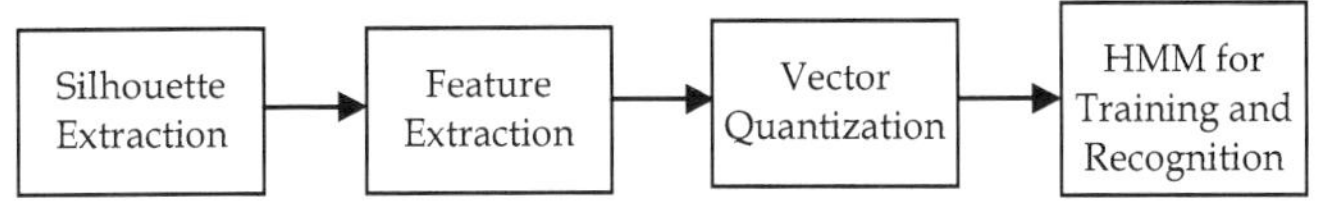

Fig. 1. Silhouette-based human activity recognition system using HMM.

2.1. Silhouette Extraction

A simple Gaussian probability distribution function is used to remove background from a
recent frame and to extract a Region of Interest (ROI). To extract the ROI, the background
subtracted difference image is converted to binary using a threshold that is experimentally
determined on the basis of subtraction result. Fig. 2 shows a generation of ROI from a
sample frame and Fig. 3 a couple of sequences of generalized ROIs for walking and running.

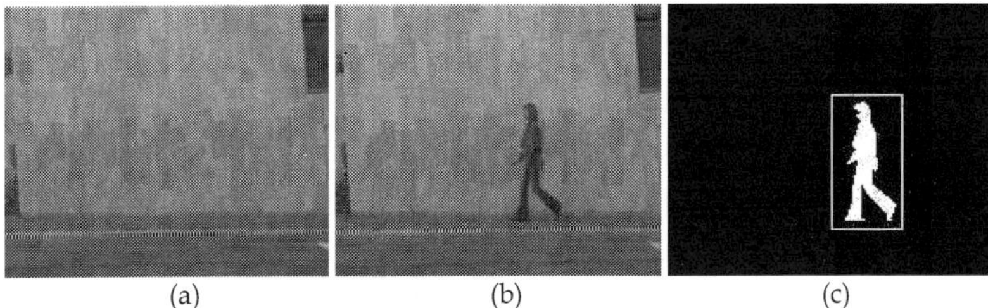

Fig. 2. (a) A Background image, (b) a frame from a walking sequence, and (c) a ROI
indicated with the rectangle.

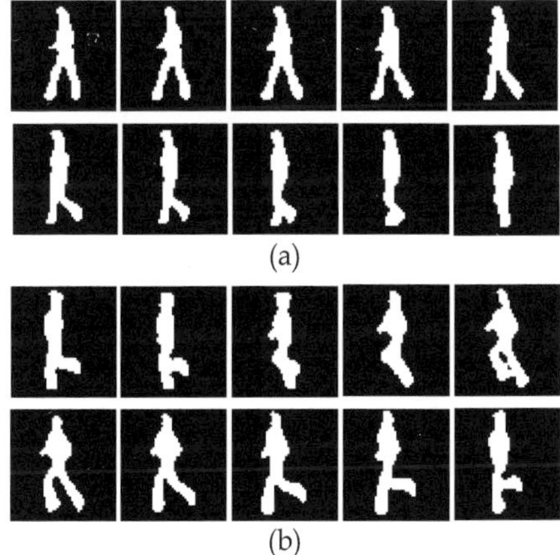

Fig. 3. Generalized ROIs or silhouettes from image sequences of (a) walking and (b) running.

To apply feature extraction on human activity binary silhouettes, every normalized ROI
image is represented as a row vector in a raster scan fashion where the dimension of the
vector is equal to the number of pixels in the entire image. Some preprocessing steps are

necessary before applying a feature extraction algorithm on the images. The first preprocessing step is to make all the training vectors as zero mean. Then the feature extraction algorithm is applied on the zero mean input vectors.

2.2. Feature Extraction Using PCA

PCA is a popular method to approximate original data in the lower dimensional feature space. The fundamental approach is to compute the eigenvectors of the covariance data matrix Q and then approximation is done using the linear combination of top eigenvectors. The covariance matrix of the sample training image vectors and the PCs of the covariance matrix can be calculated respectively as

$$Q = \frac{1}{T} \sum_{i=1}^{T} (\tilde{X}_i \tilde{X}_i^T) \tag{1}$$

$$E^T Q E = \Lambda \tag{2}$$

where E represents the matrix of orthonormal eigenvectors and Λ diagonal matrix of the eigenvalues. E reflects the original coordinate system onto the eigenvectors where the eigenvector corresponding to the largest eigenvalue indicates the axis of largest variance and the next largest one is the orthogonal axis of largest one indicating second largest variance and so on. Usually, the eigenvalues that are close to zero values carry negligible variance and hence can be excluded. So, the several m eigenvectors corresponding to the largest eigenvalues can be used to define the subspace. Thus the full dimensional silhouette image vectors can be easily represented in the reduced dimension.

However, PCA is a second order statistics-based analysis to represent global information such as average faces or eigenfaces in the case of face recognition. After applying PCA on human silhouettes of different activities, it produces global features representing frequently moving parts of human body in all activities. Fig. 4 shows 30 basis images after PCA is applied on 600 images of four activities: namely walking, running, right hand waving, and both hand waving. The basis images are the resized form of eigenvectors and normalized in gray scale. Fig. 5 shows top 150 eigenvalues corresponding to the first 150 eigenvectors where 600 silhouette image vectors are considered for PCA.

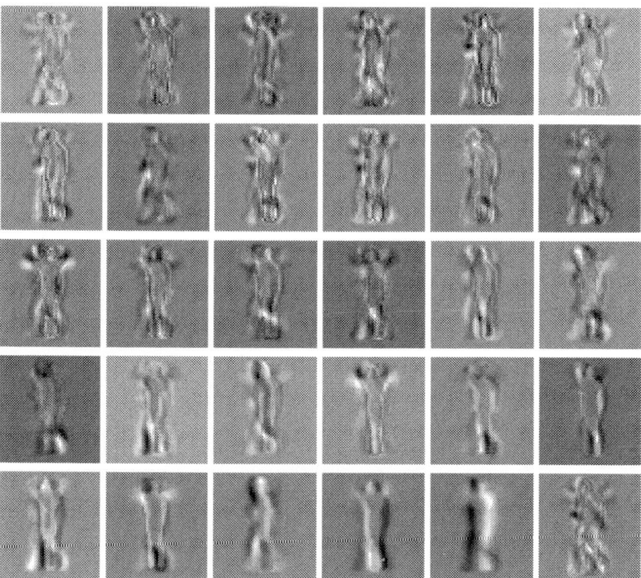

Fig. 4. Thirty PCs of all the images of the four activities.

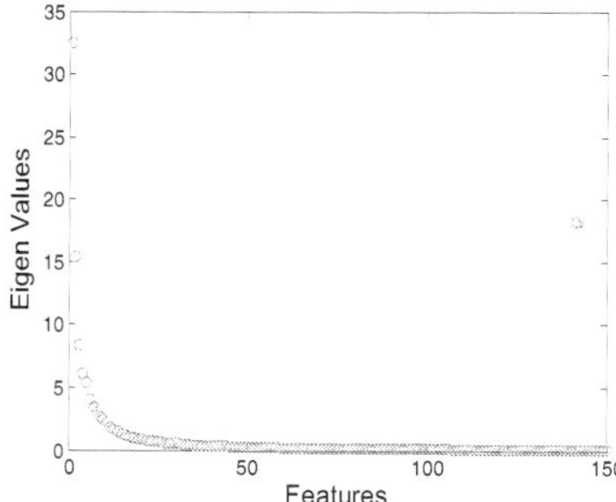

Fig. 5. Hundred and fifty top eigenvalues of the training silhouette images of the four activities.

2.3. Feature Extraction Using ICA

ICA finds the statistically independent basis images. The basic idea of ICA is to represent a set of random observed variables using basis function where the components are statistically independent. If S is collection of basis images and X is collection of input images then the relation between X and S is modeled as

$$X = MS \tag{3}$$

where M represents an unknown linear mixing matrix of full rank.

An ICA algorithm learns the weight matrix W, which is inverse of mixing matrix M. W is used to recover a set of independent basis images S. The ICA basis image focuses on local feature information rather than global information as in PCA. ICA basis images show the local features of the movements in activity such as open or closed legs for running. Fig. 6 shows 30 ICA basis images for all activities. Before applying ICA, PCA is used to reduce the dimension of the image data. ICA is performed on E_m as follows.

$$S = WE_m^T \tag{4}$$

$$E_m^T = W^{-1}S \tag{5}$$

$$X_r = VW^{-1}S \tag{6}$$

where V is projection of the images X on E_m and X_r the reconstructed original images. The independent component representation I_i of ith silhouette vector $\tilde{X}_i$ from an activity image sequence can be expressed as

$$I_i = \tilde{X}_i E_m W^{-1}. \tag{7}$$

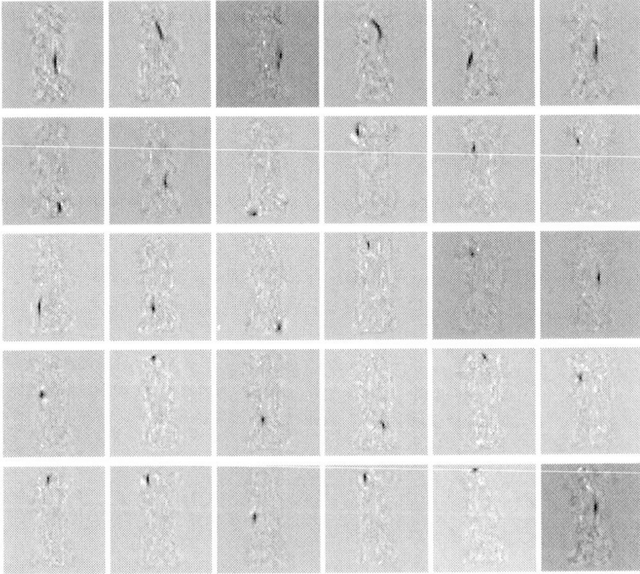

Fig. 6. Thirty ICs of all the images of the four activities.

2.4. Feature Extraction Using LDA on the IC Features

LDA produces an optimal linear discriminant function which maps the input into the classification space based on which the class identification of the samples can be decided

(Kwak & Pedrycz, 2007). The within scatter matrix, S_W and the between scatter matrix, S_B are computed by the following equations:

$$S_B = \sum_{i=1}^{c} G_i(\overline{m_i} - \overline{\overline{m}})(\overline{m_i} - \overline{\overline{m}})^T \tag{8}$$

$$S_W = \sum_{i=1}^{c} \sum_{m_k \in C_i} (m_k - \overline{m_i})(m_k - \overline{m_i})^T \tag{9}$$

where G_i is the number of vectors in i^{th} class C_i. c is the number of classes and in our case, it represents the number of activities. $\overline{\overline{m}}$ represents the mean of all vectors, $\overline{m_i}$ the mean of the class C_i and m_k the vector of a specific class. The optimal discrimination matrix D_{LDA} is chosen from the maximization of ratio of the determinant of the between and within class scatter matrix as

$$D_{LDA} = \arg \max_{D} \frac{\left| D^T S_B D \right|}{\left| D^T S_W D \right|} \tag{10}$$

where D_{LDA} is the set of discriminant vectors of S_W and S_B corresponding to the $(c-1)$ largest generalized eigenvalues λ and can be obtained via solving

$$S_B d_i = \lambda_i S_W d_i. \tag{11}$$

The LDA algorithm looks for the vectors in the underlying space to create the best discrimination among different classes. Thus the extracted ICA representations of the binary silhouettes of different activities can be extended by LDA. The feature vectors using LDA on the IC features can be represented as

$$F_i = I_i D_{LDA}^T. \tag{12}$$

Fig. 7 shows the 3-D representation of the binary silhouette features after applying on three ICs that are chosen on the basis of top kurtosis values. Fig. 8 demonstrates the 3-D plot of LDA on the IC features of the silhouettes of four classes where 150 ICs are taken. Fig. 8 shows a good separation among the representation of the silhouettes of different classes.

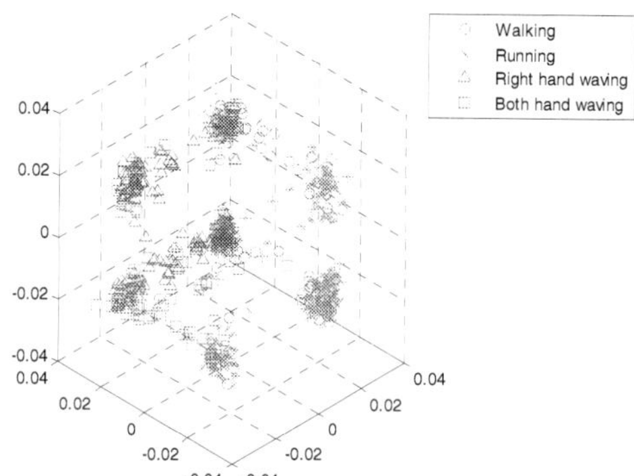

Fig. 7. 3-D plot of the IC features of 600 silhouettes of the four activities.

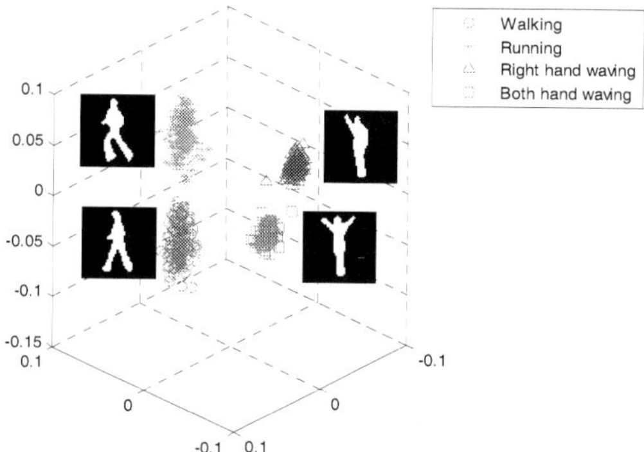

Fig. 8. 3-D plot of the LDA on the IC features of 600 silhouettes of the four activities.

2.5. Vector Quantization

We symbolize the feature vectors before applying them to train or recognize by HMM. An efficient codebook of vectors can be generated using vector quantization from the training vectors. In our experiment, we have used two vector quantization algorithms: namely ordinary K-means clustering (Kanungu et al., 2000) and Linde, Buzo, and Gray (LBG)'s clustering algorithm (Linde et al., 1980). In both of them, first initial selection of centroids is obtained. In the case of K-means clustering, until a convergence criterion is met, for every sample it seeks the nearest centroid, assign the sample to the cluster, and compute the center of that cluster again. However, in the case of LBG, recomputation is done after assigning all samples to new clusters. In LBG, initialization is done by splitting the centroid of whole dataset. It starts with the codebook size of one and recursively splits into two codewords. After splitting, optimization of the centroids is done to reduce the distortion. Since it follows the binary splitting method, the size of the codebook must be power of two. In the case of K-means, the overall performance varies due to the selection of the initial random centroids. On the contrary, LBG starts from splitting the centroid of entire dataset, thus there is less variation in its performance.

When a codebook is designed, the index numbers of the codewords are used as symbols to apply on HMM. As long as a feature vector is available then index number of the closest codeword from the codebook is the symbol for that replace. Hence every silhouette image is going to be assigned a symbol. If there are K image sequences of T length then there will be K sequences of T length symbols. The symbols are the observations, O. Fig. 9 shows the codebook generation and symbol selection from the codebook using the IC features.

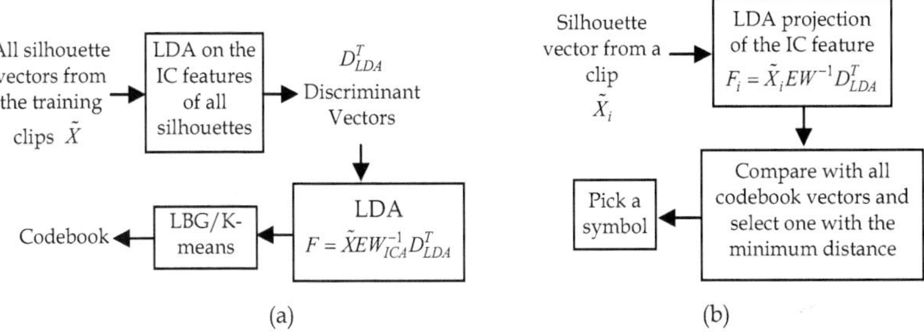

Fig. 9. Steps for (a) codebook generation and (b) symbol selection using LDA on the IC features.

2.6. HMM for Activity Modeling, Training, and Recognition

HMM has been applied extensively to solve a large number of problems including speech recognition (Lawrence & Rabiner, 1989). It has been adopted in the human activity research field as well in (Niu & Abdel-Mottaleb, 2004; Niu & Abdel-Mottaleb, 2006; Yamato et al., 1992; Nakata, 2006; Sun et al., 2002). Once human activities are represented in features then HMM can be applied effectively for human activity recognition as it is a most suitable technique for recognizing time sequential feature information. Silhouette features are converted to a sequence of symbols that are corresponding to the codewords of the codebook obtained by vector quantization. In learning HMM, the symbol sequences obtained from the training image sequences of distinct activity are used to optimize the corresponding HMM. Each activity is represented by a distinct HMM. In recognition, the symbol sequence is applied to all HMMs and one is chosen that gives the highest likelihood. An HMM is a collection of finite states connected by transitions. Every state is characterized by two types of probabilities: namely transition probability and symbol observation probability. A generic HMM can be expressed as $H = \{\Xi, \pi, A, B\}$ where Ξ denotes possible states, π the initial probability of the states, A the transition probability matrix between hidden states where state transition probability a_{ij} represents the probability of changing state from i to j, and B observation symbols' probability from every state where the probability $b_j(O)$ indicates the probability of observing the symbols O from state j. If the number of activities is N then there will be a dictionary $(H_1, H_2, ..., H_N)$ of N trained models. We used the Baum-Welch algorithm for HMM parameter estimation (Iwai et al., 1997) according to (13) to (16).

$$\xi_t(i, j) = \frac{\alpha_t(i) a_{ij} b_j(O_{t+1}) \beta_{t+1}(j)}{\sum_{i=1}^{q} \sum_{j=1}^{q} \alpha_t(i) a_{ij} b_j(O_{t+1}) \beta_{t+1}(j)} \tag{13}$$

$$\xi_t(i, j) = \frac{\alpha_t(i) a_{ij} b_j(O_{t+1}) \beta_{t+1}(j)}{\sum_{i=1}^{q} \sum_{j=1}^{q} \alpha_t(i) a_{ij} b_j(O_{t+1}) \beta_{t+1}(j)} \tag{14}$$

$$\hat{a}_{ij} = \frac{\sum_{t=1}^{T-1} \xi_t(i, j)}{\sum_{t=1}^{T} \gamma_t(i)} \tag{15}$$

$$\hat{b}_j(d) = \frac{\sum_{\substack{t=1 \\ O_t = d}}^{T-1} \gamma_t(j)}{\sum_{t=1}^{T} \gamma_t(j)} \tag{16}$$

where $\xi_t(i, j)$ is the probability of staying in a state i at time t and a state j at time $t+1$. $\gamma_t(i)$ represents the probability of staying in the state i at time t. α and β are the forward and backward variables respectively. $\hat{a}_{ij}$ represents the estimated transition probability from the state i to the state j and $\hat{b}_j(d)$ the estimated observation probability of symbol d from the state j. q is the number of states in the model.

Four-state left-to-right HMM was chosen for each activity. In the case of observation matrix B, the possible number of observations from every state is the number of codebook vectors. Fig. 10 shows the transition probabilities of a walking HMM before and after training with the codebook size of 32. To test a sequence O, the appropriate HMM is one that gives the highest likelihood. The likelihood of the sequence O at time t for an HMM H can be represented as

$$P(O \mid H) = \sum_{i=1}^{q} \alpha_t(i). \tag{17}$$

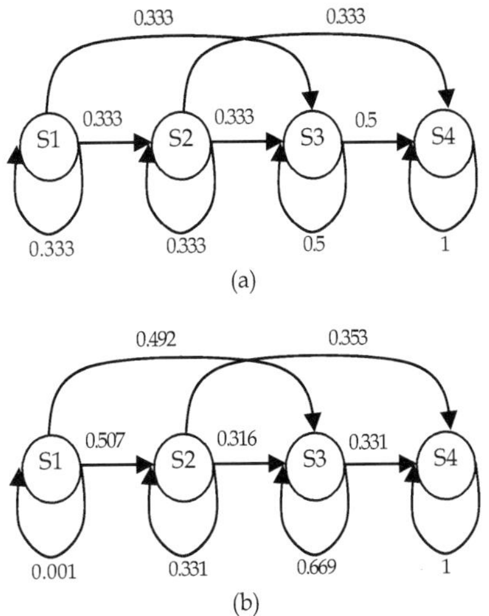

Fig. 10. A walking HMM (a) before and (b) after training.

3. Experiments and Discussion

In our silhouette-based recognition approaches, we used two different kinds of inputs:
namely binary (Uddin et al., 2008a) and depth (Uddin et al., 2008b). The binary silhouette
pixels contain a flat distribution of the intensity (i.e., 0 or 1). On the contrary, the depth
silhouette contains variable pixel intensity distribution based on the distance of human body
parts to the camera.

3.1. Recognition Using Binary Silhouettes

We recognized four activities using the IC features of the binary silhouettes through HMM:
namely walking, running, right hand waving, and both hand waving. Every sequence
consisted of 10 images. A total of 15 sequences from each activity were used to build the
feature space. Thus, the whole database consisted of a total of 600 images. After applying
ICA and PCA, 150 features were taken in the feature space.

We further extended the IC features by LDA for more robust feature representation. Thus,
several tests were performed with different features using LBG with the codebook size of 32
where LDA on the IC features showed superior recognition rate. A total of 160 sequences
were used for testing the models. Table 1 lists the recognition results using the different
features: namely PCA, LDA on the PC features, ICA, and LDA on the IC features.

Approach	Activity	Recognition Rate	Mean	Standard Deviation
PCA	Walking	100%	87.26	8.90
	Running	82.5		
	RHW*	80		
	BHW**	88		
LDA on the PC features	Walking	100	89.87	8.37
	Running	87.5		
	RHW	80		
	BHW	92		
ICA	Walking	100	96.13	4.48
	Running	92.5		
	RHW	100		
	BHW	92		
LDA on the IC features	Walking	100	99.5	1
	Running	100		
	RHW	100		
	BHW	98		

*RHW=Right Hand Waving   **BHW=Both Hand Waving

Table 1. Recognition result using different feature extraction approaches on the binary silhouettes.

3.2. Recognition Using Depth Silhouettes

Basically, binary silhouettes reflect only the silhouette contour information. On the other hand, regarding the depth-based silhouettes, pixel values are set based on the distance to the camera and hence can represent more activity information than binary. Fig. 11 shows a sample depth image of walking and running respectively where the near parts of human body from the camera have brighter pixel intensity values than the far ones. Thus, the depth silhouettes can represent the human body better than binary by differentiating the major body parts by means of different intensity values based on the distance to camera (Uddin et al., 2008b). In this work, we employed LDA on the IC features of the depth silhouettes to recognize six different activities (i.e., walking, running, skipping, boxing, sitting up, and standing down) through HMM and obtained much improvement over the binary silhouette-based approach using the same feature extraction technique. The recognition results using both the binary and depth silhouette-based approaches are shown in Table 2.

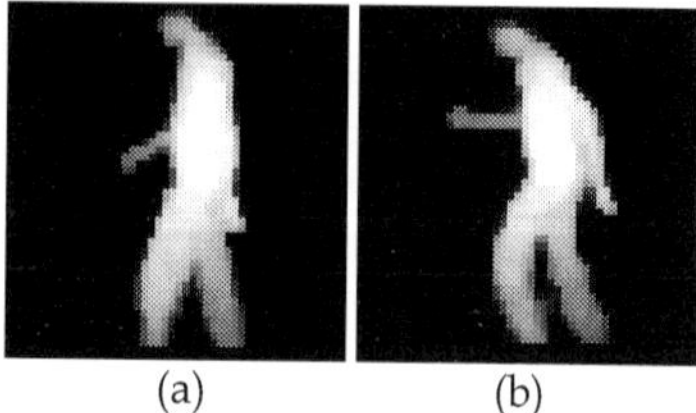

(a)   (b)

Fig. 11. Sample depth silhouette of (a) walking and (b) running.

Features	Activity	Recognition Rate with HMM	Mean	Standard Deviation
LDA on the IC features of the binary silhouettes	Walking	84	91.33	8.17
	Running	96		
	Skipping	88		
	Boxing	100		
	Sitting	84		
	Standing	100		
LDA on the IC features of the depth silhouettes	Walking	96	96.67	4.68
	Running	96		
	Skipping	88		
	Boxing	100		
	Sitting Up	100		
	Standing Down	100		

Table 2. Recognition result using LDA on the IC features of the binary and depth silhouettes.

4. Conclusion

In this chapter, we have presented novel approaches for binary and depth silhouette-based human activity recognition using ICA and LDA in combination with HMM. LDA on the binary IC feature-based approach outperforms PCA, ICA, and LDA on the PC feature-based approaches, achieving 99.5% recognition rate for the four activities. Using depth silhouettes, the recognition further improves from 91.33% to 96.67% in the overall recognition of the six different activities.

5. Acknowledgement

This work was supported by the MKE (Ministry of Knowledge Economy), Korea, under the ITRC (Information Technology Research Center) support program supervised by the IITA (Institute of Information Technology Advancement) (IITA 2008-(C1090-0801-0002)).

6. References

Bartlett, M.; Movellan, J. & Sejnowski, T. (2002). Face Recognition by Independent Component Analysis, *IEEE Transactions on Neural Networks*, Vol., 13, pp. 1450-1464.

Ben-Arie, J.; Wang, Z.; Pandit, P. & Rajaram, S. (2002). Human Activity Recognition Using Multidimensional Indexing, *IEEE Transactions on Pattern Analysis and Machine Intelligence Archive*, Vol., 24(8), pp. 1091-1104.

Carlsson, S. & Sullivan, J. (2002). Action Recognition by Shape Matching to Key Frames, *IEEE Computer Society Workshop on Models versus Exemplars in Computer Vision*, pp. 263-270.

Cohen, I. & Lim, H. (2003). Inference of Human Postures by Classification of 3D Human Body Shape, *IEEE International Workshop on Analysis and Modeling of Faces and Gestures*, pp. 74-81.

Iwai, Y.; Hata, T. & Yachida, M. (1997) Gesture Recognition Based on Subspace Method and Hidden Markov Model, *Proceedings of the IEEE/RSJ International Conference on Intelligent Robots and Systems*, pp. 960-966.

Kanungu, T.; Mount, D. M.; Netanyahu, N.; Piatko, C.; Silverman, R. & Wu, A. Y. (2000). The analysis of a simple k-means clustering algorithm, *Proceedings of 16th ACM Symposium On Computational Geometry*, pp. 101-109.

Kwak, K.-C. & Pedrycz, W. (2007). Face Recognition Using an Enhanced Independent Component Analysis Approach, *IEEE Transactions on Neural Networks*, Vol., 18(2), pp. 530-541.

Kwon, O. W. & Lee, T. W. (2004). Phoneme recognition using ICA-based feature extraction and transformation, *Signal Processing*, Vol., 84(6), pp. 1005–1019.

Lawrence, R. & Rabiner, A. (1989). Tutorial on Hidden Markov Models and Selected Applications in Speech Recognition, *Proceedings of the IEEE*, 77(2), pp. 257-286.

Linde, Y.; Buzo, A. & Gray, R. (1980). An Algorithm for Vector Quantizer Design, *IEEE Transaction on Communications*, Vol., 28(1), pp. 84–94.

Mckeown, M. J.; Makeig, S.; Brown, G. G.; Jung, T. P.; Kindermann, S. S.; Bell, A. J. & Sejnowski, T. J. (1998) Analysis of fMRI by decomposition into independent spatial components, *Human Brain Mapping*, Vol., 6(3), pp. 160–188.

Nakata, T. (2006). Recognizing Human Activities in Video by Multi-resolutional Optical Flow, *Proceedings of International Conference on Intelligent Robots and Systems*, pp. 1793-1798.

Niu, F. & Abdel-Mottaleb M. (2004).View-Invariant Human Activity Recognition Based on Shape and Motion Features, *Proceedings of the IEEE Sixth International Symposium on Multimedia Software Engineering*, pp. 546-556.

Niu, F. & Abdel-Mottaleb, M. (2005). HMM-Based Segmentation and Recognition of Human Activities from Video Sequences, *Proceedings of IEEE International Conference on Multimedia & Expo*, pp. 804-807.

Robertson, N. & Reid, I. (2006). A General Method for Human Activity Recognition in Video, *Computer Vision and Image Understanding*, Vol., 104(2), pp. 232 - 248.

Sun, X.; Chen, C. & Manjunath, B. S. (2002). Probabilistic Motion Parameter Models for Human Activity Recognition, *Proceedings of 16th International Conference on Pattern recognition*, pp. 443-450.

Yamato, J.; Ohya, J. & Ishii, K. (1992). Recognizing Human Action in Time-Sequential Images using Hidden Markov Model, *Proceedings of IEEE International Conference on Computer Vision and Pattern Recognition*, pp. 379-385.

Yang, J.; Zhang, D. & Yang, J. Y. (2005). Is ICA Significantly Better than PCA for Face Recognition?. *Proceedings of IEEE International Conference on Computer Vision*, pp. 198-203.

Uddin, M. Z.; Lee, J. J. & Kim T.-S. (2008a) Shape-Based Human Activity Recognition Using Independent Component Analysis and Hidden Markov Model, *Proceedings of The 21st International Conference on Industrial, Engineering and Other Applications of Applied Intelligent Systems*, pp. 245-254.

Uddin, M. Z.; Lee, J. J. & Kim, T.-S. (2008b). Human Activity Recognition Using Independent Component Features from Depth Images, *Proceedings of the 5th International Conference on Ubiquitous Healthcare*, pp. 181-183.

15

A Closed-Loop Method for Bio-Impedance Measurement with Application to Four and Two-Electrode Sensor Systems

Alberto Yúfera and Adoración Rueda
Instituto de Microelectrónica de Sevilla (IMS),
Centro Nacional de Microelectrónica (CNM)
University of Seville
Spain

1. Introduction and Motivation

Impedance is a useful parameter for determining the properties of matter. Today, many research goals are focused to measure the impedance of biological samples. Several are the major benefits of measuring impedances in medical and biological environment: first, most biological parameters and processes as glucose concentration (Beach, 2005), tissue impedance evolution (Yúfera et al., 2005), cell-growth tax (Huang, 2004), toxicological analysis (Radke, 2004), bacterial detection (Borkholder, 1998), etc, can be monitored using its impedance as marker. Second, the bio-impedance measurement is a non-invasive technique and third, it represents a relatively cheap technique at labs. Electrical Impedance Tomography (EIT) in bodies (Holder, 2005), and Impedance Spectroscopy (IS) of cell cultures (Giaever, 1993) are two examples of the impedance utility for measuring biological and medical parameters.

For the problem of measuring any given impedance Z_x, with magnitude Z_{xo} and phase ϕ, several methods have been reported. Commonly, these methods require excitation and processing circuits. Excitation is usually done with AC current sources, while processing steps are based on coherent demodulation principle (Ackmann, 1984) or synchronous sampling (Pallas et al., 1993), leading to excellent results. In both, processing circuits must be synchronized with input signals, as a requirement for the technique to work, obtaining the best noise performance when proper filter functions (HP and LP) are incorporated. Block diagrams for both are illustrated in Figures 1 (a) and (b) respectively. The main drawback for the Ackmann method is that the separated channels for in-phase and quadrature components must be matched to avoid large phase errors. Synchronous sampling proposed by Pallas avoids two channels and demodulation, by selecting accurate sampling times, and adding a high pass filter in the signal path to prevent low-frequency noise and sampler interferences. These measurement principles work as feed-forward systems: the signal generated on Z_x is amplified and then processed. In general, for an impedance measurement process based on electrodes, one of the main drawbacks on excitation circuit design is imposed by the need of using electrodes and its electrical performance, which is frequency dependent, having low frequency impedance values in the MΩ range. Also, applied voltage to electrodes must be amplitude limited to guarantee its correct biasing region, generally some tens of mV.

This work presents a Closed-loop method for Bio-Impedance Measurement (CBIM) based on the application of AC voltage signals, with constant amplitude, to impedance under test (ZUT). The proposed method can be applied to electrode-based sensor systems, solving the electrode frequency dependence problem by including electrode electrical models in the circuit design equations, in such a way that enables the circuit derived for measuring impedance of specific biological samples. In this chapter we develop the idea of using feedback for measuring impedances and propose the circuits employed for adapting the excitation signal to ZUT and electrodes. The CBIM method allows the possibility of considering the electrode performance at the initial phase of an experiment where the electrode characteristics (size, material, etc.) are selected depending on the biological material to be tested and the sensitivity required by the experiment. The magnitude and phase impedance are obtained directly from the proposed circuits using easy to acquire signals: a DC voltage, for magnitude, and a duty cycle of a digital signal, for phase. The proposed method is implemented with CMOS circuits, showing through electrical simulations the correct performance for a wide frequency and load ranges. The possibility of integrated CMOS electrodes also opens the door to fully lab-on-chip systems. The CBIM technique represents an alternative method for measuring, using two and four electrode setups, in techniques such as Electric Cell-substrate Impedance Spectroscopy (ECIS) and Electrical Impedance Tomography (EIT), respectively, and some examples are developed in the chapter.

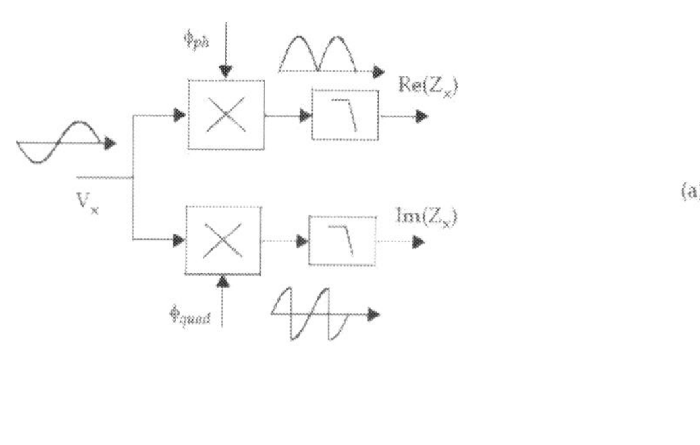

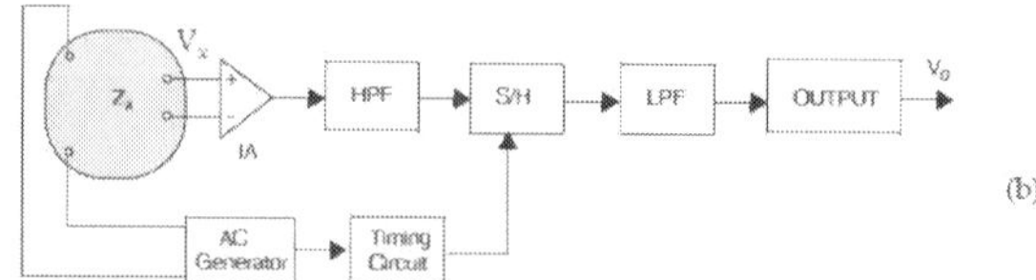

Fig. 1. (a) Synchronous demodulation. (b) Synchornous sampling.

The proposed content of the chapter is the following. The second section presents the CBIM method, its main blocks, system design equations and limitations in terms of its functional block parameters and the system specifications. The third section describes the CMOS circuits implementing the system: topology, design equations and performance limitations (design issues) for each circuit and related to the global system. The fourth section is dedicated to electrical simulation exercises of some examples to validate the proposed method. The fifth section relies on the CBIM application on a four-electrode system. Real electrode models are incorporated to the system design process and simulations. Finally, in the sixth section, a two-electrode system for cell culture applications is analysed from two perspectives: first, considering a single-cell location problem, and second, dealing with a bi-dimensional array of sensors (electrodes). This approach allows the achievement of an alternative technique for real-time monitoring and imaging cell cultures. An example of this approach is included.

2. Proposed Closed-Loop Method for Bio-Impedance Measurement

A general process for measuring a given impedance Z_x (with magnitude Z_{xo} and phase ϕ) is based on the application of an input signal (current or voltage) to create a response signal (voltage or current) and then, to extract from this its components (real and imaginary parts or magnitude and phase). This concept is illustrated on Fig. 2(a), with a current source i_x as excitation signal. This is generally an AC signal of a given amplitude (i_{xo}) and frequency (ω). Z_s considers the path resistance from source to load, and usually includes parasitic resistances from the set-up and the electrode impedance. The latter has a large magnitude and frequency dependency in the range of interest. Signal $V_x(t)$ is the voltage response obtained by applying $i_x(t)$ in series with the impedance under test (ZUT). The amplified voltage, $V_o(t)$, is processed to obtain the impedance components. Excitation and processing are usually performed by different circuits, though connected by synchronized signals.
The Z_x impedance can also be measured with a feedback system, as illustrated in Fig. 2(b), by introducing a new block, ZF. The signal excitation will depend on the amplifier output and hence on the ZUT. This idea is used to design an alternative method for impedance measurement using the feedback principle. The targets imposed to ZF feedback block are:

1) to generate the i_x excitation signal.
2) to provide the measurement of magnitude and phase.

Meanwhile, a main specification is set: *the voltage amplitude at impedance under test, V_x, must be constant*. This condition is known as the potentiostat (Pstat) condition for impedance measurement and means to setting constant and limited the voltage amplitude V_{xo} "seen" by the ZUT (Yúfera et al., 2008). From the system in Fig. 2b, voltage at Z_x has a constant amplitude, hence changes in magnitude Z_{xo} must modify the amplitude of the applied current, i_{xo}. The current i_x fits its amplitude to preserve constant the voltage amplitude on Z_x and holds the information about the Z_x magnitude. This current must be generated by the ZF block. As a consequence, the amplitude at the instrumentation amplifier (IA) output voltage is constant. The discrimination between signals with different phases are observed in terms of its delays ϕ in the voltage,

$$V_o = V_o(Z_x \alpha) = V_{ia} \sin(\omega t + \phi)_{xo}$$
(1)

being α_{ia} the instrumentation amplifier gain.

In conclusion, when feedback is applied in a system for measuring a given impedance in Pstat conditions (as aforementioned), the amplitude of the excitation current, i_{xo}, has the information about the magnitude of the ZUT, while its phase shift, ϕ, must be extracted from the constant amplitude signal in eq. (1). The measurement strategy for Z_x can benefit from the resulting conditions. A change from the method proposed in (Pallas et al., 1993) is that the magnitude and phase can be obtained directly from two different signals, being possible to separate circuit optimization tasks for both signals.

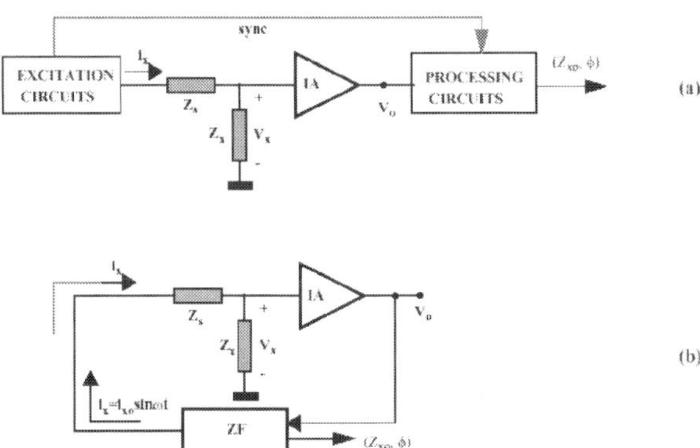

Fig. 2. (a) Basic concept for measuring the Z_{xo} and ϕ components of Z_x. (b) Proposed idea for measuring Z_x using a feedback system.

3. Basic Circuit Blocks

3.1 System Specifications

For the measurement of the impedance magnitude, Z_{xo}, it will be considered that the excitation signal is an AC current, with amplitude i_{xo} and frequency ω. The proposed circuit block diagram for ZF is shown in Fig.3. Three main components are included: an AC-to-DC converter or rectifier, an error amplifier, and a current oscillator with programmable output current amplitude. The rectifier works as a full wave peak-detector, sensing the biggest (lowest) amplitude of V_o. This functionality allows to control the output voltage swing at the instrumentation voltage acting as an envelop detector. Its result is a DC voltage, V_{dc}, with low rippley, directly proportional to the amplitude of the instrumentation amplifier output voltage, and with an α_{dc} gain ($V_{dc}=\alpha_{dc}.\alpha_{ia}V_{xo}$). The error amplifier (EA) will compare the DC signal with a voltage reference, V_{ref}, giving its amplified difference: $V_m=\alpha_{ea}.(V_{dc}-V_{ref})$. The voltage V_{ref} represents the constant voltage reference required to work in the Pstat mode, and can be interpreted as a calibration constant. The full rectifier output voltage must approach as near to V_{ref} as possible. The current oscillator generates the AC current to excite the ZUT. It is composed by a external AC voltage source, V_s, an operational transconductance amplifier (OTA), with g_m transconductance, and a voltage multiplier with K constant. The voltage source V_s, $V_{so}.\sin\omega t$, is multiplied by V_m, and then current converted with the OTA. The equivalent transconductance from the magnitude voltage, V_m, to the excitation current, i_x, is called G_m and will depend on the AC voltage amplitude, V_{so}, the K multiplier constant and the g_m of the OTA. The equivalent transconductance for the current oscillator is defined as $G_m = g_m.V_{so}.K$. A simple analysis of the full system gives the following expression for the voltage amplitude at the ZUT,

$$V_{xo} = \frac{Z_{xo}.G_m.\alpha_{ea}.V_{ref}}{1 + Z_{xo}.G_m.\alpha_{ea}.\alpha_{ia}.\alpha_{dc}} \tag{2}$$

being α_{ia}, α_{dc}, α_{ea} the gains of the instrumentation amplifier, rectifier and error amplifier, respectively, and G_m the equivalent transconductance of the current oscillator. For the condition,

$$Z_{xo}.G_m.\alpha_{ea}.\alpha_{ia}.\alpha_{dc} \gg 1 \tag{3}$$

the voltage at ZUT has the amplitude,

$$V_{xo} = \frac{V_{ref}}{\alpha_{ia}.\alpha_{dc}} \tag{4}$$

This voltage remains constant if α_{ia} and α_{dc} are also constants. Hence, the Pstat condition is fulfilled if the condition in eq. (3) is true. On the other hand, considering the relationship between the current i_x and the voltage V_m ($i_{xo}=G_m.V_m$), the impedance magnitude can be expressed as,

$$Z_{xo} = \frac{V_{xo}}{G_m.V_m} \tag{5}$$

Equation (5) means that by measuring the **magnitude voltage V_m**, the magnitude Z_{xo} can be calculated, since V_{xo} and G_m are known from eq. (4) and design parameters. For example, for a electrode with $V_{xo} = 50mV$ and $Z_{xo} = 100k\Omega$, the measures with $G_m=0.1\mu S$ gives $V_m = 50mV$ and $i_{xo} = 5nA$. If the load is divided by five, the V_m changes to 250mV and $i_{xo} = 25nA$.

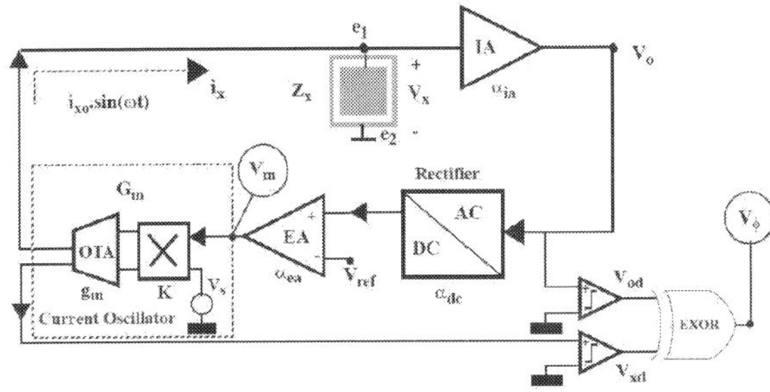

Fig. 3. Circuit blocks for impedance sensing.

For the measurement of the phase ϕ, we will consider the oscillator has an output voltage in phase with the i_x current. This signal can be squared or converted into a digital voltage signal, to be used as time reference or sync signal (V_{xd}). The V_o voltage can be also converted into a squared waveform (V_{od}) by means of a voltage comparator. If both signals feed the input of an EXOR gate, a digital signal will be obtained, the **phase voltage V_ϕ**, whose duty cycle, δ, is directly proportional to the phase of Z_x.

3.2 CMOS circuits

In the following we will give some details on the actual design considerations for CMOS circuits in Fig. 3. All circuits presented here have been designed in 0.35μm, 2P4M technology from Austria Micro-System (AMS) foundry (http://www.austriamicrosystems.com).

3.2.1 Instrumentation Amplifier

The instrumentation amplifier circuit schematic is represented in Fig. 4. It is a two-stage amplifier. A trans-conductance input stage, and a trans-resistance output stage, where filtering functionality has been included. The pass-band frequency edges were designed according to the frequency range common for impedance measurements and spectroscopy analysis. The low-pass filter corner was set at approximately 1MHz frequency, with R_2 and C_2 circuit elements, while high-pass filter corner at 100Hz, using output voltage feedback and G_{mhp} and C_1 circuit elements for its implementation. Input stage transistors have been designed to reduce the influence of electrode noise (Sawigun et al., 2006). The frequency response, magnitude and phase, are illustrated in Figures 5 (a) and (b) respectively, by using an input voltage with 10mV of amplitude.

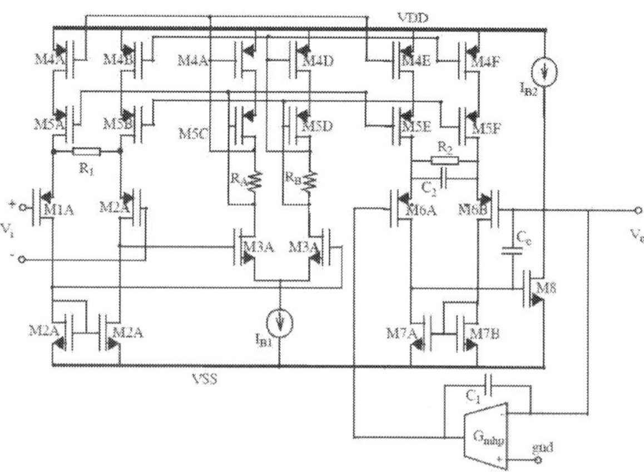

Fig. 4. Instrumentation amplifier.

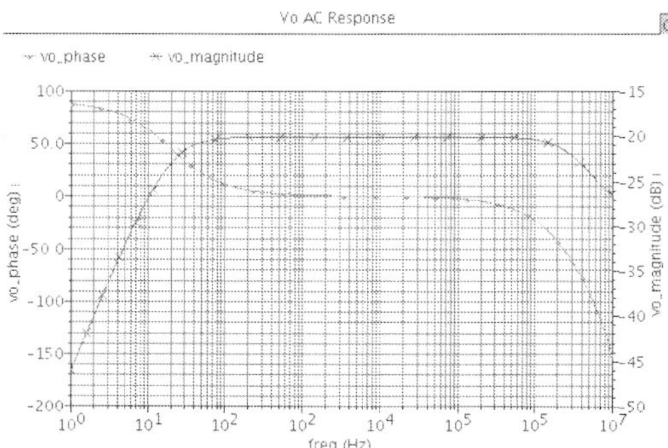

Fig. 5. Instrumentation amplifier frequency response: magnitude and phase responses for a differential input voltage of 10mV.

3.2.2 Rectifier

The full wave rectifier (positive and negative peak-detectors) in Fig. 6 is based on pass transistors (MP, MN) to load the capacitor C_r at the nearest voltage of V_o. The two comparators detect if the input signal is higher (lower) than V_{op} (V_{om}) in each instant, to charge the C_r capacitors. The discharge process of C_r is done by current sources, I_{dis}, and has been set to 1mV in a time period. Figure 7 illustrates the waveforms obtained by electrical simulations for the upper and lower rectified signals at 10 kHz. In this case, for C_r=20pF, I_{dis} has been set to 200 pA. For spectroscopy analysis, when frequency changes in a given range, the discharge current must be programmed for each frequency to fulfil the estimated 1mV voltage ripple in steady-state for the rectifier output voltage. The Comparator schematic is shown at the end of this section.

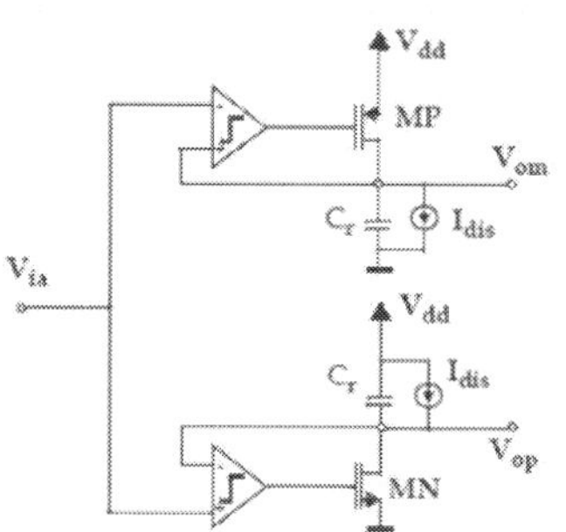

Fig. 6. Full wave rectifier schematic.

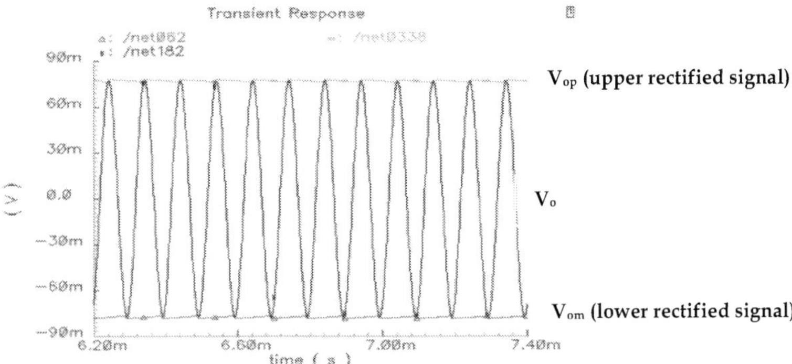

Fig. 7. Rectifier upper (V_{op}) and lower (V_{om}) output voltage waveforms. The sinusoidal signal is the Instrumentation Amplifier output voltage.

3.2.3 Error Amplifier

The first stage is a differential-to-single gain amplifier for conversion of both output voltages delivered by the full-wave rectifier. The second stage compares the result with V_{ref} and amplifies the difference to create the voltage magnitude signal, V_m, which has the information about impedance magnitude. For that, a two-stage operational amplifier is employed. One of the objectives of the system is to set at the input of the operational amplifier a voltage signal V_{dc} as near as possible to voltage V_{ref}.

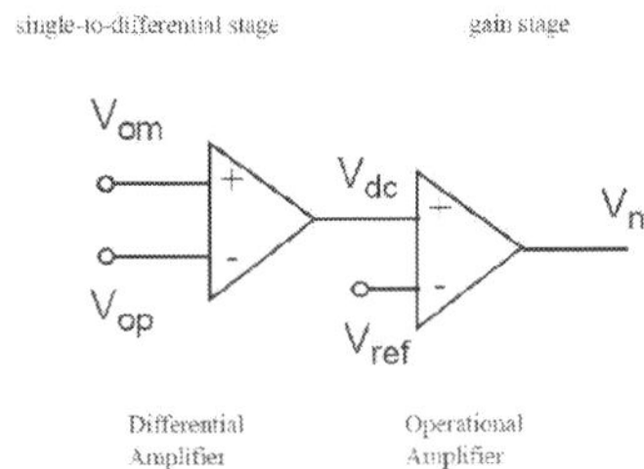

Fig. 8. Error Amplifier.

3.2.4 Current control circuit

For i_x amplitude programming, a four-quadrant multiplier and an **OTA** were designed. Both are placed in series as shown in Fig. 9. In this configuration, the external AC voltage generator is first multiplied by the voltage magnitude V_m. The result is later on converted to AC current for load excitation.

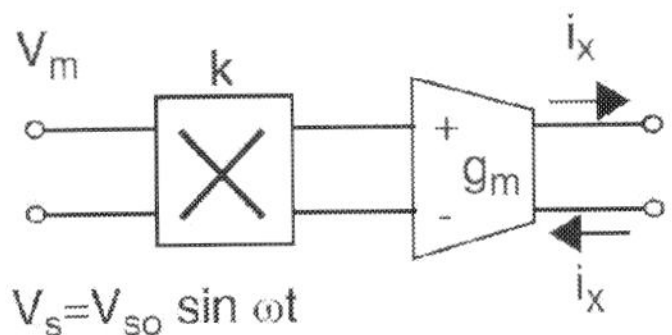

Fig. 9. The delivered AC current to electrodes (i_x) has an amplitude given by i_{xo} = (k $g_m V_{so}$).V_m, in which $G_m = k g_m V_{so}$ can be considered as the equivalent trans-conductance from V_m input voltage to i_x output current. The amplitude of i_x can be programmed with the V_m voltage.

The schematic of the multiplier circuit is shown in Fig. 10. It has two inputs that are employed for external AC voltage generator, V_s, and the voltage magnitude, V_m. The multiplier output waveforms ($V_m \times V_s$) are shown in Fig. 11. In this figure, the AC signal V_s, has 200mV of amplitude at 10 kHz frequency, and it is multiplied by a DC signal, V_m, in the range of [0,200mV]. The differential output is given by

$$V_{out} = V_{out1} - V_{out2} = 2R\sqrt{k_n k_p} V_m V_s = K V_m V_s \qquad (6)$$

Being K the constant of the multiplier, and k_n and k_p the trans-conductance parameter for M1 and M6 transistors.

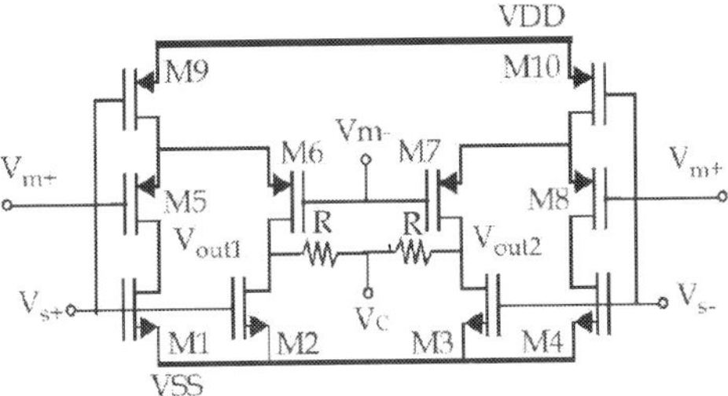

Fig. 10. Circuit schematic for the multiplier.

$$V_m \times V_s = K V_{so} V_m \sin \omega t$$

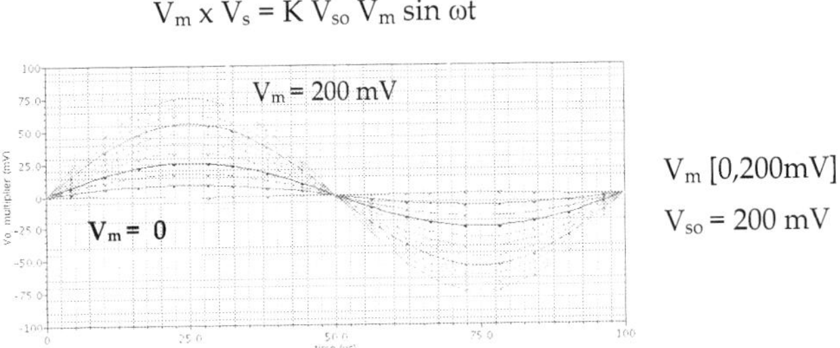

Fig. 11. Waveforms for the multiplier output voltage.

The operational transconductance amplifier employed has the schematic in Fig. 12. The cascode output stage has been chosen to reduce the load effect due to large ohmic values in loads (Z_{xo}). Typical output resistances for cascode output stages are bigger than 100MΩ, so errors expected due to load resistance effects will be small.

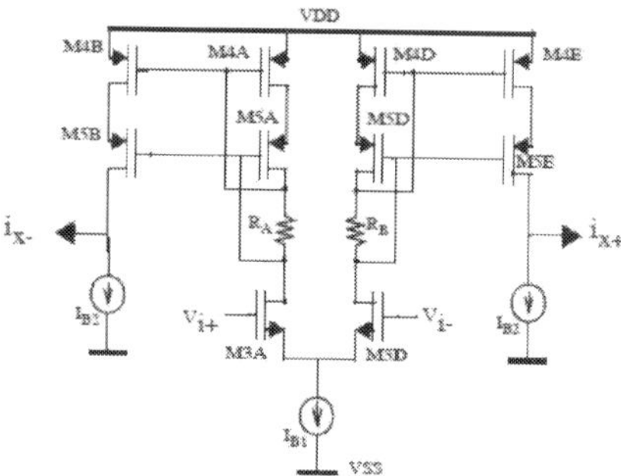

Fig. 12. Operational Transconductance Amplifier (OTA) CMOS schematic.

3.2.5 Comparator

The voltage comparator selected is shown in Fig. 13. A chain of inverters have been added at its output for fast response and regeneration of digital levels.

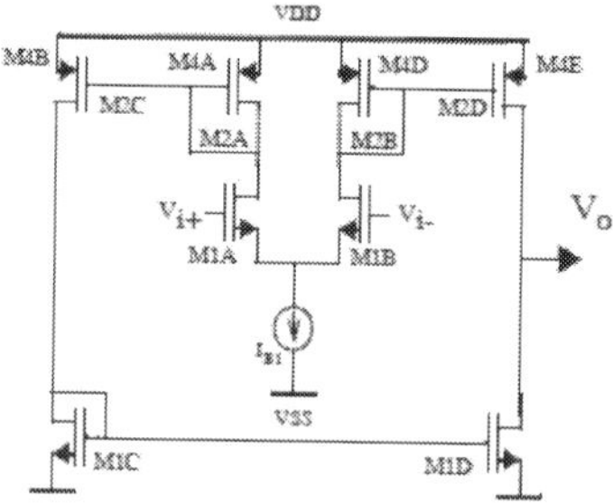

Fig. 13. Comparator schematic.

With the data employed, the voltage applied to load composed by the measurement set-up and load under test, V_x, has amplitude of 8mV. In electrode based measures, V_{xo} has typically low and limited values (tens of mV) to control its expected electrical performance (Borkholder, 1998) to secure a non-polarisable performance of the interface between an electrode and the electrolyte or biological material in contact with it. This condition can be preserved by design thanks to the voltage limitation imposed by the Pstat operation mode.

3.3 System Limitations

Due to the high gain of the loop for satisfying the condition in eq. (3), it is necessary to study the stability of the system. In steady-state operation, eventual changes produced at the load can generate variations at the rectifier output voltage that will be amplified α_{ea} times. If ΔV_{dc} is only 1 mV, changes at the error amplifier output voltage will be large, of 500mV (for α_{ea} =500) leading to out-of-range for some circuits. To avoid this, some control mechanisms should be included in the loop. We propose to use a first order low-pass filter at the error amplifier output. This LPF circuit shown in Fig. 14 acts as a delay element, avoiding an excessively fast response in the loop, by including a dominant pole. For a given ΔV_{dc} voltage increment, the design criterium is to limit, in a time period of the AC signal, the gain of the loop below unity. This means that instantaneous changes in the error amplifier input voltage cannot be amplified with a gain bigger than one in the loop, avoiding an increasing and uncontrolled signal. The opposite will cause the system to be unstable. To define parameters in the first order filter, we analize the response of the loop to a ΔV_{dc} voltage increment. If we cut the loop between the rectifier and the error amplifier, and suppose an input voltage increment of ΔV_{dc}, the corresponding voltage response at the rectifier output will be given by the expresion,

$$\Delta V_{dc,out} = G_m.\alpha_{dc}.\alpha_{ea}.\alpha_{ia}.Z_{xo}.(1-e^{-t/\tau})\Delta V_{dc} \tag{7}$$

For a gain below unity, it should be set that, in a period of time t = T, the output voltage increment of the rectified signal is less than the corresponding input voltage changes, $\Delta V_{dc,out} < \Delta V_{dc}$, leading to the condition,

$$1 < G_m.\alpha_{dc}.\alpha_{ea}.\alpha_{ia}.Z_{xo}.(1-e^{-T/\tau}) \tag{8}$$

Which means a time constant condition given by,

$$\tau < \frac{T}{\ln(\frac{\alpha_o}{\alpha_o - 1})} \tag{9}$$

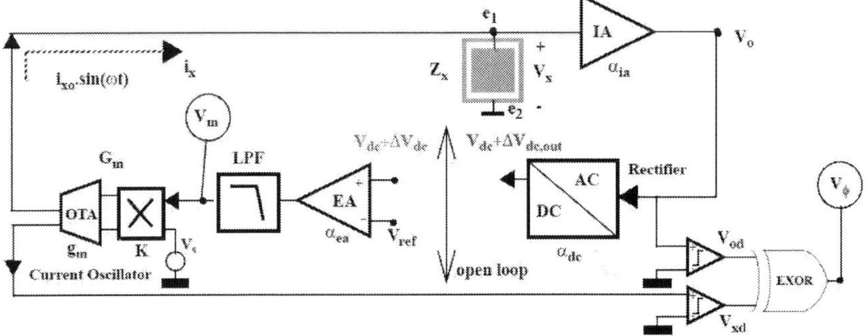

Fig. 14. Open loop system for the steady-state stability analysis.

being $\alpha_o = Z_{xo}.G_m.\alpha_{ia}.\alpha_{dc}.\alpha_{ea}$ the closed-loop gain of the system. This condition makes filter design dependent on ZUT through the paramenter Z_{xo} or impadance magnitude to be measured. So the Z_{xo} value should be quoted in order to apply the condition in eq. (9) properly. For example, if we take $\alpha_o = 100$, for a 10 kHz working frequency, the period of time is T=0.1 ms, and $\tau < 9.94991$ ms. For a $C_F = 20pF$ value, the corresponding $R_F = 500M\Omega$. Preserving by design large α_o values, which are imposed by eq. (3), the operation frequency will define the values of time constant τ in LPF.

Another problem will be the start-up operation when settling a new measurement. In this situation, the reset is applied to the system by initializing to zero the filter capacitor. All measures start from $V_m=0$, and several periods of time are required to set its final steady-state. This is the time required to load the capacitors C_r at the rectifier up to their steady-state value. When this happens, the closed-loop gain starts to work. This can be observed at the waveforms in Fig. 15, where the settling transient for the upper-lower output voltages of the rectifier are represented. When signals find a value of 80mV, the loop starts to work. The number of periods required for the settlig process is N_c. We have taken a conservative value in the range [20,40] for N_c in the automatic measurement presented in section 6. This number depends on the charge-discarge C_r capacitor process, which during settling process is limited to a maximum of 1 mV in a signal period, since the control loop is not working yet. The N_c will define the time required to perform a measurement: T. N_c. In biological systems, time constants are low and N_c values can be selected without strong limitations. However, for massive data processing such as imaging system, where a high number of measurements must be taken to obtain a frame, an N_c value requires an optimun selection.

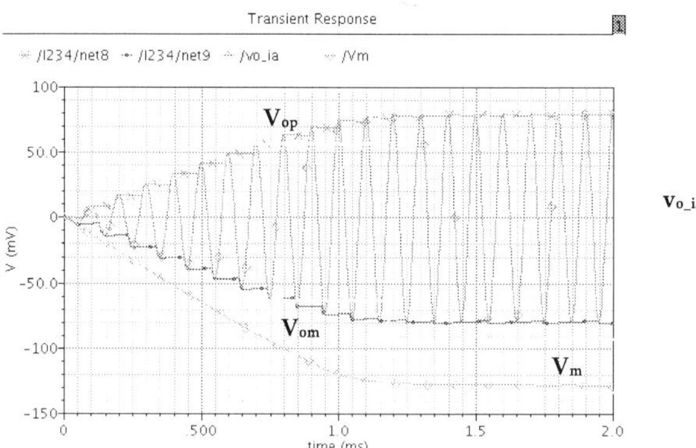

Fig. 15. Settling time transient from $V_m=0$ to its steady-state, $V_m=-128.4mV$. The upper and lower rectifier output voltages detect the increasing (deceasing) signal at the output amplifier during a settling period of about $N_c=15$ cycles of the AC input signal. After that, feedback loop gain starts to work, making the amplifier output voltage constant.

4. Simulation Results

4.1 Resistive and capacitive loads

Electrical simulations were performed for resistive and capacitive loads to demonstrate the correct performance of the measurement system. Initially, a 10kHz frequency was selected, and three types of loads: resistive ($Z_x = 100k\Omega$), RC in paralell ($Z_x = 100k\Omega||159pF$) and capacitive ($Z_x = 159pF$). The system parameters were set to satisty $\alpha_o = 100$, being $\alpha_{ia} = 10$, $\alpha_{dc} = 0.25$, $\alpha_{ea} = 500$, $G_m = 1.2uS$, and $V_{ref} = 20mV$. Figure 16 shows the waveforms obtained, using the electrical simulator Spectre, for the instrumentation amplifier output voltage V_o ($\alpha_{ia}.V_x$) with the corresponding positive and negative rectified signals (V_{op} and V_{om}), the current at the load, i_x, and the signals giving the information about the measurements: magnitude voltage, V_m, and phase voltage, V_ϕ, for the three loads. The amplifier output voltage V_o is nearly constant and equal to 80mV for all loads, fulfilling the Pstat condition ($V_{xo} = V_o/\alpha_{ia} = 8mV$), while i_x has an amplitude matched to the load. The V_m value gives the expected magnitude of Z_{xo} using eqs. (4) and (5) in all cases, as the data show in Table 1. The measurement duty-cycle allows the calculus of the Z_x phase. The 10kHz frequency has been selected because the phase shift introduced by instrumentation amplifier is close to zero, hence minimizing its influence on phase calculations. This and other deviations from ideal performance derived from process parameters variations should be adjusted by calibration. Errors in both parameters are within the expected range (less than 1%) and could be reduced by increasing the loop gain value.

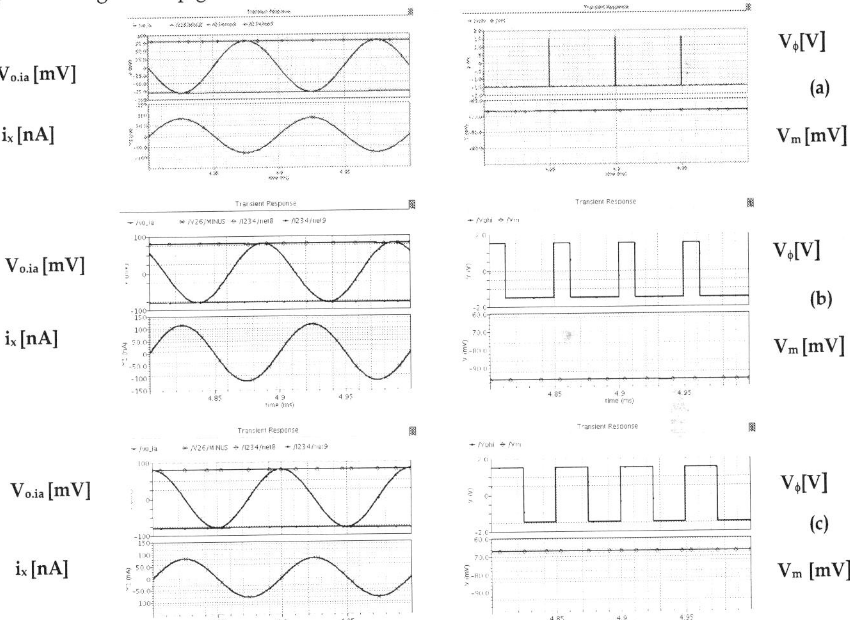

Fig. 16. Simulated waveforms for Z_x: (a) 100kΩ, (b) 100kΩ | |159pF, and (c) 159pF, showing the amplifier output voltage ($V_{o,ia}$), load current (i_x), and voltages for measurements: voltage magnitude: V_m and voltage phase: V_ϕ.

Another parallel RC load has been simulated. In this case, the working frequency has been changed to 100kHz, being $C_x = 15.9pF$, and the values of R_x in the range [10kΩ, 1MΩ], using $G_m=1.6\mu S$. The results are listed in Table 2 and represented in Fig. 17. It could be observed an excellent match with the expected performance.

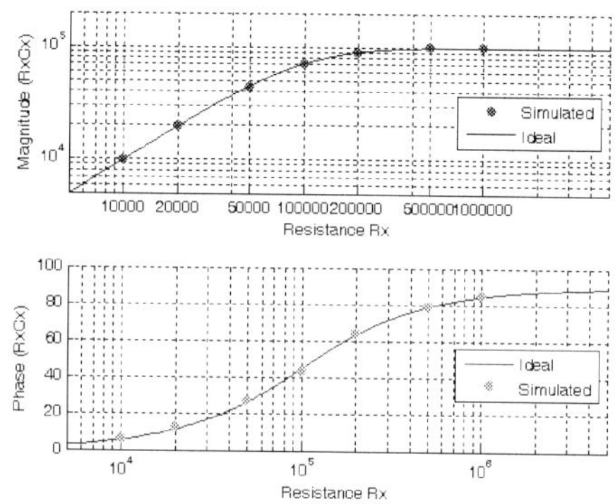

Fig. 17. Magnitude and phase for $R_x || C_x$, for $C_x = 15.9pF$ and R_x belongs to the range [10 kΩ, 1 MΩ], at 100 kHz frequency. Dots correspond to simulated results.

Z_x	V_m [mV]	δ	Z_{xo}[kΩ]		ϕ[$°$]	
	sim	sim	sim	teo	sim	teo
Case R	67.15	0.005	99.28	100.0	0.93	0
Case RC	94.96	02.47	70.20	70.70	44.44	45
Case C	67.20	0.501	99.21	100.0	90.04	90

Table 1. Simulation results at 10kHz for several RC loads.

R_x [kΩ]	V_m [mV]	δ	V_{xo}[mV]	Z_{xo}[kΩ]	ϕ[$°$]
10	491.0	0.24	7.8	9.92	6.34
20	251.2	0.40	7.8	19.43	12.1
50	112.7	0.83	7.9	43.60	27.6
100	69.7	1.34	7.9	70.80	43.6
200	55.2	1.85	7.9	89.53	64.3
500	50.4	2.27	7.9	97.97	79.4
1000	49.7	2.42	7.9	99.35	84.8

Table 2. Simulation results for $R_x || C_x$ load. (C_x=15.9pF, f=100kHz, ϕ_{IA}(100kHz)=-2.3$°$, G_m=1.6uS.

5. Four-Electrode System Applications

A **four wire system** for Z_x measurements is shown in Figures 18 (a) and (b). This kind of set-up is useful in electrical impedance tomography (EIT) of a given object (Holder, 2005), decreasing the electrode impedance influence (Z_{e1}-Z_{e4}) on the output voltage (V_o) thanks to the instrumentation amplifier high input impedance. Using the same circuits described before, the electrode model in (Yúfera et al., 2005), and a 100kΩ load, the waveforms in

Fig. 19 are obtained. The voltage at Z_x load matches the amplitude of V_{xo}=8mV, and the calculus of the impedance value at 10kHz frequency (Z_{xo}=99.8kΩ and ϕ=0.2°) is correct. The same load is maintained in a wide range of frequencies (100Hz to 1MHz) achieving the magnitude and phase listed in Table 3. The main deviations are present at the amplifier bandpass frequency edges due to lower and upper -3dB frequency corners. It can be observed the phase response measured and the influence due to amplifier frequency response in Fig. 5.

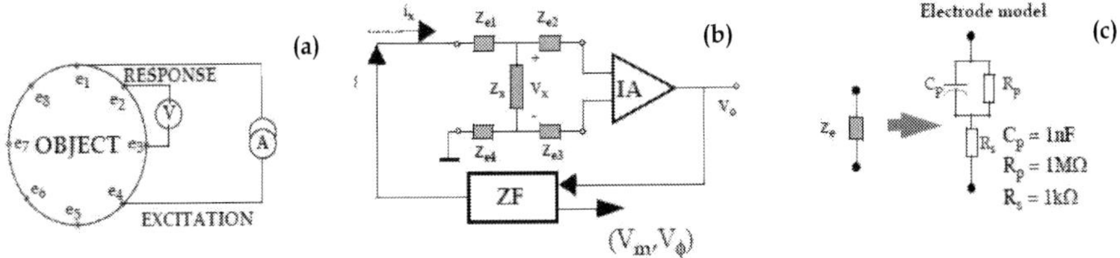

Fig. 18. (a) Eight-electrode configuration for Electrical Impedance Tomography (EIT) of an object. (b) Four-electrode system: Z_{ei} is the impedance of the electrode i. (c) Electrical model for the electrode model.

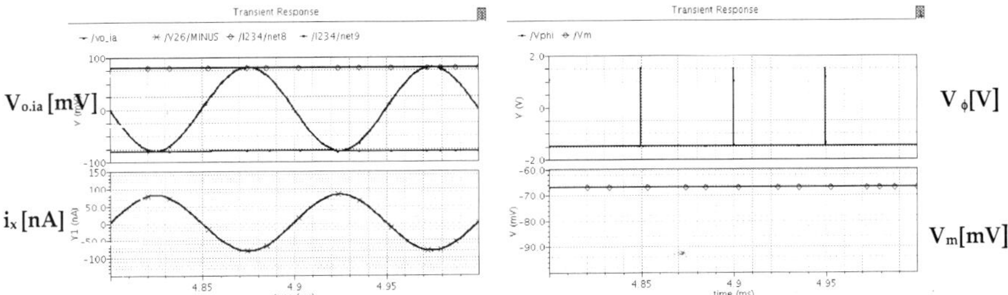

Fig. 19. Four-electrode simulation results for Z_x=100kΩ at 10 kHz frequency.

Frequency [kHz]	Z_{xo}[kΩ]		ϕ[°]	
	sim	teo	sim	teo
0.1	96.17	92.49	11.70	13.67
1	99.40	100.00	1.22	1.90
10	99.80	100.00	-0.20	-0.12
100	99.70	100.00	-4.10	-3.20
1000	95.60	96.85	-40.60	-32.32

Table 3. Simulation results for four-electrode setup and Z_x=100kΩ.

6. Two-Electrode System Applications

A two-electrode system is employed in Electric Cell substrate Impedance Spectroscopy (ECIS) (Giaever et al., 1992) as a technique capable of obtaining basic information on single or low concentration of cells (today, it is not well defined if two or four electrode systems are better for cell impedance characterization (Bragos et al., 2007)). The main drawback of two-wire systems is that the output signal corresponds to the series of two electrodes and the load, being necessary to extract the load from the measurements (Huang et al., 2004). Figures 20 (a) and (b) show a two-electrode set-up in which the load or sample (100kΩ) has been measured in the frequency range of [100Hz,1MHz]. The circuits parameters were adapted to satisfy the condition $Z_{xo}G_m\alpha_{ia}\alpha_{dc}\alpha_{ea}=100$, since Z_{xo} will change from around 1MΩ to 100kΩ when frequency goes from tens of Hz to MHz, due to electrode impedance dependence. The simulation data obtained are shown in Table 4. At 10kHz frequency, magnitude Z_{xo} is now 107.16kΩ, because it includes two-electrodes in series. The same effect occurs for the phase, being now 17.24°. The results are in Table 4 for the frequency range considered. The phase accuracy observed is better at the mid-bandwidth.

In both cases, the equivalent circuit described in Huang (2004) has been employed for the electrode model. This circuit represents a possible and real electrical performance of electrodes in some cases. In general, the electric model for electrodes will depend on the electrode-to-sample and/or medium interface (Joye et al., 2008) and should be adjusted to each measurement test problem. In this work a real and typical electrode model has been used to validate the proposed circuits.

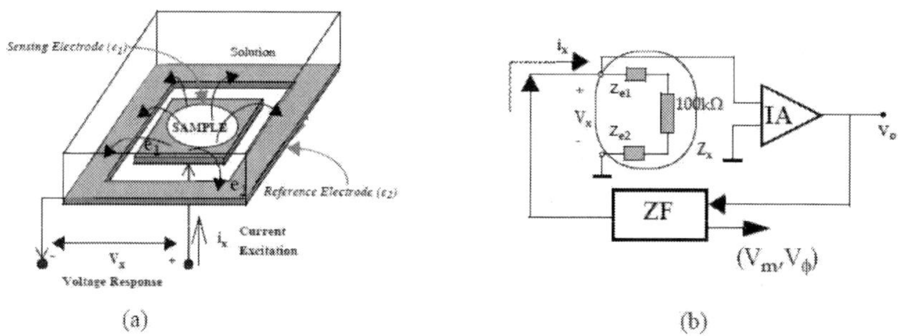

(a) (b)

Fig. 20. (a) Two-electrode system with a sample on top of electrode 1 (e_1). (b) Equivalent circuit employed for an R_{SAMPLE}=100kΩ. Z_x includes Z_{e1}, Z_{e2} and R_{SAMPLE} resistance.

Frequency [kHz]	Z_{xo}[kΩ]		$\phi[°]$	
	Sim	Teo	Sim	Teo
0.1	1058.8	1087.8	-40.21	-19.00
1	339.35	344.70	-56.00	-62.88
10	107.16	107.33	-17.24	-17.01
100	104.80	102.01	-6.48	-5.09
1000	104.24	102.00	-37.80	-32.24

Table 4. Simulation results for two-electrode set-up and Z_x=100kΩ.

6.1 Cell location applications

The cell-electrode model: An equivalent circuit for modelling the electrode-cell interface performance is a requisite for electrical characterization of the cells on top of electrodes.

Fig. 21 illustrates a two-electrode sensor useful for the ECIS technique: e_1 is called sensing electrode and e_2 reference electrode. Electrodes can be fabricated in CMOS processes using metal layers (Hassibi et al., 2006) or adding post-processing steps (Huang et al., 2004). The sample on e_1 top is a cell whose location must be detected. The circuit models developed to characterize electrode-cell interfaces (Huang, 2004) and (Joye, 2008) contain technology process information and assume, as main parameter, the overlapping area between cells and electrodes. An adequate interpretation of these models provides information about: a) *electrical simulations*: parameterized models can be used to update the actual electrode circuit in terms of its overlapping with cells. b) *imaging reconstruction*: electrical signals measured on the sensor can be associated to a given overlapping area, obtaining the actual area covered on the electrode from measurements done.

In this work, we selected the electrode-cell model reported by Huang et al. This model was obtained by using finite element method simulations of the electromagnetic fields in the cell-electrode interface, and considers that the sensing surface of e_1 could be totally or partially filled by cells. Figure 22 shows this model. For the two-electrode sensor in Fig. 21, with e_1 sensing area A, $Z(\omega)$ is the impedance by unit area of the empty electrode (without cells on top). When e_1 is partially covered by cells in a surface A_c, $Z(\omega)/(A-A_c)$ is the electrode impedance associated to non-covered area by cells, and $Z(\omega)/A_c$ is the impedance of the covered area. R_{gap} models the current flowing laterally in the electrode-cell interface, which depends on the electrode-cell distance at the interface (in the range of 10-100nm). The resistance R_s is the spreading resistance through the conductive solution. In this model, the signal path from e_1 to e_2 is divided into two parallel branches: one direct branch through the solution not covered by cells, and a second path containing the electrode area covered by the cells. For the empty electrode, the impedance model $Z(\omega)$ has been chosen as the circuit illustrated in Fig. 22(c), where C_p, R_p and R_s are dependent on both electrode and solution materials. Other cell-electrode models can be used (Joye et al., 2008), but for those the measurement method proposed here is still valid. We have considered for e_2 the model in Fig 22(a), not covered by cells. Usually, the reference electrode is common for all sensors, being its area much higher than e_1. Figure 23 represents the impedance magnitude, Z_{xoc}, for the sensor system in Fig. 21, considering that e_1 could be either empty, partially or totally covered by cells.

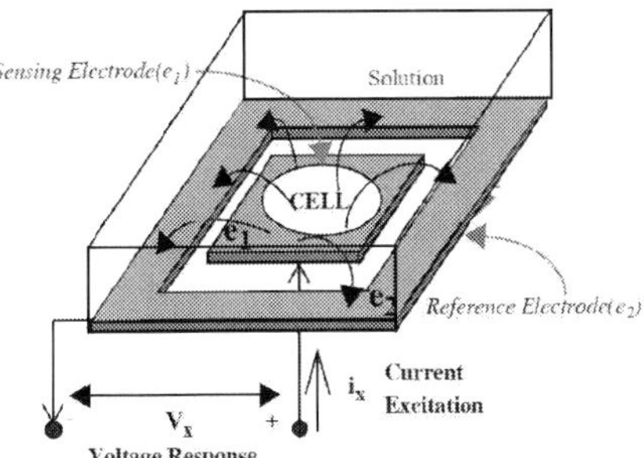

Fig. 21. Basic concept for measuring with the ECIS technique using two electrodes: e_1 or sensing electrode and e_2 or reference electrode. AC current i_x is injected between e_1 and e_2, and voltage response V_x is measured from e_1 to e_2, including effect of e_1, e_2 and sample impedances.

The parameter *ff* is called *fill factor*, being zero for A_c=0 (empty electrode), and 1 for A_c=A (full electrode). We define Z_{xoc} (*ff*=0) = Z_{xo} as the impedance magnitude of the sensor without cells.

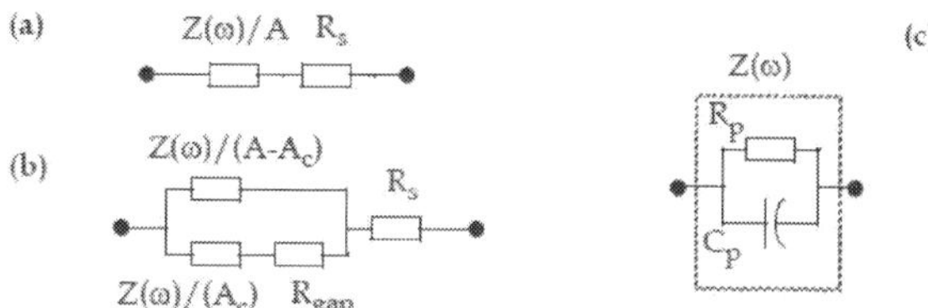

Fig. 22. Electrical models for (a) e_1 electrode without cells and, (b) e_1 cell-electrode. (c) Model for $Z(\omega)$.his work.

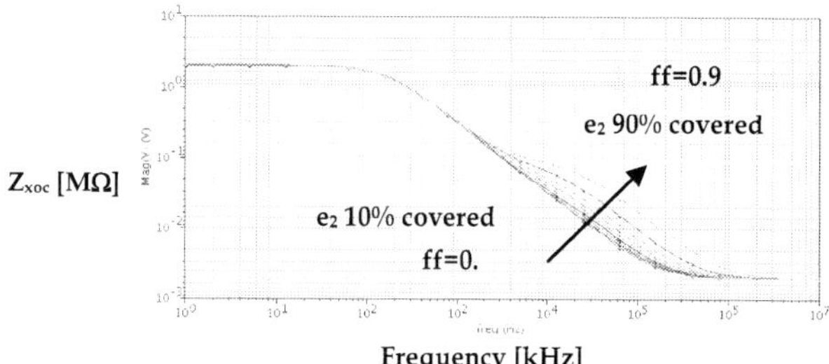

Fig. 23. Sensor impedance magnitude when the fill factor parameter (*ff*) changes. C_p=1nF, R_p=1MΩ, R_s=1kΩ and R_{gap}=100kΩ.

Absolute changes on impedance magnitude of e_1 in series with e_2 are detected in a [10 kHz, 100 kHz] frequency range as a result of sensitivity to area covered on e_1. Relative changes can inform more accurately on these variations by defining a new figure-of-merit called r (Huang et al., 2004), or *normalized impedance magnitude*, by the equation,

$$r = \frac{Z_{xoc} - Z_{xo}}{Z_{xo}} \tag{10}$$

Where r represents the relative increment of the impedance magnitude of two-electrode system with cells (Z_{xoc}) relative to the two-electrode system without them (Z_{xo}). The graphics of r versus frequency is plotted in Fig. 24, for a cell-to-electrode coverage *ff* from 0.1 to 0.9 in steps of 0.1. We can identify again the frequency range where the sensitivity to cells is high, represented by r increments. For a given frequency, each value of the normalized impedance r can be linked with its *ff*, being possible to detect the cells and to estimate the sensing electrode covered area, A_c. For imaging reconstruction, this work proposes a new CMOS system to measure the r parameter for a given frequency, and detect the corresponding covering area on each electrode according to sensitivity in Fig 24.

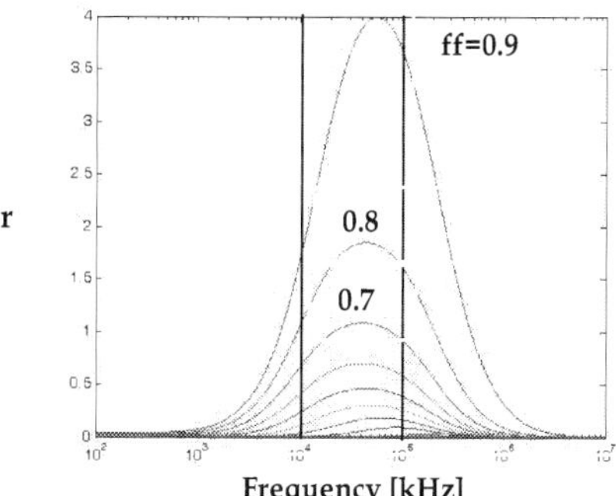

Fig. 24. Normalized magnitude impedance r for ff= 0.1 to 0.9 in steps of 0.1.

6.2 2D image applications

To test the proposed method for impedance sensing, we have chosen a simulation case with an 8x8 two-electrode array. The sample input to be analysed is a low density MCF-7 epithelial breast cancer cell culture shown in Fig. 25(a). In this image some areas are covered by cells and others are empty. Our objective is to use the area parametrized electrode-cell model and the proposed circuits to detect their location. The selected pixel size is 50µm x 50µm, similar to cell dimensions. Figure 25(a) shows the grid selected and its overlap with the image. We associate a squared impedance sensor, similar to the one described in Fig. 21, to each pixel in Fig. 25(a) to obtain a 2D system description valid for electrical simulations. An optimum pixel size can be obtained by using design curves for normalized impedance r and its frequency dependence. Each electrical circuit associated to each e_1 electrode in the array was initialized with its corresponding fill factor (ff). The matrix in Fig 25(b) is obtained in this way. Each electrode or pixel is associated to a number in the range [0,1] (ff) depending on its overlap with cells on top. These numbers were calculated with an accuracy of 0.05 from the image in Fig.25(a). The ff matrix represents the input of our system to be simulated. Electrical simulations of the full system were performed at 10kHz (midband of the IA) to obtain the value of the voltage magnitude V_m in eq. (4) for all electrodes. Pixels are simulated by rows, starting from the leftmost bottom (pixel 1) to the right-most top (pixel 64). When measuring each pixel, the voltage V_m is reset to zero and then 25 cycles (N_c) are reserved to find its steady-state, where V_m value becomes constant and is acquired. The waveforms obtained for the amplifier output voltage $\alpha_{ia}V_x$, voltage magnitude, V_m, and excitation current i_x are represented in Fig. 26. It is observed that the voltage at the sensor, V_x, has always the same amplitude (8mV), while the current decreases with ff. The V_m signal converges towards a DC value, inversely proportional to the impedance magnitude. Steady-state values of V_m are represented in Fig. 27 for all pixels. These are used to calculate their normalized impedances r using eqs. (10) and (5).

To have a graphical 2D image of the fill factor (area covered by cells) in all pixels, Fig. 28 represents the 8x8 ff-maps, in which each pixel has a grey level depending on its fill factor value (white is empty and black full). In particular, Fig. 28(a) represents the ff-map for the input image in Fig. 25(b). Considering the parameterized curves in Fig. 24 at 10kHz frequency, the fill factor parameter has been calculated for each electrode, using the V_m simulated data from Fig. 26 and the results are represented in Fig. 28(b). The same simulations have been performed at 100kHz, obtaining the *ff*-map in Fig. 28(c). As Fig. 24 predicts, the best match with the input is found at 100kHz since normalized impedance is more sensitive and the sensor has a higher dynamic range at 100kHz than at 10kHz. In both cases, the errors obtained in the *ff* values are below 1%, therefore matching with the input is excellent. The total time required to acquired data for a full image or frame will depend on the measuring frequency, the number of cycles reserved for each pixel (N_c=25 for reported example) and the array dimension (8x8). For reported simulations 160ms and 16ms for frame, working at 10kHz and 100kHz, respectively, are required. This frame acquisition time is enough for real time monitoring of cell culture systems.

pixel 64

0.30	0.40	0.15	0	0.10	0.15	0	0
0.20	0	0	0.20	0.50	0.55	0.35	0.40
0.35	0.10	0.15	0.30	0	0.05	0.10	0.10
[illegible]	0	0.20	0.20	0.40	0.30	0.30	0.15
0	0	0.05	0.10	0.60	0.50	0	0.25
0.40	0	0.05	0.30	0.50	0.30	0	0.05
0.80	0.05	0	[illegible]	0.90	0.30	0	0.45
0.90	0.20	0	0.50	0.10	0	0.05	0.15

pixel 1

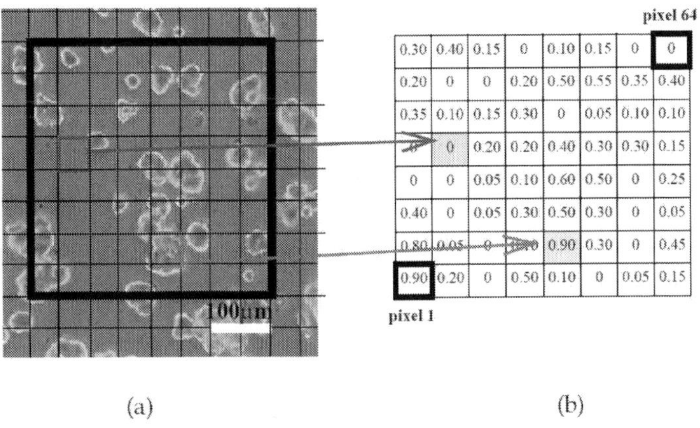

(a) (b)

Fig. 25. (a) 8x8 pixel area selection in epithelial breast cancer cell culture. (b) Fill factor map (*ff*) associated to each electrode (pixel).

pixel empty

65.3	61.0	66.6	67.8	67.7	67.7	67.8	67.8
67.2	67.6	67.7	55.0	55.0	51.5	63.5	61.0
63.5	67.8	67.5	65.2	67.8	67.8	67.7	67.7
67.8	67.8	67.2	67.2	61.0	65.2	65.2	67.7
67.8	67.8	67.6	67.7	48.1	55.0	67.8	66.4
61.0	67.8	67.5	65.1	55.1	65.3	67.7	67.7
32.8	67.8	67.8	67.6	25.0	65.3	67.8	58.2
25.0	67.2	67.8	55.0	67.7	67.8	67.7	67.6

pixel 90% full

Fig. 26. 2D matrix of values for V_m [mV] in steady-state obtained from electrical simulations at 10 kHz frequency.

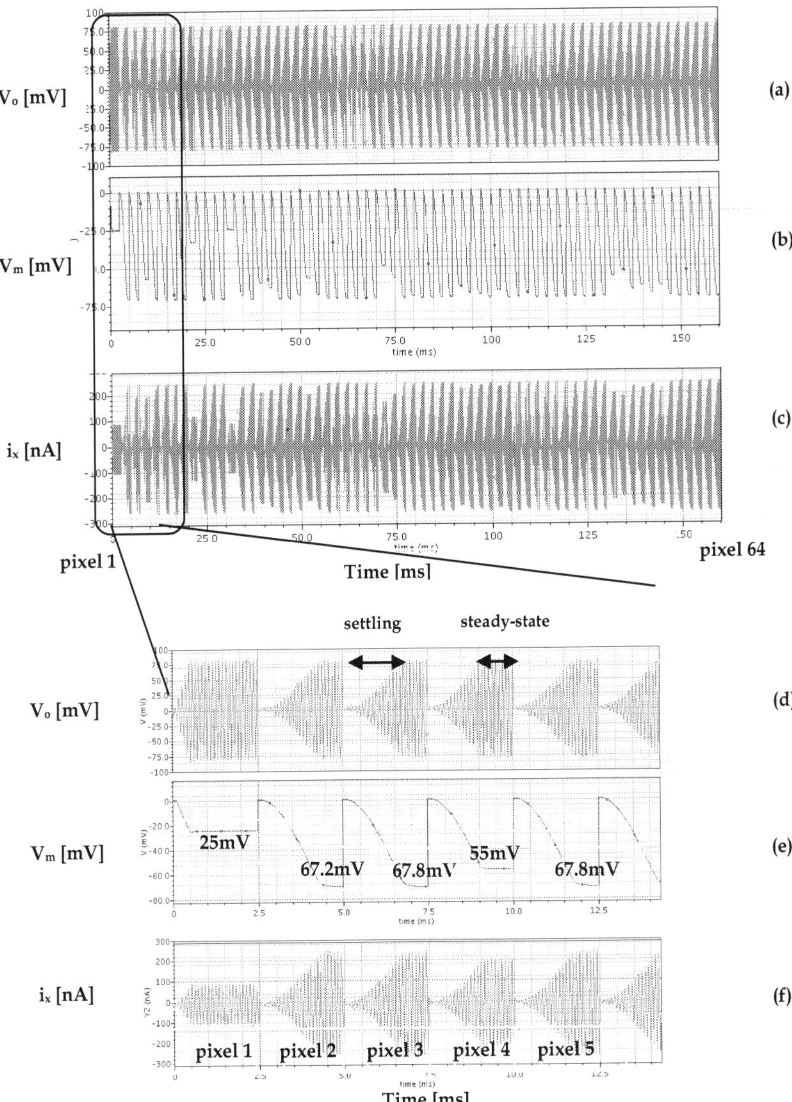

Fig. 27. Simulated waveforms for (a) $\alpha_{ia}V_x = 10V_x$, (b) V_m and (c) i_x signals for the 64 electrodes at 10 kHz. (d-f) Zoom for the first five pixels of (a-c) waveforms.

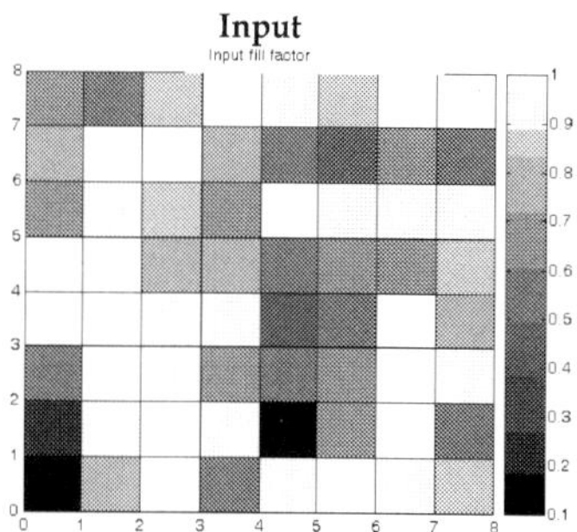

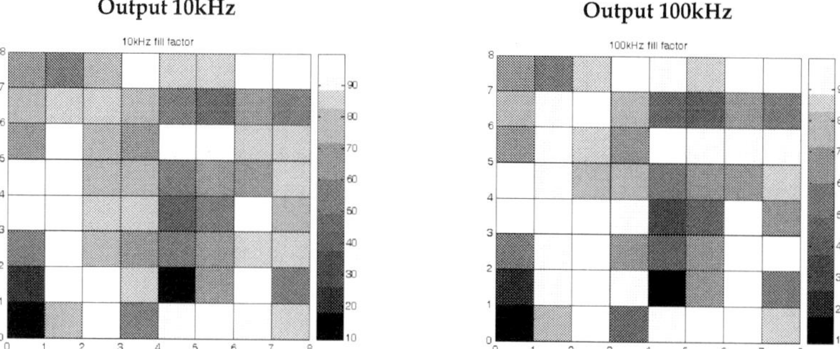

Fig. 28. 2D diagram of the fill factor maps for 8x8 pixels: (a) ideal input. Image reconstructed from simulations at (b) 10 kHz and (c) 100 kHz.

7. Conclusions

This work reports novel front-end circuits for impedance measurement based on a proposed closed-loop configuration. The system has been developed on the basis of applying an AC voltage with constant amplitude to the load under test. As a result, the proposed technique allows to perform excitation and read-out functionalities by the same circuits, delivering magnitude and phase impedance in two independent signals, easy to acquired: a constant DC signal and a digital signal with variable duty-cycle, respectively.

The proposed CMOS circuits to implement the system have been correctly validated by electrical simulation taking into account several types of resistive and capacitive loads, working at different frequencies.

A number of biomedical applications relying on impedance detection and monitoring can benefit from our proposed CBIM system in several ways: the necessity of taking/performing measurements using electrodes proves the usefulness of the proposed system because there is the possibility of limiting the voltage amplitude on the electrodes, biasing a given electrode-solution interface at the non-polarizable region, optimum for neural signal recording, for example. Also, the possibility of the simultaneous implementation of an electrode sensor and CMOS circuits in the same substrate enables the realization of fully integrated system or lab-on-chips (LoC). This fact should be tested in future works.

Standard two- and four-electrode based systems have been tested to demostrate the feasibility of the proposed system. The results for the four-wire set-up are accurate in all the frequency band, except at the corner bandwidth of the instrumentation amplifier, where its magnitude and phase responses are the main error sources. Electrical Impedance Tomography is an excellent candidate to employ the proposed impedance measurement system.

The application of CBIM to a two-wire set-up enables the proposed system for impedance sensing of biological samples to be useful for 2D imaging. An electrical model based on the overlapping area is employed in both system simulation and image reconstruction for electrode-cell characterization, allowing the incorporation of the electrode design process on the full system specifications. Electrical simulations have been done to reproduce the ECIS technique, giving promising results in cell location and imaging, and enabling our system for other real-time applications such as cell index monitoring, cell tracking, etc. In future works, precise cell electrode model, optimized sensing circuits and design trade-off for electrode sizing will be further explored for a real experimental imaging system.

8. Acknowledgements

This work is in part supported by the Spanish founded Project: TEC2007-68072/ TECATE, *Técnicas para mejorar la calidad del test y las prestaciones del diseño en tecnologías CMOS submicrométricas.*

9. References

Ackmann, J. (1993). Complex Bioelectric Impedance Measurement System for the Frequency Range from 5Hz to 1MHz. *Annals of Biomedical Engineering*, Vol. 21, pp. 135-146

Beach, R. D. et al., (2005). Towards a Miniature In Vivo Telemetry Monitoring System Dynamically Configurable as a Potentiostat or Galvanostat for Two- and Three-Electrode Biosensors. *IEEE Transactions on Instrumentation and Measurement*, Vol. 54, No. 1, pp. 61-72

Yúfera, A. et al., (2005). A Tissue Impedance Measurement Chip for Myocardial Ischemia Detection. *IEEE Transaction on Circuits and Systems: Part I. Regular papers*, Vol. 52, No. 12, pp. 2620-2628

Huang, X. (2004). Impedance-Based Biosensor Arrays. *PhD. Thesis*, Carnagie Mellon University

Radke, S. M. et al., (2004). Design and Fabrication of a Micro-impedance Biosensor for Bacterial Detection. *IEEE Sensor Journal*, Vol. 4, No. 4, pp. 434-440

Borkholder, D. A. (1998). Cell-Based Biosensors Using Microelectrodes. *PhD Thesis*, Stanford University

Giaever, I. et al., (1996). Use of Electric Fields to Monitor the Dynamical Aspect of Cell Behaviour in Tissue Culture. *IEEE Transaction on Biomedical Engineering*, Vol. BME-33, No. 2, pp. 242-247

Holder, D. (2005). Electrical Impedance Tomography: Methods, History and Applications, Philadelphia: IOP

Pallás-Areny, R. and Webster, J. G. (1993). Bioelectric Impedance Measurements Using Synchronous Sampling. *IEEE Transaction on Biomedical Engineering*, Vol. 40, No. 8, pp: 824-829. Aug

Zhao, Y. et al., (2006). A CMOS Instrumentation Amplifier for Wideband Bio-impedance Spectroscopy Systems. *Proceedings of the International Symposium on Circuits and Systems*, pp. 5079-5082

Ahmadi, H. et al., (2005). A Full CMOS Voltage Regulating Circuit for Bio-implantable Applications. *Proceeding of the International Symposium on Circuits and Systems*, pp. 988-991

Hassibi, A. et al., (2006). A Programmable 0.18μm CMOS Electrochemical Sensor Microarray for Bio-molecular Detection. *IEEE Sensor Journal*, Vol. 6, No. 6, pp. 1380-1388

Yúfera, A. and Rueda, A. (2008). A Method for Bio-impedance Measure with Four- and Two-Electrode Sensor Systems. *30th Annual International IEEE EMBS Conference*, Vancouver, Canada, pp. 2318-2321

Sawigun, C. and Demosthenous, A. (2006). Compact low-voltage CMOS four-quadrant analogue multiplier. *Electronics Letters*, Vol. 42, No. 20, pp. 1149-1150

Huang, X., Nguyem, D., Greve, D. W. and Domach, M. M. (2004). Simulation of Microelectrode Impedance Changes Due to Cell Growth. *IEEE Sensors Journal*, Vol. 4, No 5, pp. 576-583

Yúfera, A. and Rueda, A. (2009). A CMOS Bio-Impedance Measurement System. *12th IEEE Design and Diagnostic of Electronics Circuits and Systems*, Liberec, Czech Republic, pp. 252-257

Romani, A. et al., (2004). Capacitive Sensor Array for Location of Bio-particles in CMOS Lab-on-a-Chip. *International Solid Stated Circuits Conference (ISSCC)*, 12.4

Medoro, G. et al., (2003). A Lab-on-a-Chip for Cell Detection and Manipulation. *IEEE Sensor Journal*, Vol. 3, No. 3, pp: 317-325

Manaresi, N. et al (2003). A CMOS Chip for individual Cell Manipulation and Detection. *IEEE Journal of Solid Stated Circuits*, Vol. 38, No. 12, pp: 2297-2305. Dec

Joye, N. et al (2008). An Electrical Model of the Cell-Electrode Interface for High-Density Microelectrode Arrays. *30th Annual International IEEE EMBS Conference*, pp: 559-562

Bragos, R. et al., (2006). Four *Versus* Two-Electrode Measurement Strategies for Cell Growing and Differentiation Monitoring Using Electrical Impedance Spectroscopy. *28th Annual International IEEE EMBS Conference*, pp: 2106-2109

16

Characterization and enhancement of non-invasive recordings of intestinal myoelectrical activity

Y. Ye-Lin[1], J. Garcia-Casado[1], Jose-M. Bueno-Barrachina[2],
J. Guimera-Tomas[1], G. Prats-Boluda[1]and J.L. Martinez-de-Juan[1]
[1]*Instituto Interuniversitario de Investigación en Bioingeniería y Tecnología Orientada al Ser Humano, Universidad Politécnica de Valencia, Spain*
[2]*Instituto de Tecnología Eléctrica, Universidad Politécnica de Valencia, Spain*

1. Intestinal motility

Intestinal motility is a set of muscular contractions, associated with the mixing, segmentation and propulsion actions of the chyme, which is produced along the small intestine (Weisbrodt 1987). Therefore, intestinal motility is basic for the process of digesting the chyme that is coming from the stomach.

Under physiological conditions, intestinal motility can be classified in two periods: fasting motility and postprandial motility. In the fasting state, the small intestine is not quiescent, but it is characterized by a set of organized contractions that form a pattern named Interdigestive Migrating Motor Complex (IMMC) (Szurszewski 1969). This pattern of contractile activity has a double mission: to empty the content that is being poured by the stomach and to prevent the migration of germs and bacteria in the oral way (Szurszewski 1969; Weisbrodt 1987). The IMMC has a length between 90 and 130 minutes in humans and between 80 and 120 minutes in dogs. Attending to the motor activity degree of the intestine, the IMMC cycle can be divided in three phases (Szurszewski 1969; Weisbrodt 1987): phase I of quiescence, which is characterized by the absence of contractile activity; phase II of irregular contractile activity; and phase III of maximal frequency and intensity of bowel contractions. Phase III is band of regular pressure waves lasting for about 5 min and migrates aborally from the proximal small intestine to the terminal ileum. It is usually generated at the duodenum, although it can be generated at any point between the stomach and the ileum. Migration is a prerequisite for the phase III. The velocity of migration is 5-10 cm/min in the proximal small intestine and it decreases gradually along the small intestine to 0.5-1 cm/min in the ileum (Szurszewski 1969; Weisbrodt 1987). The IMMC is cyclic at fast and it is interrupted after the food ingestion, which involves the appearance of the postpandrial motility. The postpandrial pattern is characterized by an irregular contractile activity similar to the phase II of the IMMC. In figure 1, it can be appreciated a complete IMMC cycle from minute 55 until minute 155, and the appearance of the postpandrial motility pattern occurred immediately after the ingestion of food.

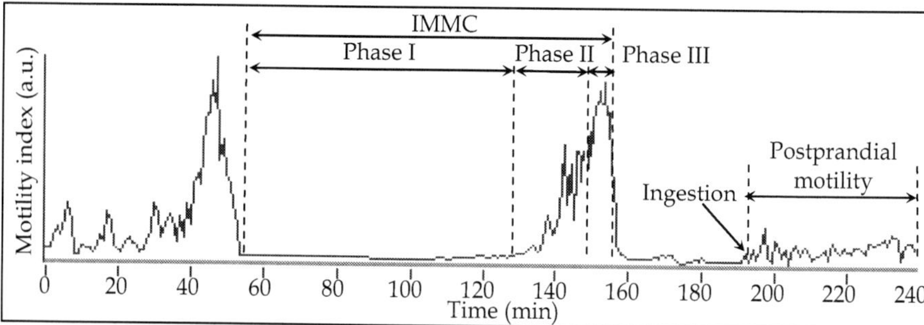

Fig. 1. Time evolution of intestinal motility index recorded from canine jejunum in fasting state and after ingestion (minute 190).

Many pathologies such as irritable bowel syndrome, mechanical obstruction, bacterial overgrowth or paralytic ileum are associated with intestinal motor dysfunctions (Camilleri et al. 1998; Quigley 1996). These dysfunctions show a high prevalence: between 10% and 20% of European and American population suffers from functional bowel disorders and irritable bowel syndrome (Delvaux 2003). Because of that, the study of the intestinal motility is of great clinical interest.

2. Recording of intestinal motility

The main problem in monitoring the intestinal activity is the anatomical difficult access to the small bowel. Traditionally, intestinal motility measurement has been performed by means of manometric techniques, because these are low cost techniques and they are a direct measurement of the intestinal contractions. However, this method presents a series of technical and physiological problems (Byrne & Quigley 1997; Camilleri et al. 1998), and its non-invasiveness is still a controversial issue.

Nowadays, non-invasive techniques for the intestinal motility monitoring are being developed such as: ultrasound based techniques (An et al. 2001), intestinal sounds (Tomomasa et al. 1999), bioelectromagnetism based techniques (Bradshaw et al. 1997), and myoelectrical techniques (Bradshaw et al. 1997; Chen et al. 1993; Garcia-Casado et al. 2005). The utility of the intestinal sounds recording sounds so as to determinate the intestinal motility has been questioned, because it is better corresponded to the intestinal transit associated with the propulsion movements rather than to the intestinal contractions (Tomomasa et al. 1999). The ultrasound techniques have been validated for the graphical visualization and the quantitative analysis of both the peristaltic and non-peristaltic movements of the small intestine (An et al. 2001), but they do not closely represent the intestinal motility. On the other hand, both the myoelectrical and the magnetical studies have demonstrated the possibility of picking up the intestinal activity on the abdominal surface (Bradshaw et al. 1997), providing a very helpful tool for the study of the gastrointestinal motor dysfunctions. However, the clinical application of the magnetic techniques is limited by the high cost of the devices (Bradshaw et al. 1997), and the development of the myoelectrical techniques is still in the experimental stage.

At the present chapter, the study of the intestinal activity is focused on the myoelectrical techniques. These techniques are based on the recording of the changes of muscular cell's membrane potential and the associated bioelectrical currents, since they are directly related to the small intestine smooth muscle contractions.

3. Intestinal myoelectrical activity

The electroenterogram (EEnG) is the myoelectrical intestinal signal originated by the muscular layers and it can be recorded on the intestinal serous wall. The EEnG is composed by two components: slow waves (SW), which is a pacemaker activity and does not represent the intestinal motility; and action potentials, also known as spike bursts (SB). These SB only appear at the plateau of the slow wave when the small intestine contracts, showing the presence and the intensity of the intestinal contraction (Martinez-de-Juan et al. 2000; Weisbrodt 1987). The relationship between the intestinal pressure and the SB activity is widely accepted (Martinez-de-Juan et al. 2000; Weisbrodt 1987). This relationship can be appreciated in figure 2, the presence of SB (trace b) is directly associated with the increments on the intestinal pressure (trace a). It can also be observed that the SW activity is always present, even when no contractions occur.

Nowadays, the hypothesis that the SW activity is generated by the interstitial cells of Cajal is widely accepted (Horowitz et al. 1999). These cells act as pacemaker cells since they possess unique ionic conductances that trigger the SW activity, whilst smooth muscle cells may lack the basic ionic mechanisms which are necessary to generate the SW activity (Horowitz et al. 1999). However, smooth muscle cells respond to the depolarization and repolarization cycle imposed by the interstitial cells of Cajal. The responses of smooth muscle cells are focused on the regulation of L-type Ca^{2+} current, which is the main source of Ca^{2+} that produce the intestinal contraction (Horowitz et al. 1999). Therefore, the frequency of the SW determines the maximal rhythm of the intestinal mechanical contraction (Weisbrodt 1987). The SWs are usually generated in the natural pacemaker that is localized at the duodenum, and they propagate from the duodenum to the ileum. The SW frequency is approximately constant at

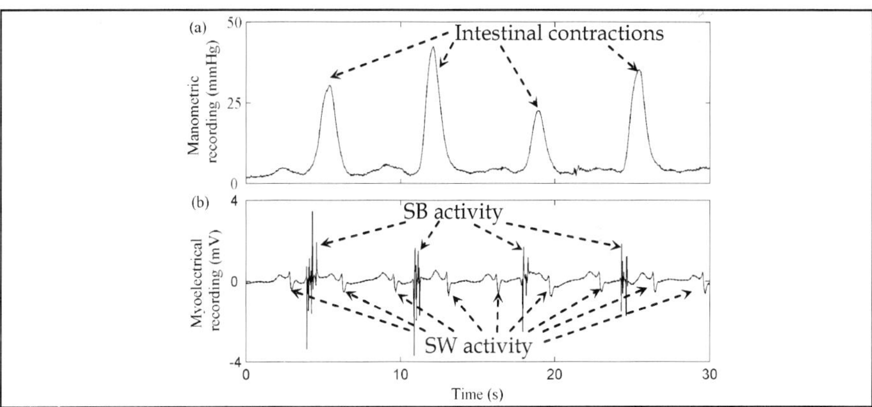

Fig. 2. Simultaneous recording of bowel pressure (a) and internal myoelectrical activity (b) in the same bowel loop from a non-sedated dog.

each point of the intestine although it decreases in distal way (Diamant & Bortoff 1969). In dogs this frequency ranges from approximately 19 cycles per minute (cpm) at the duodenum to 11 cpm at the ileum (Bass & Wiley 1965). In humans the SW frequency is around 12 cpm at upper duodenum and of 7 cpm at the terminal ileum.

With regard to the SB, they are generated by the smooth muscle cells which are responsible for the intestinal mechanical contraction (Horowitz et al. 1999). The smooth muscle of the small intestine is controlled by the enteric nervous system, and it is influenced by both the extrinsic autonomic nerves of the nervous system and the hormones (Weisbrodt 1987). Unlike the SW activity, the SB activity does not present a typical repetition frequency, but it is characterized for distributing its energy in the spectrum over 2 Hz in the internal recording of the EEnG (Martinez-de-Juan et al. 2000).

The internal recording of EEnG provides a signal of 'high' amplitude, i.e. in the order of mV, which is almost free of physiological interferences. The employment of this technique has obtained promising results for the characterization of different pathologies such as: intestinal ischemia (Seidel et al. 1999), bacterial overgrowth in acute pancreatitis (Van Felius et al. 2003), intestinal mechanical obstruction (Lausen et al. 1988), irritable bowel syndrome (El-Murr et al. 1994). However, the clinical application of internal myoelectrical techniques is limited, given that surgical intervention is needed for the implantation of the electrodes.

4. Surface EEnG recording

Surface EEnG recording can be an alternative method to non-invasively determine the intestinal motility. Logically, the morphology and the frequency spectrum of the intestinal myoelectrical signals recorded on the abdominal surface are affected by the different abdominal layers, which exercise an insulating effect between the intestinal sources and the external electrodes (Bradshaw et al. 1997).

4.1 Non-invasive recording and characterization of slow wave activity

In 1975, in an experiment designed to measure the gastric activity using surface electrodes, Brown found a component of frequency of 10-12 cpm, superposed on 3 cpm gastric electrical activity (Brown et al. 1975). They believed that the component of 10-12 cpm was of intestinal origin. Later, by means of the analysis of the simultaneous external and internal EEnG recordings, it was confirmed that it is possible to detect the intestinal SW on the human abdominal surface (Chen et al. 1993). In this last work, bipolar recording of surface signal was conducted using two monopolar contact electrodes which were placed near the umbilicus with a spacing distance of 5 cm. Figure 3 shows 5 min of the external EEnG signal (electrodes 3-4), simultaneously recorded with the gastric activity (electrodes 1-2) and the respiration signal. The external EEnG signal presents an omnipresent frequency peak of 9-12 cpm, which coincides with the typical value of the repetition rate of the human intestinal SW (12 cpm at the duodenum and 7 cpm at the ileum). The simultaneous recording of respiration signal allowed rejecting breathing as a possible source of this frequency peak.

The possibility of picking up the intestinal SW activity on the abdominal surface has been reasserted by other authors (Bradshaw et al. 1997; Chang et al. 2007; Garcia-Casado et al. 2005). The myoelectrical signal recorded on the abdominal surface of patients with total gastrectomy presented a dominant frequency of 10.9 ± 1.0 cpm in fasting state and 10.9 ± 1.3 cpm in postprandial state (Chang et al. 2007). In animal models it has been proven

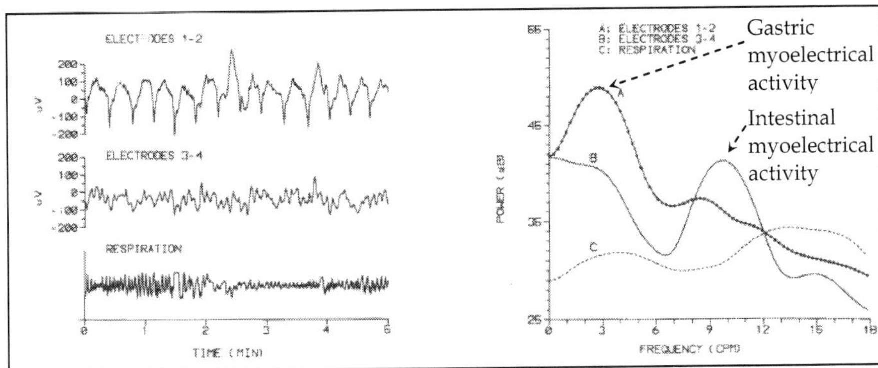

Fig. 3. Five minutes of external gastric (electrode 1-2) and intestinal (electrode 3-4) myoelectrical signal, simultaneously recorded with the respiration signal (bottom trace). The right trace shows the power spectral density of these signals (Chen et al. 1993).

that the dominant frequency of the external myoelectrical intestinal signal coincides with the repetition rate of the internal intestinal SW both in physiological conditions (Garcia-Casado et al. 2005) and in pathological conditions (Bradshaw et al. 1997).

Unlike the internal myoelectrical signal, the amplitude of the external record shows a great variation from 30 to 330 μV among subjects (Chen et al. 1993), since this amplitude depends on a set of factors such as the body mass index of the subject and the recording conditions (preparation of the skin, the contact of the electrode with the skin and the distance from the source of activity). Some authors evaluated the reliability of the information contained in the external recording of the electrogastrogram (EGG), which is a very similar signal to the intestinal myoelectrical signal (Mintchev & Bowes 1996). In that study, the following parameters of EGG signals were analyzed: the amplitude, the frequency, the time shift between different channels recorded simultaneously and the waveform. They concluded that the signal frequency is the unique consistent and trustworthy parameter of the external myoelectrical recording (Mintchev & Bowes 1996). Because of that, the analysis of the SW activity of the external EEnG is usually focused on obtaining the dominant frequency of the signal, which allows determining the intestinal SW repetition rate.

To obtain the dominant frequency of the external EEnG signal, some researchers have used non-parametric spectral estimation techniques (Chen et al. 1993; Garcia-Casado et al. 2005). These studies have showed the utility of these techniques for the identification of the intestinal SW activity on the abdominal surface. By means of these non-parametric techniques it has also been determined that the energy associated with the intestinal SW is concentrated between 0.15 and 2 Hz in the animal model (Garcia-Casado et al. 2005). Nevertheless, these techniques present some disadvantages: the selection of the window length to be used in the analysis has an important repercussion on the frequency resolution and on the stationarity of the signal. Other authors proposed the use of parametric techniques based on autoregressive models (Bradshaw et al. 1997; Moreno-Vazquez et al. 2003; Seidel et al. 1999) or on autoregressive moving average models (Chen et al. 1990; Levy et al. 2001) to obtain the frequency of the external signal. The advantage of these techniques with respect to the non-parametric techniques is that they enable to determine the dominant frequency of the signal with better frequency resolution even with a shorter window of analysis. Nevertheless, the application of these techniques present some practical limitations: the information related to the power associated with each frequency is not trustworthy. In short, it is advisable to use parametric techniques in order to identify the peak frequencies of the signal, whereas if the aim is to study the energy distribution of the signal in the frequency domain, non-parametric spectral analysis is more appropriate.

4.2. Non-invasive recording and characterization of spike bursts activity

The first works that studied the possibility of recording the SB activity of gastrointestinal origin non-invasively, were conducted analyzing the gastric SW in the external recordings (Atanassova et al. 1995; Chen et al. 1994). They stated that the presence of the SB in the internal recordings increases the amplitude of the external gastric SW (Atanassova et al. 1995), and it also leads to an increase in the instability of the power of the dominant frequency associated with the external gastric SW (Chen et al. 1994). Nevertheless, these hypotheses were refuted by other authors, causing a great controversy (Mintchev & Bowes 1996). They believed that the increase of the amplitude of the surface SW activity is due to the minor distance between the myoelectrical signal of origin and the surface electrodes associated with the stomach distension when the SB are present (Mintchev & Bowes 1996), rather than being directly related to the contractile activity of the stomach.

Very few works about external recordings of gastrointestinal activity have focused their studies out of the SW frequency band (Akin & Sun 1999; Garcia-Casado et al. 2005). In Akin's work, it was shown that the energy associated with gastric SB activity ranges from 50-80 cpm by means of spectral analysis in an animal model (50-80 cpm) (Akin & Sun 1999). The correlation study of the internal and external signal energy in that frequency range showed a high correlation index (around 0.8) (Akin & Sun 1999). Regarding to the intestinal myoelectrical signal, only a few works have been found that study the two components of the surface electroenterogram (EEnG) and not only the SW intestinal activity (Garcia-Casado et al. 2005; Ye et al. 2008). In both works, it was carried out a comparative study of the internal and external recordings of intestinal myoelectrical signal from dogs. Bipolar external recording was obtained using two monopolar contact electrodes placed on the abdominal surface. Figure 4 shows the simultaneous recording of internal (top traces) and surface signals (bottom traces) in a period of rest and in a period of maximum contractile activity. In the period of rest, 9 slow waves in 30 s can be observed both in the internal and in the external recording. On the other hand, in the period of maximum contractile activity which corresponds to the phase III of the IMMC, in the internal recording it can be observed that every SW is accompanied by a superposed SB, whereas in the external recording a high frequency component of low amplitude is superposed to the SW activity (fig. 4 right, bottom trace). Since it is not synchronized with the cardiac activity, and the SB activity is the high frequency component of EEnG recording (Martinez-de-Juan et al. 2000), these high frequency components on the external EEnG recording are believed to be associated with the intestinal SB activity (Garcia-Casado et al. 2005).

In order to study the intestinal SB activity on the surface recording, time-frequency analysis have been proposed to obtain simultaneous information both on spectral content and on time intervals (Garcia-Casado et al. 2002). These studies showed that Choi-Williams distribution is the best time-frequency distribution in order to identify the presence of SB,

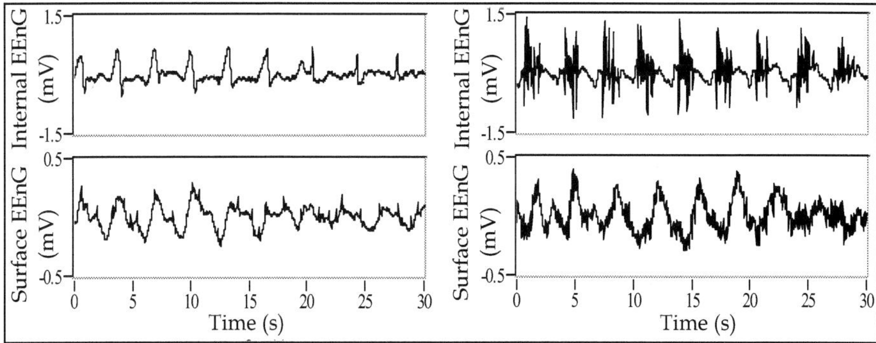

Fig. 4. Simultaneous recording of canine intestinal myoelectrical activity in fasting state during a period of rest (left traces) and during a period of maximum contractile activity (right traces). Signals are recorded in the intestinal serosa (top traces) and on abdominal surface (bottom traces) (Garcia-Casado et al. 2005).

whereas spectrogram is more useful in order to quantify the SB activity (Garcia-Casado et al. 2002). Other studies defend that non-parametric spectral techniques also can be used to study the external EEnG signal (Garcia-Casado et al. 2005), since it can be assumed the hypothesis of the stationarity of the signal if the size of the window is sufficiently small. Based on these non-parametric techniques, it has been shown that the energy of the intestinal SB activity of the external recording is concentrated between 2 and 20 Hz (Garcia-Casado et al. 2005). Therefore, the energy in this frequency band of the external EEnG, also named as SB energy, could be of great utility to quantify in a non-invasive way the intestinal motor activity (Garcia-Casado et al. 2005).

Nevertheless, the study of Garcia-Casado presents certain limitations from the medical point of view: a segment of intestine was sutured to the internal abdominal wall so as to obtain a reference pattern for the intestinal activity of the external recording (Garcia-Casado et al. 2005). In spite of the fact that the small intestine has natural adherences to the abdominal internal wall, the above mentioned artificial attachment might improve the electrical contact between the surface electrodes and the intestine (Bradshaw et al. 1997). Therefore, it can be expected that the signal-to-interference ratio of the external recording would be decreased if this artificial attachment was eliminated. On the other hand, the elimination of the artificial attachment would also have another consequence: there is no longer knowledge of the intestinal segment whose activity is being picked up on the external recording.

The latest studies have focused their efforts on the comparison between the external and internal recording of the canine intestinal myoelectrical signal in fasting state, but without the artificial attachment of an intestinal segment to the internal abdominal wall (Ye et al. 2008). Figure 5 shows the evolution of the SB energy of the external recording (trace a) with the intestinal motility index (IMI) of the different internal channels (traces b-d) acquired simultaneously in fasting state. In these figures, it is possible to identify two complete cycles of the IMMC in the different internal channels. The SB energy in the external recording shows two periods of maximum intensity (about the minute 85 and minute 167), that are probably related to the periods of maximum contractile activity of the jejunum (in the

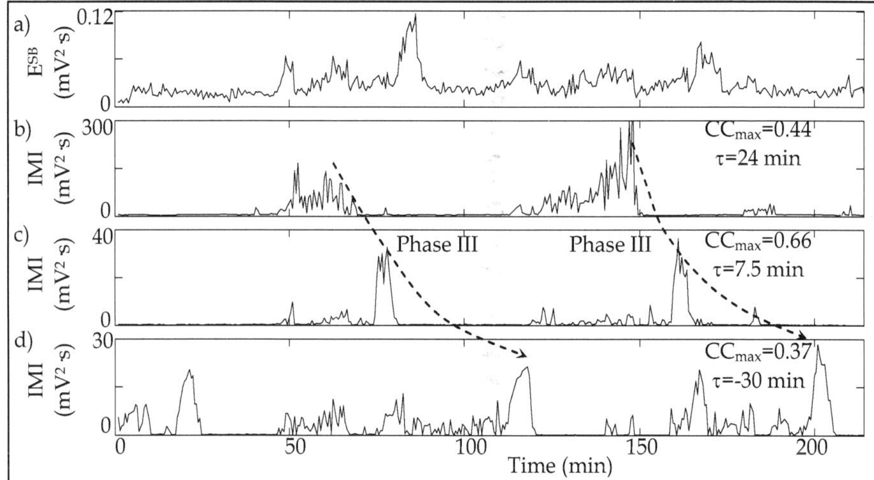

Fig. 5. Intestinal motility indicators of canine external and internal EEnG recording acquired simultaneously in fasting state: a) Surface. b) Duodenum. c) Jejunum. d) Ileum. It is also indicated the maximum value of the cross-correlation function (CC$_{max}$) between the SB energy of external recording and the internal IMI and its corresponding time lag τ.

minutes 78 and 160). This time lag is probably due to the disagreement of the recording area between the external and internal recordings. Since the phase III of the IMMC propagates in the distal way in fasting state, the external electrodes might be recording the intestinal activity from one segment of intestine located approximately 35 cm distally to the jejunum internal recording. In this context, the use of the cross-correlation function allows to make the adjustment of the possible delay, and thus reflect the relationship between the SB energy of the external recording with the internal IMI. In this case, the maximum value of the cross-correlation function (0.66) is obtained with the IMI of the jejunum channel when adjusting a delay of 7.5 minutes. The results of these preliminary studies confirm the possibility of picking up the intestinal SB activity on the abdominal surface recordings of the EEnG under physiological conditions without the need of artificial attachments (Ye et al. 2008). This means a great advance in the study of the intestinal motility by means of the non-invasive myoelectrical techniques.

4.3. Limitations of external EEnG recording

In the previous sections, it has been shown that both components of the intestinal myoelectrical activity can be recorded on the abdominal surface, and that spectral parameters are very useful to characterize these components: the dominant frequency of the signal to determine the frequency of the intestinal pacemaker, i.e. the SW; the SB energy to determine the intensity of the possible intestinal contractions. Nevertheless, the surface EEnG still presents some difficulties for its clinical application. First, the myoelectrical intestinal signal recorded on abdominal surface is a very small amplitude signal (Bradshaw et al. 1997; Chen et al. 1993; Garcia-Casado et al. 2005; Prats-Boluda et al. 2007), especially in the SB frequency range (Garcia-Casado et al. 2005), due to the insulating effect of the abdominal layers and to spatial filtering (Bradshaw et al. 1997). However, the major problem of the surface recording of the myoelectrical signal resides in the presence of strong interferences: electrocardiogram (ECG), respiration, movement artifacts, components of very low frequency and other interferences of minor relevancy (Chen et al. 1993; Garcia-Casado et al. 2005; Liang et al. 1997; Prats-Boluda et al. 2007; Verhagen et al. 1999). The presence of these interferences may impede the obtaining of trustworthy parameters derived from the external myoelectrical recordings which define the intestinal activity. This is a common problem in the non-invasive recording of the gastric, colonic, uterine and intestinal activities. In the case of the surface EEnG, the amplitude of these interferences can be of the same order of magnitude or even higher than the amplitude of the target signal. Consequently, the identification and the elimination of these interferences are of great importance in order to extract useful information from the surface EEnG. Next it is briefly described the different interferences that can appear in the surface EEnG recording:

- **Electrocardiogram (ECG):** ECG interference concerns principally the high frequency components of the external EEnG i.e. the SB, since the SB activity recorded on abdominal surface are of very low amplitude (Garcia-Casado et al. 2006). Conventional filters cannot be used for the elimination of ECG interference since its spectrum is overlapped with that of the SB.

- **Respiration:** The respiration affects mainly the SW activity due to its similarity in frequency (Chen et al. 1993; Lin & Chen 1994). The origin of this interference can be due to the variation of the distance between the surface electrodes and the intestinal sources, and also due to the variation of the contact impedance between the electrodes and the skin (Ramos et al. 1993). The presence of the respiratory interference depends strongly on the recording conditions, precisely on the fixation of the contact electrodes, on the position of the electrodes and on the position of the subject in study.

- **Components of very low frequency:** In the external EEnG recording, it can often be observed components whose frequency is below the lowest frequency of the intestinal pacemaker (Chen et al. 1993; Garcia-Casado et al. 2005; Prats-Boluda et al. 2007). Its origin may be due to the use of an inappropriate signal conditioning and digitalization system (Mintchev et al. 2000), to the variation of the contact impedance between the surface electrodes and the skin, or to the bioelectric activity of other organs with a slower dynamics (Chen et al. 1993). In this respect, the gastric activity whose frequency is around 3 cpm might be the principal source of the very low frequency interferences in the study of the human surface EEnG (Chen et al. 1993).

- **Artifacts:** The artifacts consist of abrupt changes on the amplitude of the external myoelectrical signal. Its occurrence is intermittent and unpredictable and they can completely distort the signal power spectrum (Verhagen et al. 1999). Liang et al. showed in their studies that the morphology of the artifacts in external myoelectrical recordings is diverse and depends on the kind of movement, being its amplitude in the time domain very high compared to that of the target signal (Liang et al. 1997). In addition, the presence of artifacts usually provokes a considerable increase in the spectral content, especially in the high frequency range (Liang et al. 1997).

In short, all these interferences must be somehow eliminated before the analysis of the external EEnG signal in order to be able to obtain more robust parameters that characterize the intestinal activity from the non-invasive myoelectrical recordings.

5. Enhancement of surface EEnG recordings

In the past years, there have been developed diverse signal processing techniques for the interferences reduction on the biomedical signals which can be suitable for being applied to the external EEnG signals, such as adaptive filtering, independent component analysis (ICA), or empirical mode decomposition (EMD).

Given the peculiarity of the intestinal EEnG signal, i.e., that the energies of the SW activity and the SB activity are distributed in different frequency ranges, this section is divided into two subsections, one for each of these frequency bands: the low frequency band where the intestinal SW activity is contained, and high frequency band where the SB activity spreads its energy.

5.1. Study of the EEnG in the low frequency band

From the first studies that have validated the possibility of recording the intestinal myoelectrical activity on abdominal surface, diverse techniques have been proposed for the interferences' reduction in the low frequency range. The aim of these techniques is to cancel respiration and components of very low frequency, and to extract the intestinal SW activity contained in the external EEnG signal. The final goal is to improve the quality of the external EEnG signal and to bring the non-invasive myoelectrical techniques closer to the clinical application. Among these interferences, the respiratory interference has received special attention of diverse researchers, given its similarity in frequency with the intestinal SW activity.

5.1.1 Adaptive filtering

The fundamental idea of adaptive filtering is the following one: it is given a primary signal which is a mixture of the target signal and the interference, and a reference signal which can be an estimation of the interference (interference canceller structure), an estimation of the target signal (signal-enhancer structure), or an estimation of the occurrence in the time (Ferrara & Widrow 1981). In agreement with a pre-established target function, for example the minimizations of the expected value of the output signal in the interference canceller structure, the parameters of the filter are changed by means of an adaptive algorithm. The result of this process is the obtaining of an output signal that turns out to be the best estimation of the target signal with minimal interferences content. Adaptive filtering has been widely used for the interferences' reduction contained in the biomedical signals.

With regard to the intestinal signals, diverse authors have used this technique to eliminate the respiratory interference contained in the external EEnG. Precisely, different configurations have been used: in time domain (Prats-Boluda et al. 2007); in frequency domain (Chen & Lin 1993); and in discrete cosine transform (Lin & Chen 1994). In the first work, the authors implemented adaptive filtering with the LMS (least minimum square) algorithm (Prats-Boluda et al. 2007). In this case, the reference signal is a filtered version of the external EEnG signal. Specifically, a band-pass filter in the respiration frequency range was used. The cut-off frequencies are obtained from the simultaneously recorded respiration signal. Figure 6 shows 120 s of the respiration signal (trace a) and of the external EEnG before and after the application of adaptive filtering, and their corresponding power spectral densities (PSDs). In this figure it is possible to observe that the respiratory interference is highly attenuated after the adaptive filtering, although a remaining component of the interference can still be observed in the processed signals.

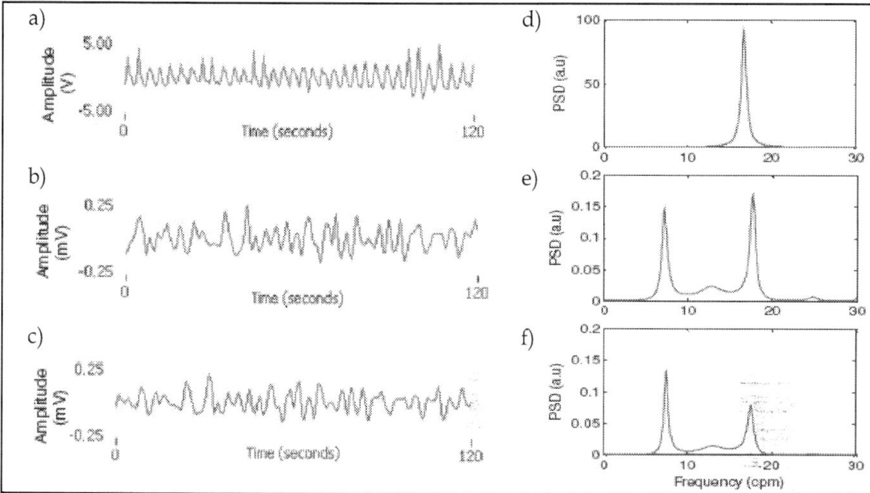

Fig. 6. a) Respiration signal. b) Original EEnG signal recorded on the human abdominal surface c) Processed signal by means of adaptive filtering. e-f) PSD of the signals that are depicted on the left-hand side (Prats-Boluda et al. 2007).

Other authors have used transform-domain adaptive filtering for the elimination of the respiratory interference from the external EEnG recording. This technique consists in applying both to the primary signal (external EEnG) and to the reference signal (respiration signal), the Fourier's transform (Chen & Lin 1993) or the discreet cosine transform (Lin & Chen 1994), before obtaining the target function and adjusting the filter weights. These studies concluded that the application of adaptive filtering allows improving considerably the quality of the external recording of the human EEnG. Figure 7 shows the original external EEnG signal and the filtered one by means of adaptive filtering based on the discrete cosine transform, and its corresponding PSDs in the low frequency range. In that work, the reference signal of the adaptive filter is an estimation of the target signal, which is obtained by band-pass filtering the external EEnG signal. In this figure it is possible to observe that the intestinal components (8-12 cpm) have not been affected by the signal processing, whereas the non-desired components have been attenuated more than 20 dB (Lin & Chen 1994).

The results of these studies show that the effectiveness of the adaptive filtering technique to cancel the interference strongly depends on the reference signal (Chen & Lin 1993; Lin & Chen 1994; Prats-Boluda et al. 2007). In this respect, the frequency of the respiratory interference contained in the surface EEnG may be identical to that of the recorded respiration signal, but the waveform and phase can be different. This can severely reduce the adaptive filtering capacity to suppress the respiratory interference of the surface EEnG, if the respiration signal is used as the reference signal in a time-domain adaptive filter. In addition, the respiratory interference is not usually present in the external EEnG recording

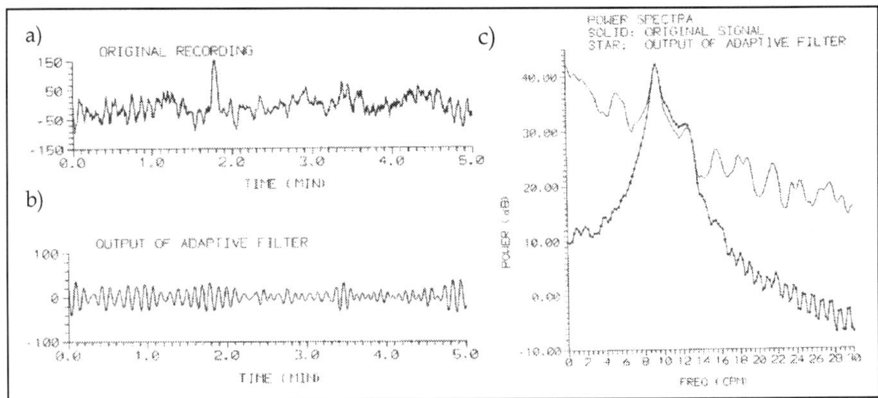

Fig. 7. a) Original external EEnG recording. b) Processed signal by means of adaptive filetering based on discrete cosine transform. c) PSD of original signal (solid line) and that of processed signal (line with stars) (Lin & Chen 1994).

during the whole recording session. In fact, it could have great variations in its intensity for adjacent segments. This can impede the selection of the adaptive filter parameters: the order of the filter and the step size. In these cases, the extracted interference might differ from the interference which is really contained in the external myoelectrical record, and therefore the resultant signal might contain remaining interference, or the components of the target signal may be distorted (Prats-Boluda et al. 2007).

5.1.2 Independent component analysis (ICA)

This technique departs from the hypothesis that the observed or recorded signals are the result of an unknown mixing process of the source signals which are supposed to be mutually independent. Independent component analysis (ICA) consists in extracting a set of statistically independent components from a set of observed signals based on statistical learning of the data, without any previous knowledge of the source signals and the mixing matrix (Hyvarinen et al. 2001). In the biomedical signals context, it is usually considered that the mixing process is instantaneous and linear, assuming that the observed signals in the different channels are a simple linear combination of the attenuated source signals (James & Hesse 2005).

The ICA algorithm has found application in diverse fields of engineering, among them the identification of the signal components and the reduction of interferences contained in the biomedical signals. To the knowledge of the authors, it has not been found any work that has used this technique to improve the quality of the external EEnG signal. Nevertheless, the results found in the literature with regard to the gastric signal, suggest us that the ICA could also be applied to the intestinal myoelectrical signals. This is the reason why the ICA has been included in the present chapter.

With respect to the myoelectrical gastric signal, the ICA has been used by diverse authors for the reduction of respiratory interference in order to recover the gastric SW activity of the external records (Liang 2001; Wang et al. 1999). These authors state that, when a few number of external EGG recordings is available, it is only possible to recover one signal of gastric origin in the output of the ICA algorithm, whereas the respiratory interference and other noises are concentrated in other channels (Liang 2001; Wang et al. 1999). Figure 8a-b shows an example of the application of ICA to a segment of EGG signal recorded on the human abdominal surface. Figure 8a shows 3 external channels of the original EGG record. After the application of the ICA algorithm, 3 independent components (ICs) have been obtained which can be observed in the fig. 8b. It is possible to appreciate that the respiration and other noises are concentrated in the channels 2 and 3 of the output, whereas the channel 1 of output, which presents less respiratory interference, corresponds to the gastric SW activity contained in the original signals. Nevertheless, the channels 2 and 3 of the output can also contain gastric SW activity. Consequently, the ICA can be a useful tool to identify the dominant frequency of the SW activity, but it is not suitable to improve the signal - interference ratio of every external channel (Wang et al. 1999).

Some authors propose the identification of the gastric SW activity in each of the channels in a multichannel record of the external EGG (3 external channels) by means of the combined method based on ICA and adaptive filtering (Liang 2005). This combined method consists in using the output signal of the ICA algorithm, as reference signal for the implementation of adaptive filtering to each of the external channels. This technique proved to improve the quality of every channel of the external EGG (Liang 2005). This combined method also benefits from the maximum possible independence among the different output signals of the ICA algorithm, which might potentially improve the signal quality obtained by means of adaptive filtering (Liang 2005). Figure 8c shows the signals filtered by means of the combined method based in ICA and adaptive filtering. The presence of the gastric SW activity in three external channels can be observed more clearly than in the original signals.

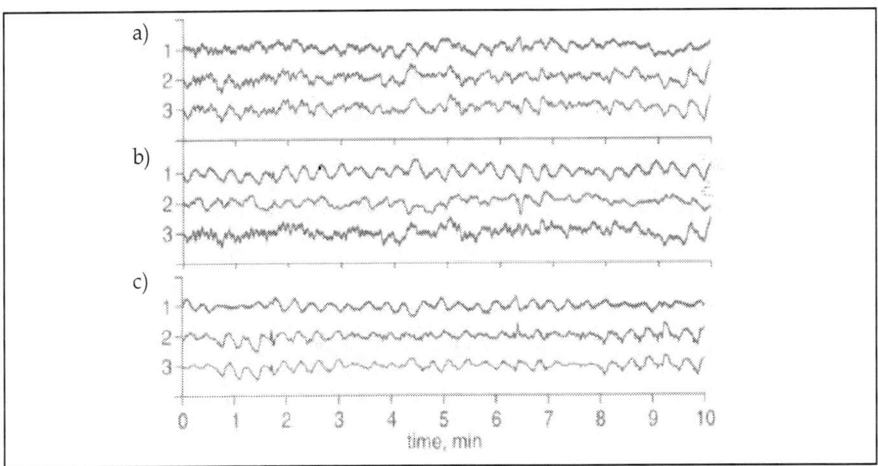

Fig. 8. Extraction of the gastric SW activity from multichannel surface EGG signal by means of a combined method based on ICA and adaptive filtering. a) 3 channels of original external EGG signals recorded simultaneously. b) Independent components estimated by the ICA algorithm (output of ICA). c) Processed signal after the application of adaptive filtering, using the channel 1 of the output of the ICA algorithm as reference signal (Liang 2005).

The constrained ICA has also been proposed for the extraction of the gastric SW activity from the external EGG recordings (Peng et al. 2007). In this work it has been used 4 channels of external EGG, and a piezoelectric sensor placed near the navel to record the abdomen movement and the cardiac activity. The last signal will be used as reference signal to the elimination of the respiratory and cardiac interferences (Peng et al. 2007). The results of that study show that the constrained ICA allows to extract the gastric SW activity with less interference of high frequency, i.e. cardiac interference, than the conventional ICA method, thanks to the restriction of "as far as possible" to the reference signals (Peng et al. 2007).

Other authors defend that the increase of the number of simultaneously recorded channels enables improving the separability of the different components contained in the original signals (Liang 2001). In a recent study, it has been determined by means of the dynamic analysis, that a minimum of 6 simultaneously recorded channels are required for the correct separation of the different components contained in the multichannel recording of the EGG in healthy subjects (Matsuura et al. 2007). In this context, other authors who used 19 channels of surface magnetogastrogram (MGG) proved that the ICA algorithm allows the extraction of the respiratory interference, the ECG interference, the artifacts and the gastric SW activity, improving in this way the quality of the non-invasive recordings of gastric activity (Irimia & Bradshaw 2005).

All the above mentioned works which were carried out on non-invasive recordings of gastric activity show the potential of ICA-based techniques to reduce the interferences in the low frequency range which are present in the external EEnG recordings, although to the author's knowledge, there are have not been published studies which confirm this fact. In addition, the minimal number of simultaneously recorded channels which are needed to separate the different components contained in the external EEnG signal is still to be determined. In this respect, possible future works should consider that, given the low spatial resolution of external bipolar EEnG recording, every channel might be recording the myoelectrical activity of more than one intestinal handle. This would mean that the activity of a higher number of source signals is being recorded, and therefore it might needed an even higher number of recording channels for a correct separation of the sources.

5.1.3 Empirical mode decomposition (EMD)

The empirical mode decomposition (EMD) algorithm was proposed initially for the study of fluid mechanics by Huang et al. (Huang et al. 1998), and soon found applications in biomedical signals processing both for the characterization of the signals and for the elimination of interferences contained in these signals (Liang et al. 2000; Maestri et al. 2007). This technique does not need any previous knowledge of the signal and it consists of expanding any complicated signal in a finite number of oscillatory functions, called intrinsic mode functions (IMFs). An IMF is defined as any function that has the same number of extrema (local maximums and minimums) as the number of zero crossings, and that has a local mean of zero (Huang et al. 1998). The IMFs defined in this way are symmetrical with regard to the zero axis, and they have a unique local frequency. This is, the different IMFs extracted from a signal do not share the same frequency at the same time (Huang et al. 1998).

The IMFs can be interpreted as adaptive basis functions which are directly extracted from the signal. Therefore, the EMD method is suitable for the analysis of the signals obtained from non-linear and non-stationary processes (Huang et al. 1998). This is a principal advantage of EMD over the Fourier's transform, in which the basis functions are linear combinations of sinusoidal waves. In comparison with Wavelet analysis, the IMFs obtained by the EMD method, which represent the dynamic processes masked inside the original signal, have usually better physical interpretation of the process (Huang et al. 1998).

With regard to the gastrointestinal signals, the EMD has been used for the reduction of the interferences contained in the external EGG recordings (Liang et al. 2000), and in the external EEnG recordings (Ye et al. 2007). In the latter work, the EMD method was used to analyze the external EEnG recordings obtained from anesthetized dogs (assisted respiration with mechanical ventilation fixed to 27 cpm), in order to reduce the interferences in the low frequency range and to improve the quality of the external EEnG signals (Ye et al. 2007).

In figure 9 it is shown an example of the application of the EMD to 1 minute of external EEnG signal. The preprocessed external EEnG signal appears in the trace a). Its corresponding PSD between 0 and 1 Hz (trace h) shows two clear peaks: at 0.20 Hz and at 0.45 Hz. The 0.20 Hz component is probably associated with the intestinal SW activity, since this frequency is within the frequency range of the intestinal SW rate. The 0.45 Hz component probably corresponds to the respiratory interference given the coincidence with the respiration frequency (27 cpm), and in addition it cannot be a harmonic of the intestinal SW activity. The decomposition of this signal by means of the EMD algorithm has given rise to 4 IMFs and a residual signal (traces b-f), their corresponding PSDs are depicted on the right-hand side. In these figures it is possible to observe that every IMF has different frequency components. Especially, the first extracted IMF fits to the most rapid variation of the original signal. As the process of decomposition advances, the mean frequency of the IMFs diminishes gradually. In this case, the spectral analysis has identified the IMF_2 component as the respiratory interference, and the residual signal r_4 as an interference of very low frequency. Therefore, the processed signal (trace g) is obtained adding the IMF_1, IMF_3 and IMF_4. A comparison of the original signal with the processed one, allows us to affirm that the application of the EMD method has considerably reduced the interferences in the low frequency range, making easy to identify the myoelectrical signal of intestinal origin that is contained in the original signal.

The application of the EMD method allows to improve significantly the signal-to-interference (S/I) ratio. Furthermore, this improvement owes principally to the attenuation of the energy associated with the interferences, whereas the energy associated with the target signal remains almost constant (Ye et al. 2007). Thanks to the reduction of the interferences by means of the EMD method, the variability of the dominant frequency of the external EEnG signal is also considerably diminished. These results show that the EMD method is a very helpful tool to improve the quality of the external EEnG recordings, and therefore it is possible to extract more trustworthy parameters that permit to identify non-invasively the intestinal SW activity. Nevertheless, this study still presents some limitations, for example ,the respiration is assisted and fixed (0.45 Hz) (Ye et al. 2007). When recording in physiological conditions, the respiration frequency might change during the session which could complicate the identification of the respiratory interference in the different IMFs obtained from the EMD algorithm. In this respect, the simultaneous recording of the respiration signal would be of great help in order to obtain a reference of the breathing frequency, and hence to correctly identify and eliminate this interference on the external signal. Also, the applicability of the EMD method to the human external EEnG recordings in physiological conditions has to be checked in future studies.

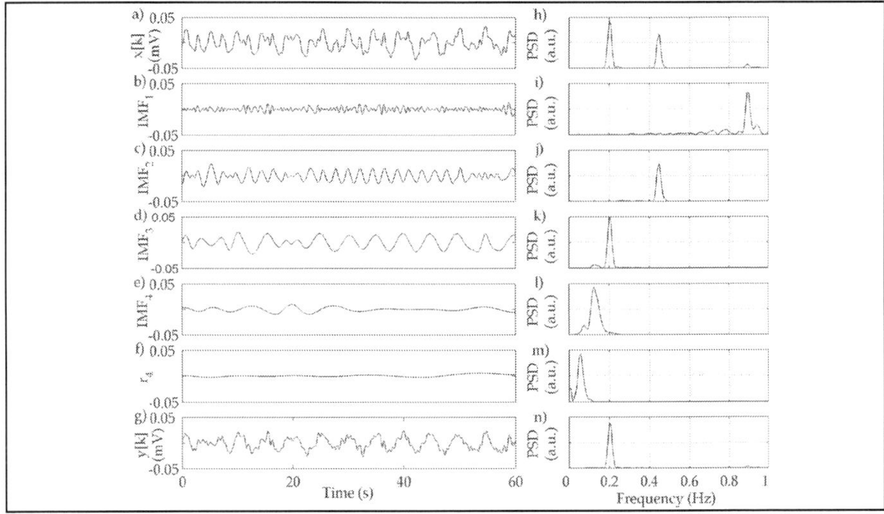

Fig. 9. Application of the EMD method to 1 minute of surface EEnG recording with strong respiration interference (0.45 Hz). a) Original EEnG recording after preprocessing x[k] (low pass filter with cut-off frequency at 2 Hz). b-f). b-f) Outputs of the EMD method: four IMFs and one residual signal. g) Processed signal y[k]: sum of IMF_1, IMF_3 y IMF_4. h-n) PSD of the signals that are depicted on the left-hand side (Ye et al. 2007). The PSD of the processed signal is represented at the same scale of the original signal

5.2 Study of the EEnG in the high frequency band

Given the small amplitude of the intestinal SB activity when recorded on abdominal surface, and the strong interferences that are present in the high frequency range which mainly are the ECG interference and movement artifacts, several techniques have been developed for the reduction of these interferences. These interferences should be removed so as to improve the quality of the external EEnG signal for the correct identification and quantification of the SB activity in a non-invasive way. It should be emphasized here that very few works have been found that are related to the reduction of these interferences (ECG and artifacts) in the intestinal signal, since the majority of the authors have focused their studies on the intestinal SW activity and in these cases the high frequency interferences can be eliminated by conventional low-pass filtering (Bradshaw et al. 1997; Chen & Lin 1993; Lin & Chen 1994; Seidel et al. 1999).

5.2.1 Adaptive filtering

Adaptive filtering has been used for the reduction of the ECG interference contained in the canine external EEnG recording (Garcia-Casado et al. 2006). In that study, a technique based on synchronized averaging has been used to estimate the ECG interference of the external EEnG. Precisely, the interference estimator is obtained by averaging a number of windows of the external EEnG recording using the onset of the R wave of the ECG as synchronizing event. This procedure is similar to the obtaining of event-related potentials. Once the estimation of ECG's interference is obtained, it is used as the reference signal for the implementation of an adaptive filter based on the LMS algorithm for the elimination of this interference (Garcia-Casado et al. 2006).

Figure 10 shows 10s of the original external EEnG signal and after being processed by means of the adaptive filter in a period of rest (traces a and b), and in a period of maximum contractile activity (traces c and d). In these figures it can be observed that the application of the adaptive filter allows reducing the ECG interference contained in the external EEnG signal both in periods of rest and of maximum contractile activity; whereas both components of the myoelectrical intestinal activity (SW and SB) are minimally affected by the signal processing (Garcia-Casado et al. 2006). The reduction of the interference has enabled improving the ECG's signal-to-interference ratio significantly (Garcia-Casado et al. 2006). These results confirm that adaptive filtering can be a tool of great help to reduce ECG interference and to improve the quality of the external EEnG recordings.

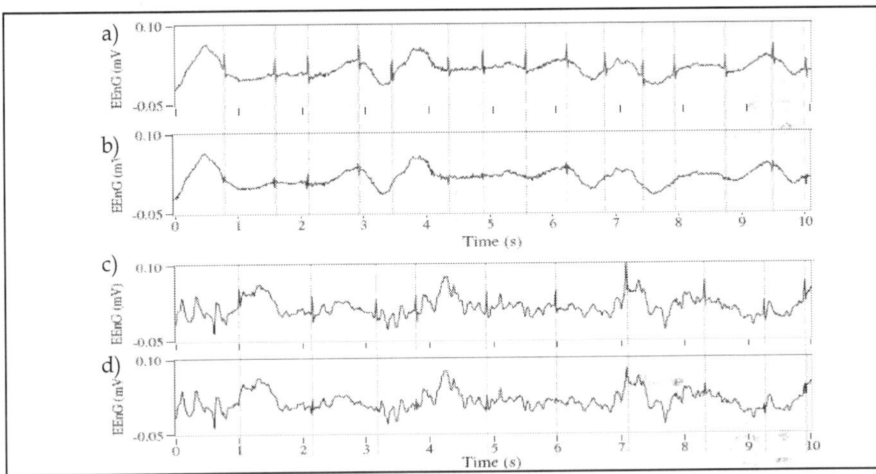

Fig. 10. a-b) Original external EEnG signal during a period of rest and the processed signal by adaptive filtering respectively. c-d) Original external EEnG signal during a period of maximum contractile activity and after being processed by adaptive filtering respectively. (Garcia-Casado et al. 2006). Signals were recorded from conscious dogs in fasting state. Fiducial points of the R-wave are marked with a vertical broken line.

5.2.2 Combined method based on EMD and ICA

In a recent study, a combined method based on EMD and ICA has been proposed to reduce both the ECG interference and the movement artifacts in the high frequency range of the multichannel recordings of the external EEnG (Ye et al. 2008). This combined method consists in firstly analyzing separately each of 4 simultaneous recordings of external EEnG by means of the EMD algorithm. Later, there are selected those IMFs (results of the EMD algorithm) whose mean frequency is revealed to be higher than 1 Hz by means of spectral analysis. This procedure usually results in a variable number of IMFs which contain the information of high frequency components (>1 Hz). These IMFs obtained from 4 external channels will be analyzed together by means of the ICA algorithm in order to obtain the independent components (Ye et al. 2008). Subsequently, the interferences associated to ECG and movement artifacts are identified in the outputs of the ICA algorithm. Finally, the processed signals are reconstructed without the identified interferences by means of an inverse process.

In figure 11 it is shown an example of the application of the combined method to a window of external EEnG signals in a period of rest. In the original signals of external EEnG recordings (traces b-e), it can be observed a low frequency component (3-4 cycles in 15s) which is associated with the intestinal SW activity. It can also be appreciated the presence of strong ECG interference in the channels 1 and 2 (traces b and c), which is synchronized with the simultaneously recorded ECG signal (trace a). On the other hand, the ECG interference in the channels 3 and 4 (traces d and e) is weak. Finally, it can also be appreciated in the original signals the appearance of movement artifacts in the 4 external channels around the second 10. The signals processed by means of the combined method are shown in traces g-j. A comparison of the original signals with the processed ones allows deducing that the application of the combined method has cancelled both ECG interference and movement artifacts from the original signals, without affecting the intestinal myoelectrical activity.

The application of the combined method to a window of external EEnG signals in a period of maximal contractile activity appears in figure 12. Again, it can be observed the presence of a low frequency activity in the 4 external channels (traces b-e), that probably corresponds to the intestinal SW activity. In these traces it is also possible to observe the presence of components of high frequency and low amplitude which are superposed to the intestinal SW activity, which are possibly associated with the intestinal SB activity. The appearance of these components of high frequency impedes the visual identification of ECG interference in the external EEnG signal. In this case, the ECG interference can only be clearly appreciated in the channel 2 (trace c). The signals processed by means of the combined method are shown in traces g-j. Again, the application of the combined method has eliminated the ECG interference contained in the original signals, whereas the intestinal myoelectrical activity has been minimally affected.

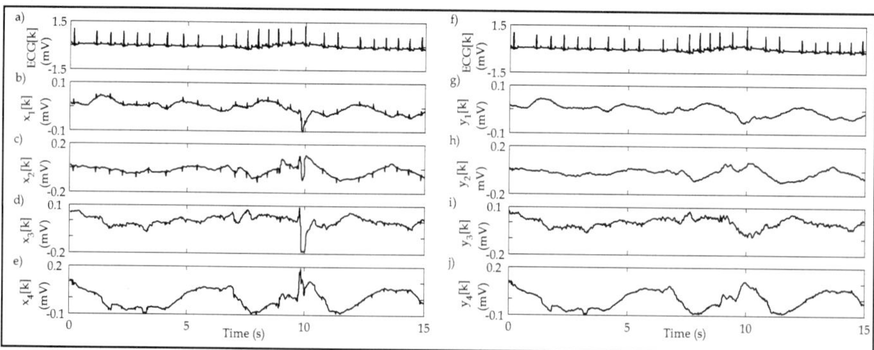

Fig. 11. Application of the combined method based on EMD and ICA to multichannel surface EEnG recording; the window length of the analysis is 30s. a) and f) ECG signal. b-e) original signals of 4 surface EEnG channels ($x_1[k]$-$x_4[k]$) during a period of rest. It can be appreciated the appearance of movement artifacts around the second 10. g-j) Processed signals $y_1[k]$-$y_4[k]$. Signals were recorded from conscious dogs in fasting state.

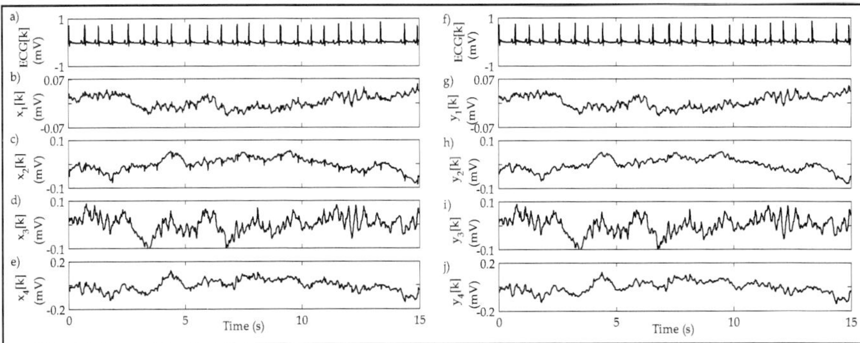

Fig. 12. Application of the combined method based on EMD and ICA to multichannel surface EEnG recording; the window length of the analysis is 30s. a) and f) ECG signal. b-e) original signals of 4 surface EEnG channels ($x_1[k]$-$x_4[k]$) during a period of maximum contactile activity. g-j) Processed signals $y_1[k]$-$y_4[k]$. Signals were recorded from conscious dogs in fasting state.

The results of that study indicate that the application of the combined method allows to significantly improve the signal-to- ECG interference of the external EEnG recordings, and to reduce the variability of the non-invasive indicator of the intestinal motility (Ye et al. 2008). This is due to the fact that the combined method enables achieving an improvement on the separation of the different components contained in the original signal when compared to the conventional ICA method. The difference between both techniques lies in the reduction of the number of sources which are present in the original signals by restricting the frequency band of analysis (over 1 Hz), and also by using a higher number of virtual channels due to the decomposition of the original signals into multiple oscillatory functions using the EMD algorithm. When compared to conventional EMD method, if only EMD was used, the SB activity could be mixed with interferences of similar instant frequencies in the same IMFs, whereas the combined method takes advantage of the capacity of the ICA algorithm to separate these independent components. This preliminary study shows the potential of the use of the combined method based on EMD and ICA to improve the quality of the external EEnG recording. The application of this method permits to obtain more robust non-invasive parameters which measure the internal intestinal motility.

6. Futures perspectives

The results from recent works suggest the possibility of detecting both components of the intestinal myoelectrical activity in the external recording of EEnG in animal model (Garcia-Casado et al. 2005; Ye et al. 2008). Future studies on animal models might test the possibility of the non-invasive myoelectrical techniques to diagnose different pathologies related to intestinal activity dysfunctions. On the other hand, other recent studies suggest the possibility of recording the human gastric SB activity in the external recordings of the magnetogastrogram (Irimia et al. 2006). Based on these works, we believe that the intestinal SB activity might also be detected in the external myoelectrical records of humans. Future researches should extend the analysis of the external EEnG signals from humans out of the range of the intestinal SW activity, and to focus their efforts on the frequency band of the intestinal SB activity in order to check the possibility of detecting not only the pacemaker activity but also the contractile activity on abdominal surface of humans.

In this chapter, it has been presented a review on the different techniques used for the elimination of interferences contained in the EEnG external recordings. Among them, it has to be outlined the EMD method to cancel the interferences in the low frequency range, and the combined method based on EMD and ICA to reduce the interferences in the high frequency range. The analysis of quantitative parameters which allow evaluating the reduction of these interferences, has validated the applicability of these techniques to improve the quality of the canine external EEnG. By means of the application of these techniques, more robust parameters of the intestinal activity from the external recordings can be obtained. Specifically, it diminishes considerably the variability of the dominant frequency and of the intestinal motility index. The previously mentioned signal processing techniques could be easily adapted to be applied to the non-invasive recordings of the intestinal myoelectrical activity from humans. Fundamentally the frequency bands should be adjusted to the human EEnG characteristics. All this, in order to bring the non-invasive myoelectrical techniques closer to their future clinical application.

Besides the development of signal processing techniques, which turns out to be indispensable to improve the quality of the external EEnG, different research groups are developing techniques to record the Laplacian of the potential so as to improve the spatial resolution of conventional bipolar and monopolar recordings (Li et al. 2005; Prats-Boluda et al. 2007). Theoretically, the Laplacian of the potential is proportional to the second derivative of the orthogonal current density to the surface of the body (He & Cohen 1992). The Laplacian technique could be considered to be similar to a filter that assigns higher weights to the orthogonal bioelectric dipoles adjacent to the measuring surface, and attenuates the bioelectrical interferences which propagate tangentially to the abdominal surface (He & Cohen 1992). Recent studies have demonstrated that the signal-to-ECG interference ratio of the discrete approximation to the Laplacian recording of the EEnG is significantly higher than that of bipolar EEnG recordings (Prats-Boluda et al. 2007). At present, active electrodes which obtain a direct estimation of the Laplacian potential by concentric rings are being developed. The use of these Laplacian electrodes would improve the spatial resolution of the non-invasive recordings of the intestinal myoelectrical activity. These recordings, together with the above mentioned signal processing techniques, would permit to derive more robust non-invasive parameters that characterize the intestinal SW and SB activity.

Finally, the development of pattern classifiers which enable discriminating with better accuracy physiological and pathological conditions from myoelectrical recordings is another key point for the future clinical application of this technique. In respect to this, the application of neural networks and support vector machines to the external EGG signals has demonstrated its utility to detect delayed gastric emptying (Chen et al. 2000; Liang & Lin 2001). Future studies should concentrate in adapting these pattern classifiers to distinguish the external EEnG signals in different pathological conditions from healthy conditions.

7. Conclusion

Both the SW activity and the intestinal SB activity can be recorded on the abdominal surface, which suggests that the EEnG recordings on the abdominal surface would be an alternative method for the non-invasive monitoring of the intestinal activity. Nevertheless, the external EEnG signal is very weak, and in addition it is contaminated by a set of interferences (ECG, artifacts, respiration and components of very low frequency). The presence of these interferences impedes the extraction and interpretation of parameters that characterize the intestinal myoelectrical activity based on its non-invasive record. In this respect, the application of modern signal processing techniques turns out to be indispensable to reduce these interferences, and to improve the quality of the external recordings of the EEnG. In parallel, advances in signal recording and instrumentation techniques like the Laplacian recording of the potential also might contribute to the enhancement of the raw EEnG external signals, by permitting to obtain external signals with less physiological interference and with better spatial resolution. Thanks to the development of the signal processing techniques and to the improvement in the instrumentation techniques, it is possible to obtain robust parameters of the intestinal SW and SB activity derived from the surface EEnG recordings that bring these non-invasive myoelectrical techniques closer to their clinical application.

8. References

Akin, A. & Sun, H. H. (1999), Time-frequency methods for detecting spike activity of stomach, *Med. Biol. Eng Comput.*, vol. 37, No. 3, pp. 381-390, ISBN. 0140-0118.

An, Y. J., Lee, H., Chang, D., Lee, Y., Sung, J. K., Choi, M., & Yoon, J. (2001), Application of pulsed Doppler ultrasound for the evaluation of small intestinal motility in dogs, *J. Vet. Sci.*, vol. 2, No. 1, pp. 71-74.

Atanassova, E., Daskalov, I., Dotsinsky, I., Christov, I., & Atanassova, A. (1995), Noninvasive Electrogastrography .2. Human Electrogastrogram, *Archives of Physiology and Biochemistry*, vol. 103, No. 4, pp. 436-441, ISBN. 1381-3455.

Bass, P. & Wiley, J. N. (1965), Electrical and Extraluminal Contractile-Force Activity of Duodenum of Dog, *Am. J. Dig. Dis.*, vol. 10, No. 3, pp. 183-200, ISBN. 0002-9211.

Bradshaw, L. A., Allos, S. H., Wikswo, J. P., & Richards, W. O. (1997), Correlation and comparison of magnetic and electric detection of small intestinal electrical activity, *Am. J. Physiol. -Gastroint. Liver Physiol.*, vol. 35, No. 5, p. G1159-G1167, ISBN. 0193-1857.

Brown, B. H., Smallwood, R. H., Duthie, H. L., & Stoddard, C. J. (1975), Intestinal Smooth-Muscle Electrical Potentials Recorded from Surface Electrodes, *Medical & Biological Engineering*, vol. 13, No. 1, pp. 97-103, ISBN. 0025-696X.

Byrne, K. G. & Quigley, E. M. M. (1997), Antroduodenal manometry: An evaluation of an emerging methodology, *Dig. Dis.*, vol. 15, pp. 53-63, ISBN. 0257-2753.

Camilleri, M., Hasler, W. L., Parkman, H. P., Quigley, E. M. M., & Soffer, E. (1998), Measurement of gastrointestinal motility in the GI laboratory, *Gastroenterology*, vol. 115, No. 3, pp. 747-762, ISBN. 0016-5085.

Chang, F. Y., Lu, C. L., Chen, C. Y., Luo, J. C., Lee, S. D., Wu, H. C., & Chen, J. Z. (2007), Fasting and postprandial small intestinal slow waves non-invasively measured in subjects with total gastrectomy, *J Gastroenterol. Hepatol.*, vol. 22, No. 2, pp. 247-252.

Chen, J. D. & Lin, Z. (1993), Adaptive cancellation of the respiratory artifact in surface recording of small intestinal electrical activity, *Comput. Biol. Med.*, vol. 23, No. 6, pp. 497-509.

Chen, J. D., Lin, Z., & Mccallum, R. W. (2000), Noninvasive feature-based detection of delayed gastric emptying in humans using neural networks, *IEEE Trans. Biomed. Eng*, vol. 47, No. 3, pp. 409-412.

Chen, J. D., Richards, R. D., & Mccallum, R. W. (1994), Identification of Gastric Contractions from the Cutaneous Electrogastrogram, *American Journal of Gastroenterology*, vol. 89, No. 1, pp. 79-85, ISBN. 0002-9270.

Chen, J. D., Schirmer, B. D., & Mccallum, R. W. (1993), Measurement of Electrical-Activity of the Human Small-Intestine Using Surface Electrodes, *IEEE Trans. Biomed. Eng.*, vol. 40, No. 6, pp. 598-602, ISBN. 0018-9294.

Chen, J. D., Vandewalle, J., Sansen, W., Vantrappen, G., & Janssens, J. (1990), Adaptive Spectral-Analysis of Cutaneous Electrogastric Signals Using Autoregressive Moving Average Modeling, *Med. Biol. Eng Comput.*, vol. 28, No. 6, pp. 531-536, ISBN. 0140-0118.

Delvaux, M. (2003), Functional bowel disorders and irritable bowel syndrome in Europe, *Aliment. Pharmacol. Ther.*, vol. 18 Suppl 3, pp. 75-79.

Diamant, N. E. & Bortoff, A. (1969), Nature of the intestinal low-wave frequency gradient, *Am. J. Physiol.*, vol. 216, No. 2, pp. 301-307.

El-Murr, M., Kimura, K., Ellsberg, D., Yamazato, M., Yoshino, H., & Soper, R. T. (1994), Motility of isolated bowel segment Iowa model III, *Dig. Dis. Sci.*, vol. 39, No. 12, pp. 2619-2623.

Ferrara, E. R. & Widrow, B. (1981), Multichannel Adaptive Filtering for Signal Enhancement, *IEEE Trans. Acoustics Speech and Signal Processing*, vol. 29, No. 3, pp. 766-770, ISBN. 0096-3518.

Garcia-Casado, J., Martinez-de-Juan, J. L., & Ponce, J. L. (2006), Adaptive filtering of ECG interference on surface EEnGs based on signal averaging, *Physiol. Meas.*, vol. 27, No. 6, pp. 509-527, ISBN. 0967-3334.

Garcia-Casado, J., Martinez-de-Juan, J. L., & Ponce, J. L. (2005), Noninvasive measurement and analysis of intestinal myoelectrical activity using surface electrodes, *IEEE Trans. Biomed. Eng.*, vol. 52, No. 6, pp. 983-991.

Garcia-Casado, J., Martinez-de-Juan, J. L., Silvestre, J., Saiz, J., & Ponce, J. L. (2002), Identification of surface recordings of electroenterogram through time-frequency analysis, *4th International Workshop on Biosignal Interpretation*, Como, Italy.

He, B. & Cohen, R. J. (1992), Body surface Laplacian ECG mapping, *IEEE Trans. Biomed. Eng*, vol. 39, No. 11, pp. 1179-1191.

Horowitz, B., Ward, S. M., & Sanders, K. M. (1999), Cellular and molecular basis for electrical rhythmicity in gastrointestinal muscles, *Annu. Rev. Physiol*, vol. 61, pp. 19-43.

Huang, N. E., Shen, Z., Long, S. R., Wu, M. L. C., Shih, H. H., Zheng, Q. N., Yen, N. C., Tung, C. C., & Liu, H. H. (1998), The empirical mode decomposition and the Hilbert spectrum for nonlinear and non-stationary time series analysis, *Proc. Roy. Soc. LOND A MAT*, vol. 454, No. 1971, pp. 903-995, ISBN. 1364-5021.

Hyvarinen, A., Karhunen, J., & Oja, E. (2001), *Independent component analysis*, New York: John Wiley & Sons.

Irimia, A. & Bradshaw, L. A. (2005), Artifact reduction in magnetogastrography using fast independent component analysis, *Physiol. Meas.*, vol. 26, No. 6, pp. 1059-1073.

Irimia, A., Richards, W. O., & Bradshaw, L. A. (2006), Magnetogastrographic detection of gastric electrical response activity in humans, *Physics in Medicine and Biology*, vol. 51, No. 5, pp. 1347-1360, ISBN. 0031-9155.

James, C. J. & Hesse, C. W. (2005), Independent component analysis for biomedical signals, *Physiol Meas.*, vol. 26, No. 1, p. R15-R39, ISBN. 0967-3334.

Lausen, M., Reichenbacher, D., Ruf, G., Schoffel, U., & Pelz, K. (1988), Myoelectric activity of the small bowel in mechanical obstruction and intra-abdominal bacterial contamination, *Eur. Surg. Res.*, vol. 20, No. 5-6, pp. 304-309.

Levy, J., Harris, J., Chen, J., Sapoznikov, D., Riley, B., De La, N. W., & Khaskelberg, A. (2001), Electrogastrographic norms in children: toward the development of standard methods, reproducible results, and reliable normative data, *J. Pediatr. Gastroenterol. Nutr.*, vol. 33, No. 4, pp. 455-461.

Li, G., Wang, Y., Lin, L., Jiang, W., Wang, L. L., Lu, C., & Besio, W. G. (2005), Active Laplacian Electrode for the data-acquisition system of EHG, *Journal of Physics: Conference series.*, vol. 13, pp. 330-335.

Liang, H. L. (2001), Adaptive independent component analysis of multichannel electrogastrograms, *Med. Eng. Phys.*, vol. 23, No. 2, pp. 91-97, ISBN. 1350-4533.

Liang, H. L. (2005), Extraction of gastric slow waves from electrogastrog rams: combining independent component analysis and adaptive signal enhancement, *Med. Biol. Eng. Comput.*, vol. 43, No. 2, pp. 245-251, ISBN. 0140-0118.

Liang, H. L. & Lin, Z. (2001), Detection of delayed gastric emptying from electrogastrograms with support vector machine, *IEEE Trans. Biomed. Eng*, vol. 48, No. 5, pp. 601-604.

Liang, H. L., Lin, Z., & Mccallum, R. W. (2000), Artifact reduction in electrogastrogram based on empirical mode decomposition method, *Med. Biol. Eng. Comput.*, vol. 38, No. 1, pp. 35-41.

Liang, J., Cheung, J. Y., & Chen, J. D. Z. (1997), Detection and deletion of motion artifacts in electrogastrogram using feature analysis and neural networks, *Ann. Biomed. Eng.*, vol. 25, No. 5, pp. 850-857, ISBN. 0090-6964.

Lin, Z. Y. & Chen, J. D. Z. (1994), Recursive Running DCT Algorithm and Its Application in Adaptive Filtering of Surface Electrical Recording of Small-Intestine, *Med. Biol. Eng. Comput.*, vol. 32, No. 3, pp. 317-322, ISBN. 0140-0118.

Maestri, R., Pinna, G. D., Porta, A., Balocchi, R., Sassi, R., Signorini, M. G., Dudziak, M., & Raczak, G. (2007), Assessing nonlinear properties of heart rate variability from short-term recordings: are these measurements reliable?, *Physiol Meas.*, vol. 28, No. 9, pp. 1067-1077.

Martinez-de-Juan, J. L., Saiz, J., Meseguer, M., & Ponce, J. L. (2000), Small bowel motility: relationship between smooth muscle contraction and electroenterogram signal, *Med. Eng. Phys.*, vol. 22, No. 3, pp. 189-199.

Matsuura, Y., Yokoyama, K., Takada, H., & Shimada, K. (2007), Dynamics analysis of electrogastrography using Double-Wayland algorithm, *Conf Proc.IEEE Eng Med.Biol.Soc.*, pp. 1973-1976.

Mintchev, M. P. & Bowes, K. L. (1996), Extracting quantitative information from digital electrogastrograms, *Med. Biol. Eng. Comput.*, vol. 34, No. 3, pp. 244-248, ISBN. 0140-0118.

Mintchev, M. P., Rashev, P. Z., & Bowes, K. L. (2000), Misinterpretation of human electrogastrograms related to inappropriate data conditioning and acquisition using digital computers, *Dig. Dis. Sci.*, vol. 45, No. 11, pp. 2137-2144.

Moreno-Vazquez, J. J., Martinez-de-Juan, J. L., Garcia-Casado, J., & Ponce, J. L. (2003), Autoregressive Spetral Analysis of Electroenterogram (EEnG) for Basic Electric Rhythm Identification, *Conf.Proc.IEEE Eng Med.Biol.Soc.*, pp. 2539-2542 Cancun, México.

Peng, C., Qian, X., & Ye, D. T. (2007), Electrogastrogram extraction using independent component analysis with references, *Neural comput. & Applic.*, vol. 16, No. 6, pp. 581-587.

Prats-Boluda, G., Garcia-Casado, J., Martinez-de-Juan, J. L., & Ponce, J. L. (2007), Identification of the slow wave component of the electroenterogram from laplacian abdomianl surface recording in Humans, *Physiol. Meas.*, vol. 28, pp. 1-19.

Quigley, E. M. (1996), Gastric and small intestinal motility in health and disease, *Gastroenterol. Clin. North Am.*, vol. 25, No. 1, pp. 113-145.

Ramos, J., Vargas, M., Fernández, M., Rosell, J., & Pallás-Areny, R. (1993), A system for monitoring pill electrode motion in esophageal ECG, *Conf Proc. IEEE Eng Med.Biol.Soc.*, pp. 810-811 San Diego.

Seidel, S. A., Bradshaw, L. A., Ladipo, J. K., Wikswo, J. P., Jr., & Richards, W. O. (1999), Noninvasive detection of ischemic bowel, *J. Vasc. Surg.*, vol. 30, No. 2, pp. 309-319.

Szurszewski, J. H. (1969), A Migrating Electric Complex of the Canine Small Intestine, *Am. J. Physiol.* pp. 1757-1763.

Tomomasa, T., Morikawa, A., Sandler, R. H., Mansy, H. A., Koneko, H., Masahiko, T., Hyman, P. E., & Itoh, Z. (1999), Gastrointestinal sounds and migrating motor complex in fasted humans, *Am. J. Gastroenterol.*, vol. 94, No. 2, pp. 374-381, ISBN. 0002-9270.

Van Felius, I. D., Akkermans, L. M., Bosscha, K., Verheem, A., Harmsen, W., Visser, M. R., & Gooszen, H. G. (2003), Interdigestive small bowel motility and duodenal bacterial overgrowth in experimental acute pancreatitis, *Neurogastroenterol. Motil.*, vol. 15, No. 3, pp. 267-276.

Verhagen, M. A. M. T., Van Schelven, L. J., Samsom, M., & Smout, A. J. P. M. (1999), Pitfalls in the analysis of electrogastrographic recordings, *Gastroenterology*, vol. 117, No. 2, pp. 453-460, ISBN. 0016-5085.

Wang, Z. S., Cheung, J. Y., & Chen, J. D. Z. (1999), Blind separation of multichannel electrogastrograms using independent component analysis based on a neural network, *Med. Biol. Eng. Comput.*, vol. 37, No. 1, pp. 80-86, ISBN. 0140-0118.

Weisbrodt, N. W. (1987), Motility of the small intestine, in *Physiology of the Gastrointestinal Tract (Vol.1)*,pp. 631-633, Raven Press, New York.

Ye, Y., Garcia-Casado, J., Martinez-de-Juan, J. L., Alvarez Martinez, D., & Prats-Boluda, G. (2008), Quantification of Combined Method for Interferences Reduction in Multichannel Surface Electroenterogram, *Conf.Proc.IEEE Eng Med.Biol.Soc.*, pp. 3612-3615 Vancouver, Canada.

Ye, Y., Garcia-Casado, J., Martinez-de-Juan, J. L., & Ponce, J. L. (2007), Empirical mode decomposition: a method to reduce low frequency interferences from surface electroenterogram, *Med. Biol. Eng Comput.*, vol. 45, No. 6, pp. 541-551.

17

New trends and challenges in the development of microfabricated probes for recording and stimulating of excitable cells

Dries Braeken and Dimiter Prodanov
Bioelectronic Systems, IMEC vzw, Kapeldreef 75, 3001 Leuven
Belgium

I. Methods for the Recording of Electrical Signals from Cells in vitro and in vivo

1. Methods for the Recording of Electrical Activity from Cells In Vitro

1.1 Introduction

Excitable cells such as nerve cells communicate via signals transferred under the form of electrical potentials, the so-called action potentials. The communication is transmitted from one cell to another via numerous interconnections called synapses. This communication is critical for the life of higher organisms. Electrical activity of these cells can be studied using primary cell cultures, immortalized cell lines and acute slice preparations that are mostly brought in contact with a surface for adhesion or growth promotion. The study of single or groups of cells in these preparations is called 'in vitro' research. The study of the conduction of this electrical activity 'in vitro' and its impairment is of great importance in the development of new therapies for various neurological disorders such as Alzheimer's and Parkinson's disease, and epilepsia. Methods for studying action potentials can be conducted outside (extracellular recordings) or inside the cell (intracellular recordings).

The recording of the intracellular membrane potential requires either impaling the cell membrane with a sharp glass micro-electrode or establishing electrical access to the cell with a glass patch pipette. Extracellular recordings use either fixed or movable glass or insulated metal/metaloxide electrodes, positioned on the outside of the cell. In the following, a brief historical overview of the development of these techniques will be given, and new techniques based on micro-fabrication that gained a growing attention recently will be discussed.

The recording of the intracellular membrane potential provides the most precise description of the electrical behavior of a cell and, therefore, it requires specialized techniques. The use of sharp glass micro-electrodes for intracellular recordings is a challenging method and mostly limited to recordings in large cells from invertebrates. By impaling the cell with the sharp tip of the glass pipette, holding a Ag/AgCl electrode connected to a voltage follower, changes in the intracellular membrane potential can be measured. In addition, the pipette is usually filled with a high concentrated salt solution (KCl) to decrease the electrical resistance. The first studies on action potentials were performed on neurons of invertebrates using these intracellular glass micro-electrodes (Hodgkin (1939)).

1.2 Extracellular Recording

Although intracellular recordings provide the measurement of the intracellular potential of a cell, they are in any case invasive to the cell and its membrane. These recordings are, therefore, always limited in time. This rules out some investigations of important communication processes, such as late phase long-term potentiation (LTP) recordings. Potential changes of the membrane of a cell can also be measured from the outside of the membrane without making any physical contact to the cell. Glass micro-electrodes or thin, insulated metal electrodes can be used for extracellular recording of the membrane potential. Ionic movements across cell membranes are detected by placing a recording electrode close to the cell. The extracellular signal recorded upon the firing of an action potential is characterized by a brief, alternating voltage between the recording electrode and a ground electrode. Extracellular recordings with a glass electrode are thus advantageous in the investigation of long-term processes, such as LTP. Because the electrode is in close proximity but not in direct contact with the cell, the recordings are usually stable and not liable to mechanical instabilities. Although activity can be detected at the level of a single cell, recordings usually reflect the averaged response of a population of cells.

Despite the non-invasiveness of this method, the throughput of this type of experiments is rather low. The researcher has to manually bring the electrodes close to the cell membrane to be able to perform the recordings. With the progress in micro-fabrication techniques, planar micro-electrodes were developed that were able to record extracellularly from cultured cells grown on top of the electrode area. Planar micro-electrodes have been used as substrates for the culture support and non-invasive recording of cells, and electrical activity of single cells and networks of cells have been monitored successfully. In 1972, Thomas *et al.* described the first attempt to record electrical activity from cultured cells using a micro-electrode array (MEA) (Thomas et al. (1972)). They used gold-plated nickel electrodes on a glass substrate passivated with patterned photoresist. Embryonic chick heart cells were cultured in a glass chamber. Electrical activity was recorded extracellularly from the contracting heart cells simultaneously from many electrodes. Gross *et al.* used a similar system to record extracellular electrical responses from explanted neural tissue from the snail *Helix pomatia* (Gross et al. (1977)). Pine *et al.* were the first to report electrical recordings of dissociated neurons (superior cervical ganglia of neonatal rats) (Pine (1980)). Moreover, they combined the traditional method of intracellular recording using a glass micro-pipette with extracellular recording using a metal micro-electrode. Combining both techniques enables validation and calibration of the extracellular micro-electrode recording with the vast amount of information from intracellular recordings. These successes led to many groups using planar micro-electrodes for cultured cells (Droge et al. (1986); Eggers et al. (1990); Gross (1979); Gross et al. (1977); Martinoia et al. (1993); Novak & Wheeler (1986); Pine (1980); Thomas et al. (1972)).

The simultaneous stimulation and recording of cells is a logical next step and several researchers have already succeeded in stimulation and recording of embryonic chick myocytes cultured on planar micro-electrode arrays (Connolly et al. (1990); Israel et al. (1984)). In 1992, Jimbo and Kawana further expanded the possibilities with these systems by stimulation of neurites that were guided by micro-channels (Jimbo & Kawana (1992)). The same group later reported the simultaneous recording of electrical activity and intracellular [Ca^{2+}] using fluorescent dyes, showing the combination of optical and electrical techniques (Jimbo et al. (1993)).

1.3 Active Multitransistor Arrays

Although micro-electrode arrays are of growing interest in electrophysiological and pharmacological research, there are still shortcomings in these devices. The most abundant disadvantages are the low signal quality and the small amount of electrodes on the chip, which are both technological aspects. Most micro-electrode arrays are passive arrays that only amplify the signal once it is led through wires connecting the electrodes. The capacitive load that is introduced in this way attenuates the signal significantly. The small amount of electrodes is based on the used micro-fabrication technology used in these systems. Technological improvements over the years, however, made it possible to address these shortcomings. In 1991, Fromherz *et al.* reported recordings of extracellular field potentials from Retzius cells from the leech *Hirundo medicinalis* measured by an integrated transistor (Fromherz et al. (1991)). Here, the neuron was directly coupled to the gate of a field effect transistor that consisted of silicon dioxide. The validation of the measured potentials was performed by injecting a micro-electrode, which both stimulated the cell and monitored the intracellular voltage. Fromherz *et al.* used this system to further investigate the physics behind the coupling of the neuron and the transistor using an array of transistors below the neuron, as well as the capacitive stimulation of the neuron through the oxide layer (Fromherz et al. (1993); Fromherz & Stett (1995)). Recently, the same group showed the possibility of capacitive stimulation of specific ion channels using field effect transistors and recombinant HEK293 cells (Kupper et al. (2002)). In general, dense arrays of transistors, called multi-transistor arrays, have been used in increasing frequency for the recording of electrical activity from different cell types (Ingebrandt et al. (2001); Kind et al. (2002); Lorenzelli et al. (2003); Martinoia & Massobrio (2004); Martinoia et al. (2001); Meyburg et al. (2006)).

1.3.1 Cell-Chip Coupling

While these sensors show high signal-to-noise ratios, integration of read-out functionality and the possibility for downscaling, which makes these systems superior to passive MEA systems, this technology is still in an experimental phase and, therefore, very expensive. Furthermore, another crucial design and fabrication problem is the need for a biocompatible system. Most materials that are typically used in integrated circuitries are not optimized for use in liquids and with cultured cells. Both MEAs and arrays of FETs have been mostly used for recording from acute slices and large cells from invertebrates. Although some examples of extracellular recordings of mammalian cells have been demonstrated, single-cell addressability of small, mammalian cells remains challenging.

1.3.2 Recent Advances in Multitransistor Arrays

The electrical coupling between the cell membrane and the chip is mainly based on the contact between the lipid bilayer and the surface of the chip and the most important factor responsible for signal strength attenuation. Parameters that influence the cell-chip coupling are the distance between cell membrane and electrode and the electrical resistance that exists in this gap. The distance between the cell membrane and the surface was characterized extensively by Braun *et al.*, using fluorescent dye molecules to stain the membrane on silicon chips with microscopic oxide terraces (Braun & Fromherz (2004)). Using HEK293 cells on chips coated with fibronectin, the measured distance was ~70 nm, independent of the electrical resistivity of the bath (Gleixner & Fromherz (2006)). Later, the same group used fluorescence interference contrast microscopy to calculate the distance between the cell membrane and chip surface. The separation between membrane and surface is caused by proteins in the membrane (glycocalyx) and the surface coating on the chip. This gap could be narrowed down to 20 nm, when snail neurons were used on a laminin fragment that was anchored to the surface (Schoen & Fromherz (2007)). The electrical coupling between the chip surface and the cell depends on the electrical resistance of this thin layer between the oxide and the lipid bilayer. Fromherz *et al.* used a technique with alternating voltages applied to the chip to map this electrical resistance. The resistance and the capacitances of the surface (metal oxide) and membrane determine the voltage across the attached membrane. In normal culture medium, the sheet resistance was determined to be $\sim$10 MΩ. When the gap was 20 nm, the estimated resistance was $\sim$1.5 GΩ. The conclusion of these experiments was that the space between the cell membrane and the chip surface which was filled with cell medium, created a conductive sheet that prevented an effective interaction by direct electrical polarization. The resistance that exists in this gap is often referred to as the seal resistance (R_{seal}). One of the most important challenges in MEA recording is increasing the value of this seal resistance.

To enhance the signal-to-noise ratio when recording with MEAs, attempts have been made to hold or guide the cells. For example, if the cell can be positioned precisely on top of the sensor, the distance between the cell and the sensor surface can be decreased. Lind *et al.* proved this after performing a finite element analysis model of the extracellular action potential, whereby cells surrounded by extracellular fluid were compared with cells in grooves and cubic pits. The signal could be improved by as much as 700% when the extracellular space was confined by the external structures (Lind et al. (1991)). These modeling results were later confirmed by recordings of neurons from the snail *Lymnaea stagnalis*, cultured in a 10 μm wide, 1 μm deep groove (Breckenridge et al. (1995)).

In the Bioelectronic Systems Group of the Interuniversity Micro-Electronics Center (IMEC) in Leuven, Belgium, a multidisciplinary research team works towards the fabrication of micro-structured electrode arrays with three-dimensional electrodes. The concept lays in the fact that if the electrodes are small enough, the cell membrane will engulf the electrodes, creating a strong interaction between the membrane and the electrode surface. This would eventually lead to a stronger electrical coupling because of a higher electrical resistance in the gap between cell and chip. Preliminary data suggest strong engulfment of the electrode by the cell membrane, as could be observed by immunohistochemical actin filament staining and focused ion beam scanning electron microscopy (Figure 1)(Braeken et al. (2008); Huys et al. (2008); Van Meerbergen et al. (2008)). Moreover, the electrodes are spaced very close to each other, which allows for single cell recording and stimulation. However, this feature is highly dependent on the technology level that is used.

2. Methods for Recording of Electrical Activity from Cells In Vivo

2.1 Introduction

Understanding of the neural codes and the development of brain-computer interfaces for the normal and injured nervous system would require simultaneous selective recording and stimulation at multiple locations along the sensory-motor circuits. At present, there are several technological platforms that are capable of scaling to such recording and stimulation modalities.

The probes designed for deep brain recording need to penetrate the soft meninges and the underlying brain matter. Therefore, most of the designs implement either sharp tips or specialized add-ons for insertion. On the other hand, probes for surface recording, such as the surface arrays and the cuff electrodes, are flexible and are designed to adapt to the surface of the brain sulci or the nerves, respectively.

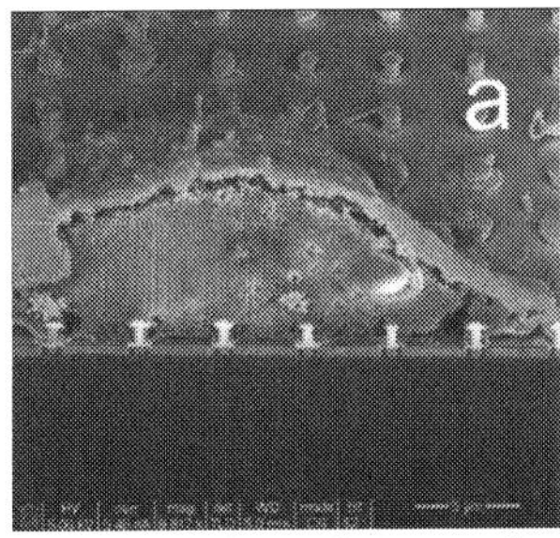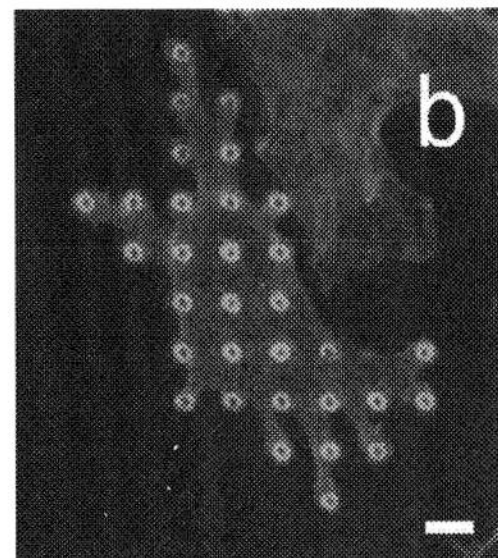

Fig. 1. Micro-structured electrode arrays developed in IMEC, Belgium. a) Focused ion beam scanning micrograph of a neuroblastoma cell on a nail bed. b) Actin filament staining of a single cardiomyocyte on a nail bed. Scale bar is 3 μm. ©IMEC. *All rights reserved.*

2.2 Silicone-based Probes

The first silicon-based electrode arrays for 'in vivo' recording were developed by Wise, Starr, and Angell in 1970 (Wise & Angell (1975); Wise et al. (1970)). They introduced the use of *integrated circuit* (IC) technology to develop micro-electrodes.

2.2.1 The Michigan probe

BeMent et al. (1986) reported for the first time the development of a micro-fabricated micro-electrode array from silicon having many recording contacts. These probes have evolved into the devices commonly known as the Michigan probes. Michigan probes are supported and distributed by the Center for Neural Communication Technology (CNCT) since 1994. There are multiple designs already disseminated through CNCT. Some of them are commercially available from the company NeuroNexus Technology.

The Michigan probes are based on a silicon substrate, the thickness and shape of which are precisely defined using boron etch-stop micro-machining. The substrate supports an array of conductors that are insulated by thin-film dielectrics. Openings through the upper dielectrics are inlaid with metal to form the electrode sites for contact with the tissue, and the bond pads for connection to the external world. The Michigan probe has also been modified for 3D configuration. Arrays of planar, comb-like multi-shank structures have been assembled into 3D arrays. Such three-dimensional structures can be constructed from the two-dimensional components using micro-assembly techniques. The procedure is based on inserting multiple two-dimensional probes into a silicon micro-machined platform that is intended to lay on the cortical surface. The Michigan probe process is compatible with the inclusion of on-chip CMOS (complementary metal-oxide semiconductor) circuitry for signal conditioning and multiplexing. Such active arrays were also validated in neural recording experiments. Bai & Wise (2001) reported the fabrication of "active" electrodes with monolithically integrated CMOS circuitry. High density probes for massively parallel recording, with on-chip preamplifiers to remove movement-related artifacts and reduce the weight of the headgear for small animals, were used to record simultaneously from the soma and dendrites of the same neurons (Csicsvari et al. (2003)).

2.2.2 The Utah Electrode Array

The group of Dr. Richard Normann at the University of Utah, USA, developed a micro-electrode array referred to as the Utah Electrode Array. The Utah Array has a matrix of densely-packed penetrating shafts, which are between 1 and 1.5 mm long and project from a very thin (200 μm) glass/silicon composite substrate and are separated from each other by 400 μm. The device is formed from a monocrystalline block of silicon using a diamond dicing saw and chemical sharpening (Nordhausen et al. (1996)). It provides a multichannel interface with the cortex. The resulting silicon shafts are electrically isolated from one another with a glass frit and from the surrounding tissue with deposited polyimide or silicon nitride. The tip-most 50 to 100 μm of each shaft is coated with platinum to form the recording contact. Interconnection to the electrode sites is accomplished by bonding either individual, insulated 25 μm-thick wires or a polyimide ribbon cable having many individual leads to bond pads on the top of the array. The Utah array was originally designed with the goal to serve as an interface for a human cortical visual prosthesis (Branner & Normann (2000)). Performed experiments demonstrated numerous issues in favor of such an approach. Nevertheless, the device turned to be a successful research tool in animal experimentation. For example, it was used for acute and chronic recordings in the cat cortex (Maynard et al. (1997); Rousche & Normann (1998)). A modified design was also tested in cat peripheral nerve (Branner & Normann (2000); Branner et al. (2001)). The design of the Utah array was used for human motor cortical prosthesis spun-off in the company Cyberkinetics. There is an ongoing clinical trial authorized by FDA in five severely disabled patients to determine the usability of the technology (Hochberg et al. (2006)).

2.3 European designs

In Europe, there are co-ordinated efforts to build integrated probes for recording, stimulation and local drug delivery. Among the leading centers are IMTEK in Germany, Twente University in the Netherlands, IMEC in Belgium and EPFL in Switzerland. The devices are based on silicon micro-technology and are compatible with a CMOS process.
Several types of multi-electrode probes have been recently designed and fabricated at IMEC. Musa et al. (2008) reported the fabrication of single-shank passive probes for cortical recording. The probe implements a planar array of electrode contacts of varying sizes (4, 10, 25 and 50 μm). In some configurations, an additional larger reference electrode is placed close to the electrode array. Another probe design contains crescent-shaped electrodes. Two of the configurations are shown in Figure 2.
The devices produced in collaboration by IMTEK and IMEC[1] are based on the principle of modular assembly. The probes consist of needle-like structures made of silicon realized using deep reactive ion etching (Ruther et al. (2008)). The first generation devices come as single-shaft probes available in two lengths: 4 mm and 8 mm, each with cross-sections of 120 x 100 μm. In both cases, the probes have a row of nine equidistantly spaced, planar electrodes. The second generation of devices comprises comb-like rows of four probes, each of them with the same dimensions and number of electrodes as in the first generation. This two-dimensional array can be provided with a guide wire or with a thumbtack structure for insertion purposes. Another version of the device contains two such rows assembled in a back-to-back fashion.
Norlin et al. (2002) demonstrated the manufacture of a probe with 32 recording sites[2]. The silicon probes consist of 8 shafts with a minimal cross-section of 20 μm x 20 μm. The shafts

---

[1] part of the Neuroprobes research consortium
[2] part of the VSAMUEL research consortium

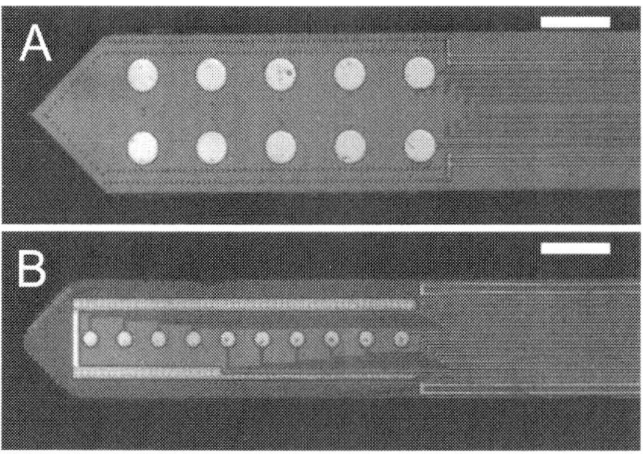

Fig. 2. First generation IMEC recording and stimulation probes

A – NP50 configuration. The probe contains 10 disk electrode sites arranged in a square lattice with diameters of 50 μm. The spacing between contacts is 100 μm. The tip angle is 90°. B – NP25 configuration. The probe contains a linear array of 10 disk electrode sites with diameters of 25 μm. The spacing between contacts is 50 μm. The tip angle is 90°. The shafts are long 2 mm; the cross-section is 200 x 200 μm. The active interface is realized from **Pt**. The probes are insulated with *Parylene C*. The fabrication approach is fully scalable. The fabrication process can be easily adapted to produce longer probes. Scale bars are 100 μm. *©IMEC. All rights reserved.*

taper to very sharp tips (4°). Each of the shafts carries four **Ir** micro-electrodes (10 μm x 10 μm) as recording sites on their side.

Rutten et al. (1995) reported the fabrication of a 3D needle array with 128 recording sites on one electrode placed on the tip of a needle intended to serve as interface to peripheral nerves. The different lengths of the needles allowed selective stimulation of different volumes in peripheral nerves.

2.4 Non silicon-based hard substrates

Silicon-on-Insulator SOI electrodes can be also produced using silicon-on-insulator (SOI) technology (Cheung (2007)). SOI wafers use an insulating oxide layer to separate a thin silicon device layer (1 to 100 μm) from the thick silicon of the backside (about 500 μm thick). The SOI wafer gives excellent control over the final probe thickness. The buried oxide acts as an etch stop during a backside deep RIE of the silicon wafer. The same group presented SOI-based probes with integrated microfluidic channels, which permitted localized injections of chemical substances of very small volumes.

Ceramic-based The insulator ceramic (alumina, Al_2O_3) has been used as a substrate to reduce crosstalk between adjacent connecting lines (Burmeister & Gerhardt (2001); Burmeister et al. (2000)). Ceramic is a mechanically strong material which allows for development of micro-electrodes that can access much deeper brain structures (up to 5 – 6 cm versus 2 – 4 mm for silicon). Precise placement of the micro-electrode in tissue without flexing or breaking can be achieved. Individual devices have to be cut from the wafer either by a diamond saw or by a laser. Numerous four- and five-site platinum micro-electrodes on ceramic substrates have been developed. Some designs are used for electrochemical measurements of neurotransmitters (Barbosa et al. (2008); Pomerleau et al. (2003)).

One of the very attractive features of the planar photo-engraved probes is the ability to customize design for specific experiments. The substrate can have any two-dimensional shape with single or multiple shanks, electrode sites can be of any surface area and can be placed anywhere along the shank(s) at any spacing, tips can be made very sharp or blunt, and features such as holes or channels can also be included.

2.5 Flexible substrates

The fabrication processes of flexible probes so far employed polyimide, parylene (DuPont) and benzocyclobutene as substrate materials. Polyimide films have been also used as top insulators for cortical micro-electrodes. Micro-electrodes less than 20 μm thick have been constructed with the use of parylene (Rousche et al. (2001)).

Polyimide probes have also been seeded with bioactive molecules such as neural growth factor (NGF) near the recording sites (Rousche et al. (2001)) with the idea to encourage neurite growth toward the active interface and to improve the stability in time (Metz et al. (2001)).

Benzocyclobutene can be used as an alternative to polyimide in the fabrication of neural interfaces. For example, Lee, He & Wang (2004) reported the fabrication of benzocyclobutene coated neural implants with embedded microfluidic channels (Lee, He & Wang (2004); Lee, Clement, Massia & Kim (2004)).

An important development direction in Europe is the development of flexible electrodes for cortical (Myllymaa et al. (2009); Rubehn et al. (2009)) and peripheral nerve recording (Navarro et al. (2001); Stieglitz & Meyer (1999)). Developed electrodes have been based on polyimide as carrier material.

Polymer-based implants using polyimide as both the structural and insulation material have been micro-machined with multilayer metallization for both acute and chronic nerve recording. Hybrid polyimide cuff electrodes embedded in silicone guidance channels have been fabricated for electrical stimulation of peripheral nerves (Stieglitz et al. (2005)). Polyimide sieve electrodes have been used in the regeneration and functional re-innervation of sensory and motor nerve fibers (Rodríguez et al. (2000)).

Rubehn et al. (2009) reported the fabrication of a micro-machined 252-channel ECoG (electrocorticogram)-electrode array made of a thin polyimide foil substrate enclosing sputtered platinum electrode sites and conductor paths. The array was designed to chronically interface the visual cortex of the macaque.

3. Commercialized Micro-electrode Arrays

Only recently, micro-electrode arrays are being increasingly used. However, valuable research was performed much earlier. The reason for earlier commercialization were the limitations of the computing technology available at that time. Because of their recent accessibility and affordability, interest in MEA systems has been renewed. Indeed, multi-electrode recordings accelerate the collection of sample sizes needed for valuable statistical analyses in drug screening assays. Today, MEAs suitable for routine electrophysiological recordings to monitor the activity of neuronal and cardiac populations *in vitro* are commercially available. Well-known manufacturers of these systems include Multichannel Systems, AlphaMed, Ayanda Biosystems and BioCell-Interface.

Most of the clinical neuronal probes used at present are fabricated by Medtronic. The Michigan probe was commercialized in the company NeuroNexus Technology.

4. Biomedical Applications of Micro-fabricated Arrays

4.1 Planar Micro-Electrode Array Systems

Micro-electrode arrays are fastly gaining interest as research instruments for the investigation of various disorders and diseases or the study of fundamental communication processes. Because they do not require highly trained personnel, various tissue preparations can be applied to the electrode surfaces, including acute slices of brain, retina and heart and primary dissociated cell cultures of different regions of the heart and central nervous system.

The biomedical applications are related to these preparations and can be classified into two categories: neuronal and cardiac. Neuronal electrophysiological research with micro-electrode arrays is conducted in various domains of neuroscience, for example long term potentiation from acute slice preparations (Dimoka, Courellis, Gholmieh, Marmarelis & Berger (2008); Dimoka, Courellis, Marmarelis & Berger (2008)) or organotypic slice cultures (Cater et al. (2007); Haustein et al. (2008)), electroretinograms (Wilms & Eckhorn (2005)) and microERGs (Rosolen et al. (2008; 2002)) and recordings from cortical, hippocampal or striatal primary cell cultures for various studies including network plasticity (Chiappalone et al. (2008); Wagenaar et al. (2006)) and memory processing and network activity (Baruchi & Ben-Jacob (2007); Pasquale et al. (2008)). Micro-electrode arrays are also widely used to study electrophysiological properties of the heart, such as gap junction functionality and impulse conduction (Reisner et al. (2008)), arrhythmias (Ocorr et al. (2007)) and experimental stem-cell derived cardiac research (Gepstein (2008); Mauritz et al. (2008)).

4.2 Neuroprosthetic and Neuromodulatory Applications

4.2.1 Development of Neuroprosthetic applications

The development of neural prostheses was influenced to a great extent by the successful clinical application of the cardiac pacemakers (review in Prodanov et al. (2003)).

In the 1970s, after two decades of continuous technological development, the pacemakers were adopted on a great scale in clinical practice. Similar was the case of the *respiratory pacemakers*, which were developed in parallel for patients suffered from cervical spinal cord injury. Stimulation of the phrenic nerves causes constriction of the diaphragm and inspiration. The first attempts to pace the diaphragm with implanted electrodes were carried out in 1948 – 1950 by Sarnoff et al. (1950). One of the most important prerequisites for the clinical acceptance of this technique was the introduction of the long-term electrical stimulation by the radio-frequency inductive method around the end of the 1950s (Glenn et al. (1964)). The first commercial phrenic nerve pacers were introduced in the early 1980s. *Restoration of hearing* was successfully introduced in the late 1950s based on the previous observations of Gersuni & Volokhov (1937). The proof of principle was demonstrated in the intraoperative experiments of Djourno & Eyries (1957) who stimulated the inner ear by an implanted electrode coupled inductively to an outside coil that was in turn connected to a microphone. The actual usefulness of the first experimental device was very limited since the patient could recognize only few words from the transmitted signal (*papa, maman*, and *allo*). The indications and contraindications for this implantation were elaborated in a broad debate between the clinicians and the pioneers of the cochlear prostheses. The general approval of the cochlear prostheses was given by FDA in 1984 after 20 years of design and trials. Over the past 20 years of clinical experience, more than 20 000 people worldwide have received cochlear implants. Cochlear implantation has a profound impact on hearing and speech perception in postlingually deafened adults. Most individuals demonstrate significantly enhanced speech reading capabilities during daily life. To restore the lost functions of the paralyzed leg muscles, experiments were performed for the first time in 1961 by Liberson et al. (1961). The system was developed to compensate for the "drop foot" problem in hemiplegic stroke patients. The "drop foot" stimulation systems activate the nerve fibers in the peroneal nerve with the net effect of flexion in the tarsal joint.

From the presented cases, it is apparent that the successfully applied neural prostheses so-far have been developed for systems, which have either uniform topographic mapping, such as the phrenic or peroneal nerves, and/or inherent ability to learn the stimulation pattern - for example the auditory prostheses.

In contrast, in other sensory and motor systems so-derived principles apply to a limited extent and the performance of the neural prostheses is lower. For example, the usefulness of the *motor neural prostheses* is still insufficient for general clinical use. Motor tasks require orchestrated activation of many muscles, which in turn requires selective stimulation of only defined parts of the nerves or muscle groups. Existing leg and hand neuroprostheses are still far from providing such level of functional selectivity without extensive surgery. Steps towards improving the expected selectivity of stimulation were made by investigation of the topographic mapping of some peripheral nerves and spinal roots in rats (Prodanov (2006); Prodanov & Feirabend (2007; 2008); Prodanov et al. (2007)). However, those results still need to be translated to men. Other examples are some of the *hand prostheses and orthoses*. Most of the proposed implantable systems require extensive surgery in order to interface the hand nerves at several locations to improve selectivity. The surface stimulation systems need to combine several stimulation channels to provide an acceptable level of selectivity. The neuroprostheses have demonstrated improvement of the grasping function in clinical trials including stroke or spinal cord injury subjects. However, the grasp strategies that can be provided with the existing neuroprostheses for grasping are very limited and can only be used for a restricted set of grasping and holding tasks (review in Prodanov et al. (2003)).

Visual prostheses have been developed for the last 30 years (review in Prodanov et al. (2003)). Major research lines were focused on the development of cortical prostheses (Brindley & Lewin, 1968; Dobelle & Mladejovsky, 1974; Normann et al., 2001); retinal prostheses (review in Zrenner (2002)) and optic nerve prostheses (Veraart et al. (1998)). The results in the field demonstrate that generating perception of light patterns in blind people is feasible. However, true object recognition still can not be achieved. The *surface cortical microstimulation* (Brindley & Lewin (1968); Dobelle & Mladejovsky (1974)) could not provide useful images because of its limited spatial resolution and the fading of the induced phosphenes (sensations of light). Subsequent human trials with *penetrating cortical implants* (i.e. Utah arrays; see section 2.2.2) were more promising (Dobelle (2000); Normann et al. (1996); Schmidt et al. (1996)), but diminished neuronal excitation and the stability of spatial resolution were still unsolved problems even using high-resolution intracortical electrode arrays (Normann et al. (2001)). The group of Veraart at Université Catholique Louvain (UCL), Brussels, demonstrated that by stimulation of the optic nerve to have the patient recognize single spots of light (Veraart et al. (1998)).

In the end of the 1980s, several North American, Australian and European teams (Eckmiller (1997)) started developing retinal prostheses. Notably, these are the groups of M. Humayun (John Hopkins University) (Schmidt et al. (1996)) and that of J. Rizzo (Harvard University) (Rizzo et al. (2003)) in association with the Massachusetts Institute of Technology, which develop epiretinal implants. The epiretinal implant has no light-sensitive elements. In the epiretinal configuration a tiny camera-like sensor is positioned either outside the eye or within an intraocular plastic lens that replaces the natural lens of the eye. An alternative type of retinal prosthesis is the *subretinal implant* developed by Chow & Chow (1997) in Chicago and

Zrenner et al. (1997) in Tübingen. The Tübingen subretinal device is implanted between the pigment epithelial layer and the outer layer of the retina. The device consists of thousands of light-sensitive microphotodiodes equipped with micro-electrodes assembled on a very thin plate. The light falling on the retina generates currents in the photodiodes, which then activate the micro-electrodes and stimulate the retinal sensory neurons. Epiretinal and subretinal implants depend on the uniform topographic mapping of the retina. If the provided stimulation can trigger learning phenomena in the visual system, we could anticipate another successful clinical application.

4.2.2 Development of Neuromodulatory applications

Deep brain stimulation (DBS) and vagus nerve stimulation (VNS) can be regarded as examples for fast-developing neuromodulatory applications. DBS will be used further also to illustrate some of the challenges in the development of neural interfaces with the brain.

VNS uses an implanted battery-powered signal generator, which stimulates the left vagus nerve in the neck via a pair of spiral cuff-electrodes connected through a lead wire also implanted under the skin. In the case of VNS, the first experimental demonstrations of an anticonvulsant effect of VNS were made in 1980s (reviews in George et al. (2000) and Groves & Brown (2005)). So far the FDA approved the use of VNS as an adjunctive therapy for epilepsy in 1997 and for treatment resistant depression in 2005. Ongoing experimental investigations include various anxiety disorders, Alzheimer's disease, migraines (Groves & Brown (2005)), and fibromyalgia. Current implantable systems (notably the NCP system of Cyberonics Ltd) provide non-selective stimulation, which activates all A_α nerve fibers. Since the vagus nerve projects to three major brain stem nuclei [3], which in turn relay to other brain stem nuclei, such as the *reticular formation*, the *parabrachial nucleus* and the *locus coeruleus*, the effects induced by the electric stimulation of the vagus A_α nerve fibers are multiple and most probably interact with each other. Therefore, the beneficial effects of VNS most probably develop by plastic changes in all affected subsystems, i.e. a learning phenomenon.

Deep brain stimulation is a surgical treatment involving the implantation of electrodes in the brain, which are driven through a battery-powered programmable stimulator. Current versions of the therapy use high-frequency stimulation trains (i.e. in the range 80 – 130 Hz), which can modulate certain parts of the the motor circuits in the basal ganglia.

In 1991, two groups independently reported beneficial effects of thalamic stimulation for tremor suppression (Benabid et al. (1991); Blond & Siegfried (1991)). DBS is considered already as a standard and accepted treatment for Parkinson's disease (Deep Brain Stimulation in Parkinson's Disease Group, 2001), essential tremor, dystonia, and cerebellar outflow tremor (recent overview in Baind et al. (2009)). In the USA, the FDA approved DBS as a treatment for essential tremor in 1997, for Parkinson's disease in 2002 and for dystonia in 2003. There are undergoing clinical trials for epilepsy, depression, obsessive-compulsive disorder, and minimally conscious states (review in Montgomery & Gale (2008)). DBS offers important advantages over the irreversible effects of ablative procedures, including the reversibility of the surgical outcome and the ability to adjust stimulation parameters post-operatively to optimize therapeutic benefit for the patient while minimizing adverse effects (Johnson et al. (2008)).

The mechanisms of action of DBS are still subject to debate arising from conflicting sets of experimental observations. Early hypotheses proposed that stimulation mimicked the outcome of ablative surgeries by inhibiting neuronal activity at the site of stimulation, i.e. "functional

---

[3] *n. dorsalis n. vagi* (efferent), *n. tractus solitarii* (afferent), *n. ambiguus* (afferent)

ablation". This comprises the direct inhibition hypothesis. Several possibilities have been proposed to explain this view including (i) depolarization blockade, (ii) synaptic inhibition, (iii) neurotransmitter depression, and (iv) stimulation of presynaptic terminals with neurotransmitter release (see McIntyre et al. (2004)). Recent studies have challenged this hypothesis (reviews in Johnson et al. (2008); Montgomery & Gale (2008)), suggesting that, although somatic activity near the DBS electrode may exhibit substantial inhibition or complex modulation patterns, the output from the stimulated nucleus follows the DBS pulse train by direct axonal excitation. The intrinsic activity is thus overridden by more regular high-frequency activity that is induced by the stimulation. A number of alternative hypotheses about the mechanisms of DBS are offered in literature (Montgomery & Gale (2008)). These include (i) indirect inhibition of the stimulated nucleus possibly through thalamo-cortical loops; (ii) increased regularity of *globus pallidus internus* firing by decrease of the information content of the network output due to the regularity of the stimulation; and (iii) resonance effects through stimulation via reentrant loops. None of proposed hypothesis is entirely supported by the existing experimental evidence. However, in view of the recent experimental evidence, the direct inhibition hypothesis seems least probable.

If the same considerations apply also for neuromodulation, two similar principles of development can be stated. The successful neuromodulatory systems will be appplied in areas with uniform or discrete topology (for example the vagus nerve) and the overall effect of the applied stimulation should affect generic/systemic control mechanisms.

II. Biocompatibility of Micro-fabricated Devices

5. Introduction

When combining non-biological entity with living, biological matter, interaction between both is inevitable. When interfacing biological elements, whether they are peptides, proteins, cells or tissues, with non-biological elements, a new interface or situation is created. This interface situation is an interaction between two completely different milieus and, therefore, it is a crucial element for an optimal functioning of both. This interaction can either influence the role of both the biological and non-biological element in a manner that can change the original state of that element, and therefore, it can not be neglected. In this part, we will introduce the interfacing problems that originate from the contact between biological samples and tissues and non-biological materials present in implants and other bioelectronic devices. Biocompatibility issues and challenges will be presented for both in vivo and in vitro conditions, and future challenges and directions will be discussed.

Biocompatibility is extensively debated in biomaterials science and bioelectronic interfacing, but its definition is questionable and very broad. Because many different situations in biomedical engineering exist where biocompatibility is an issue, the uncertainty about the mechanisms and conditions is a serious impediment to the development of new techniques in biomedical and nanobiological research.

Biocompatibility refers to the ability of a material to perform with an appropriate host response in a speficic situation. This definition states that a material as such can not just exist inside a tissue or close to a biological organism, but has to fulfill three major requirements: (i) the response it evokes has to be appropriate for the application, (ii) the nature of the response to a certain material and (iii) its appropriateness may vary from one situation to another (Williams (1987; 2008a;b)). However, this definition is very general and so self-evident that it does not lead to an advancing knowlegde of biocompatibility. It is more likely that one concept cannot apply to all material-biological element reactions in the widely spread applications such as brain implants, tissue engineering, prosthesis, biosensors or micro-electrode arrays. The nature of material itself plays a large role in the evoked response in the biological element. Some major material variables are material composition, micro- (or nano)-structure, morphology, hydrophobicity or hydrophilicity, porosity, surface chemical and topographical composition, surface electronic properties, corrosion parameters and metal ion toxicity. These parameters can all influence the functioning of the biological element (Williams (2008a)).

6. Biocompatibility of In Vitro Devices

6.1 Cytotoxicity

Although the degree of biocompatibility is much more complex at the level of implantable materials and devices, in vitro biocompatibility cannot be neglected, especially because of the growing amount of new materials and technologies. In the following, biocompatibility will be described in the specific situation of micro-electrode arrays, a fast growing field in bioelectronics. Micro-electrode arrays can consist of many different materials, for which some general cytotoxicity is known, but for others, very little information is available.

Cytotoxicity is strongly dependent on the type of cell or cell culture that is used. A material which is toxic for one type of cell is not necessarily toxic for another, or the lethal concentration (LC50) can be vastly different. Therefore, a cytotoxicity test should always be designed for the final situation were the system will be used. It is clear that immortalized cancer cell lines are more robust to cytotoxic agents than fresh, primary cell preparations (e.g., Olschlager et al. (2009)). It is, therefore, important that the biocompatibility test is carefully designed. For obvious reasons, cell cultures of excitable cells are interesting for cultivation on micro-electrode arrays. These cell cultures mostly include preparations of the heart (embryonic artrial, ventricular or whole heart cultures) and the central nervous system (embryonic cortical, hippocampal, spinal cord cultures) and retinal neuronal cultures. Viability assays for these cell cultures include visual microscopic inspection, trypan blue staining, cell death (apoptosis and necrosis) assays using fluorescent microscopy, bioluminescence imaging and cytofluorometry. At present, there is a variety of standardized ready-to-use assays available to investigate cell proliferation, adhesion and survival.

copper toxicity Materials used in modern micro-fabrication are typically chosen based on their durability, ease of processing, conductivity and price. However, this mostly appears to be at odds with their biocompatible properties. Although most commercialized micro-electrode arrays are fabricated with biocompatible materials including borosilicate glass, platinum, gold, titanium (nitride), and several metal oxides, more advanced technologies require unexplored materials. One of the most important materials used in advanced complementary metal oxide semiconductor (CMOS) technology is copper. Copper is a cheap material with excellent conducting properties which is relatively easy to process in micro-fabrication tools.

Because copper can migrate fast through other materials, it can cause problems in bio-electronic devices. Copper (Cu) is an essential trace element found in small amounts in a variety of cells and tissues with the highest concentrations in the liver. Cu ions can exist in both an oxidized, cupric (Cu^{2+}), or reduced, cuprous (Cu^+), state. Copper functions as a co-factor and is required for structural and catalytic properties of a variety of important enzymes, including cytochrome c oxidase, tyrosinase, and Cu-Zn superoxidase dismutase. Copper is known to be a highly cytotoxic material. Several reports show the role of reactive oxygen species (ROS) in cell death induced by heavy metals (Houghton & Nicholas (2009)). Both cupric and cuprous ions can participate in oxidation and reduction reactions. In the presence of superoxide or reducing agents such as ascorbic acid, Cu^{2+} can be reduced to Cu^+, which is capable of catalyzing the formation of hydroxyl radicals from hydrogen peroxide. This is called the Haber-Weiss reaction, whereby copper catalyzes the formation of ROS by peroxidation of membranous lipids. The hydroxyl radical is the most powerful oxidizing radical likely to arise in biological systems, and is capable of reacting with practically every biological molecule (Buettner & Oberley (1979)). It can initiate oxidative damage by abstracting the hydrogen from an amino-bearing carbon to form a carbon-centered protein radical and from an unsaturated fatty acid to form a lipid radical (Powell et al. (1999)). Copper is cabable of inducing DNA strand breaks and oxidation of bases (Kawanishi et al. (2002)).

6.2 Interface Layers for Cell-based Biosensors

Another important aspect of in vitro biocompatibility is the growth of cell cultures on top of electrode surfaces. To perform successful experiments with cells on micro-electrode arrays, cells must adhere, grow and maintain on the surface of electrodes. Although some cells, such as immortalized fibroblast cell lines, can adhere easily to most surfaces, most cells need an interface layer to be present to adhere. The following describes straightforward methods for the adhesion and growth of various cell cultures.

An interface layer must mimic the normal environment of the biological element, creating optimal conditions for optimal functioning of the hybrid device. Although there are various strategies to construct interface layers, not all of them are suitable for cell-based biosensor technology. Self-assembled monolayers (SAMs) offer a reproducible manner of interfacing cells with sensor materials. Extracellular matrix peptides, polymers or proteins are also often used to attract and adhere cells. The enhancement of cell attachment and spreading through surface functionalization is a crucial parameter in the optimization of the functioning of cell-based micro-electrode arrays.

6.2.1 Self-Assmbled Monolayers

Characterized by high temperatures and the formation of a monolayer, chemisorption is often used in the formation of SAMs. They provide a convenient, flexible and simple system that tailors the interfacial properties of metals, metal oxides and semiconductors. Self-assembled monolayers are organic assemblies formed by the adsorption of molecular constituents deposited from solution or vapor onto a solid surface. They organize spontaneously into crystalline structures. However, the experimental conditions for their development need to be strictly controlled to ensure clean, complete monolayer formation. The molecules that form SAMs have a chemical functionality, or 'headgroup', with a specific affinity for a substrate. In many cases, the headgroup also has a high affinity for the surface and displaces other adsorbed organic materials (Love et al. (2005)). The headgroup-substrate pair is typically used to define the individual SAM system. The most common examples are thiols (R-SH, where R denotes the rest of the molecule) on metals (e.g., gold, platinum) or silane-based molecules on metal/semiconductor oxides (e.g., silicon dioxide, tantalum pentoxide). Self-assembled monolayers are structurally well-ordered, and are therefore an ideal substrate for the binding of various extracellular matrix proteins. The proteins adsorbed on top of these layers can be structured and immobilized with a large density to promote attachment, spreading and migration of cells.

Self-assembled monolayers can be also engineered to prevent non-specific adsorption of proteins (Frederix et al. (2004)). The majority of applications that have been reported make use of polyethylene glycol or derivates, which excludes protein adsorption through mechanisms that depend on the conformational properties of highly solvated polymer layers. Another approach of SAMs for the adhesion of cells is the use of monolayers that present peptide fragments from extracellular proteins such as fibronectin. These peptides are ligands for some of the integrin family cell-surface receptors, which are an important class of receptors found on all cellular surfaces and that mediate attachment of cells to the extracellular matrix (Critchley (2000)). Many different peptides fragments have been used over the years to promote cell adhesion to electrode surfaces or chip surfaces (Huang et al. (2009); Tsai et al. (2009); Van Meerbergen et al. (2008)).

6.2.2 Extracellular Matrix Proteins and Polymers

Extracellular matrix proteins that are often used for cell adhesion are laminin, fibronectin, and collagen. These proteins directly bind to integrin receptors on the outside of the cell membrane (Critchley (2000)). In this way, they communicate in a direct way with the cytoskeleton of the cell, responsible for cell adhesion and spreading on surfaces. Although not inherently biological, many polymers have been used as well to promote cell adhesion, including poly-L/D-lysine, poly-L-ornithine and polyethyleneimine. The principle of cell adhesion using these artificial ligands is based upon the strong electrostatic binding of the cell membrane to the surface (Hategan et al. (2004)). The main advantage and the direct reason of their success is the availability and price of these synthetic molecules.

7. Biocompatibility of Implantable Devices

7.1 Regulatory Aspects

The selection and evaluation of materials and devices intended for use in humans requires a structured program of assessment to establish appropriate levels of biocompatibility and safety. Current regulations, whether in accordance with the US FDA (ISO 10993-1/EN 30993 standard, since 1995), the International Organization for Standardization (ISO), or EU regulation bodies (The EU Council Directive - 93/42/EEC), as part of the regulatory clearance process require conduction of adequate safety testing of the finished devices through pre-clinical and clinical phases (Bollen & Svendsen (1997)). An extensive account on the biocompatibility can be found in the standard ISO 10993-1/EN 30993. An implant can be considered biocompatible if it gives negative results on the following tests:

cytotoxicity The aim of in vitro cytotoxicity tests is to detect the potential ability of a device to induce sublethal or lethal effects on mammal cells (mostly on fibroblast cultures). Three main types of cell-culture assays have been developed: the elution test, the direct-contact test, and the agar diffusion test.

sensitisation The sensitization test recognizes a possible sensitization reaction (allergic contact dermatitis) induced by a device, and is required by the ISO 10993-1 standard for all device categories.

genotoxicity Genetic toxicity tests are used to investigate materials for possible mutagenic effects–that is, damage to the genes or chromosomes of the test organism (e.g. bacteria or mammal cells).

implantation Implantation tests are designed to assess any localized effects of a device designed to be used inside the human body. Implantation testing methods essentially attempt to imitate the intended conditions of use.

carcinogenicity The objective of long-term carcinogenicity studies is to observe test animals over a major portion of their life span to detect any development of neoplastic lesions (tumor induction) during or after exposure to various doses of a test substance.

skin irritation The ISO 10993-10 standard describes skin-irritation tests for both single and cumulative exposure to a device. Skin-irritation tests of medical devices are performed either with two extracts obtained with polar and nonpolar solvents or with the device itself.

intracutaneous reactivity The intracutaneous reactivity test is designed to assess the localized reaction of tissue to the presence of a given substance.

acute systemic toxicity is the adverse effect occurring within a short time after administration of a single dose of to the presence of given substances. ISO 10993-1 requires that the test for acute systemic toxicity be considered for all device categories that indicate blood contact. For this test, extracts of medical devices are usually administered intravenously or intraperitoneally in rabbits or mice.

subchronic and chronic toxicity tests are carried out after initial information on toxicity has been obtained by acute testing, and provides data on possible health hazards likely to arise from repeated exposures over a limited time.

As can be seen from Figure 4, undesirable interactions affecting biocompatibility can occur in most of the levels of the issue tree. For example, implants may be subject to continuous attacks by hydrolytic enzymes or free radicals produced by macrophages and/or cell lysis (Salthouse (1976)). Stability of implanted material is important not only for a stable function but also because degradation products may be harmful to the host organism. An overview on the biological reactions to implanted materials can be found in Ratner et al. (1996).

While the ISO standard addresses the general bio-compatibilty requirements of a medical device, it does not address specifically the interactions on the active tissue-device interface.

7.2 Interactions on the Active Interface
7.2.1 Chemical Properties of the Active Interface

Appropriate implant materials should be as chemically inert as possible. If chemical reactions are to be expected, they should be minimal and all resulting products should be inert. Candidate materials for use in neuroprotheses pass very rigorous testing since they must remain inert not only passively but also when subjected to electrical stimulation and when placed in contact with the biological tissue.

According to the literature the following criteria should be considered when choosing material for an implanted electrode: (i) the intensity of the tissue response, (ii) eventual occurrence of allergic response, (iii) electrode-tissue impedance, (iv) radiographic visibility and (v) MRI safety (Geddes & Roeder (2003)).

For electrodes that make Ohmic contact with tissues, **Au, Pt, Pt-Ir** alloys, **W**, and **Ta** are recommended as materials for the active interface (Geddes & Roeder (2003); Heiduschka & Thanos (1998)). The use of some metals should be avoided because of vigorous tissue reactivity. These pure metals are notably **Fe, Cu, Ag, Co, Zn, Mg, Mn**, and **Al** (Geddes & Roeder (2003)).

It can be necessary to distinguish between stimulating and recording electrodes. Good materials for *recording electrodes* are: **Pt, Ir,** and **Rh** and **Au**. Materials of choice for *stimulating*

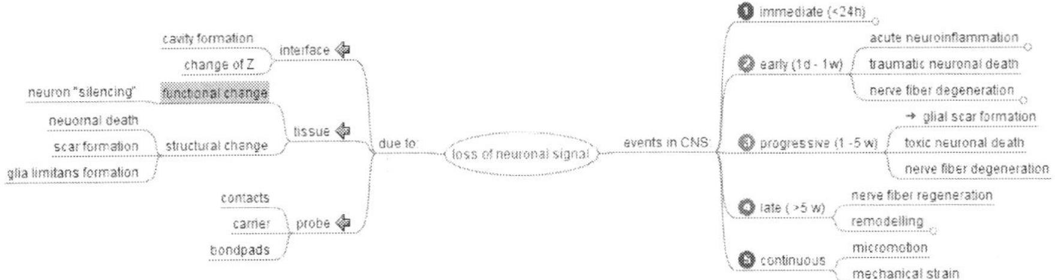

Fig. 3. Loss of signal

The **immediate effects** are caused by the mechanical interaction of the device with the brain tissue during implantation. These are notably *vascular damage, hemorrhage* and *brain edema*.
During the **progressive phase**, the acute inflammation, cell death and nerve fiber degeneration predominate. The inflammation process is driven by the complement complex activation, the extravasation of neutrophils and mononuclear cells and the secretion of cytokines. The **late effects** involve gliosis or chronic inflammation and the tissue remodeling. Some processes, notably the micromotion and mechanical strain, act **continuously** during all stages.

electrodes are **Pt**, **Pt-Ir** alloys, **W**, and **Rh**. For capacitive stimulating electrodes, tantalum pentoxide (Ta_2O_5) has the highest dielectric constant, followed by iridium oxide (IrO_2). Aluminum oxide (Al_2O_3) is a candidate with a lower dielectric constant.
Glassy carbon or carbon fibers are also used as electrode materials, and they are biocompatible and stable, though they have a higher roughness than metals. Among the currently studied conducting polymers, polypyrrole (*PPy*) and poly-3,4-ethylenedioxythiopentane (*PEDOT*) appear the best candidates for materials. They provide interesting opportunities to incorporate other substances, for example peptides or growth factors, during the process of polymerisation in order to improve biocompatibility in vivo. Interesting candidates for materials are the nano-structured materials and notably the carbon nanotubes.

7.2.2 Biotic-abiotic Reactions

As recognized by many groups in the field, one of the central issues in favor of a closed-loop implantable system is the uncertain performance of the recording function in chronic conditions (Berger et al. (2007)). This can be attributed to causes related to the device, to the tissue or to the active interface (Figure 3). While it is generally believed that the brain tissue response to chronically implanted silicon micro-electrode arrays contributes to recording instability and failure, the underlying mechanisms are unclear. From the side of the tissue the loss of signal can be caused by several biological processes, which are part of the response to implantation. The loss of sources could occur due to neuronal cell death or spatial shift. *Neuronal cell death* can occur early after implantation when some neurons close to the insertion track die due to the trauma. At a later stage, some neurons can die due to the continuing process of neuroinflammation. It has been shown that activated macrophages migrate to the device-tissue interface and suggested that the presence of such devices are a persistent source of inflammatory stimuli (i.e. classical "foreign body" reaction). Since macrophages can be a source of neurotoxic cytokines, they could potentially induce cell death in the surrounding neurons. The effect of the activated macrophages on the quality of electrophysiological recording is still largely unexplored. In addition to the persistence of inflammatory cells, studies have observed significant reductions in nerve fiber density and neuronal cell bodies in the tissue immediately surrounding implanted electrodes (Biran et al. (2005); Edell et al. (1992)). The *spatial shift* can also occur in different times after implantation. Early after implantation, the resorption of the local tissue edema can retract the tissue surrounding the active interface. This could result in liquid pocket, which can serve as a shunt for the neuronal signal.

At a later stage, the neuroinflammatory events lead to the formation of dense mesh of astrocytes and extracellular matrix proteins, which form together the glial scar. The formation of the glial scar (gliosis) is a complex reactive process involving the interaction between several types of cells, notably astrocytes and activated microglia. During this process the cells change substantially the composition, the morphology and the functional properties of the extracellular matrix. Detailed overviews of the process can be found in (Stichel & Müller (1998),Michael et al. (2008) and Polikov et al. (2005)). These observations motivated hypotheses that astrogliotic encapsulation contributes to the failure of such devices to maintain connectivity with adjacent neurons due to increase of the active interface impedance possibly by increase of the diffusion path (Syková (2005)). This scar may serve as a spatial barrier (low pass filter) for the neuronal signal. The hyperthrophy of the extracellular matrix could retract the remaining neurons out of the optimal recording distance (Polikov et al. (2005)).

7.2.3 Nervous tissue reaction to electrical stimulation

Electrical stimulation of nervous tissue could result in neuronal excitation, metabolic changes and/or cell damage. In general, low-intensity suprathreshold stimulation will result in excitation and transient changes of the cell metabolism and gene expression. On the other hand, prolonged and high-intensity electrical stimulation could result in cell damage and eventual death.

Suprathreshold electric stimulation of the peripheral or the cranial nerves results in increased expression of the so-called *immediate early genes* (IEG), such as *c-fos*, in the neuronal cell bodies anatomically connected with the stimulated region (Liang & Jones (1996)). For example, brief unilateral electrical stimulation of the cochlear nerve (120-250 μA, 5 Hz, 30 min) in anaesthetized rats with a biphasic current resulted in increased expression of c-Fos in the ipsilateral ventral and in the dorsal cochlear nuclei bilaterally (Nakamura et al. (2003)). Intracochlear electrical stimulation using a cochlear implant led to changes in the phosphorylation state of the cAMP response element binding protein (CREB) and the expression of *c-Fos* and *Egr-1* in the auditory brainstem nuclei in a tonotopical pattern (Illing et al. (2002)).

Electrical stimulation at high intensities results in damage of the nervous tissue. Analyzing previous results of Agnew & McCreery (1990); McCreery et al. (1990; 1992); Shannon (1992) presented an empirical model explaining the safety limits of electrical stimulation parameters. However, the model gives little physical and physiological insight into the mechanisms of damage. Butterwick et al. (2007) established that for electrodes having diameters larger than the distance to target cells the current density determined the damage threshold and small electrodes (diameters less than 200 μm), acted as point sources and the total current determined the damage threshold. The width of the safe therapeutic window (i.e., the ratio of damage threshold to stimulation threshold) depended on pulse duration. The damage threshold current density on large electrodes scaled with pulse duration as approximately $1/\sqrt{T_{pulse}}$. The threshold current density for repeated exposure on the retina varied between $61\ mA/cm^2$ at 6 ms to $1.3\ A/cm^2$ at 6 μs.

The neuronal injury originating from electrical stimulation can occur by several mechanisms:

Electrochemical injury, which can result from the production of substances on the electrodes, for example local changes in pH or diffusion of toxic ions into the electrolyte. Brummer

& Turner (1972) have shown that the rate of production of compounds by electrochemical reactions and the type of compounds produced are directly related to the charge density[4].

Cell injury resulting from electroporation A possible mechanism for electrical damage is electroporation or electropermeabilization. Recently, Butterwick et al. (2007) claimed that electroporation is the mechanism which underlines retinal damage during microelectrode stimulation. During electroporation, the applied pulses of electric field create transient hydrophilic pores in the cell membrane of different sizes (Krassowska & Filev (2007); Smith et al. (2004)) and different life times.

Excitotoxic neuronal injury, which is caused by the excitatory neurotransmitter glutamate through its NMDA receptors. This view is supported also by the finding that the NMDA receptor antagonist MK-801 (dizocilpine) is a neuroprotective factor during prolonged electrical stimulation (Agnew et al. (1993)). The mechanism of the induced neuronal cell death is necrotic.

III. Challenges and Issues in the Development of Micro-fabricated Devices

Issues in the development of neural prostheses are interrelated and frequently arise due to contradicting feature requirements. For example, the perfect DBS system should provide stimulation on-demand in order to maximize the lifetime of operation and minimize the amount of transferred charge and the amount of cell damage (Section 7.2.3). This implies the presence of recording functionality and software able to distinguish between normal and pathological neuronal circuit activity in the relevant signal bands (e.g., action potentials and/or local field potentials). Implementation of such software implies certain active signal processing that should occur in the implant, which would lead to the increase of the power consumption. Then the question would be whether such approach can actually increase the lifetime of the battery. Such ideal device should also deliver highly selective electrical stimulation in order to minimize the unwanted stimulation of other brain circuits. The electrode tissue interface should be stable for the whole lifetime of the device (possibly several decades).

Micro-fabricated devices that can be used in vitro for the recording and stimulation from single cells should on the one hand interfere minimally with the cells positioned on top of the electrodes, but on the other hand, a good coupling between the cell and the chip is desired. Although recent advances in micro-fabrication and computing technology have created many opportunities, the challenges that we face in the development of such devices remain critical. In the following, issues related to the development of both in vitro and in vivo systems are highlighted, and some future directions and perspectives are suggested.

Issues in the development of implantable systems can be conceptualized in the diagram shown in Figure 4. These can be conveniently classified as issues related to the active interface, the overall device, the biological system and issues stemming from deficiencies in the knowledge base. On the level of the **active interface,** there are several interrelated biophysical, chemical and biological processes that can result in changes of the electrical coupling of the active interface. Such changes of the active interface are manifested by changes of the electrical impedance and eventual loss of the neuronal signal. This is especially valid for the implantable prostheses, but also true in in vitro systems.

The bio-physico-chemical interactions on the active interface can include release of metal ions or molecules into the extracellular space (due to corrosion of the metal electrode surfaces or

---

[4] the charge transferred per unit area of the electrode surface

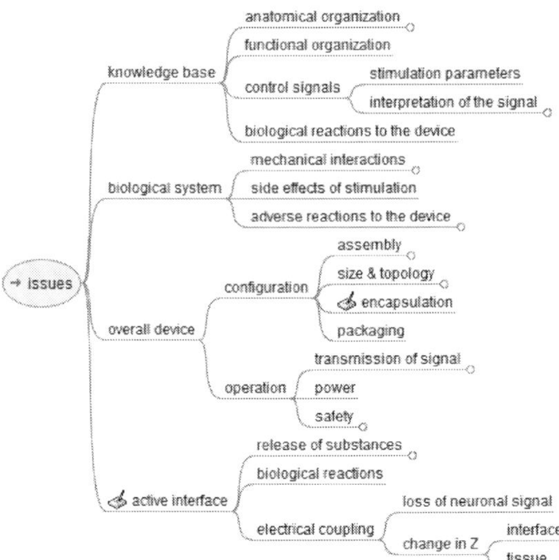

Fig. 4. Issues related to the development of micro-fabricated devices.

depolymerisation in case of polymeric electrodes) and biochemical reactions with the surrounding cells and extracellular matrix. While the biophysical and chemical aspects of those processes have been established, the biochemical and pathophysiogcial aspects are still under investigation. Notably, our understanding of the evolution of the encapsulation process (gliosis) and its influence on the recording capabilities and the eventual loss of signal, are incomplete.

On the level of the biological system (e.g. the **human body**), it is important to note the aspects of mechanical interactions, the side effects of stimulation and the overall biocompatibility. The *mechanical interactions* between the device and the body and notably the micro-motions are caused by the respiration and heartbeats and the strain of the leads that can be caused by directed movements (e.g., by the head, neck, etc.). Other potential issues can be related to the general biocompatibility of the device. This evolved into a set of regulatory requirements (section 7). Some issues can be grouped around the undesired effects of the electrical stimulation, e.g. excitation or inhibition of other neuronal circuits, which can lead to undesired physiological and/or behavioral effects.

As discussed in section 7, direct cytotoxicity is an important factor in the development of in vitro devices. Leakage of metal ions from materials used in devices and their diffusion in the cell medium leads to toxicity problems. Materials used in innovative and advanced technologies, therefore, need to be investigated on the cellular level before implementation. Different from implantable devices, in vitro devices require sophisticated surface chemistries that have to be characterized for specific materials and applications. Hence, cell adhesion and growth is a key factor in these devices.

On the level of the **knowledge base** there are deficiencies in the understanding of the functional organization of the brain, the detailed mapping of the anatomical connectivity and the control signals. The control signals which are delivered through the active interface in many types of neural prostheses are unclear. Notable exceptions for this are the auditory cochlear prostheses, which exploit the sonotopic organization of the cochlea, the cardiac pacemakers, the phrenic stimulator and the foot drop stimulator. Current DBS systems for Parkinson's disease rely on the high frequency stimulation, which can result in blocking of certain mid-brain pathways. The encoding of the kinematic information in these structures is still unknown. Dissociated cell cultures lose their anatomical connectivity and structure when seeded on substrates in vitro. The 'new' situation that exists on these surfaces is interesting in terms of communication between individual cells and their function in advanced networks. However, the translation of these processes to the in vivo situation is not always straightforward and challenging.

On the level of the **overall device** several types of issues can be grouped in the categories of configuration and operation. Issues related to the *configuration* can be related to the assembly, the size and topology of the device, the encapsulation and the packaging of the device. Devices have to be packaged in a way that prevents leakage of the environment, which contains high salt and protein concentrations, to the chip. These packages have to be leakage-proof on the one hand and non-toxic for the cell culture or tissue on the other hand.

Issues related to the *operation* of the device can be grouped under the power, safety and communication of the device. The operation has to be compatible with cell cultures or in vivo environments, which in this case has to be in agreement with certain regulations. One other important aspect of the safety of operation are the interactions with other equipment, for example MRI.

8. References

Agnew, W. F. & McCreery, D. B. (eds) (1990). *Neural Prostheses: Fundamental Studies*, Prentice Hall Advanced Reference Series, Prentice Hall, Englewood Cliffs.

Agnew, W. F., McCreery, D. B., Yuen, T. G. & Bullara, L. A. (1993). MK-801 protects against neuronal injury induced by electrical stimulation, *Neuroscience* 52: 45–53.

Bai, Q. & Wise, K. D. (2001). Single-unit neural recording with active microelectrode arrays., *IEEE Trans Biomed Eng* 48(8): 911–920.

Baind, P., Aziz, T., Liu, X. & Nandi, D. (eds) (2009). *Deep Brain Stimulation*, Oxford University Press, Oxford, UK.

Barbosa, R. M., Lourenco, C. F., Santos, R. M., Pomerleau, F., Huettl, P., Gerhardt, G. A. & Laranjinha, J. (2008). In vivo real-time measurement of nitric oxide in anesthetized rat brain., *Methods Enzymol* 441: 351–367.

Baruchi, I. & Ben-Jacob, E. (2007). Towards neuro-memory-chip: imprinting multiple memories in cultured neural networks., *Phys Rev E Stat Nonlin Soft Matter Phys* 75(5 Pt 1): 050901.

BeMent, S. L., Wise, K. D., Anderson, D. J., Najafi, K. & Drake, K. L. (1986). Solid-state electrodes for multichannel multiplexed intracortical neuronal recording, *IEEE Trans. Biomed. Eng.* 33: 230–241.

Benabid, A. L., Pollak, P., Gervason, C., Hoffmann, D., Gao, D. M., Hommel, M., Perret, J. E. & de Rougemont, J. (1991). Long-term suppression of tremor by chronic stimulation of the ventral intermediate thalamic nucleus., *Lancet* 337(8738): 403–406.

Berger, T., Chapin, J., Gerhardt, G., McFarland, D., Principe, J., Soussou, W., Taylor, D. & Tresco, P. (2007). International assessment of research and development in brain-computer interfaces, *Technical report*, WTEC.

Biran, R., Martin, D. C. & Tresco, P. A. (2005). Neuronal cell loss accompanies the brain tissue response to chronically implanted silicon microelectrode arrays., *Exp Neurol* **195**(1): 115–126.

Blond, S. & Siegfried, J. (1991). Thalamic stimulation for the treatment of tremor and other movement disorders., *Acta Neurochir Suppl (Wien)* **52**: 109–111.

Bollen, L. S. & Svendsen, O. (1997). Regulatory guidelines for biocompatibility safety testing, *Medical Plastics and Biomaterials* pp. 1–16.

Braeken, D., Jans, D., Rand, D., Huys, R., Van Meerbergen, B., Loo, J., Borghs, G., Callewaert, G. & Bartic, C. (2008). Local electrical stimulation of cultured embryonic cardiomyocytes with sub-micrometer nail structures., *Conf Proc IEEE Eng Med Biol Soc* **2008**: 4816–4819.

Branner, A. & Normann, R. A. (2000). A multielectrode array for intrafascicular recording and stimulation in sciatic nerve of cats, *Brain Res. Bull.* **51**(4): 293–306.

Branner, A., Stein, R. B. & Normann, R. A. (2001). Selective stimulation of cat sciatic nerve using an array of varying-length microelectrodes., *J Neurophysiol* **85**(4): 1585–1594.

Braun, D. & Fromherz, P. (2004). Imaging neuronal seal resistance on silicon chip using fluorescent voltage-sensitive dye, *Biophys J* **87**(2): 1351–1359.

Breckenridge, L. J., Wilson, R. J., Connolly, P., Curtis, A. S., Dow, J. A., Blackshaw, S. E. & Wilkinson, C. D. (1995). Advantages of using microfabricated extracellular electrodes for in vitro neuronal recording, *J Neurosci Res* **42**(2): 266–276.

Brindley, G. S. & Lewin, W. S. (1968). The visual sensations produced by electrical stimulation of the medial occipitalcortex, *J. Physiol. (Lond)* **194**: 54–5P.

Brummer, S. B. & Turner, M. (1972). Electrochemical aspects of neuromuscular stimulation, *Technical report*, National Academy of Sciences, Washington, DC.

Buettner, G. R. & Oberley, L. W. (1979). The production of hydroxyl radical by tallysomycin and copper(ii)., *FEBS Lett* **101**(2): 333–335.

Burmeister, J. J. & Gerhardt, G. A. (2001). Self-referencing ceramic-based multisite microelectrodes for the detection and elimination of interferences from the measurement of l-glutamate and other analytes., *Anal Chem* **73**(5): 1037–1042.

Burmeister, J. J., Moxon, K. & Gerhardt, G. A. (2000). Ceramic-based multisite microelectrodes for electrochemical recordings., *Anal Chem* **72**(1): 187–192.

Butterwick, A., Vankov, A., Huie, P., Freyvert, Y. & Palanker, D. (2007). Tissue damage by pulsed electrical stimulation, *Biomedical Engineering, IEEE Transactions on* **54**(12): 2261–2267.

Cater, H. L., Gitterman, D., Davis, S. M., Benham, C. D., Morrison, B. & Sundstrom, L. E. (2007). Stretch-induced injury in organotypic hippocampal slice cultures reproduces in vivo post-traumatic neurodegeneration: role of glutamate receptors and voltage-dependent calcium channels., *J Neurochem* **101**(2): 434–447.

Cheung, K. (2007). Implantable microscale neural interfaces., *Biomed Microdevices* **9**(6): 923–938.

Chiappalone, M., Massobrio, P. & Martinoia, S. (2008). Network plasticity in cortical assemblies., *Eur J Neurosci* **28**(1): 221–237.

Chow, A. Y. & Chow, V. Y. (1997). Subretinal electrical stimulation of the rabbit retina, *Neurosci. Lett.* **225**: 13–16.

Connolly, P., Clark, P., Curtis, A. S. G., Dow, J. A. T. & W., W. C. D. (1990). An extracellular microelectrode array for monitoring electrogenic cells in culture, *Biosens Bioelectron* **5**(3): 223–234.

Critchley, D. R. (2000). Focal adhesions - the cytoskeletal connection, *Curr Opin Cell Biol* **12**(1): 133–139.

Csicsvari, J., Henze, D. A., Jamieson, B., Harris, K. D., Sirota, A., Barthó, P., Wise, K. D. & Buzsáki, G. (2003). Massively parallel recording of unit and local field potentials with silicon-based electrodes., *J Neurophysiol* **90**(2): 1314–1323.

Dimoka, A., Courellis, S. H., Gholmieh, G. I., Marmarelis, V. Z. & Berger, T. W. (2008). Modeling the nonlinear properties of the in vitro hippocampal perforant path-dentate system using multielectrode array technology., *IEEE Trans Biomed Eng* **55**(2 Pt 1): 693–702.

Dimoka, A., Courellis, S. H., Marmarelis, V. Z. & Berger, T. W. (2008). Modeling the nonlinear dynamic interactions of afferent pathways in the dentate gyrus of the hippocampus., *Ann Biomed Eng* **36**(5): 852–864.

Djourno, A. & Eyries, C. (1957). Prothese auditive par excitation electrique a distance du nerf sensoriela l'aide d'un bodinage inclus a demeure, *Presse Med.* **35**: 14–17.

Dobelle, W. H. (2000). Artificial vision for the blind by connecting a television camera to thevisual cortex, *ASAIO J.* **46**: 3–9.

Dobelle, W. H. & Mladejovsky, M. G. (1974). Phosphenes produced by electrical stimulation of human occipital cortex,and their application to the development of a prosthesis for the blind, *J. Physiol. (Lond)* **243**: 553–576.

Droge, M. H., Gross, G. W., Hightower, M. H. & Czisny, L. E. (1986). Multielectrode analysis of coordinated, multisite, rhythmic bursting in cultured cns monolayer networks, *Journal Of Neuroscience* **6**(6): 1583–1592.

Eckmiller, R. (1997). Learning retina implants with epiretinal contacts., *Ophthalmic Res* **29**(5): 281–289.

Edell, D. J., Toi, V. V., McNeil, V. M. & Clark, L. D. (1992). Factors influencing the biocompatibility of insertable silicon microshafts in cerebral cortex., *IEEE Trans Biomed Eng* **39**(6): 635–643.

Eggers, M. D., Astolfi, D. K., Liu, S., Zeuli, H. E., Doeleman, S. S., McKay, R., Khuon, T. S. & Ehrlich, D. J. (1990). Electronically wired petri dish - a microfabricated interface to the biological neuronal network, *Journal Of Vacuum Science And Technology B* **8**(6): 1392–1398.

Frederix, F., Bonroy, K., Reekmans, G., Laureyn, W., Campitelli, A., Abramov, M. A., Dehaen, W. & Maes, G. (2004). Reduced nonspecific adsorption on covalently immobilized protein surfaces using poly(ethylene oxide) containing blocking agents, *J Biochem Biophys Methods* **58**(1): 67–74.

Fromherz, P., Muller, C. O. & Weis, R. (1993). Neuron transistor: Electrical transfer function measured by the patch-clamp technique, *Phys Rev Lett* **71**(24): 4079–4082.

Fromherz, P., Offenhausser, A., Vetter, T. & Weis, J. (1991). A neuron-silicon junction: a retzius cell of the leech on an insulated-gate field-effect transistor, *Science* **252**(5010): 1290–1293.

Fromherz, P. & Stett, A. (1995). Silicon-neuron junction: Capacitive stimulation of an individual neuron on a silicon chip, *Phys Rev Lett* **75**(8): 1670–1673.

Geddes, L. A. & Roeder, R. (2003). Criteria for the selection of materials for implanted electrodes., *Ann Biomed Eng* **31**(7): 879–890.

George, M. S., Sackeim, H. A., Rush, A. J., Marangell, L. B., Nahas, Z., Husain, M. M., Lisanby, S., Burt, T., Goldman, J. & Ballenger, J. C. (2000). Vagus nerve stimulation: a new tool for brain research and therapy., *Biol Psychiatry* **47**(4): 287–295.

Gepstein, L. (2008). Experimental molecular and stem cell therapies in cardiac electrophysiology., *Ann N Y Acad Sci* **1123**: 224–231.

Gersuni, G. & Volokhov, A. (1937). On the effect of alternating currents on the cochlea, *J. Physiol. (Lond).* **89**: 113–121.

Gleixner, R. & Fromherz, P. (2006). The extracellular electrical resistivity in cell adhesion, *Biophys J* **90**(7): 2600–2611.

Glenn, W. W., Hageman, J. H., Mauro, A., Eisenberg, L. & Harvard, S. F. B. M. (1964). Electrical stimulation of excitable tissue by radiofrequency transmission, *Ann. Surg.* **160**: 338–350.

Gross, G. W. (1979). Simultaneous single unit recording invitro with a photoetched laser deinsulated gold multi-micro-electrode surface, *IEEE Transactions On Biomedical Engineering* **26**(5): 273–279.

Gross, G. W., Rieske, E., Kreutzberg, G. W. & Meyer, A. (1977). New fixed-array multi-microelectrode system designed for long-term monitoring of extracellular single unit neuronal-activity invitro, *Neurosci Lett* **6**(2-3): 101–105.

Groves, D. A. & Brown, V. J. (2005). Vagal nerve stimulation: a review of its applications and potential mechanisms that mediate its clinical effects., *Neurosci Biobehav Rev* **29**(3): 493–500.

Hategan, A., Sengupta, K., Kahn, S., Sackmann, E. & Discher, D. E. (2004). Topographical pattern dynamics in passive adhesion of cell membranes, *Biophys J* **87**(5): 3547–3560.

Haustein, M. D., Reinert, T., Warnatsch, A., Englitz, B., Dietz, B., Robitzki, A., Rubsamen, R. & Milenkovic, I. (2008). Synaptic transmission and short-term plasticity at the calyx of held synapse revealed by multielectrode array recordings., *J Neurosci Methods* **174**(2): 227–236.

Heiduschka, P. & Thanos, S. (1998). Implantable bioelectric interfaces for lost nerve functions, *Prog. Neurobiol.* **55**: 433–461.

Hochberg, L. R., Serruya, M. D., Friehs, G. M., Mukand, J. A., Saleh, M., Caplan, A. H., Branner, A., Chen, D., Penn, R. D. & Donoghue, J. P. (2006). Neuronal ensemble control of prosthetic devices by a human with tetraplegia., *Nature* **442**(7099): 164–171.

Hodgkin, A. L. (1939). The relation between conduction velocity and the electrical resistance outside a nerve fibre, *J Physiol* **94**(4): 560–570.

Houghton, E. A. & Nicholas, K. M. (2009). In vitro reactive oxygen species production by histatins and copper(i,ii)., *J Biol Inorg Chem* **14**(2): 243–251.

Huang, J., Grater, S. V., Corbellini, F., Rinck, S., Bock, E., Kemkemer, R., Kessler, H., Ding, J. & Spatz, J. P. (2009). Impact of order and disorder in rgd nanopatterns on cell adhesion., *Nano Lett* **9**(3): 1111–1116.

Huys, R., Braeken, D., Van Meerbergen, B., Winters, K., Eberle, W., Loo, J., Tsvetanova, D., Chen, C., Severi, S., Yitzhaik, S., Spira, M., Shappir, J., Callewaert, G., Borghs, G. & Bartic, C. (2008). Novel concepts for improved communication between nerve cells and silicon electronic devices, *Solid-State Electronics* **52**(4): 533–539.

Illing, R. B., Michler, S. A., Kraus, K. S. & Laszig, R. (2002). Transcription factor modulation and expression in the rat auditory brainstemfollowing electrical intracochlear stimulation, *Exp. Neurol.* **175**: 226–244.

Ingebrandt, S., Yeung, C. K., Krause, M. & Offenhausser, A. (2001). Cardiomyocyte-transistor-hybrids for sensor application, *Biosens Bioelectron* **16**(7-8): 565–570.

Israel, D., Barry, W. H., Edell, D. J. & Mark, R. G. (1984). An array of microelectrodes to stimulate and record from cardiac-cells in culture, *American Journal Of Physiology* **247**(4): H669–H674.

Jimbo, Y. & Kawana, A. (1992). Electrical-stimulation and recording from cultured neurons using a planar electrode array, *Bioelectrochemistry And Bioenergetics* **29**(2): 193–204.

Jimbo, Y., Robinson, H. P. C. & Kawana, A. (1993). Simultaneous measurement of intracellular calcium and electrical-activity from patterned neural networks in culture, *IEEE Transactions On Biomedical Engineering* **40**(8): 804–810.

Johnson, M. D., Miocinovic, S., McIntyre, C. C. & Vitek, J. L. (2008). Mechanisms and targets of deep brain stimulation in movement disorders., *Neurotherapeutics* **5**(2): 294–308.

Kawanishi, S., Hiraku, Y., Murata, M. & Oikawa, S. (2002). The role of metals in site-specific dna damage with reference to carcinogenesis., *Free Radic Biol Med* **32**(9): 822–832.

Kind, T., Issing, M., Arnold, R. & Muller, B. (2002). Electrical coupling of single cardiac rat myocytes to field-effect and bipolar transistors, *IEEE Trans Biomed Eng* **49**(12 Pt 2): 1600–1609.

Krassowska, W. & Filev, P. D. (2007). Modeling electroporation in a single cell., *Biophys J* **92**(2): 404–417.

Kupper, J., Prinz, A. A. & Fromherz, P. (2002). Recombinant kv1.3 potassium channels stabilize tonic firing of cultured rat hippocampal neurons, *Pflugers Arch* **443**(4): 541–547.

Lee, K., He, J. & Wang, L. (2004). Benzocyclobutene (bcb) based neural implants with microfluidic channel., *Conf Proc IEEE Eng Med Biol Soc* **6**: 4326–4329.

Lee, K.and He, J., Clement, R., Massia, S. & Kim, B. (2004). Biocompatible benzocyclobutene (bcb)-based neural implants with micro-fluidic channel., *Biosens Bioelectron* **20**(2): 404–407.

Liang, F. & Jones, E. G. (1996). Peripheral nerve stimulation increases Fos immunoreactivity without affectingType II Ca^{2+}/Calmodulin-dependent protein kinase, Glutamicacid Decarboxylase, or $GABA_A$ receptor gene expression in cat spinalcord, *Exp. Brain Res.* **111**: 326–336.

Liberson, W. T., Holmquest, H. J., Scot, D. & Dow, M. (1961). Functional electrotherapy: Stimulation of the peroneal nerve synchronizedwith the swing phase of the gait of hemiplegic patients, *Arch. Phys. Med. Rehabil.* **42**: 101–105.

Lind, R., Connolly, P., Wilkinson, C. D. W. & Thomson, R. D. (1991). Finite-element analysis applied to extracellular microelectrode design, *Sensors And Actuators B-Chemical* **3**(1): 23–30.

Lorenzelli, L., Margesin, B., Martinoia, S., Tedesco, M. T. & Valle, M. (2003). Bioelectrochemical signal monitoring of in-vitro cultured cells by means of an automated microsystem based on solid state sensor-array, *Biosens Bioelectron* **18**(5-6): 621–626.

Love, J. C., Estroff, L. A., Kriebel, J. K., Nuzzo, R. G. & Whitesides, G. M. (2005). Self-assembled monolayers of thiolates on metals as a form of nanotechnology., *Chem Rev* **105**(4): 1103–1169.

Martinoia, S., Bove, M., Carlini, G., Ciccarelli, C., Grattarola, M., Storment, C. & Kovacs, G. (1993). A general-purpose system for long-term recording from a microelectrode array coupled to excitable cells, *Journal Of Neuroscience Methods* **48**(1-2): 115–121.

Martinoia, S. & Massobrio, P. (2004). Isfet-neuron junction: circuit models and extracellular signal simulations, *Biosens Bioelectron* **19**(11): 1487–1496.

Martinoia, S., Rosso, N., Grattarola, M., Lorenzelli, L., Margesin, B. & Zen, M. (2001). Development of isfet array-based microsystems for bioelectrochemical measurements of cell populations, *Biosens Bioelectron* **16**(9-12): 1043–1050.

Mauritz, C., Schwanke, K., Reppel, M., Neef, S., Katsirntaki, K., Maier, L. S., Nguemo, F., Menke, S., Haustein, M., Hescheler, J., Hasenfuss, G. & Martin, U. (2008). Generation of functional murine cardiac myocytes from induced pluripotent stem cells., *Circulation* **118**(5): 507–517.

Maynard, E. M., Nordhausen, C. T. & Normann, R. A. (1997). The utah intracortical electrode array: a recording structure for potential brain-computer interfaces., *Electroencephalogr Clin Neurophysiol* **102**(3): 228–239.

McCreery, D. B., Agnew, W. F., Yuen, T. G. & Bullara, L. (1990). Charge density and charge per phase as cofactors in neural injury induced by electrical stimulation., *IEEE Trans Biomed Eng* **37**(10): 996–1001.

McCreery, D. B., Yuen, T. G., Agnew, W. F. & Bullara, L. A. (1992). Stimulation with chronically implanted microelectrodes in the cochlear nucleus of the cat: histologic and physiologic effects., *Hear Res* **62**(1): 42–56.

McIntyre, C. C., Savasta, M., Walter, B. L. & Vitek, J. L. (2004). How does deep brain stimulation work? present understanding and future questions., *J Clin Neurophysiol* **21**(1): 40–50.

Metz, S., Holzer, R. & Renaud, P. (2001). Polyimide-based microfluidic devices., *Lab Chip* **1**(1): 29–34.

Meyburg, S., Goryll, M., Moers, J., Ingebrandt, S., Bocker-Meffert, S., Luth, H. & Offenhausser, A. (2006). N-channel field-effect transistors with floating gates for extracellular recordings, *Biosens Bioelectron* **21**(7): 1037–1044.

Michael, T. F., S., J. & T.J. (2008). Cns injury, glial scars, and inflammation: Inhibitory extracellular matrices and regeneration failure., *Exp Neurol* **209**(2): 294–301.

Montgomery, E. B. & Gale, J. T. (2008). Mechanisms of action of deep brain stimulation (dbs)., *Neurosci Biobehav Rev* **32**(3): 388–407.

Musa, S., Welkenhuysen, M., Huys, R., Eberle, W., van Kuyck, K., Bartic, C., Nuttin & Borghs, G. (2008). Planar 2d-array neural probe for deep brain stimulation and recording, *Proc. of the 4th European Conference of IFMBE*, Vol. 22, Antwerp, Belgium, pp. 2421 – 2425.

Myllymaa, S., Myllymaa, K., Korhonen, H., Töyräs, J., Jääskeläinen, J. E., Djupsund, K., Tanila, H. & Lappalainen, R. (2009). Fabrication and testing of polyimide-based microelectrode arrays for cortical mapping of evoked potentials., *Biosens Bioelectron* **24**(10): 3067–3072.

Nakamura, M., Rosahl, S. K., Alkahlout, E., Gharabaghi, A., Walter, G. F. & Samii, M. (2003). C-fos immunoreactivity mapping of the auditory system after electrical stimulationof the cochlear nerve in rats, *Hearing Res.* **184**: 75–81.

Navarro, X., Valderrama, E., Stieglitz, T. & Schüttler, M. (2001). Selective fascicular stimulation of the rat sciatic nerve with multipolar polyimide cuff electrodes., *Restor Neurol Neurosci* **18**(1): 9–21.

Nordhausen, C. T., Maynard, E. M. & Normann, R. A. (1996). Single unit recording capabilities of a 100 microelectrode array., *Brain Res* **726**(1-2): 129–140.

Norlin, P., Kindlundh, M., Mouroux, A., Yoshida, K. & Hofmann, U. (2002). A 32-site neural recording probe fabricated by drie of soi substrates, *J. Micromech. Microeng.* **12**: 414—419.

Normann, R. A., Warren, D. J., Ammermuller, J., Fernandez, E. & Guillory, S. (2001). High-resolution spatio-temporal mapping of visual pathways using multi-electrode arrays., *Vision Res* **41**(10-11): 1261–1275.

Normann, R., Maynard, E., Guillory, K. & Warren, D. (1996). Cortical implants for the blind, *IEEE Spectrum* **33**(5): 54–59.

Novak, J. L. & Wheeler, B. C. (1986). Recording from the aplysia abdominal-ganglion with a planar microelectrode array, *IEEE Transactions On Biomedical Engineering* **33**(2): 196–202.

Ocorr, K., Reeves, N. L., Wessells, R. J., Fink, M., Chen, H.-S. V., Akasaka, T., Yasuda, S., Metzger, J. M., Giles, W., Posakony, J. W. & Bodmer, R. (2007). Kcnq potassium channel mutations cause cardiac arrhythmias in drosophila that mimic the effects of aging., *Proc Natl Acad Sci U S A* **104**(10): 3943–3948.

Olschlager, V., Schrader, A. & Hockertz, S. (2009). Comparison of primary human fibroblasts and keratinocytes with immortalized cell lines regarding their sensitivity to sodium dodecyl sulfate in a neutral red uptake cytotoxicity assay., *Arzneimittelforschung* **59**(3): 146–152.

Pasquale, V., Massobrio, P., Bologna, L. L., Chiappalone, M. & Martinoia, S. (2008). Self-organization and neuronal avalanches in networks of dissociated cortical neurons., *Neuroscience* **153**(4): 1354–1369.

Pine, J. (1980). Recording action-potentials from cultured neurons with extracellular micro-circuit electrodes, *Journal Of Neuroscience Methods* **2**(1): 19–31.

Polikov, V. S., Tresco, P. A. & Reichert, W. M. (2005). Response of brain tissue to chronically implanted neural electrodes., *J Neurosci Methods* **148**(1): 1–18.

Pomerleau, F., Day, B. K., Huettl, P., Burmeister, J. J. & Gerhardt, G. A. (2003). Real time in vivo measures of l-glutamate in the rat central nervous system using ceramic-based multisite microelectrode arrays., *Ann N Y Acad Sci* **1003**: 454–457.

Powell, S. R., Gurzenda, E. M., Wingertzahn, M. A. & Wapnir, R. A. (1999). Promotion of copper excretion from the isolated rat heart attenuates postischemic cardiac oxidative injury., *Am J Physiol* **277**(3 Pt 2): H956–62.

Prodanov, D. (2006). *Morphometric analysis of the rat lower limb nerves. Anatomical data for neural prosthesis design*, PhD thesis, Twente University, Enschede, The Netherlands.

Prodanov, D. & Feirabend, H. K. P. (2007). Morphometric analysis of the fiber populations of the rat sciatic nerve, its spinal roots, and its major branches., *J Comp Neurol* **503**(1): 85–100.

Prodanov, D. & Feirabend, H. K. P. (2008). Automated characterization of nerve fibers labeled fluorescently: Determination of size, class and spatial distribution., *Brain Res* **1233**: 35–50.

Prodanov, D., Marani, E. & Holsheimer, J. (2003). Functional Electric Stimulation for sensory and motor functions: Progressand problems, *Biomed. Rev.* **14**: 23–50.

Prodanov, D., Nagelkerke, N. & Marani, E. (2007). Spatial clustering analysis in neuroanatomy: applications of different approaches to motor nerve fiber distribution., *J Neurosci Methods* **160**(1): 93–108.

Ratner, B. D., Hoffman, A., Lemons, J. E. & Schoen, F. J. (1996). *Biomaterials Science - An Introduction to Materials in Medicine*, Academic Press, New York.

Reisner, Y., Meiry, G., Zeevi-Levin, N., Barac, D. Y., Reiter, I., Abassi, Z., Ziv, N., Kostin, S., Shaper, J., Rosen, M. R. & Binah, O. (2008). Impulse conduction and gap junctional remodeling by endothelin-1 in cultured neonatal rat ventricular myocytes., *J Cell Mol Med* .

Rizzo, J., Wyatt, J., Loewenstein, J., Kelly, S. & Shire, D. (2003). Methods and perceptual thresholds for short-term electrical stimulationof human retina with microelectrode arrays, *Invest Ophthalmol. Vis. Sci.* **44**: 5355–5361.

Rodríguez, F. J., Ceballos, D., Schüttler, M., Valero, A., Valderrama, E., Stieglitz, T. & Navarro, X. (2000). Polyimide cuff electrodes for peripheral nerve stimulation., *J Neurosci Methods* **98**(2): 105–118.

Rosolen, S. G., Kolomiets, B., Varela, O. & Picaud, S. (2008). Retinal electrophysiology for toxicology studies: applications and limits of erg in animals and ex vivo recordings., *Exp Toxicol Pathol* **60**(1): 17--32.

Rosolen, S. G., Rigaudiere, F. & Lachapelle, P. (2002). A practical method to obtain reproducible binocular electroretinograms in dogs., *Doc Ophthalmol* **105**(2): 93–103.

Rousche, P. J. & Normann, R. A. (1998). Chronic recording capability of the utah intracortical electrode array in cat sensory cortex., *J Neurosci Methods* **82**(1): 1–15.

Rousche, P. J., Pellinen, D. S., Pivin, D. P. J., Williams, J. C., Vetter, R. J. & Kipke, D. R. (2001). Flexible polyimide-based intracortical electrode arrays with bioactive capability., *IEEE Trans Biomed Eng* **48**(3): 361–371.

Rubehn, B., Bosman, C., Oostenveld, R., Fries, P. & Stieglitz, T. (2009). A mems-based flexible multichannel ecog-electrode array., *J Neural Eng* **6**(3): 036003.

Ruther, P., Aarts, A., Frey, O., Herwik, S., Kisban, S., Seidl, K., Spieth, S., Schumacher, A., Koudelka-Hep, M., Paul, O., Stieglitz, T., Zengerle, R. & Neves, H. (2008). The NeuroProbes project – multifunctional probe arrays for neural recording and stimulation, *Proc. of the 13th Annual Conf. of the IFESS*, Vol. 53 of *Biomed. Tech.*, Freiburg, Germany, pp. 238 – 240.

Rutten, W. L., Frieswijk, T. A., Smit, J. P., Rozijn, T. H. & Meier, J. (1995). 3D neuro-electronic interface devices for neuromuscular control: Designstudies and realisation steps, *Biosens. Bioelectron.* **10**: 141–153.

Salthouse, T. N. (1976). Cellular enzyme activity at the polymer-tissue interface: a review, *J Biomed. Mater. Res.* **10**: 197–229.

Sarnoff, S. J., Gaensler, E. A. & Maloney, J. V. (1950). Electrophrenic respiration: the effectiveness of contralateral ventialtionduring activity of one phrenic nerve, *J. Thoracic. Surg.* **19**: 929.

Schmidt, E. M., Bak, M. J., Hambrecht, F. T., Kufta, C. V., K.O'Rourke, D. & Vallabhanath, P. (1996). Feasibility of a visual prosthesis for the blind based on intracorticalmicrostimulation of the visual cortex, *Brain* **119 (Pt 2)**: 507–522.

Schoen, I. & Fromherz, P. (2007). The mechanism of extracellular stimulation of nerve cells on an electrolyte-oxide-semiconductor capacitor, *Biophysical Journal* **92**(3): 1096–1111.

Shannon, R. V. (1992). A model of safe levels for electrical stimulation., *IEEE Trans Biomed Eng* **39**(4): 424–426.

Smith, K. C., Neu, J. C. & Krassowska, W. (2004). Model of creation and evolution of stable electropores for dna delivery., *Biophys J* **86**(5): 2813–2826.

Stichel, C. C. & Müller, H. W. (1998). The cns lesion scar: new vistas on an old regeneration barrier., *Cell Tissue Res* **294**(1): 1–9.

Stieglitz, T. & Meyer, J. U. (1999). Implantable microsystems. polyimide-based neuroprostheses for interfacing nerves., *Med Device Technol* **10**(6): 28–30.

Stieglitz, T., Schuettler, M. & Koch, K. P. (2005). Implantable biomedical microsystems for neural prostheses., *IEEE Eng Med Biol Mag* **24**(5): 58–65.

Syková, E. (2005). Glia and volume transmission during physiological and pathological states., *J Neural Transm* **112**(1): 137–147.

Thomas, C. A., Springer, P. A., Okun, L. M., Berwaldn.Y & Loeb, G. E. (1972). Miniature microelectrode array to monitor bioelectric activity of cultured cells, *Experimental Cell Research* **74**(1): 61.

Tsai, W. B., Chen, R. P., Wei, K. L., Chen, Y. R., Liao, T. Y., Liu, H. L. & Lai, J. Y. (2009). Polyelectrolyte multilayer films functionalized with peptides for promoting osteoblast functions., *Acta Biomater* .

Van Meerbergen, B., Jans, K., Loo, J., Reekmans, G., Braeken, D., Chong, S., Bonroy, K., Maes, G., Borghs, G., Engelborghs, Y., Annaert, W. & Bartic, C. (2008). Peptide-functionalized microfabricated structures for improved on-chip neuronal adhesion., *Conf Proc IEEE Eng Med Biol Soc* **2008**: 1833–1836.

Veraart, C., Raftopoulos, C., Mortimer, J. T., Delbeke, J., Michaux, D. P. G., Vanlierde, A., Parrini, S. & Wanet-Defalque, M. C. (1998). Visual sensations produced by optic nerve stimulation using an implantedself-sizing spiral cuff electrode, *Brain Res.* **813**: 181–186.

Wagenaar, D. A., Pine, J. & Potter, S. M. (2006). An extremely rich repertoire of bursting patterns during the development of cortical cultures., *BMC Neurosci* **7**: 11.

Williams, D. F. (1987). *Definitions in Biomaterials*, Elsevier, Amsterdam, chapter 4, p. 54.

Williams, D. F. (2008a). On the mechanisms of biocompatibility., *Biomaterials* **29**(20): 2941–2953.

Williams, D. F. (2008b). The relationship between biomaterials and nanotechnology., *Biomaterials* **29**(12): 1737–1738.

Wilms, M. & Eckhorn, R. (2005). Spatiotemporal receptive field properties of epiretinally recorded spikes and local electroretinograms in cats., *BMC Neurosci* **6**: 50.

Wise, K. D. & Angell, J. B. (1975). A low-capacitance multielectrode probe for use in extracellular neurophysiology., *IEEE Trans Biomed Eng* **22**(3): 212–219.

Wise, K. D., Angell, J. B. & Starr, A. (1970). An integrated-circuit approach to extracellular microelectrodes., *IEEE Trans Biomed Eng* **17**(3): 238–247.

Zrenner, E. (2002). Will retinal implants restore vision?, *Science* **295**(5557): 1022–1025.

Zrenner, E., Miliczek, K. D., Gabel, V. P., Graf, H. G., Haemmerle, E. G. H., Hoefflinger, B., Kohler, K., Nisch, W., Stett, M. S. A. & Weiss, S. (1997). The development of subretinal microphotodiodes for replacement of degeneratedphotoreceptors, *Ophthalmic Res.* **29**: 269–280.

18

Skin Roughness Assessment

Lioudmila Tchvialeva[a], Haishan Zeng[a,b], Igor Markhvida[a],
David I McLean[a], Harvey Lui[a,b] and Tim K Lee[a,b]
[a]*Laboratory for Advanced Medical Photonics and Photomedicine Institute,*
Department of Dermatology and Skin Science,
University of British Columbia and Vancouver Coastal Health Research Institute,
Vancouver, Canada
[b]*Cancer Control and Cancer Imaging Departments,*
British Columbia Cancer Research Centre,
Vancouver, Canada

1. Introduction

The medical evaluation and diagnosis of skin disease primarily relies on visual inspection for specific lesional morphologic features such as color, shape, border, configuration, distribution, elevation, and texture. Although physicians and other health care professionals can apply classification rules to visual diagnosis (Rapini, 2003) the overall clinical approach is subjective and qualitative, with a critical dependence on training and experience. Over the past 20 years a number of non-invasive techniques for measuring the skin's physical properties have been developed and tested to extend the accuracy of visual assessment alone. Skin relief, also referred to as surface texture or topography, is an important biophysical feature that can sometimes be difficult to appreciate with the naked eye alone. Since the availability of quantification tools for objective skin relief evaluation, it has been learned that skin roughness is influenced by numerous factors, such as lesion malignancy (Connemann et al., 1995; Handels et al., 1999; del Carmen Lopez Pacheco et al., 2005; Mazzarello et al., 2006), aging (Humbert et al., 2003; Lagarde et al., 2005; Li et al., 2006a; Fujimura et al., 2007), diurnal rhythm and relative humidity (Egawa et al., 2002), oral supplement (Segger & Schonlau, 2004), cosmetics and personal care products (Korting et al., 1991; Levy et al., 2004; Kampf & Ennen, 2006; Kim et al., 2007; Kawada et al., 2008), laser remodeling (Friedman et al., 2002a), and radiation treatment (Bourgeois et al., 2003).

Two early surveys (Fischer et al., 1999; Leveque, 1999) reviewing assessment methods for topography were published a decade ago. In this chapter, we update current research techniques along with commercially-available devices, and focus on the state-of-the-art methods. The first part of the chapter analyzes indirect replica-based and direct *in-vivo* techniques. Healthy skin roughness values obtained by different methods are compared, and the limitations of each technique are discussed. In the second part, we introduce a novel approach for skin roughness measurement using laser speckle. This section consists of a survey on applying speckle for opaque surfaces, consideration of the theoretical relationship between polychromatic speckle contrast and roughness, and a critical procedure for eliminating volume-scattering from semi-transparent tissues. Finally we compare roughness values for different body sites obtained by our technique to other *in-vivo* methods. Limitations of each technique and their practical applicability are discussed throughout the chapter.

2. Skin surface evaluation techniques

According to the International Organization for Standardization (ISO), methods for surface texture measurement are classified into three types: line profiling, areal topography, and area-integrating (International Organization for Standardization Committee, 2007). Line-profiling uses a small probe to detect the peaks and valleys and produces a quantitative height profile $Z(x)$. Areal topography methods create 2 dimensional $Z(x,y)$ topographic images. To compare surfaces, we have to analyse and calculate statistical parameters from the 2D maps. On the other hand, area-integrated methods capture an area-based signal and relate it directly to one or more statistical parameters without detailed point-by-point analysis of the surface.

ISO defines a set of parameters characterizing the roughness, which is the variation of the Z coordinate (height) from the mathematical point of view. We will discuss three of them: arithmetical mean deviation R_a, root mean square (rms) deviation R_q, and maximum height of profile R_z. Line profiling and areal topography methods commonly use R_a, which is the average of the absolute values $|Z - <Z>|$ within the sampling region and $<Z>$ is the average surface height. Theoretical formulations of the area-integrating methods mostly utilize $R_q = (<(Z - <Z>)^2>)^{1/2}$,which is a statistical measure of the Z variation within the sampling region. The parameters R_a and R_q are highly correlated, for example $R_a \approx 1.25\ R_q$ when Z has a Gaussian distribution. Some applications employ the maximum height of the profile (R_z), which is defined as the distance between the highest peak and the lowest valley within a sampling region.

From the technical point of view, skin roughness can be measured directly (*in-vivo*) or indirectly from a replica. Replica-based methods were the first to be developed and implemented, and are still commonly used today despite the recent advancements in *in-vivo* techniques and devices. Therefore, we discuss both approaches in the following section.

2.1 Replica-based methods

Replica-based methods require two-steps. Skin surface has to be imprinted and a skin replica is produced. Roughness measurement is then performed on the replica. The most commonly used material for the replica is silicone rubber (Silfo®, Flexico Developments Ltd., UK). Silicon dental rubber (Silasoft®, Detax GmbH & Co., Gemany) (Korting, et al., 1991), polyvinylsiloxane derivative (Coltene®, Coltène/Whaledent Ltd., UK) (Mazzarello, et al., 2006), and silicon mass (Silaplus®, DMG, Gamany) (Hof & Hopermann, 2000) have also been used. The comparison between Flexico and DMG silicones revealed a good agreement (Hof & Hopermann, 2000).

The range of skin topography dictates the choice of technical approaches for the assessment. According to the classification given in (Hashimoto, 1974), the surface pattern of the human skin can be divided into primary structure, which consists of primary macroscopic, wide, deep lines or furrows in the range of 20 µm to 100 µm, secondary structure formed by finer, shorter and shallower (5 µm - 40 µm) secondary lines or furrows running over several cells, tertiary structure lines (0.5 µm) that are the borders of the individual horny cells, and quaternary lines (0.05 µm) on individual horny cells surfaces. The range of the skin roughness value, as expected, is mainly determined by the primary and secondary structures which are in the order of tens of microns. These structures can be examined by mechanical profilometry with a stylus. The tertiary and quaternary structures do not visibly contribute to the roughness parameters, but causes light to be reflected diffusively. In order to evaluate these fine structures, optical techniques should be employed (Hocken et al., 2005).

2.1.1 Line Profile – contact method

Mechanical profilometry is a typical line-profiling approach. The stylus tip follows the surface height directly with a small contacting force. The vertical motion on the stylus is converted to an electrical signal, which is further transformed into the surface profile $Z(x)$. The smallest vertical resolution is 0.05 µm (Hof & Hopermann, 2000). The best lateral resolution is 0.02 µm, which is limited by the size of the stylus tip. The finite tip size causes smoothing in valleys (Connemann et al., 1996) but peaks can be followed accurately. The stylus may damage or deform the soft silicone rubber. Nevertheless, due to its high accuracy and reliability, mechanical profilometry is still in use since an early study reported in the 1990s (Korting, et al., 1991).

2.1.2 Areal Topography - optical techniques

Microphotography is the easiest way to image skin texture and works well with the anisotropy of skin furrows (Egawa, et al., 2002) or the degree of skin pattern irregularity (Setaro & Sparavigna, 2001). In a study (Mazzarello, et al., 2006), surface roughness is presented as a non-ISO parameter by the standard deviation of the grey level of each pixel in a scanning electron microscopy image. In optical shadow casting (Gautier et al., 2008), a skin replica is illuminated by a parallel light beam with at a non-zero incident angle and the cast shadow length is directly related to the height of the furrows. Surface mapping can be done by simple trigonometric calculations (del Carmen Lopez Pacheco, et al., 2005). However, this method cannot detect relief elements located inside the shadowed areas. Its resolution depends on the incident angle and is lower than other optical methods. Some microphotography studies reported extreme values. For example the value R_a averaged over different body sites has been reported as high as 185.4 µm (del Carmen Lopez Pacheco, et al., 2005), which was by an order of magnitude greater than the commonly accepted values (Lagarde, et al., 2005). Another study on forearm skin (Gautier, et al., 2008) reported a very low R_z value, 8.7 µm, which was by an order of magnitude lower than the common range (Egawa, et al., 2002). Currently, microphotography is primarily used for wrinkle evaluation.

Optical profilometry is based on the autofocus principle. An illumination-detection system is focused on a flat reference plane. Any relief variation will result in image defocusing and decrease the signal captured by a detector. Automatic refocusing is then proceeded by shifting the focusing lens in the vertical direction. This shift is measured at each point (x,y) and then converted to surface height distribution $Z(x,y)$. The presicion of laser profilometers

(Connemann, et al., 1995; Humbert, et al., 2003) is very high: vertical resolution of 0.1 µm (up to 1 nm) with a measurement range of 1 mm, and lateral resolution of 1 µm with a horizontal range up to 4 mm. However this performance requires about 2 hours of sampling time for a 2 mm × 4 mm sample (Humbert, et al., 2003). In addition, a study showed that the roughness value is sensitive to the spatial frequency cut-off and sampling interval during the signal processing (Connemann, et al., 1996). The new confocal microscopy approach used by (Egawa, et al., 2002) reduces the sampling time to a few minutes. However, the new approach inherits the same disadvantages in signal processing with regards to the wavelength cut-off and sampling interval.

The light transmission method records the change of transparency of thin (0.5 mm) silicone replicas (Fischer, et al., 1999). The thickness of relief is calculated according to the Lambert-Beer Law for the known absorption of the transmitted parallel light. The advantages of this method are the relatively short processing time (about 1 min), and good performance: vertical resolution is 0.2 µm with a range of 0.5 mm, and lateral resolution is 10 µm with a horizontal range up to 7.5 mm. A commercial device is available. However, making thin replicas requires extra attention over a multi-step procedure. Analyzing the gray level of the transmission image provides relative, but not the standard ISO roughness parameters (Lee et al., 2008). Furthermore, volume-scattered light introduces noise that must be suppressed by a special image processing step (Articus et al., 2001).

The structured light and triangulation technique combines triangulation with light intensity modulation using sinusoidal functions (Jaspers et al., 1999). Triangulation methodology uses three reference points: the source, surface, and image point. Variation along the height of the surface points alters their positions on the detector plane. The shift is measured for the entire sample and is transformed to a Z(x,y) map. The addition of modulated illumination light intensity (fringe projection) allows the use of a set of micro photos with different fringe widths and avoids point-to-point scanning. The acquisition time drops to a few seconds. This technique has been applied to skin replica micro-relief investigation in many studies (Lagarde, et al., 2005; Li, et al., 2006a; Kawada, et al., 2008).

2.1.3 Area-integrating methods

Industrial application of area-integrating methods has been reported (Hocken, et al., 2005), but the technique has not been applied for skin replicas prior to our laser speckle method, which will be described in detail in the second half of this chapter. Although the laser speckle method is designed for *in-vivo* measurement, it can be used for skin replicas.

2.2 *In-vivo* methods

Because replica-based methods are inconvenient in clinical settings and susceptible to distortions during skin relief reproduction, direct methods are preferable. However, data acquisition speed is one of the critical criteria for *in-vivo* methods. Many replica-based methods such as mechanical profilometry, optical profilometry, and light transmission cannot be applied *in-vivo* to skin because of their long scanning times. A review article (Callaghan & Wilhelm, 2008) divided the existing *in-vivo* methods into three groups: videoscopy (photography), capacitance mapping, and fringe projection methods. Videoscopy provides 2D grayscale micro (Kim, et al., 2007) or macro (Bielfeldt et al., 2008) photographs for skin texture analysis. Capacitive pixel-sensing technology (SkinChip®, (Leveque & Querleux, 2003), an area-integrating surface texture method, images a small area of about 50 µm and exposes skin pores, primary and secondary lines, and wrinkles, etc. Unfortunately, both approaches are unable to quantify roughness according to the ISO standards and therefore they are rarely applied. To the best of our knowledge, the only technique widely used today for *in-vivo* skin analysis is fringe projection areal topography.

2.2.1 Fringe projection

The first in-vivo line profiling optical device based on the triangulation principle was introduced in (Leveque & Querleux, 2003). The lateral resolution and vertical range were designed to be 14 µm and 1.8 mm, respectively. The scanning time was up to 5 mm/sec. However, the device was not commercialized because it was too slow for analyzing area roughness and not portable. After combining this triangulation device with illumination by sinusoidal light (fringe pattern projection), and recording several phase-shifted surface images, the acquisition time was reduced to less than 1 second; commercial area topography systems was now feasible. Currently, two such devices are available on the market: PRIMOS® (GFMesstechnik GmbH, Berlin, Germany) and DermaTOP® (Breuckmann, Teltow, Germany). The main difference between them is in how the fringe patterns are produced: the PRIMOS® uses micro-mirrors with different PRIMOS® models available according to sampling sizes (Jaspers, et al., 1999), while DermaTOP® uses a template for the shadow projection and offers the option of measuring different sized areas using the same device (Lagarde et al., 2001). Similar performances are reported by both systems. DermaTOP® shows the highest performance for measuring an area of 20 × 15 mm². It achieves 2 µm for vertical resolution and 15 µm for lateral resolution with an acquisition time less than 1 second (Rohr & Schrader, 1998). The PRIMOS® High Resolution model examines a 24 × 14 mm² area in 70 ms with a vertical resolution of 2.4 µm, and lateral resolution of 24 µm (Jacobi et al., 2004). The drawbacks for fringe projection are interference of back scattering from skin tissue volume effects, micro movement of the body which deforms the fringe image and concern over the accuracy due to moderate resolution.

2.2.2 Comparing replica and *in-vivo* skin roughness results

Evaluating devices that measure skin roughness requires the consideration of a reference gold standard for the "true" skin roughness. The skin is difficult to study *in-vivo* and therefore the first roughness measurements were simply done on skin replicas with the assumption that they were faithful reproductions. Unfortunately replicas represent low pass filters due to the material viscosity that causes some loss of finer relief structure, ultimately leading to lower replica roughness values than direct *in-vivo* roughness measurements (Hof & Hopermann, 2000). This effect was reported in (Rohr & Schrader, 1998; Hof & Hopermann, 2000; Friedman et al., 2002b). The uncertainty introduced by replicas in roughness measurements was estimated as 10% (Lagarde, et al., 2001). In Figure 1 we plot the literature data for replica roughness and *in-vivo* roughness for three body sites. The arithmetical mean roughness was measured by PRIMOS® (Hof & Hopermann, 2000; Friedman, et al., 2002b; Rosén et al., 2005) and DermaTOP® (Rohr & Schrader, 1998), directly and from replicas of the same area.

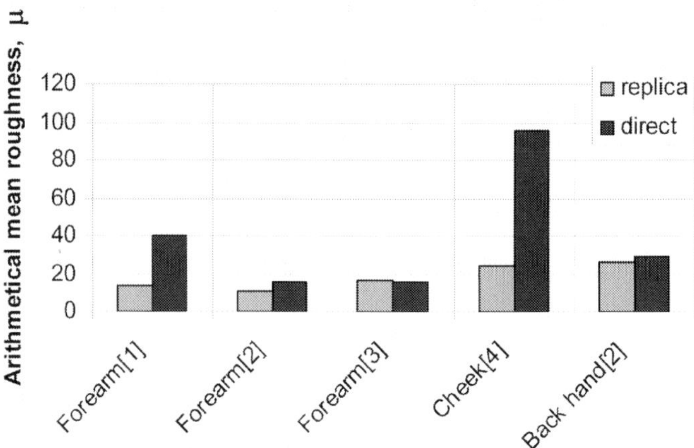

Fig. 1. Direct *in-vivo* roughness (■ direct) and replica roughness (□ replica) for three different body sites. [1]: (Rohr & Schrader, 1998); [2]: (Hof & Hopermann, 2000); [3]: (Rosén et al., 2005); [4]: (Friedman et al., 2002b).

The first three column pairs depict roughness data taken from volar forearm skin. As reported by (De Paepe et al., 2000; Lagarde, et al., 2001; Egawa, et al., 2002; Lagarde, et ai., 2005) the skin roughness of the volar forearm has more consistent characteristics and does not vary significantly with age or gender: by only from 13% (Jacobi, et al., 2004) up to 20% (De Paepe, et al., 2000). Comparing the three different studies, we observed that the spread of the replica roughness is close to 20%, whereas the variability of the *in-vivo* roughness substantially exceeds the upper bound of 20%. Figure 1 also shows a large difference between *in-vivo* roughness and replica roughness in a study involving forearm skin (Rohr & Schrader, 1998) which was conducted with DermaTOP®, and another study of the cheek (Friedman, et al., 2002b) measured by PRIMOS®. These large discrepancies may have many different causes including those of replica and *in-vivo* methods indicated in the previous sections, but they also suggest that further investigations in the area of *in-vivo* skin micro-relief measurement are required.

3. In-vivo skin roughness measured by speckle

In this section, we introduce a novel approach to skin roughness assessment by laser speckle. When surface profiling is not necessary, speckle techniques are popular in industry for surface assessment because the techniques deploy a low cost and simple imaging device which allows a fast sampling time. Speckle methods are classified as an area-integrating optical technique for direct measurements. We first examine various speckle techniques used in industrial applications, and classify them according to their designated roughness range. Then we discuss the adaptation of the technique to *in-vivo* skin measurement.

3.1 Speckle application for opaque surfaces

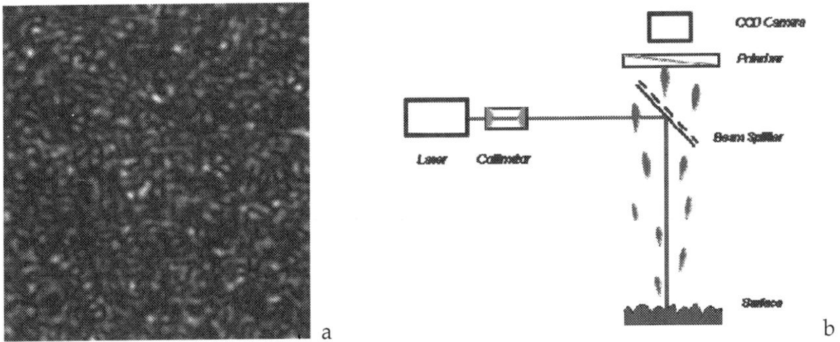

Fig. 2. Speckle pattern (a) and optical setup for speckle measurements (b)

Speckle is a random distribution of intensity of coherent light that arises by scattering from a rough surface.

Fig. 2 shows a typical speckle pattern (a) and an optical setup (b) for obtaining the speckle signal, which in turn contains information about roughness.

Speckle theories for roughness measurement were established a couple of decades ago and were reviewed in (Briers, 1993). However these theories had not been developed into practical instruments in the early years due to technical issues. Recent developments in light sources and registration devices have now revived interest in speckle techniques.

In general, these techniques can be categorized into two approaches: a) finding differences or similarities for two or more speckle patterns and b) analyzing the properties of a speckle pattern.

3.1.1 Correlation methods
Correlation methods analyze the decorrelation degree of two or more speckle images produced under different experimental conditions by altering the wavelength (Peters & Schoene, 1998), the angle of illumination (Death et al., 2000), or the microstructure of surfaces using different surface finishes (Fricke-Begemann & Hinsch, 2004). Although these methods hold a solid theoretical foundation, they are not suitable for *in-vivo* skin examination. One of the reasons is that internal multiply scattering contributes significantly to the total speckle decorrelation.

3.1.2 Speckle image texture analysis
The speckle photography approach analyzes features on a single speckle pattern. The analysis may include assessments of speckle elongation (Lehmann, 2002), co-occurrence matrices (Lu et al., 2006), fractal features of the speckle pattern (Li et al., 2006b), or the mean size of "speckled" speckle (Lehmann, 1999). A speckle image can be captured easily by a camera when a light source illuminates a surface and a speckle pattern is formed. The main

drawback of the approach is that the relationships between most of the texture patterns and surface roughness, except (Lehmann, 2002), were established empirically. As a result, the success of this approach entirely depends on a rigid image formation set up and a careful and detailed calibration between the texture features and surface roughness. In addition, these "ad-hoc" assessments do not conform to the ISO standards.

3.1.3 Speckle contrast techniques

Speckle contrast (see detailed definition in Section 3.2.1) is a numerical value that can be easily measured and is well-described theoretically. It depends on the properties of the light source, surface roughness and the detector. Surface parameters can be recovered from the measured contrast. (Goodman, 2006).

From a physics point of view, there are two situations that can change (decrease) the contrast of a speckle pattern. One is to decrease the path difference between the elementary scattered waves in comparison with their wavelengths. This is the so-called weak-scattering surface condition which is used in many earlier practical applications (Fujii & Asakura, 1977) based on monochromatic light. A recent modification of this method gives a useful analytical solution for speckle contrast in terms of surface roughness, aperture radius and lateral-correlation length (Cheng et al., 2002). The weak-scattering condition limits the measurable roughness to no larger than 0.3 times the illuminating wavelength. The upper limit of surface roughness can be raised by a factor of 4 for a high angle of incidence light (Leonard, 1998). However the light wavelength introduces the natural upper limit of the measurable roughness range for weak-scattering methods. There have been few attempts to increase the detection range while also achieving quantitative results at the same time. In one case, a complex two-scale surface structure was studied (Hun et al., 2006), and in another case, the results conflicted with the speckle theory (Lukaszewski et al., 1993).

The second scenario for contrast alternation is to increase the path difference of the elementary scattered waves, up to the order of the coherence length of the light source. Implementation of this technique is based on a polychromatic source of light with finite coherence. Known practical realization of this technique covers only a narrow range of few microns (Sprague, 1972).

The measurable roughness ranges reported in the literature are plotted in Figure 3. The chart shows that the majority of the existing speckle methods are sensitive to the submicron diapason. Only the angle correlation technique accessed roughness up to 20 microns. To evaluate skin, whose roughness may be up to 100 microns, a new approach is needed.

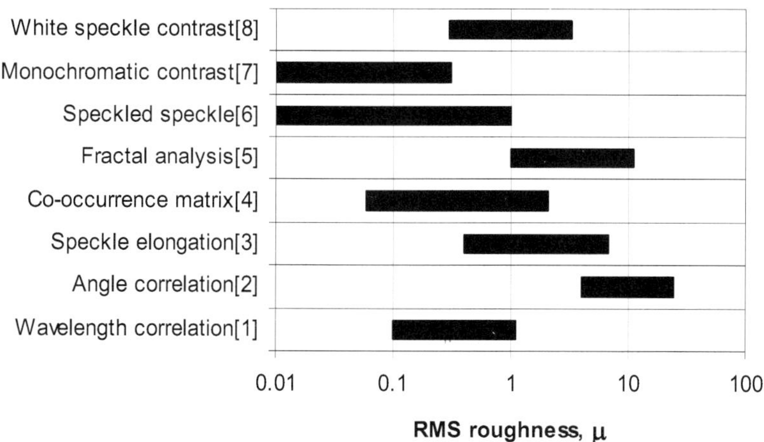

Fig. 3. Chart for roughness range achieved by existing speckle techniques. The roughness range is in a log scale. [1]: (Peters & Schoene,1998); [2]: (Death et al., 2000); [3]: (Lehmann, 2002); [4]: (Lu et al., 2006b); [5]: (Li et al., 2006b); [6]: (Lehmann, 1999); [7]: (Fujii & Asakura, 1977); [8]: (Sprague, 1972).

3.2 Skin roughness measurement by speckle contrast

The possibility of measuring roughness within the range of the coherence length of a light source was experimentally demonstrated over three decades ago (Sprague, 1972). Later the theoretical formulation of this problem, i.e., relating contrast in terms of rms surface roughness R_q with a Gaussian spectral shape light source, was described by Parry (Parry, 1984). Therefore, the problem of measuring skin roughness, ranging from 10 μm up to 100 μm, becomes one of using an appropriate light source. A typical diode laser provides a coherence length of a few tens of microns and as such is suitable for skin testing. Unfortunately, a diode lasers' resonator is typically a Fabry-Perot interferometer with a multi-peak emission spectrum (Ning et al., 1992), which violates the Gaussian spectral shape assumption of Parry's theory. Therefore, we have to find a relation between R_q and the polychromatic speckle contrast for any light source with an arbitrary spectrum.

3.2.1 Extension of the speckle detection range

Contrast C of any speckle pattern is defined as (Goodman, 2006)

$$C = \frac{\sigma_I}{<I>} \tag{1}$$

where $<...>$ denotes an ensemble averaging, and σ_I is the standard deviation of light intensity I, with $\sigma_I{}^2$ being the variance:

$$\sigma_I{}^2 = <I^2> - <I>^2. \tag{2}$$

Let us illuminate a surface with a polychromatic light source that has a finite spectrum and a finite temporal coherence length. The intensity of polychromatic speckles is the sum of the monochromatic speckle pattern intensities:

$$I(x) = \int_0^\infty F(k)\, I(x, k)\, dk, \tag{3}$$

where k is wave number, $F(k)$ is the spectral line profile of the illuminating light, and x is a vector in the observation plane. Eq. (3) implies that the registration time is much greater than the time of coherence. In other words, speckle patterns created by individual wavelengths are incoherent and we summarize them on the intensity basis. The behavior of $I(x)$ depends on many factors. In some areas of the observation plane, intensity $I(x, k)$ for all k will have the same distribution and the contrast of the resultant speckle pattern will be the same as the contrast of the single monochromatic pattern. In other areas the patterns will be shifted and their sum produces a smoothed speckle pattern with a reduced contrast. The second moment of the intensity $I(x)$ can be calculated using Eq. (3):

$$<I^2(x)> = \int_0^\infty \int_0^\infty F(k_1)F(k_2)\, <I(x, k_1)\, I(x, k_2)>\, dk_1\, dk_2. \tag{4}$$

Calculating the variance according to Eqs. (2) - (4) we obtain:

$$\sigma_I^2 = <I^2> - <I>^2 = \int_0^\infty \int_0^\infty F(k_1)F(k_2)\, [<I(x, k_1)\, I(x, k_2)> - <I(x, k_1)><I(x, k_2)>]\, dk_1 dk_2 \tag{5}$$

It has been shown in (Markhvida et al., 2007) that Eqs. (3)-(5) can be transformed to

$$C^2(R_q) = \frac{2\int_0^\infty (\int_0^\infty F(k)F(k + \Delta k)dk)\exp(-(2R_q\Delta k)^2)d\Delta k}{(\int_0^\infty F(k)dk)^2}, \tag{6}$$

Knowing the emission light source spectrum $F(k)$ and performing a simple numerical calculation of Eq. (6), the calibration curve for the contrast C vs. the rms roughness R_q can be obtained. To derive a calibration curve we performed a numerical integration of Eq. (6) with the experimental diode laser spectra converted to $F(k)$. The calculated dependencies of contrast on roughness for a blue, 405 nm, 20 mW laser (BWB-405-20E, B&WTek, Inc.) and a red, 663 nm fiber-coupled, 5 mW laser (57PNL054/P4/SP, Melles Griot Inc.) are shown in Figure 4. Analyzing the slopes of the calibration curves validates the effectiveness of both lasers up to 100 μm (unpublished observations). For a typical contrast error of 0.01, the best accuracy was estimated as 1 μm and 2 μm for the blue and red lasers, respectively. It should be noted that the calibration curve is generated using surface-reflected light and is validated for opaque surfaces. However, in the case of *in-vivo* skin testing, the majority of incident light will penetrate the skin and thus a large portion of the remitted signal is from volume backscattering. This volume effect must be removed to avoid a large systematic error.

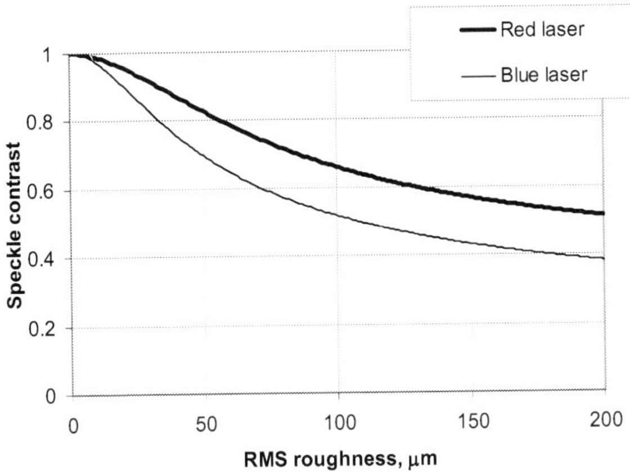

Fig. 4. The calculated contrast vs. R_q for a red and a blue diode lasers.

3.2.2 Separation of surface reflection from back-scattered light

The discrimination of light emerging from the superficial tissue from the light scattered in volume tissues is based on an assumption that the number of scatterings is correlated with the depth of penetration. The surface-reflected and subsurface scattered light is single scattered, whereas light emerging from the deeper volume is multiply-scattered. Three simple techniques for separating the single- and multiply-scattered light (spatial, polarization and spectral filtering) were recently established. Figure 5 illustrates how the filtering procedures work.

Spatial filtering relies on the property that single scattered light emerges at positions close to the illuminating spot (Phillips et al., 2005). Therefore the superficial signal can be enhanced by limiting the emerging light. Applying an opaque diaphragm centered at the incident beam allows the single scattered light from region 1 to be collected (Figure 5).

Polarization filtering is based on the polarization-maintaining property of single scattered light. When polarized light illuminates a scattering medium, the single scattered light emerging from the superficial region 1 maintains its original polarization orientation, while multiply scattered light emerging from a deeper region 2 possesses a random polarization state (Stockford et al., 2002).

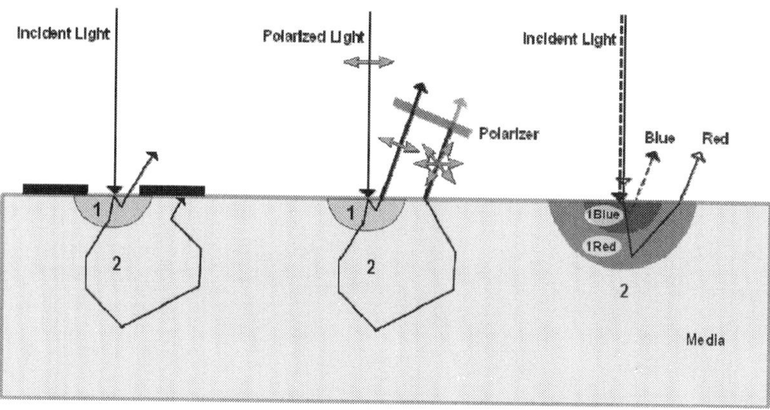

Fig. 5. Filtering principles of light propagating inside a biological tissue. Superficial and deep regions are marked as 1 and 2, respectively.

Registration of the co- and cross-linear polarizer output channels allows the determination of the degree of polarization (DOP), which is defined as:

$$DOP = \frac{<I_{\mathrm{II}}> - <I_{\perp}>}{<I_{\mathrm{II}}> + <I_{\perp}>} \tag{7}$$

where $<I_{\parallel}>$ and $<I_{\perp}>$ are the mean intensity of the co- and cross-polarized speckle patterns. Subtracting the cross-polarized pattern from the co-polarized pattern suppresses the volume scattering.

Spectral filtering (Demos et al., 2000) is based on the spectral dependence of skin attenuation coefficients (Salomatina et al., 2006). Shorter wavelengths are attenuated more heavily in a scattering medium and yield a higher output of scattered light than longer wavelengths. Therefore region 1 for the blue light is expected to be shallower than the red light, and, we should thus use the blue laser for skin roughness measurements (Tchvialeva et al., 2008).

In another study (Tchvialeva et al., 2009), we adopted the above filtering techniques for speckle roughness estimation of the skin. However, our experiment showed that the filtered signals still contained sufficient volume-scattered signals and overestimated the skin roughness. Therefore, we formulate a mathematical correction to further adjust the speckle contrasts to their surface reflection values.

3.2.3 Speckle contrast correction
The idea of speckle contrast correction for eliminating the remaining volume scattering was inspired by the experimental evidence arising from the co-polarized contrast vs. DOP as

shown in Figure 6 (Tchvialeva, et al., 2009). There is a strong correlation between the co-polarized contrast and DOP (r = 0.777, p < 0.0001).

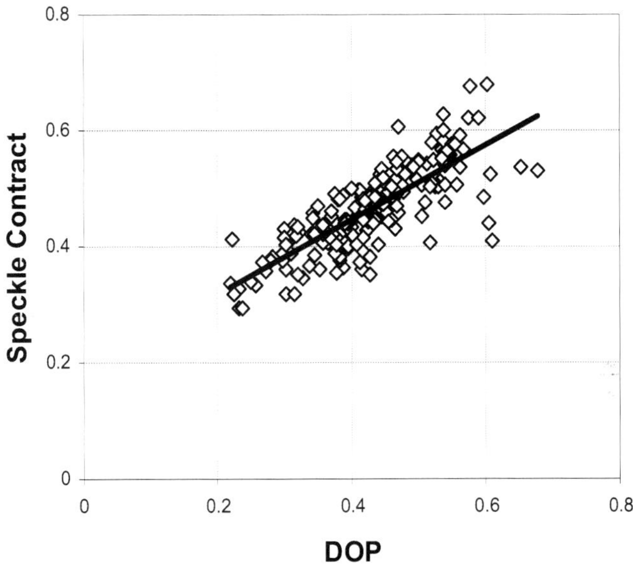

Fig. 6. The linear fit of the experimental points for co-polarized contrast vs. DOP.

We assume (at least as a first approximation) that this linear relation is valid for the entire range of DOP from 0 to 1. We also know that weakly scattered light has almost the same state of polarization as incident light (Sankaran et al., 1999; Tchvialeva, et al., 2008). If the incident light is linearly polarized (DOP = 1), light scattered by the surface should also have $DOP_{surf} = 1$. Based on this assumption, we can compute speckle contrast for surface scattered light by linearly extrapolating the data for DOP = 1. The corrected contrast is then applied to the calibration curve for the blue laser (Figure 4) and is mapped to the corrected roughness value.

3.2.4 Comparing *in-vivo* data for different body sites

To compare skin roughness obtained by our prototype with other *in-vivo* data, we conducted an experiment with 34 healthy volunteers. Figure 7 shows preliminary data for speckle roughness and standard deviation for various body sites. We also looked up the published *in-vivo* roughness values for the same body site and plot these values against our roughness measurements. Measured speckle roughness are consistent with published values. Currently, we are in the process of designing a study to compare the speckle roughness with replica roughness.

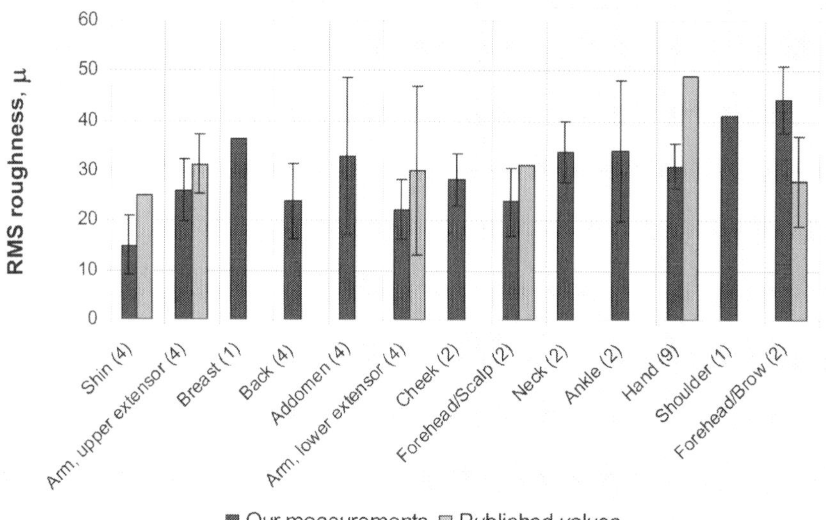

Fig. 7. In-vivo skin rms roughness obtained by our speckle device and by published values of fringe projection systems. The number of samples measured by the speckle prototype is denoted within the parentheses after the body sites.

4. Conclusion

Skin roughness is important for many medical applications. Replica-based techniques have been the *de facto* method until the recent development of fringe projection, an area-topography technique, because short data acquisition time is most crucial for *in-vivo* skin application. Similarly, laser speckle contrast, an area-integrating approach, also shows potential due to its acquisition speed, simplicity, low cost, and high accuracy. The original theory developed by Parry was for opaque surfaces and for light source with a Gaussian spectral profile. We extended the theory to polychromatic light sources and applied the method to a semi-transparent object, skin. Using a blue diode laser, with three filtering mechanisms and a mathematical correction, we were able to build a prototype which can measure rms roughness R_q up to 100 μm. We have conducted a preliminary pilot study with a group of volunteers. The results were in good agreement with the most popular fringe project methods. Currently, we are designing new experiments to further test the device.

5. References

Articus, K.; Brown, C. A. & Wilhelm, K. P. (2001). *Scale-sensitive fractal analysis using the patchwork method for the assessment of skin roughness*, Skin Res Technol, Vol. 7, No. 3, pp. 164-167

Bielfeldt, S.; Buttgereit, P.; Brandt, M.; Springmann, G. & Wilhelm, K. P. (2008). *Non-invasive evaluation techniques to quantify the efficacy of cosmetic anti-cellulite products, Skin Res Technol*, Vol. 14, No. 3, pp. 336-346

Bourgeois, J. F.; Gourgou, S.; Kramar, A.; Lagarde, J. M.; Gall, Y. & Guillot, B. (2003). *Radiation-induced skin fibrosis after treatment of breast cancer: profilometric analysis, Skin Res Technol*, Vol. 9, No. 1, pp. 39-42

Briers, J. (1993). Surface roughness evaluation. In: *Speckle Metrology, Sirohi, R. S.* (Eds), by CRC Press

Callaghan, T. M. & Wilhelm, K. P. (2008). *A review of ageing and an examination of clinical methods in the assessment of ageing skin. Part 2: Clinical perspectives and clinical methods in the evaluation of ageing skin, Int J Cosmet Sci*, Vol. 30, No. 5, pp. 323-332

Cheng, C.; Liu, C.; Zhang, N.; Jia, T.; Li, R. & Xu, Z. (2002). *Absolute measurement of roughness and lateral-correlation length of random surfaces by use of the simplified model of image-speckle contrast, Applied Optics*, Vol. 41, No. 20, pp. 4148-4156

Connemann, B.; Busche, H.; Kreusch, J.; Teichert, H.-M. & Wolff, H. (1995). *Quantitative surface topography as a tool in the differential diagnosis between melanoma and naevus, Skin Res Technol*, Vol. 1, pp. 180-186

Connemann, B.; Busche, H.; Kreusch, J. & Wolff, H. H. (1996). *Sources of unwanted variability in measurement and description of skin surface topography, Skin Res Technol*, Vol. 2, pp. 40-48

De Paepe, K.; Lagarde, J. M.; Gall, Y.; Roseeuw, D. & Rogiers, V. (2000). *Microrelief of the skin using a light transmission method, Arch Dermatol Res*, Vol. 292, No. 10, pp. 500-510

Death, D. L.; Eberhardt, J. E. & Rogers, C. A. (2000). *Transparency effects on powder speckle decorrelation, Optics Express*, Vol. 6, No. 11, pp. 202-212

del Carmen Lopez Pacheco, M.; da Cunha Martins-Costa, M. F.; Zapata, A. J.; Cherit, J. D. & Gallegos, E. R. (2005). *Implementation and analysis of relief patterns of the surface of benign and malignant lesions of the skin by microtopography, Phys Med Biol*, Vol. 50, No. 23, pp. 5535-5543

Demos, S. G.; Radousky, H. B. & Alfano, R. R. (2000). *Deep subsurface imaging in tissues using spectral and polarization filtering, Optics Express*, Vol. 7, No. 1, pp. 23-28

Egawa, M.; Oguri, M.; Kuwahara, T. & Takahashi, M. (2002). *Effect of exposure of human skin to a dry environment, Skin Res Technol*, Vol. 8, No. 4, pp. 212-218

Fischer, T. W.; Wigger-Alberti, W. & Elsner, P. (1999). *Direct and non-direct measurement techniques for analysis of skin surface topography, Skin Pharmacol Appl Skin Physiol*, Vol. 12, No. 1-2, pp. 1-11

Fricke-Begemann, T. & Hinsch, K. (2004). *Measurement of random processes at rough surfaces with digital speckle correlation, J Opt Soc Am A Opt Image Sci Vis*, Vol. 21, No. 2, pp. 252-262

Friedman, P. M.; Skover, G. R.; Payonk, G. & Geronemus, R. G. (2002a). *Quantitative evaluation of nonablative laser technology, Semin Cutan Med Surg*, Vol. 21, No. 4, pp. 266-273

Friedman, P. M.; Skover, G. R.; Payonk, G.; Kauvar, A. N. & Geronemus, R. G. (2002b). *3D in-vivo optical skin imaging for topographical quantitative assessment of non-ablative laser technology, Dermatol Surg*, Vol. 28, No. 3, pp. 199-204

Fujii, H. & Asakura, T. (1977). *Roughness measurements of metal surfaces using laser speckle, JOSA*, Vol. 67, No. 9, pp. 1171-1176

Fujimura, T.; Haketa, K.; Hotta, M. & Kitahara, T. (2007). *Global and systematic demonstration for the practical usage of a direct in vivo measurement system to evaluate wrinkles, Int J Cosmet Sci,* Vol. 29, No. 6, pp. 423-436

Gautier, S.; Xhauflaire-Uhoda, E.; Gonry, P. & Pierard, G. E. (2008). *Chitin-glucan, a natural cell scaffold for skin moisturization and rejuvenation, Int J Cosmet Sci,* Vol. 30, No. 6, pp. 459-469

Goodman, J. W. (2006). *Speckle Phenomena in Optics: Theory and Application,* Roberts and Company Publishers

Handels, H.; RoS, T.; Kreusch, J.; Wolff, H. H. & Poppl, S. J. (1999). *Computer-supported diagnosis of melanoma in profilometry, Meth Inform Med,* Vol. 38, pp. 43-49

Hashimoto, K. (1974). *New methods for surface ultrastructure: Comparative studies of scanning electron microscopy, transmission electron microscopy and replica method, Int J Dermatol,* Vol. 13, No. 6, pp. 357-381

Hocken, R. J.; Chakraborty, N. & Brown, C. (2005). *Optical metrology of surface, CIRP Annals - Manufacturing Technology,* Vol. 54, No. 2, pp. 169-183

Hof, C. & Hopermann, H. (2000). *Comparison of replica- and in vivo-measurement of the microtopography of human skin, SOFW Journal,* Vol. 126, pp. 40-46

Humbert, P. G.; Haftek, M.; Creidi, P.; Lapiere, C.; Nusgens, B.; Richard, A.; Schmitt, D.; Rougier, A. & Zahouani, H. (2003). *Topical ascorbic acid on photoaged skin. Clinical, topographical and ultrastructural evaluation: double-blind study vs. placebo, Exp Dermatol,* Vol. 12, No. 3, pp. 237-244

Hun, C.; Bruynooghea, M.; Caussignacb, J.-M. & Meyrueisa, P. (2006). Study of the exploitation of speckle techniques for pavement surface, *Proc of SPIE 6341,* pp. 63412A,

International Organization for Standardization Committee (2007). *GPS-Surface texture:areal-Part 6: classification of methods for measuring surface structure, Draft 25178-6*

Jacobi, U.; Chen, M.; Frankowski, G.; Sinkgraven, R.; Hund, M.; Rzany, B.; Sterry, W. & Lademann, J. (2004). *In vivo determination of skin surface topography using an optical 3D device, Skin Res Technol,* Vol. 10, No. 4, pp. 207-214

Jaspers, S.; Hopermann, H.; Sauermann, G.; Hoppe, U.; Lunderstadt, R. & Ennen, J. (1999). *Rapid in vivo measurement of the topography of human skin by active image triangulation using a digital micromirror device mirror device, Skin Res Technol,* Vol. 5, pp. 195-207

Kampf, G. & Ennen, J. (2006). *Regular use of a hand cream can attenuate skin dryness and roughness caused by frequent hand washing, BMC Dermatol,* Vol. 6, pp. 1

Kawada, A.; Konishi, N.; Oiso, N.; Kawara, S. & Date, A. (2008). *Evaluation of anti-wrinkle effects of a novel cosmetic containing niacinamide, J Dermatol,* Vol. 35, No. 10, pp. 637-642

Kim, E.; Nam, G. W.; Kim, S.; Lee, H.; Moon, S. & Chang, I. (2007). *Influence of polyol and oil concentration in cosmetic products on skin moisturization and skin surface roughness, Skin Res Technol,* Vol. 13, No. 4, pp. 417-424

Korting, H.; Megele, M.; Mehringer, L.; Vieluf, D.; Zienicke, H.; Hamm, G. & Braun-Falco, O. (1991). *Influence of skin cleansing preparation acidity on skin surface properties, International Journal of Cosmetic Science,* Vol. 13, pp. 91-102

Lagarde, J. M.; Rouvrais, C. & Black, D. (2005). *Topography and anisotropy of the skin surface with ageing, Skin Res Technol,* Vol. 11, No. 2, pp. 110-119

Lagarde, J. M.; Rouvrais, C.; Black, D.; Diridollou, S. & Gall, Y. (2001). *Skin topography measurement by interference fringe projection: a technical validation, Skin Res Technol*, Vol. 7, No. 2, pp. 112-121

Lee, H. K.; Seo, Y. K.; Baek, J. H. & Koh, J. S. (2008). *Comparison between ultrasonography (Dermascan C version 3) and transparency profilometry (Skin Visiometer SV600), Skin Res Technol*, Vol. 14, pp. 8-12

Lehmann, P. (1999). *Surface-roughness measurement based on the intensity correlation function of scattered light under speckle-pattern illumination, Applied Optics*, Vol. 38, No. 7, pp. 1144-1152

Lehmann, P. (2002). *Aspect ratio of elongated polychromatic far-field speckles of continuous and discrete spectral distribution with respect to surface roughness characterization, Applied Optics*, Vol. 41, No. 10, pp. 2008-2014

Leonard, L. C. (1998). *Roughness measurement of metallic surfaces based on the laser speckle contrast method, Optics and Lasers in Engineering*, Vol. 30, No. 5, pp. 433-440

Leveque, J. L. (1999). *EEMCO guidance for the assessment of skin topography. The European Expert Group on Efficacy Measurement of Cosmetics and other Topical Products, J Eur Acad Dermatol Venereol*, Vol. 12, No. 2, pp. 103-114

Leveque, J. L. & Querleux, B. (2003). *SkinChip, a new tool for investigating the skin surface in vivo, Skin Res Technol*, Vol. 9, No. 4, pp. 343-347

Levy, J. L.; Servant, J. J. & Jouve, E. (2004). *Botulinum toxin A: a 9-month clinical and 3D in vivo profilometric crow's feet wrinkle formation study, J Cosmet Laser Ther*, Vol. 6, No. 1, pp. 16-20

Li, L.; Mac-Mary, S.; Marsaut, D.; Sainthillier, J. M.; Nouveau, S.; Gharbi, T.; de Lacharriere, O. & Humbert, P. (2006a). *Age-related changes in skin topography and microcirculation, Arch Dermatol Res*, Vol. 297, No. 9, pp. 412-416

Li, Z.; Li, H. & Qiu, Y. (2006b). *Fractal analysis of laser speckle for measuring roughness, SPIE*, Vol. 6027, pp. 60271S

Lu, R.-S.; Tian, G.-Y.; Gledhill, D. & Ward, S. (2006). *Grinding surface roughness measurement based on the co-occurrence matrix of speckle pattern texture, Applied Optics*, Vol. 45, No. 35, pp. 8839–8847

Lukaszewski, K.; Rozniakowski, K. & Wojtatowicz, T. W. (1993). *Laser examination of cast surface roughness, Optical Engineering*, Vol. 40, No. 9, pp. 1993-1997

Markhvida, I.; Tchvialeva, L.; Lee, T. K. & Zeng, H. (2007). *The influence of geometry on polychromatic speckle contrast, Journal of the Optical Society of America A*, Vol. 24, No. 1, pp. 93-97

Mazzarello, V.; Soggiu, D.; Masia, D. R.; Ena, P. & Rubino, C. (2006). *Melanoma versus dysplastic naevi: microtopographic skin study with noninvasive method, J Plast Reconstr Aesthet Surg*, Vol. 59, No. 7, pp. 700-705

Ning, Y. N.; Grattan, K. T. V.; Palmer, A. W. & Meggitt, B. T. (1992). *Coherence length modulation of a multimode laser diode in a dual Michelson interferometer configuration, Applied Optics*, Vol. 31, No. 9, pp. 1322–1327

Parry, G. (1984). Speckle patterns in partially coherent light. In: *Laser Speckle and Related Phenomena, Dainty, J. C.* (Eds), pp. 77-122, Springer-Verlag, Berlin; New York

Peters, J. & Schoene, A. (1998). *Nondestructive evaluation of surface roughness by speckle correlation techniques, SPIE*, Vol. 3399, pp. 45-56

Phillips, K.; Xu, M.; Gayen, S. & Alfano, R. (2005). *Time-resolved ring structure of circularly polarized beams backscattered from forward scattering media*, Optics Express, Vol. 13, No. 20, pp. 7954-7969

Rapini, R. (2003). Clinical and Pathologic Differential Diagnosis. In: *Dermatology, Bolognia, J. L., Jorizzo, J. L. and Rapini, R. P.* (Eds), Mosby, London

Rohr, M. & Schrader, K. (1998). *Fast Optical in vivo Topometry of Human Skin (FOITS) - Comparative Investigations with Laser Profilometry*, SOFW Journal, Vol. 124, pp. 52-59

Rosén, B.-G.; Blunt, L. & Thomas, T. R. (2005). *On in-vivo skin topography metrology and replication techniques*, Phys.: Conf. Ser., Vol. 13, pp. 325-329

Salomatina, E.; Jiang, B.; Novak, J. & Yaroslavsky, A. N. (2006). *Optical properties of normal and cancerous human skin in the visible and near-infrared spectral range*, J Biomed Opt, Vol. 11, No. 6, pp. 064026

Sankaran, V.; Everett, M. J.; Maitland, D. J. & Walsh, J. T., Jr. (1999). *Comparison of polarized-light propagation in biological tissue and phantoms*, Opt Lett, Vol. 24, No. 15, pp. 1044-1046

Segger, D. & Schonlau, F. (2004). *Supplementation with Evelle improves skin smoothness and elasticity in a double-blind, placebo-controlled study with 62 women*, J Dermatolog Treat, Vol. 15, No. 4, pp. 222-226

Setaro, M. & Sparavigna, A. (2001). *Irregularity skin index (ISI): a tool to evaluate skin surface texture*, Skin Res Technol, Vol. 7, No. 3, pp. 159-163

Sprague, R. A. (1972). *Surface Roughness Measurement Using White Light Speckle*, Applied Optics, Vol. 11, No. 12, pp. 2811-2816

Stockford, I. M.; Morgan, S. P.; Chang, P. C. & Walker, J. G. (2002). *Analysis of the spatial distribution of polarized light backscattered from layered scattering media*, J Biomed Opt, Vol. 7, No. 3, pp. 313-320

Tchvialeva, L.; Zeng, H.; Lui, H.; McLean, D. I. & Lee, T. K. (2008). Comparing in vivo Skin surface roughness measurement using laser speckle imaging with red and blue wavelengths, *The 3rd world congress of noninvasive skin imaging*, pp. Seoul, Korea, May 7-10, 2008

Tchvialeva, L.; Zeng, H.; Markhvida, I.; Dhadwal, G.; McLean, L.; McLean, D. I. & Lui, H. (2009). Optical discrimination of surface reflection from volume backscattering in speckle contrast for skin roughness measurements, *Proc of SPIE BiOS 7161* pp. 71610I-716106, San Jose, Jan. 24-29, 2009

Contact

Tim K. Lee, PhD
BC Cancer Research Centre
Cancer Control Research Program
675 West 10th Avenue
Vancouver, BC
Canada V5Z 1L3
Tel: 604-675-8053
Fax: 604-675-8180
Email: tlee@bccrc.ca

19

Off-axis Neuromuscular Training for Knee Ligament Injury Prevention and Rehabilitation

Yupeng Ren, Hyung-Soon Park, Yi-Ning Wu,
François Geiger, and Li-Qun Zhang
Rehabilitation Institute of Chicago and Northwestern University
Chicago, USA

1. Introduction

Musculoskeletal injuries of the lower limbs are associated with the strenuous sports and recreational activities. The knee was the most often injured body area, with the anterior cruciate ligament (ACL), the most frequently injured body part overall (Lauder et al., Am J Prev. Med., 18: 118-128, 2000). Approximately 80,000 to 250,000 ACL tears occur annually in the U.S. with an estimated cost for the injuries of almost one billion dollars per year (Griffin et al. Am J Sports Med. 34, 1512-32). The highest incidence is in individuals 15 to 25 years old who participate in pivoting sports (Bahr et al., 2005; Griffin et al., 2000; Olsen et al., 2006; Olsen et al., 2004). Considering that the lower limbs are free to move in the sagittal plane (e.g., knee flexion/extension, ankle dorsi-/plantar flexion), musculoskeletal injuries generally do not occur in sagittal plane movements. On the other hand, joint motion about the minor axes (e.g., knee valgus/varus (synonymous with abduction/adduction), tibial rotation, ankle inversion/eversion and internal/external rotation) is much more limited and musculoskeletal injuries are usually associated with excessive loading/movement about the minor axes (or called off-axes) (Olsen et al., 2006; Yu et al., 2007; Olsen et al., 2004; Boden et al., 2000; Markolf et al., 1995; McNair et al., 1990). The ACL is most commonly injured in pivoting and valgus activities that are inherent to sports and high demanding activities, for example. It is therefore critical to improve neuromuscular control of off-axis motions (e.g., tibial rotation / valgus at the knee) in order to reduce/prevent musculoskeletal injuries.

However, there are no convenient and effective devices or training strategies which train off-axis knee neuromuscular control in patients with knee injuries and healthy subjects during combined major-axis and off-axis functional exercises. Existing rehabilitation/ prevention protocols and practical exercise/training equipment (e.g., elliptical machines, stair climbers, steppers, recumbent bikes, leg press machines) are mostly focused on sagittal plane movement (Brewster et al., 1983, Vegso et al., 1985, Decarlo et al., 1992, Howell et al., 1996, Shelbourne et al., 1995). Training on isolated off-axis motions such as rotating/abducting the leg alone in a static seated/standing position is unlikely to be practical and effective. Furthermore, many studies have shown that neuromuscular control is one of the key factors in stabilizing the knee joint and avoiding potentially injurious motions. Practically neuromuscular control is modifiable through proper training

(Myklebust et al., 2003; Olsen et al., 2005; Hewtt et al., 1999; Garaffa et al., 1996). It is therefore very important to improve neuromuscular control about the off-axes in order to reduce knee injuries and improve recovery post injury/surgical reconstruction.

The proposed training program that addresses the specific issue of off-axis movement control during sagittal plane stepping/running functional movements will be helpful in preventing musculoskeletal injuries of the lower limbs during strenuous and training and in real sports activities. Considering that ACL injuries generally do not occur in sagittal plane movement (McLean et al., 2004; Zhang and Wang 2001; Park et al. 2008), it is important to improve neuromuscular control in off-axis motions of tibial rotation and abduction. A pivoting elliptical exercise machine is developed to carry out the training which generates perturbations to the feet/legs in tibial rotations during sagittal plane elliptical movement. Training based on the pivoting elliptical machine addresses the specific issue of movement control in pivoting and potentially better prepare athletes for pivoting sports and helps facilitate neuromuscular control and proprioception in tibial rotation during dynamic lower extremity movements. Training outcome can also be evaluated in multiple measures using the pivoting elliptical machine.

2. Significance for Knee Ligament Injury Prevention/Rehabilitation

An off-axis training and evaluation mechanism could be designed to help subjects improve neuromuscular control about the off-axes external/internal tibial rotation, valgus/varus, inversion/eversion, and sliding in mediolateral, anteroposterior directions, and their combined motions (change the "modifiable" factors and reduce the risk of ACL and other lower limb injuries). Practically, an isolated tibial pivoting or frontal plane valgus/varus exercise against resistance in a seated posture, for example, is not closely related to functional weight-bearing activities and may not provide effective training. Therefore, off-axis training is combined with sagittal plane movements to make the training more practical and potentially more effective. In practical implementations, the off-axis pivoting training mechanism can be combined with various sagittal plane exercise/training machines including the elliptical machines, stair climbers, stair steppers, and exercise bicycles.

This unique neuromuscular exercise system on tibial rotation has significant potential for knee injury prevention and rehabilitation.

1) Unlike previous injury rehabilitation/prevention programs, the training components of this program specifically target major underlying mechanisms of knee injuries associated with off-axis loadings.

2) Combining tibial rotation training with sagittal plane elliptical movements makes the training protocol practical and functional, which is important in injury rehabilitation/prevention training.

3) Considering that tibial rotation is naturally coupled to abduction in many functional activities including ACL injury scenarios, training in tibial rotation will likely help control knee abduction as well. Practically, it is much easier to rotate the foot and adjust tibial rotation than to adduct the knee.

4) Training-induced neuromuscular changes in tibial rotation properties will be quantified by strength, laxity, stiffness, proprioception, reaction time, and instability (back-and-forth variations in footplate rotation) in tibial rotation. The quantitative measures will help us

evaluate the new rehabilitation/training methods and determine proper training dosage and optimal outcome (reduced recovery time post injury/surgery, alleviation of pain, etc.)

5) Success of this training program will facilitate identification of certain neuromuscular risk factors or screening of "at-risk" individuals (e.g. individuals with greater tibial rotational instability and higher susceptibility of ACL injuries); so early interventions can be implemented on a subject-specific basis.

6) The training can be similarly applied to patients post-surgery/post-injury rehabilitation and to healthy subjects for injury prevention.

7) Although this article focuses on training of the knee, the training involves ankle and hip as well. Practically, in most injury scenarios, the entire lower limb (and trunk) in involved with the feet on the ground, so the proposed exercise will likely help ankle/hip training/rehabilitation as well.

3. Pivoting Elliptical System Design

Various neuromuscular training programs have been used to prevent non-contact ACL injury in female athletes (Caraffa et al., 1996; Griffin et al., 2006; Heidt et al., 2000; Hewett et al., 2006; Mandelbaum et al., 2005; Pfeiffer et al., 2006). The results of these programs were mixed; with some showing significant reduction of injury rate and some indicating no statistical difference in the injury rate between trained and control groups. Thus it is quite necessary to design a new system or method with functional control and online assessments. More exercise information will be detected and controlled with this designing system, which will be developed with controllable strengthening and flexibility exercises, plyometrics, agility, proprioception, and balance trainings.

3.1 Pivoting Elliptical Machine Design with Motor Driven

A special pivoting elliptical machine is designed to help subjects improve neuromuscular control in tibial rotation (and thus reduce the risk of ACL injuries in pivoting sports). Practically, isolated pivoting exercise is not closely related to functional activities and may not be effective in the training. Therefore, in this method, pivoting training is combined with sagittal plane stepping movements to make the pivot training practical and functional.

The traditional footplates of an elliptical machine are replaced with a pair of custom pivoting assemblies (Figure.1). The subject stands on each of the pivoting assemblies through a rotating disk, which is free to rotate about the tibial rotation axis. The subject's shoes are mounted to the rotating disks through a toe strap and medial and lateral shoe blockers, which makes the shoe rotate together with the rotating disk while allowing the subject to get off the machine easily and safely. Each rotating disk is controlled by a small motor through a cable-driven mechanism. An encoder and a torque sensor mounted on the servomotor measure the pivoting angle and torque, respectively. A linear potentiometer is used to measure the linear movement of the sliding wheel on the ramp and thus determine the stride cycle of the elliptical movement. Practically, the pivoting elliptical machine involves the ankle and hip as well as the knee. Considering that the entire lower extremities and trunk are involved in an injury scenario in pivoting movements, it is appropriate to train the whole lower limb together instead of only training the knee. Therefore, the proposed training will be useful for the purpose of rehabilitation after ACL reconstruction with the multiple joints of the lower limbs involved. Mechanical and electrical stops plus enable switch will be used to insure safe pivoting. Selection of a small but appropriately sized motor with 5~10 Nm torque will make it safe for the off-axis loading to the knee joint and the whole lower limb.

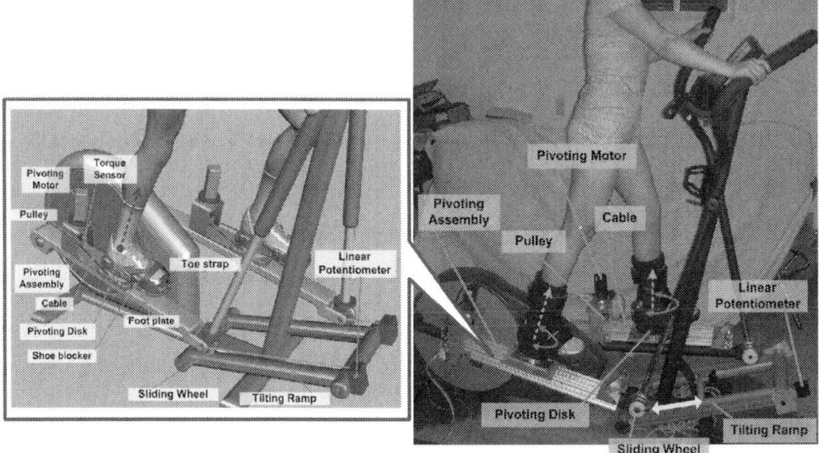

Fig. 1. A pivoting elliptical machine with controlled tibial rotation (pivoting) during sagittal stepping movement. The footplate rotation is controlled by two servomotors and various perturbations can be applied flexibly

3.2 Design Pivoting Training Strategies

The amplitude of perturbation applied to the footplate rotation during the elliptical movement starts from moderate level and increase to a higher level of perturbations, within the subject's comfort limit. The subjects are encouraged to exercise at the level of strong tibial rotation. The perturbations can be adjusted within pre-specified ranges to insure safe and proper training. If needed, a shoulder-chest harness can be used to insure subject's safety.

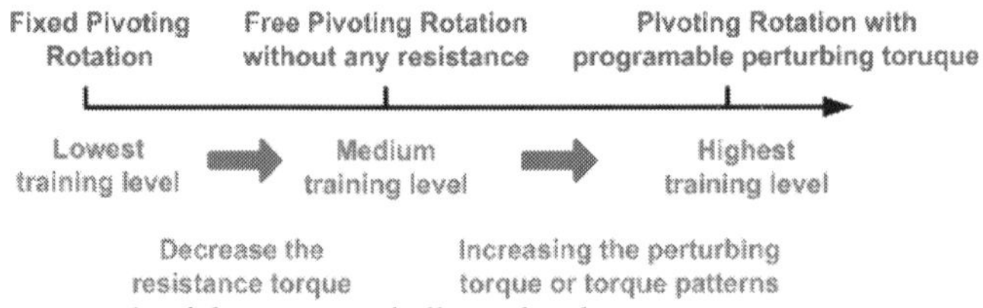

Fig. 2. the main principle of the training challenge levels

Figure 2 shows the main principle of the training challenge levels involved in the off-axis training. The flowchart will help the subject/operator decide and adjust the training/challenge levels. The subject can also reach their effective level by adjsuting the challenge level.

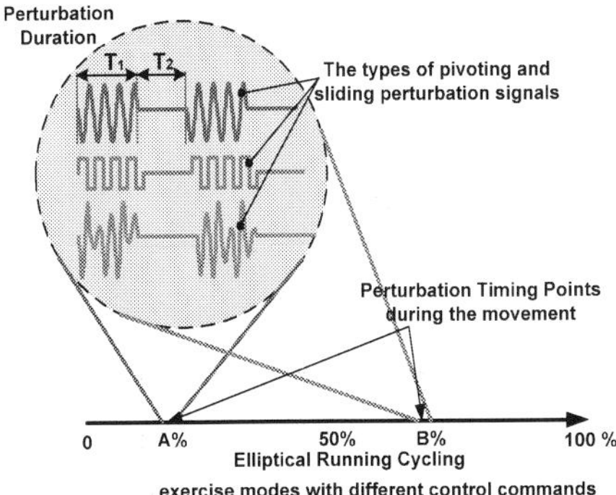

Fig. 3. Elliptical Running Cycling exercise modes with different control commands

Sinusoidal, square and noise signals will be considered to generate perturbation torque commands, which control the pivoting movements, as shown in Figure 3. The subject is asked to resist the pivoting perturbations and keep the foot at the neutral target position in the VR environment during the elliptical stepping/running movement.

The duration, interval, frequency and amplitude of each control signal are adjusted by the microcontroller. As the exercise feedback, the instability of the lower limb perturbation will be displayed on the screen. In addition, the specific perturbation timing during the stepping/running movement will be controlled according to the different percentage of the stepping/running cycling (e.g. A%, B%), as shown in Figure 3. The different torque comands will provide different intensities and levels of the lower limb exercise.

According to the the training challenge levels, two training modes have been developed. The operation parameters for the trainers and therapists would be optimized and siplimfied, so that it would be easy for the users to understand and adjust to the proper training levels. We put those optimized parameters on the control panel as the default parameters and also create a "easy-paraterm" with 10 steps for quick use.

Training Mode 1: The footplate is perturbed back and forth by tibial rotation (pivoting) torque during the sagittal plane stepping/running movement. The subject is asked to resist the foot/tibial rotation torque and keep the foot pointing forward and lower limb aligned properly while doing the sagittal movements. Perturbations are applied to both footplates simultaneously during the pivoting elliptical training. The perturbations will be random in timing or have high frequency so the subject can not predict and reaction to the individual perturbation pulses. The tibial rotation/mediolateral perturbation torque/position amplitude, direction, frequency, and waveform can be adjusted conveniently. The perturbations will be applied throughout the exercise but can also be turned on only for selected time if needed.

Training Mode 2: The footplate is made free to rotate (through back-drivability control which minimizes the back-driving torque at the rotating disks or by simply releasing the cable driving the rotating disk) and the subject needs to maintain stability and keep the foot straight during the elliptical stepping exercise. Both of the modes are used to improve neuromuscular control in tibial rotation (Fig. 4).

To make the training effective and keep subjects safe during the pivoting exercise, specific control strategies will be evaluated and implemented. Pivoting angle, resistant torque, reaction time and standard deviation of the rotating angle, those above recording information will be monitored to insure proper and safe training. The system will return to the initial posture if one of those variables is out of range or reaches the limit.

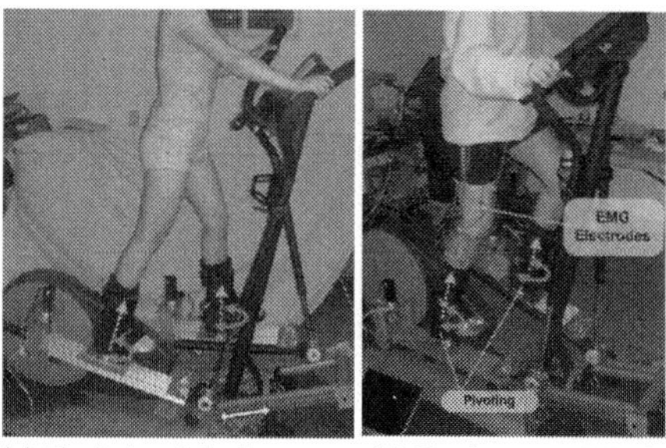

(a) Training Mode   (b) Evaluation Mode

Fig. 4. The pivoting elliptical machine with controlled tibial rotation during sagittal plane elliptical running movement. The footplate rotation is controlled by a servomotor and various perturbations are applied. The EMG measurement is measured for the evaluation.

3.3 Using Virtual Reality Feedback to Guide Trainers in Pivoting Motion

Real-time feedback of the footplate position is used to update a virtual reality display of the feet, which is used to help the subject achieve proper foot positioning (Fig. 5). A web camera is used to capture the lower limb posture, which is played in real-time to provide qualitative feedback to the subject to help keep the lower limbs aligned properly. The measured footplate rotation is closely related to the pivoting movements. The pivoting training using the pivoting device may involve ankle and hip as well as the knee. However, considering the trunk and entire lower extremities are involved in an injury scenario in pivoting sports, it is more appropriate to train the whole lower limb together instead of training the knee in isolation. Therefore, the pivot training is useful for the purpose of lower limb injury prevention and/or rehabilitation with the multiple joints involved.

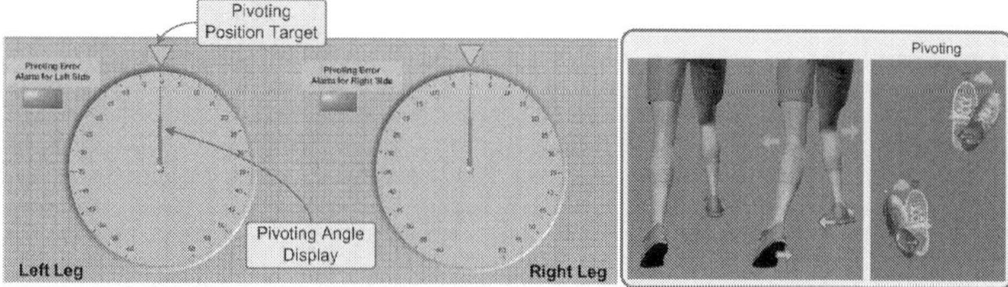

Fig. 5. Real-time feedback of the footplate position is used to update a virtual reality display of the feet, which is used to help the subject achieve proper foot positioning

A variety of functional training modes have been programmed to provide the subjects with a virtual reality feedback for lower limb exercise. The perturbation timing of pivoting movements will be adjusted in real-time to simulate specific exercise modes at the proper cycle points (e.g. A%, B%), as shown in Figure 3. According to the VR feedback on the screen, the subjects need to give the correct movement response to maintain the foot pointing forward and aligned with the target position for neuromuscular control training of the lower limbs (Fig. 5). The VR system shows both the desired and actual lower limb posture/foot positions according to signals measured in real time, the subject needs to correct their running or walking posture to track the target (Fig. 5)

4. Evaluation Method Design and Experimental Results

4.1 Evaluation Method for the neuromuscular and biomechanical properties of the low limb with the pivoting train

The neuromuscular and biomechanical properties could be evaluated as follows:

The subject will stand on the machine with the shoes held to the pivoting disks. The evaluations can be done at various lower limb postures. Two postures are selected. First, the subject stands on one leg with the knee at full extension and the contralateral knee flexed at about 45°. Measurements will be done at both legs, one side after the other. The flexed knee posture is helpful in separating the tibial rotation from femoral rotation, while the extended side provides measurements of the whole lower limb. The second posture will be the reverse of the first one. The testing sequence will be randomized to minimize learning effect. Several measures of neuromuscular control in tibial rotation could be taken at each of the postures as follows:

1. *Stiffness:* At a selected posture during the elliptical running movement, the servomotor will apply a perturbation with controlled velocity and angle to the footplate, and the resulting pivoting rotation and torque will be measured. Pivoting stiffness will be determined from the slope of the torque-angle relationship at the common positions and at controlled torque levels (Chung et al., 2004; Zhang and Wang 2001; Park et al. 2008).

2. *Energy loss:* For joint viscoelasticity, energy loss will be measured as the area enclosed by the hysteresis loop (Chung et al., 2004).

3. *Proprioception:* The footplate will be rotated by the servomotor at a standardized slow velocity and the subject will be asked to press a handheld switch as soon as she feels the movement. The perturbations will be applied randomly to the left or right leg and internal or external rotation. The subject will be asked to tell the side and direction of the slow movement at the time she presses the switch. The subject will be blind-folded to eliminate visual cues.

4. *Reaction time* to sudden twisting perturbation in tibial rotation: Starting with a relaxed condition, the subject's leg will be rotated at a controlled velocity and at a random time. The subject will be asked to react and resist the tibial rotation as soon as he feels the movement. Several trials will be conducted, including both left and right legs and both internal and external rotation directions.

5. *Stability (or instability)* in tibial rotation will be determined as the variation of foot rotation (in degrees) during the elliptical running movement.

Muscle strength will be measured while using the pivoting elliptical machine. With the pivoting disk locked at a position of neutral foot rotation, the subject will perform maximal voluntary contraction (MVC) in tibial external rotation and then in tibial internal rotation. The MVC measurements will be repeated twice for each direction.

4.2 Experimental Results: 1. Muscle activities

The subjects performed the pivoting elliptical movement naturally with rotational perturbations at both feet. The perturbations resulted in stronger muscle activities in the targeted lower limb muscles. Compared with the trial of the footplate-locked exercise (e.g. like an original elliptical exerciser), the hamstrings and gastrocnemius which have considerable tibial rotation action showed considerably increased actions during forward stepping movement with the sequence of torque perturbation pulses (Fig. 6). for example, comparing Fig. 6b. LG/MG EMG plots with Fig. 6a.

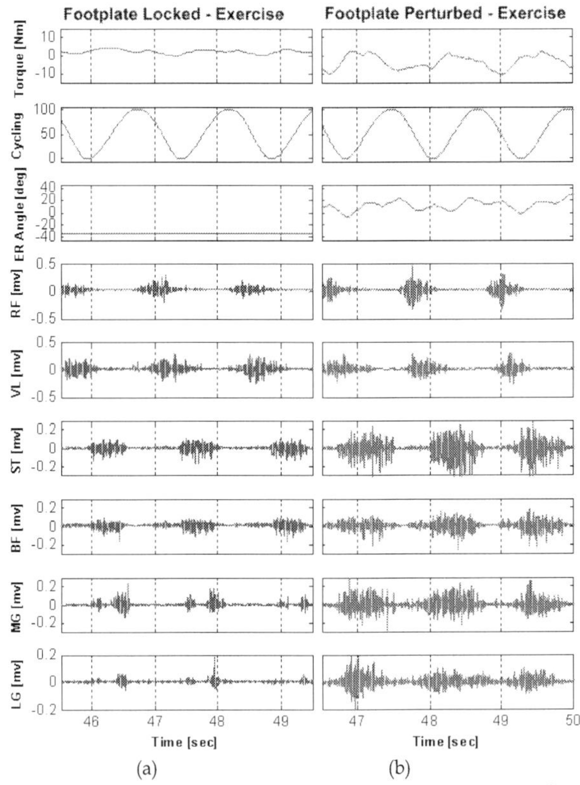

Fig. 6. A subject performed the pivoting elliptical exercise using the pivoting elliptical machine. (a) The footplates were locked in the elliptical movement. (b) The footplates were perturbed by a series of torque pulses which rotate the footplates back and forth. The subject was asked to perform the elliptical movement while maintaining the foot pointing forward. From top to bottom, the plots show the footplate external rotation torque (tibial internal rotator muscle generated torque was positive), sliding wheel position (a measurement of elliptical cycle), footplate rotation angle (external rotation is positive), and EMG signals from the rectus femoris (RF), vastus lateralis (VL), semitendinosus (ST), biceps femoris (BF), medial gastrocnemius (MG), and lateral gastrocnemius (LG).

4.3 Experimental Results: Stability in tibial rotation

Three female and 3 male subjects were tested to improve their neuromuscular control in tibial rotation (pivoting). Subjects quickly learned to perform the elliptical movement with rotational perturbations at both feet naturally. The pilot training strategies showed several training-induced sensory-motor performance improvements. Over five 30-minute training sessions, the subjects showed obvious improvement in controlling tibial rotation, as shown in the reduced rotation instability (variation in rotation) (Fig. 7).

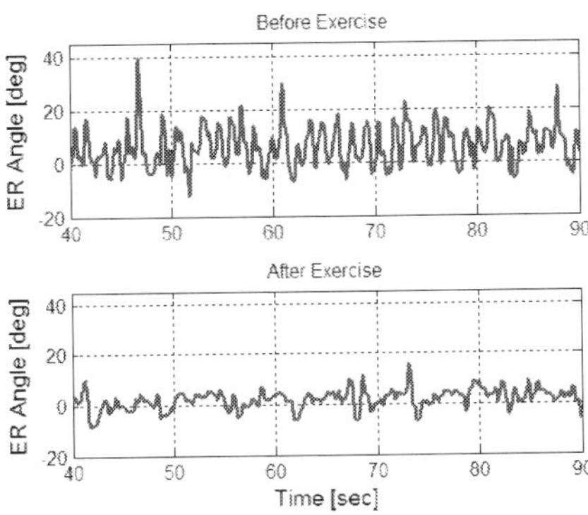

Fig. 7. Stability in tibial rotation with the footplate free to rotate during the pivoting elliptical exercise before and after 5 sessions of training using the pivoting elliptical machine. The data are from the same female subject. Notice the considerable reduction in rotation angle variation and thus improvement in rotation stability.

The pivoting disks were made free to rotate and the subject was asked to keep the feet stable and pointing forward during the elliptical movements. Standard deviation of the rotating angle during the pivoting elliptical exercise was used to measure the rotating instability, which was reduced markedly after the training (Fig. 7), and the instability reduction was obvious for both left and right legs (Fig. 8).

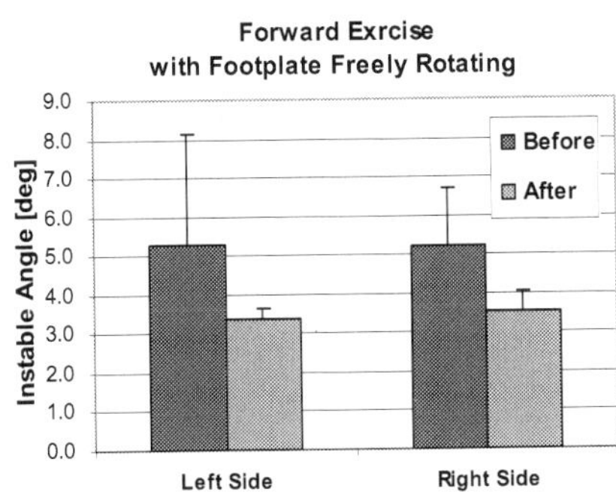

Fig. 8. Rotation instability of a female subject before and after 5 sessions of training during forward elliptical exercise with foot free to rotate. Similar results were observed in backward pivoting elliptical movements.

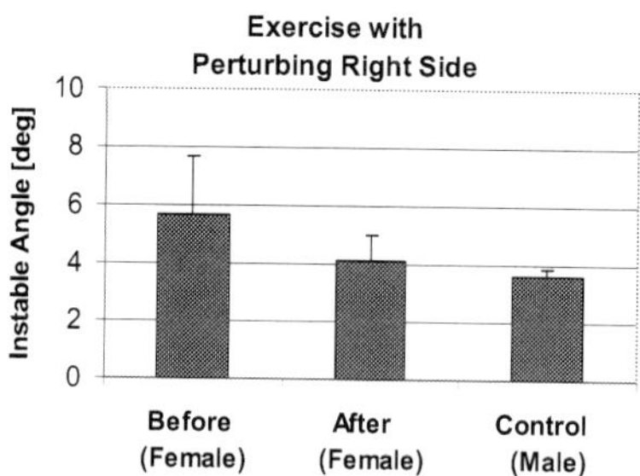

Fig. 9. Rotation instability of multiple subjects before and after 5 sessions of training during forward pivoting elliptical exercise with footplate perturbed in rotation by the servomotor.

Relevant improvement for rotation stability of the lower limb was observed when measured under external perturbation of the footplate by the motor, as shown in Fig.9, which also showed higher rotation instability of females as compared with males. The increased stability following the training may be related to improvement in tibial rotation muscle strength, which was increased after the training of multiple sessions.

4.4 Experimental Results: Proprioception and Reaction time in sensing tibia/footplate rotation

The subjects stood on the left leg (100% body load) on the pivoting elliptical machine with the right knee flexed and unloaded (0% body load). From left to right, the 4 groups of bars correspond to the reaction time for external rotating (ER) the loaded left leg, the reaction time for internal rotating (IR) the loaded left leg; the reaction time for external rotating the unloaded right leg; and the reaction time for internal rotating the unloaded right leg.

Proprioception in sensing tibia/footplate rotation also showed improvement with the training, as shown in Fig. 10. In addition, reaction time tends to be shorter for the loaded leg as compared to the unloaded one and tendency of training-induced improvement was observed (Fig. 11). Statistical analysis was not performed due to the small sample size in the pilot study.

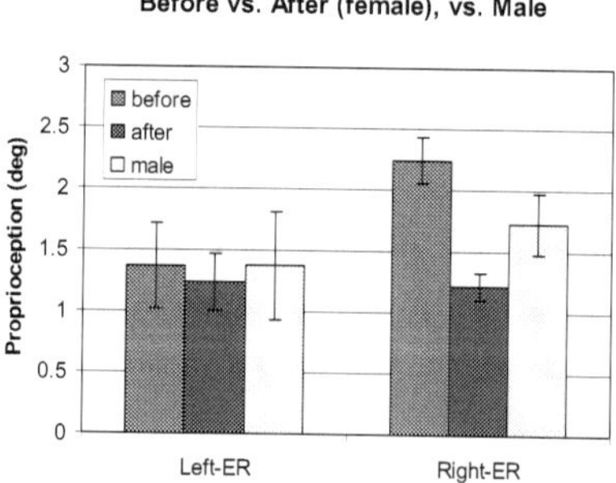

Fig. 10. Proprioception in sensing tibia/foot rotation before and after 5 sessions of training, and the males (before training only)

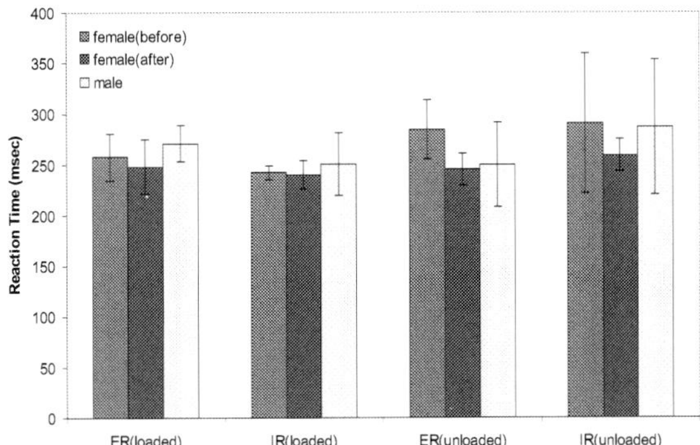

Fig. 11. Reaction time of the subjects (mean±SD) to sudden external rotation (ER) and internal rotation (IR) perturbations before and after training.

5. Discussion

A number of treatment strategies are available for ACL injuries (Caraffa et al., 1996; Griffin et al., 2006; Heidt et al., 2000; Hewett et al., 2006; Hewett et al., 1999; Mandelbaum et al., 2005; Myklebust et al., 2003; Petersen et al., 2005; Pfeiffer et al., 2006; Soderman et al., 2000). It appears that the successful programs had one or several of the following training components: traditional strengthening and flexibility exercises, plyometrics, agility, proprioception, and balance trainings. Some programs also included sports-specific technique training.

Improper neuromuscular control and proprioception are associated with ACL injuries, and therefore relevant training was conducted for ACL injury prevention and rehabilitation (Griffin et al., 2006; Caraffa et al., 1996). Griffin and co-workers reviewed some of the applied prevention approaches (the 2005 Hunt Valley Meeting). The general outcome is that neuromuscular training reduces the risk of ACL injuries significantly, if plyometrics, balance, and technique training were included.

In the current exercise machine market, the elliptical machine, stepper, and bicycle do not provide any controllable pivoting functions, therefore they are not suitable for off-axis neuromuscular training for ACL injury rehabilitation/prevention. The current clinical and research market needs a system which can not only implement the existing treatments and prevention strategies but also perform off-axis rotation training for the knee injury prevention and rehabilitation. Our controllable training system with quantitative outcome evaluation will offer various training modes including traditional strengthening and flexibility exercises, plyometrics, agility, proprioception, balance trainings and sports-specific technique training. Additionally the success of this project will offer the researchers a new tool to conduct further quantitative study in the field.

Tibial rotation training using the pivoting elliptical machine may involve ankle and hip as well as the knee. However, considering the trunk and entire lower extremities are involved in an injury scenario in pivoting sports, it is more appropriate to train the whole lower limb together instead of training the knee in isolation. Therefore, the pivot training is useful for the purpose of ACL injury prevention with the multiple joints involved.

6. References

Bahr, R. and T. Krosshaug, (2005). "Understanding injury mechanisms: a key component of preventing injuries in sport. " *Br J Sports Med,* 39(6): p. 324-9.

Boden, B. P., Dean, G. S., Feagin, J. A., Jr., and Garrett, W. E., Jr., 2000. Mechanisms of anterior cruciate ligament injury. *Orthopedics.* 23, 573-578.

Brewster, C., D. Moynes, and F. Jobe. (1983). Rehabilitation for anterior cruciate reconstruction. *J. Orthop. Sports Phys. Ther.* 5:121-126.

Caraffa, A., Cerulli, G., Projetti, M., Aisa, G., and Rizzo, A., (1996) "Prevention of anterior cruciate ligament injuries in soccer. A prospective controlled study of proprioceptive training. " *Knee Surg Sports Traumatol Arthrosc.* 4, 19-21.

Chung, S. G., van Rey, E. M., Bai, Z., Roth, E. J., and Zhang, L.-Q., 2004. Biomechanical changes in ankles with spasticity/contracture in stroke patients. *Archives of Physical medicine and Rehabilitation.* 85, 1638-1646.

Decarlo, M., K. Shelbourne, J. McCarroll, and A. Retig. (1992). Traditional versus accelerated rehabilitation following ACL reconstruction: a one-year follow-up. *J. Orthop. Sports Phys. Ther.* 15:309-316.

Griffin, L. Y., Albohm, M. J., Arendt, E. A., Bahr, R., (2006). "Understanding and Preventing Noncontact Anterior Cruciate Ligament Injuries: A Review of the Hunt Valley II Meeting, January 2005." *Am J Sports Med.* 34, 1512-1532.

Griffin, L. Y., Agel, J., Albohm, M. J., Arendt, E. A., Dick, R. W., (2000). Noncontact anterior cruciate ligament injuries: Risk factors and prevention strategies. *Journal of the American Academy of Orthopaedic Surgeons.* vol.8, 141-150.

Heidt, R. S., Jr., Sweeterman, L. M., Carlonas, R. L., Traub, J. A., and Tekulve, F. X., (2000). "Avoidance of Soccer Injuries with Preseason Conditioning." *Am J Sports Med.* 28, 659-662.

Hewett, T. E., Lindenfeld, T. N., Riccobene, J. V., and Noyes, F. R., (1999). The Effect of Neuromuscular Training on the Incidence of Knee Injury in Female Athletes: A Prospective Study. *Am J Sports Med.* 27, 699-706.

Hewett, T. E., Ford, K. R., and Myer, G. D., (2006). "Anterior Cruciate Ligament Injuries in Female Athletes: Part 2, A Meta-analysis of Neuromuscular Interventions Aimed at Injury Prevention." *Am J Sports Med.* 34, 490-498.

Howell, S. and M. Taylor, (1992). Brace-free rehabilitation, with early return to activity, for knees reconstructed with a double-looped semitendinosus and gracilis graft. *J. Bone Joint Surg.* 78A:814-823, 1996.

Mandelbaum, B. R., Silvers, H. J., Watanabe, D. S., Knarr, J. F., Thomas, S. D., Griffin, L. Y., Kirkendall, D. T., and Garrett, W., Jr., (2005). "Effectiveness of a Neuromuscular and Proprioceptive Training Program in Preventing Anterior Cruciate Ligament Injuries in Female Athletes: 2-Year Follow-up. " *Am J Sports Med.* 33, 1003-1010.

Markolf, K.L., et al., (2005). Combined knee loading states that generate high anterior cruciate ligament forces. *J Orthop Res,* 13(6): p. 930-5.

McLean, S. G., Huang, X., Su, A., and van den Bogert, A.J., (2004) "Sagittal plane biomechanics cannot injure the ACL during sidestep cutting." *Clinical Biomechanics.* 19, 828-838.

McNair, P. J., Marshall, R. N., and Matheson, J. A., 1990. Important features associated with acute anterior cruciate ligament injury. *New Zealand Medical Journal.* 14, 537-539.

Myklebust, G., Engebretsen, L., Braekken, I. H., Skjolberg, A., Olsen, O. E., and Bahr, R., (2003). Prevention of anterior cruciate ligament injuries in female team handball players: a prospective intervention study over three seasons. *Clin J Sport Med.* 13, 71-8.

Olsen, O.E., et al., (2004). Injury mechanisms for anterior cruciate ligament injuries in team handball: a systematic video analysis. *Am J Sports Med,* 32(4): p. 1002-12.

Olsen, O.E., et al., (2005). Exercises to prevent lower limb injuries in youth sports: cluster randomised controlled trial. *BMJ,* 330(7489): p. 449.

Olsen, O.E., et al., (2006). "Injury pattern in youth team handball: a comparison of two prospective registration methods". *Scand J Med Sci Sports,* 2006. 16(6): p. 426-32.

Park, H.-S., Wilson, N.A., Zhang, L.-Q., 2008. Gender Differences in Passive Knee Biomechanical Properties in Tibial Rotation. *Journal of Orthopaedic Research* 26, 937-944

Petersen, W., Braun, C., Bock, W., Schmidt, K., Weimann, A., Drescher, W., Eiling, E., Stange, R., Fuchs, T., Hedderich, J., and Zantop, T., (2005). A controlled prospective case control study of a prevention training program in female team handball players: the German experience. *Arch Orthop Trauma Surg.* 125, 614-621.

Pfeiffer, R. P., Shea, K. G., Roberts, D., Grandstrand, S., and Bond, L., (2006) "Lack of Effect of a Knee Ligament Injury Prevention Program on the Incidence of Noncontact Anterior Cruciate Ligament Injury. " *J Bone Joint Surg Am.* 88, 1769-1774.

Shelbourne, K. M. Klootwyk, J. Wilckens, and M. Decarlo. (1995). Ligament stability two to six years after anterior cruciate ligament reconstruction with autogenous patellar tendon graft and participation in accelerated rehabilitation program. *Am. J. Sports Med.* 23:575-579.

Soderman, K., Werner, S., Pietila, T., Engstrom, B., and Alfredson, H., (2000). Balance board training: prevention of traumatic injuries of the lower extremities in female soccer players? A prospective randomized intervention study. *Knee Surg Sports Traumatol Arthrosc.* 8, 356-63.

T. D. Lauder, S. P. Baker, G. S. Smith, and A. E. Lincoln, (2000). "Sports and physical training injury hospitalizations in the army," *American Journal of Preventive Medicine,* vol. 18, pp. 118–128.

Vegso, J., S. Genuario, and J. Torg. Maintenance of hamstring strength following knee surgery. Med. Sci. Sports Exerc. 17:376-379, 1985.

Yu, B. and W.E. Garrett, Mechanisms of non-contact ACL injuries. Br J Sports Med, 2007. 41 Suppl 1: p. i47-51.

Zhang, L.-Q., and Wang, G., (2001). "Dynamic and Static Control of the Human Knee Joint in Abduction-Adduction. " *J. Biomech.* 34, 1107-1115

20

Evaluation and Training of Human Finger Tapping Movements

Keisuke Shima[1], Toshio Tsuji[1], Akihiko Kandori[2],
Masaru Yokoe[3] and Saburo Sakoda[3]
[1]Graduate School of Engineering, Hiroshima University,
[2]Advanced Research Laboratory, Hitachi Ltd,
[3]Graduate School of Medicine, Osaka University
Japan

1. Introduction

The number of patients suffering from motor dysfunction due to neurological disorders or cerebral infarction has been increasing in an aging society. A survey by the Ministry of Health, Labor and Welfare in Japan revealed that the total number of patients with cerebrovascular disease is as high as approximately 137 million people [1]. In particular, Parkinson's disease (PD) is a progressive, incurable disease that affects approximately one in five hundred people (around 120,000 individuals) in the UK [2]. Assessment of its symptoms through blood tests or clinical imaging procedures such as computed tomography (CT) scanning and magnetic resonance imaging (MRI) cannot fully determine the severity of the disease. Evidence obtained from clinical semiology and the assessment of drug therapy efficacy therefore depend on the doctor's inquiries into the patient's status, or on complaints from patients themselves. For patients with such motor function impairment, it is necessary to detect the disease in its early stages by evaluation of motor function and retard its progression through movement rehabilitation training.

For assessment of neurological disorders such as PD or spinocerebellar degeneration, various assessment methods have been used including hand open-close movement, pronosupination and finger tapping movement [3]. In particular, finger tapping movements have been widely applied in clinical environments for evaluation of motor function since Holmes [4] proved that the rhythm of the movements acts as an efficient index for cerebellar function testing. The Unified Parkinson's Disease Rating Scale [3] part III (Motor) finger tapping score (UPDRS-FT) is generally used to assess the severity of PD in patients. However, this method is semiquantitative, and has drawbacks including the vagueness of the basis of evaluation for determining the course of the disease [5]. It would therefore be more practical if clinical semiology and the efficacy of drug therapy could be evaluated easily and quantitatively from finger tapping movements.

The quantification of finger tapping movements has already been extensively investigated through techniques such as evaluating tapping rhythms using electrocardiographic apparatus [6] and examining the velocity and amplitude of movements based on images measured by infrared camera [7], [8]. However, Shimoyama *et al.* [6] discussed the finger tapping rhythms only. These camera systems can capture the 3D motion of fingers, but require large and expensive equipments. Further, a compact, lightweight acceleration sensor [9], [10] and magnetic sensor [11], [12] have been utilized for movement analysis in recent years. As for the evaluation of finger tapping movements, however, only the basic analyses have been performed such as verification of the feature quantities of PD patients, which have never been used for the routine assessment of PD in clinical environments.

Motor function training has also been widely applied in clinical environments, and several efficient training methods have been reported [13]–[15]. As an example, Thaut *et al.* and Enzensberger *et al.* conducted walking training along with indicated rhythm or melody for patients recovering from strokes or those with PD. They confirmed that freezing of gait was decreased, and walking velocity and length of stride were increased. Furthermore, Olmo *et al.* discussed the effectiveness of training for PD patients using finger tapping movements in recent years [15]. Unfortunately, however, the psychological burden on the subjects was a concern due to the one-sided nature of the training, as the trainees must remain under the constant direction of the therapist and the training system. It is therefore necessary to develop a method that can lower the psychological burden and allow the trainee to enjoy the training process to enable training to be continued in daily life.

In this Chapter, we explain a novel evaluation and training method of finger tapping movements to realize a system to support diagnosis and enjoyable motor function training for use in daily life. This system measures finger movements with high accuracy using magnetic sensors [11] developed by Kandori *et al.* Ten evaluation indices consisting of feature quantities extracted on the basis of medical knowledge (such as the maximum amplitude of the measured finger taps and variations in the tapping rhythm) are computed, and radar charts of the evaluation results are then displayed in real time on a monitor. At the same time, the extracted features are discriminated using a probabilistic neural network (PNN) and allocated as operation commands for machines such as domestic appliances and a game console. The system not only allows users to train finger movements through operation of these machines, but also enables quantitative evaluation of motor functions. The user can therefore intuitively understand the features of finger tapping movements and training results.

In this Chapter, the structure and algorithm of the evaluation and training method for finger tapping movements are explained in Section 2. Sections 3 and 4 describe the experiments conducted to identify the effectiveness of the method. Finally, Section 5 concludes the Chapter and discusses the research work in further detail.

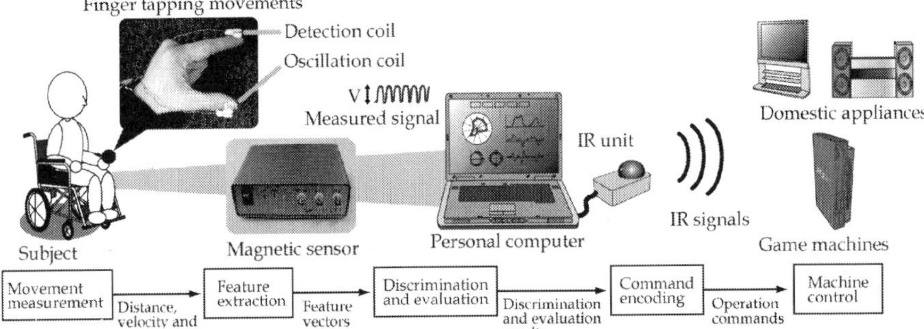

Fig. 1. Overview of the evaluation and training system for finger tapping movements

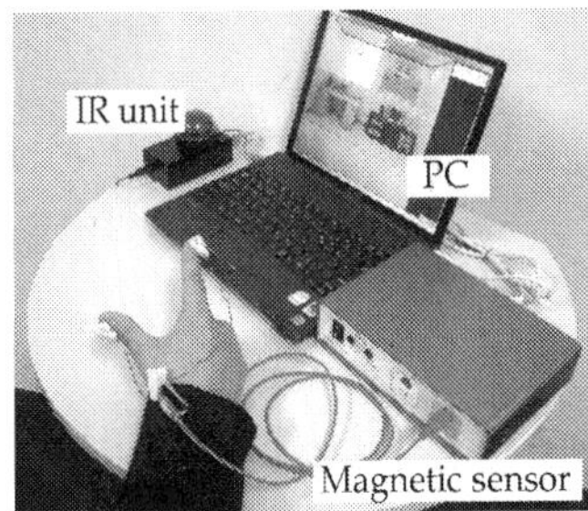

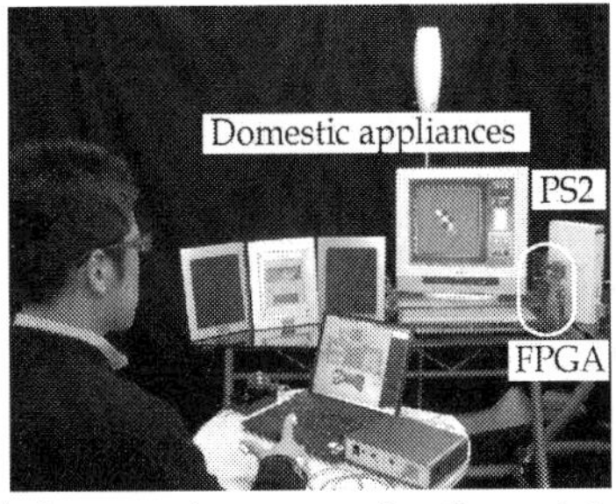

(a) Prototype system developed   (b) An operation scene using the prototype

Fig. 2. Photographs of the prototype system developed and an operation scene

2. Evaluation and training system for finger tapping movements

The measurement and evaluation system of finger tapping movements is shown in Fig. 1. It consists of a magnetic sensor for measuring finger taps and a personal computer (PC). The user conducts finger tapping movements with two magnetic sensor coils attached to the distal parts of the thumb and index finger, and the magnetic sensor then outputs voltages according to the distance between the two coils. The voltages measured are converted into values representing the distance between the two fingertips (the fingertip distance) based on a nonlinear calibration model in the PC. Further, the features of the movements measured are computed from the fingertip distance, velocity and acceleration for evaluation of the finger taps. The details of each process are explained in the following subsections. Figure 2 shows (a) the prototype developed and (b) the operation scene of Othello using the prototype.

2.1 Magnetic measurement of finger tapping movements [23]

In this system, the magnetic sensor developed by Kandori *et al.* [11] is utilized to measure finger tapping movements. The sensor can output a voltage corresponding to changes in distance between the detection coil and the oscillation coil by means of electromagnetic induction. First, the two coils are attached to the distal parts of the user's fingers, and finger

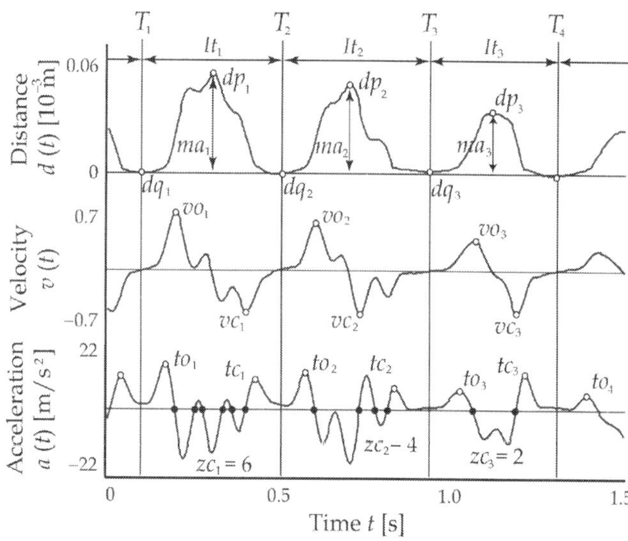

Fig. 3. Examples of the signals measured

tapping movements are measured. The fingertip distances are then obtained from the output voltage by a calibration model expressed as

$$d(t) = \alpha' \widetilde{V}(t) - \varepsilon,$$
$$\widetilde{V}(t) = V^{-\frac{1}{3}}(t),$$

(1)

where $d(t)$ denotes the fingertip distance, $V(t)$ is the measured voltage of the sensors at a given time t, and α and ε are constants computed from the calibration [12]. In the calibration process, α and ε are estimated using the linear least-square method for n values measured output voltages and the fingertip distances of each subject. The calibration process can reduce the influence of the slope of the coils and modeling errors. Further, the velocity $v(t)$ and acceleration $a(t)$ can be calculated from the fingertip distance $d(t)$ using differentiation filters [21].

2.2 Feature extraction [23]

The evaluation indices of finger tapping movements are calculated for quantitative evaluation at the feature extraction stage. This Chapter defines ten indices based on previous observations [9], [10] as follows:

   (1)   *Total tapping distance*
   (2)   *Average maximum amplitude of finger taps*
   (3)   *Coefficient of variation (CV) of maximum amplitude*
   (4)   *Average finger tapping interval*
   (5)   *CV of finger tapping interval*

(6) *Average maximum opening velocity*
(7) *CV of maximum opening velocity*
(8) *Average maximum closing velocity*
(9) *CV of maximum closing velocity*
(10) *Average zero-crossing number of acceleration*

To calculate the above indices, the contact point between the fingers is determined from $d(t)$, $v(t)$ and $a(t)$. First, the threshold M^{th} is calculated as

$$M^{th} = \begin{cases} \widetilde{M}^{th} & (\widetilde{M}^{th} \geq \varsigma) \\ \varsigma & (\widetilde{M}^{th} < \varsigma) \end{cases},$$

$$\widetilde{M}^{th} = \eta \left(\frac{1}{K}\sum_{k=1}^{K} d_k^{max} - \frac{1}{K'}\sum_{k'=1}^{K'} d_{k'}^{min} \right),$$

$$(2)$$

where ς and η are constants determined by the minimum and maximum values of all subjects' fingertip distances; d_k^{max} denotes the distance between fingertips at the kth time when $v(t) = 0$ and $a(t) < 0$ in the measurement time window, and $d_{k'}^{min}$ denotes the same at the k' th time when $v(t) = 0$ and $a(t) > 0$; and K and K' are the number of d_k^{max} and $d_{k'}^{min}$, respectively. Then, the ith time at which the distance $d_{k'}^{min}$ falls below the threshold M^{th} is defined as the contact point T_i (i = 1, 2,..., I, where I is the number of contacts between fingertips).

First, the integration of the absolute value of velocity $v(t)$ through the measurement time is signified as the total tapping distance (Index 1). As feature quantities of the ith tapping, the maximum and minimum amplitude points (dp_i, dq_i) between the interval $[T_i, T_{i+1}]$ are calculated from the measured fingertip distance $d(t)$, and the average (Index 2) and CV (Index 3) of maximum amplitudes $ma_i = dp_i - dq_i$ are computed. Further, the finger tapping interval It_i, which is the time interval between two consecutive contacts, is applied as $It_i = T_{i+1} - T_i$, and the positive and negative maximum velocity points are defined as the maximum opening velocity vo_i and the maximum closing velocity vc_i respectively. The averages and CVs of the finger tapping interval, maximum opening velocity and maximum closing velocity are then computed from all the values of It_i, vo_i, and vc_i (Indices 4–9) respectively.

In addition, zc_i, which denotes the number of zero crossings of the acceleration waveform $a(t)$, is calculated from each interval between T_i and T_{i+1}, and the numbers of zero-crossing points of acceleration zc_i are defined as the evaluation value of multimodal movements (Index 10). Here, the number of zero crossings zc_i increases in accordance with the number of extrema of $v(t)$ in a tap movement. As examples, $zc_3 = 2$ implies a smooth tap, while $zc_1 = 6$ or $zc_2 = 4$ would represent a jerky tap (see Fig. 3). Multimodal movements that have several peaks of distance in a single finger tap may be observed in PD patients due to bradykinesia and disturbances in rhythm formation. It is therefore possible to evaluate the smoothness of motion based on the number of zero crossings.

Additionally, the ith input vector $\mathbf{x}(i) = [x_1(i),...,x_5(i)]^T$ is defined as $x_1(i) = ma_i$, $x_2(i) = It_i$, $x_3(i) = vo_i$, $x_4(i) = vc_i$, and $x_5(i) = zc_i$ for discrimination of finger tapping movements using PNN.

2.3 Discrimination and evaluation [23][24]

The calculated evaluation indices of the subject are normalized based on the indices of normal subjects to enable comparison of the difference in movements. Here, it was observed from the preliminary experimental results that three evaluation indices of PD patients (i.e. average maximum amplitude, maximum opening velocity and maximum closing velocity) were smaller than those of normal elderly subjects. These indices were used to calculate the inverse number for every single tap, and the total tapping distance was converted to its inverse number. Hence, all the indices of PD patients are greater than those of normal elderly subjects.

In this system, the standard normally distributed variables x_p are converted to the mean and standard deviations of the tapping data from those of the normal subjects using Eq. 3.

$$x_p = \left(z_p - \mu_p\right)/\sigma_p \, , \tag{3}$$

Here, p corresponds to the index number, z_p is the computed value in each index, and μ_p and σ_p describe the average and standard deviation of each index in the group of normal elderly subjects respectively. $p = 1$ represents the total tapping distance, $p = 2,\ldots, 9$ signify the average and CV of maximum amplitude, finger tapping interval, maximum opening velocity and maximum closing velocity, and $p = 10$ denotes the average zero-crossing number of acceleration. Each index for the normal elderly subjects follows a normal distribution as the average becomes 0 and the standard deviation becomes 1.

The extracted features are also discriminated for operation of machines. In this Chapter, a log-linearized Gaussian mixture network (LLGMN) [22] is used as the PNN. This LLGMN is based on the Gaussian mixture model (GMM) and the log-linear model of the probability density function, and the *a posteriori* probability is estimated based on GMM by learning. Through learning, the LLGMN distinguishes movement patterns with individual differences, thereby enabling precise pattern recognition for bioelectric signals such as EMG and EEG [18]–[22].

In the training mode, the system first instructs the user to conduct K types of finger tapping movement with different features, such as the amplitude of tapping and the opening velocity. The feature vectors calculated from these movements are then input to the LLGMN as teacher vectors, and the LLGMN is trained to estimate the *a posteriori* probabilities of each movement. After the training, the system can calculate the similarity between patterns in the user's movements and trained movements as *a posteriori* probabilities by inputting the newly measured vectors to the LLGMN. In order to prevent discrimination errors, the entropy $E(t)$ (which shows the obscurity of the information) is here calculated from the LLGMN outputs. Since the output $O_k(t)$ of the LLGMN represents *a posteriori* probabilities for each movement M ($M = M_1, M_2,\ldots, M_K$), entropy is defined as

$$E(t) = -\sum_{k=1}^{K} O_k(t)\log O_k(t) \, . \tag{4}$$

If $E(t)$ is smaller than discrimination determination threshold value E_d, the movement with the highest *a posteriori* probability becomes the result of discrimination. Otherwise, if $E(t)$ exceeds E_d, discrimination is suspended as obscure movement. Thus, the finger taps conducted by the user can be classified based on their features of movement using the LLGMN.

2.4 Command encoding [24]

The finger tapping movement of the user M ($M = M_1, M_2,..., M_K$) identified through LLGMN discrimination is allocated as operation command U ($U = U_1, U_2,..., U_c$), for each machine. K denotes the number of movements conducted by the user, and C represents the number of commands required to operate machines such as gaming consoles. Here, when the number of K exceeds the total number of C, the corresponding estimated movement M_K with command U_c enables the user to directly execute commands using individual movements. However, since there are limits on the features of finger tapping movements that the user can voluntarily conduct, it is impossible to select all machine operation commands using movement M_K.

For control of domestic appliances, therefore, operation commands are arranged in a hierarchical structure to enable a range of operations by repeating the commands of execution and selection [18]. With this method, if two patterns (such as menu changes and menu selections) can be distinguished, the system can be operated appropriately.

An example of the interface screen based on GUI function for domestic appliances is shown in Fig. 4, and indicates that the screens of the three hierarchies are layered. Each hierarchy is displayed as one screen. The screen, which is suitable for use in living environments, is designed for intuitive operation. There are several selectable areas on the screen. The user can move from an upper hierarchy to a lower hierarchy by choosing the desired area, and the intended operation is then performed. As an example, Fig. 4 shows the process to turn on a television set using the two interface operations of execution and selection. First, the user repeats the execution command in the first layer, and the selection command is carried out in the area that contains the television. This action expands the first-layer selection area into the second layer, and the television, MD player and electric fan are displayed on the same screen. Once again, the user repeats the execution command and selects the television using the selection command. In the third layer, the television interface displays commands for options such as power supply, volume control and channel selection. Finally, the user selects the power supply command using the execution and selection commands.

On the other hand, in the case of game operation, commands are grouped and selected using movements. When the number K of the user movements and the required number C of commands are given, all commands are divided into G groups with (K–1) commands ($K \geq 2$). The number G becomes

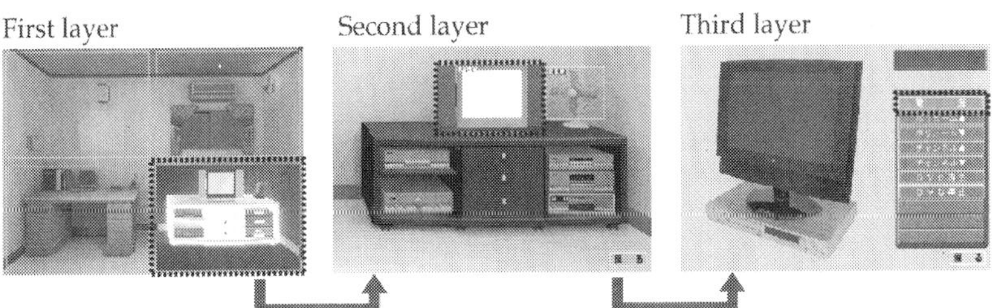

Fig. 4. GUI for domestic appliances

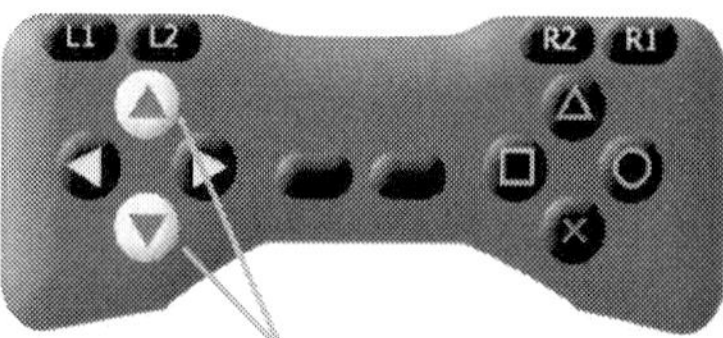

Selected command group

Fig. 5. GUI for game machines

$$G = \text{ceil}\left[C/(K-1)\right], \tag{5}$$

where ceil [*y*] is a function giving the minimum integer equal to or larger than real number *y*. The commands included in the group are freely configurable by the user, and can be set up in-line, e.g. increasing the number of commands based on the game machine in order to configure the same commands for multiple groups. The group can be changed using the remaining one of K movements allotted to each group. Based on the above techniques, the user changes groups and selects commands by repeating K movements.

Figure 5 shows an example of a GUI for game operation. This GUI uses a format similar to that of a game control pad, and the selected command group is displayed inverted. The user can therefore operate the game machine by shifting groups and selecting commands while watching the graphics on a monitor.

2.5 Machine control [24]

In general, since domestic appliances can be operated using IR communication, an IR transmitter and receiving unit [18] is utilized for the operation of each machine in this system. For domestic appliance operation, the IR signals corresponding to each command are set to the system in advance, and the user then controls each machine through selection of commands using finger tapping movements. In order for the IR unit to support the IR learning function [18], the IR signals of each appliance can be registered and deleted.

On the other hand, since gaming communication protocols differ from machine to machine, the system must be changed as needed. The game machine control circuit is therefore configured as a field-programmable gate array (FPGA) for easy reconstruction [19]. The FPGA, which is a large-scale integrated circuit (LSI), electrically reconfigures the internal circuit by rewriting the program. Less time is taken to implement the targeted circuit than through an application-specific integrated circuit (ASIC), allowing the program to be redesigned. In this system, a generation circuit to issue control signals corresponding to the selected command and a communication circuit to communicate with the game machine are implemented on an FPGA. The generation circuit uses a look-up table (LUT) to pre-store the control signals in the memory, to match the selected commands to the address in the memory, and to generate the required signal. The communication circuit includes the protocol of the individual game machine, and the control signals generated are sent to the machine according to IR signals received from the IR receiver attached to the FPGA.

2.6 Graphical output during evaluation [23]

The measured signals, computed feature quantity and indices are displayed for doctors on a graphic display during evaluation of finger tapping movements. An example of the operation of the evaluation system is shown in Fig. 6. During operation, the monitor displays the following information: (i) the measured fingertip distance $d(t)$, velocity $v(t)$ and acceleration $a(t)$; (ii) computed indices and radar charts calculated for all measurement time and at prespecified time intervals; (iii) phase-plane trajectories of $d(t)$ and $v(t)$, and $v(t)$ and $a(t)$ on a real-time basis (the phase-plane trajectories can visually describe the dynamics of motion); (iv) operation buttons; and (v) a scrollbar to allow the waveform display time and the scale of the figure to be changed. Users can also input information and observations and use them for electronic medical charts and databases, which enables comparison with previous measurement data.

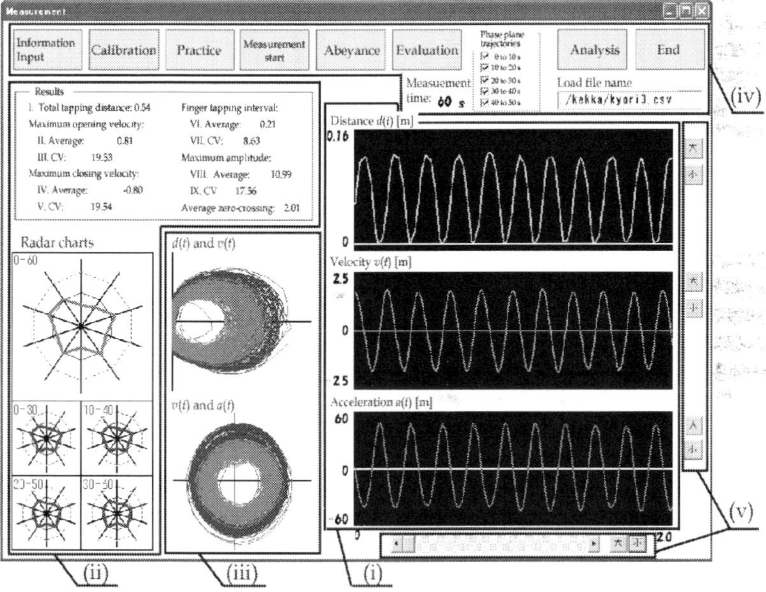

Fig. 6. Example of graphic display during evaluation [23]

3. Evaluation experiments of finger tapping movements

To verify the validity of the proposed system, it is necessary to investigate the effectiveness of the following two criteria: (i) finger tapping evaluation to assess motor function, and (ii) finger tapping training. We therefore developed the prototype, and the conducted experiments involving evaluation and discrimination of finger tapping movements, operation of domestic appliances and a game machine, and finger tapping training using the developed prototype. The effectiveness of finger tapping evaluation is explained in this section, and the validity of finger tapping training is discussed in Section 4.

In the prototype system, the control circuit of the game machine is designed using an evaluation board (RC100, Celoxica) on which the FPGA (XC2S200-5FG456) is mounted, and the circuit is described using Verilog-HDL. The operation frequency of the circuit is 2.5 [MHz], and the control signal bit width stored in the memory is 16 bits. The LUT and communication circuits are implemented based on the communication protocol of the PlayStation 2 (Sony Computer Entertainment Inc., PS2), which the user operates using finger tapping movements.

3.1 Experimental conditions

The subjects were 16 patients with PD (average age: 71.2 6.4, male: 5, female: 11) and 32 normal elderly subjects (average age: 68.2 5.0, male: 16, female: 16). The subjects were directed to assume a sitting posture at rest. The coils were attached to the distal parts of the thumb and index finger as shown in Fig. 1, and the magnetic sensor was calibrated using three calibration values of 20, 30 and 90 mm. After a brief finger tapping movement trial using both the left and right hands, the movement of each hand was measured for 60 s in compliance with instructions to move the fingers as far apart and as quickly as possible. The subjects were isolated from the electrical supply of the PC. The severities of PD in the patients were evaluated by a neuro-physician based on the finger tap test of UPDRS [3]. The investigation was approved by the local Ethics Committee, and written informed consent was obtained from all subjects. The calculated indices were standardized on the basis of values obtained from the normal elderly subjects. The parameters of analysis were $\eta = 0.1$ and $\zeta = 5$ mm, and the sampling frequency was 100 Hz.

3.2 Results and discussion

Examples of the finger tapping movements of a normal elderly subject (a) and a PD patient (UPDRS-FT 2: UPDRS part III Finger Tapping score 2) (b) are shown in Figs. 7. Figure 7 plots the measured fingertip distance $d(t)$, velocity $v(t)$ and acceleration $a(t)$. This figure shows the results of the measured data during the period from 0 to 10 s. Further, a radar chart representation of the results of the indices is shown in Fig. 8; (a) to (c) illustrate the charts of normal elderly subjects, PD patients with UPDRS-FT 1 and those with UPDRS-FT 2 respectively. The solid lines describe the average number of normal elderly subjects, and the dotted lines show double and quintuple the standard deviation (2SD, 5SD) in Fig. 8. Further, in order to verify whether each index can evaluate Parkinsonian symptoms, the indices of PD patients and normal elderly subjects were compared using a heteroscedastic t-test. Table 1 shows the test results of each evaluation index.

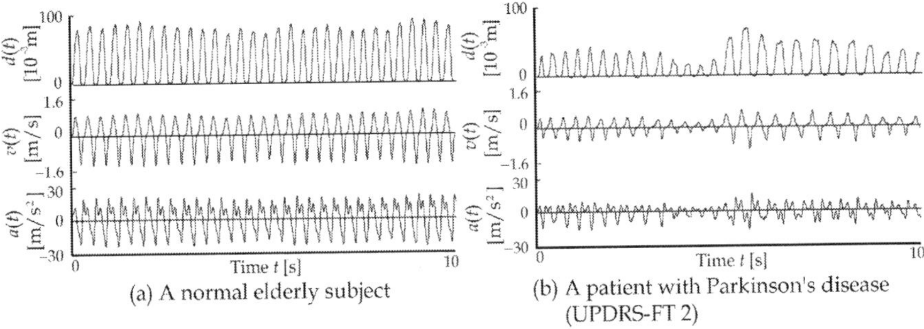

(a) A normal elderly subject

(b) A patient with Parkinson's disease (UPDRS-FT 2)

Fig. 7. Measured results of finger tapping movements [23]

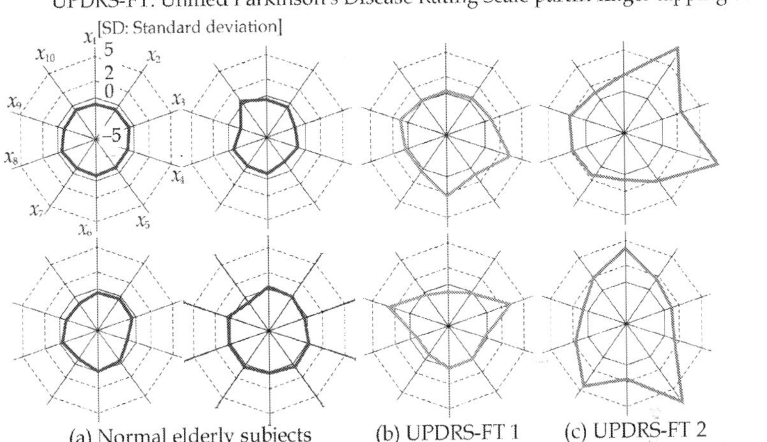

(a) Normal elderly subjects   (b) UPDRS-FT 1   (c) UPDRS-FT 2

Fig. 8. Examples of radar chart representation of the results of the evaluated indices [23]

The experiments demonstrated that the movement waveforms of PD patients and normal elderly subjects have different tapping rhythms and scales, in which PD patients show larger variation in tapping rhythm and smaller scale than normal elderly subjects (Fig. 7). Further, by plotting radar charts of the indices of movements computed and standardized on the basic values obtained from normal elderly subjects, we identified that data from normal elderly subjects lie near the average, while those in PD patients' charts become larger according to the severity of their conditions. These results lead us to the conclusion that radar charts can comprehensibly present evaluation results and features of movement. Moreover, comparison of each index of PD patients and normal elderly subjects using a t-test shows that all indices differ significantly at the 1% level (x_1 to x_3, and x_6 to x_9) or the 5% level (x_4, x_5, x_{10}), and these results denote the same tendency mentioned in [9] and [10]. In the case of evaluating the severity of PD, however, the indices differing significantly at the 1% level between UPDRS-FT 1 and -FT 2, -FT 1 and -FT 3, and -FT 2 and -FT 3 are only three

Evaluation indices	Significance probability p			
	Normal elderly and PD	UPDRS-FT1 and -FT2	UPDRS-FT1 and -FT3	UPDRS-FT2 and -FT3
x_1	2.552×10^{-4} **	3.084×10^{-2} *	1.024×10^{-2} *	1.128×10^{-1}
x_2	9.345×10^{-7} **	2.751×10^{-1}	8.976×10^{-2}	1.062×10^{-1}
x_3	1.701×10^{-5} **	4.292×10^{-5} **	2.569×10^{-3} **	2.463×10^{-1}
x_4	3.694×10^{-3} *	4.916×10^{-1} *	2.869×10^{-1}	5.172×10^{-1}
x_5	1.265×10^{-2} *	2.126×10^{-1} **	4.332×10^{-2} *	8.354×10^{-2}
x_6	1.888×10^{-10} **	1.313×10^{-1}	3.218×10^{-2} *	5.820×10^{-2}
x_7	7.564×10^{-8} **	1.107×10^{-1}	2.289×10^{-2} *	8.890×10^{-2}
x_8	1.302×10^{-11} **	1.018×10^{-1}	4.477×10^{-2} *	7.164×10^{-2}
x_9	1.943×10^{-6} **	1.988×10^{-3} **	7.016×10^{-5} **	4.491×10^{-2} *
x_{10}	1.268×10^{-2} *	1.344×10^{-1}	6.900×10^{-2}	4.695×10^{-1}

x_1: Total tapping distance x_6: Average maximum opening velocity
x_2: Average maximum amplitude x_7: CV of the maximum opening velocity
x_3: CV of the maximum amplitude x_8: Average maximum closing velocity
x_4: Average finger tapping interval x_9: CV of the maximum closing velocity
x_5: CV of finger tapping interval x_{10}: Average zero-crossing number of acceleration
CV: Coefficient of variation, ** : Significance level 1.0%, * : 5.0%

Table 1. T-test results of the evaluation indices [23]

(x_3, x_5, x_9), two (x_3, x_9) and zero, respectively. Since the number of PD experimental subjects (16) was small, it is necessary to investigate and improve the indices for accurate evaluation of the severity of PD with an increased number of subjects.

4. Finger tapping training experiments

We conducted operation experiments of the domestic appliances and a game console to identify the basic effectiveness of the proposed method for finger tapping training. In the experiments, the subjects (three healthy males, A-C, 23-25 years old) were directed to assume a sitting posture at rest. The coils were attached to the distal parts of the first finger and the index finger as shown in Fig. 1. The magnetic sensor was calibrated using three output voltages and fingertip distances (20, 30, 90 mm) (Eq. 1). The parameter for determining the contact time of the fingertips was $\beta = 0.1$, with a measurement sampling frequency of 100 [Hz]. The game used in the experiment was Othello (SUCCESS Corporation), and consent was obtained from all subjects.

4.1 Operation experiments

To examine the effects of discrimination of finger tapping movements, discrimination experiments were conducted using finger taps measured from all subjects. In the experiments, the subjects were asked to conduct two types of movement with low and high velocities ($K = 2$) during a fixed time. For LLGMN learning, 20 sets of feature vectors extracted from these movements were randomly selected, and a total of 40 sets of patterns were used as teacher vectors. The subjects were then asked to repeat two types of movement alternately, and the tapping was measured during a 20-second period. There were five trials, and the discrimination determination threshold was $E_d = 0.1$.

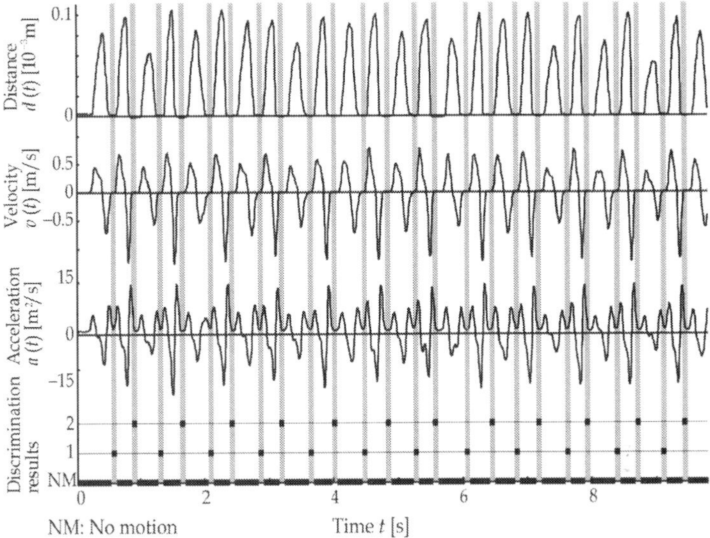

Fig. 9. An example of discrimination results [24]

An example of the results of finger tapping movement discrimination with subject A is shown in Fig. 9. This shows the plot of the measured fingertip distance $d(t)$ using a magnetic sensor, velocity $v(t)$, acceleration $a(t)$ waveforms and the discrimination results. The figure describes the results of the data measured during the interval 0–10 s. The shaded area indicates the contact time of the fingertips, and No motion (NM) in the discrimination results represents periods of no motion using Eq. 4. From the figure, it was confirmed that the subject performed low- and high-velocity movements iteratively, and that the movements were discriminated accurately by the system. The average discrimination rate of all trials with all subjects was 98.56 $\pm$ 1.15 [%].

Experiments with domestic appliances and game operation were also conducted. In these experiments, the subjects were asked to operate the machines by voluntarily performing four types of finger tapping movement ($K = 4$) related to velocity and amplitude. These were M_1 (low velocity and small amplitude), M_2 (low velocity and large amplitude), M_3 (high velocity and small amplitude) and M_4 (high velocity and large amplitude). Instructions were given to operate each machine as presented in Fig.10. Figure 11 shows examples of the results of operation ((a) domestic appliance operation; (b) game operation), and includes fingertip distance $d(t)$, velocity $v(t)$, acceleration $a(t)$ waveforms, discrimination results, layers of menu and command groups, and selected commands. The shaded area indicates the contact time of the fingertips. It should be noted that two movements (M_1 and M_2) were used for operation of domestic appliances, and four (M_1 to M_4) were used for game operation. Here, the changing of groups by game operation commands was decided based on Fig. 12 ($C = 14$). Figure 11 shows that the subjects could operate each machine using finger tapping movements with different velocities and amplitudes. We therefore concluded

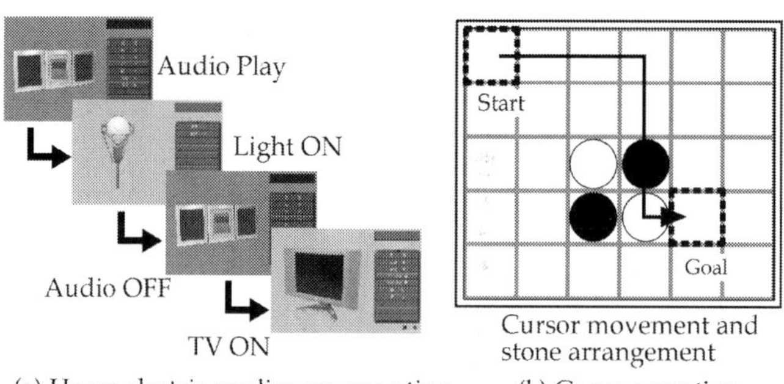

(a) Home electric appliances operation   (b) Game operation

Fig. 10. The target tasks in the experiments [24]

that the subjects were able to voluntarily conduct finger taps and operate the machines as instructed.

4.2 Example of the training experiments

To identify the effectiveness of the developed interface for motor function training, training experiments were conducted on all subjects. After a brief trial, finger tapping movement was measured for 30 s with the instruction to move the fingers while maintaining values for the maximum amplitude of finger taps, the finger tapping interval, the maximum opening velocity and the maximum closing velocity. The average of each value and half the average value of the maximum amplitude of finger taps were then used as teacher vectors of class 1 and 2 respectively, and the LLGMN was trained ($K = 2$). The subjects could therefore operate the game using two types of movement (M_1: large amplitude of finger taps; M_2: small amplitude). In other words, the subjects had to reproduce two types of trained movement for game operation. Further, they were instructed to play one game of Othello, and the movements were measured again after the game. The discrimination determination threshold was $E_d = 0.1$.

Figure 13 shows the experimental results, and plots each subject's coefficient of variation (CV) of each feature measured for 30 s before and after game operation. It is observed that the CVs of each value after the game are smaller than those before it. As the results indicate, the developed interface system is feasible for use in motor function training of finger tapping movements through game machine and domestic appliance operation.

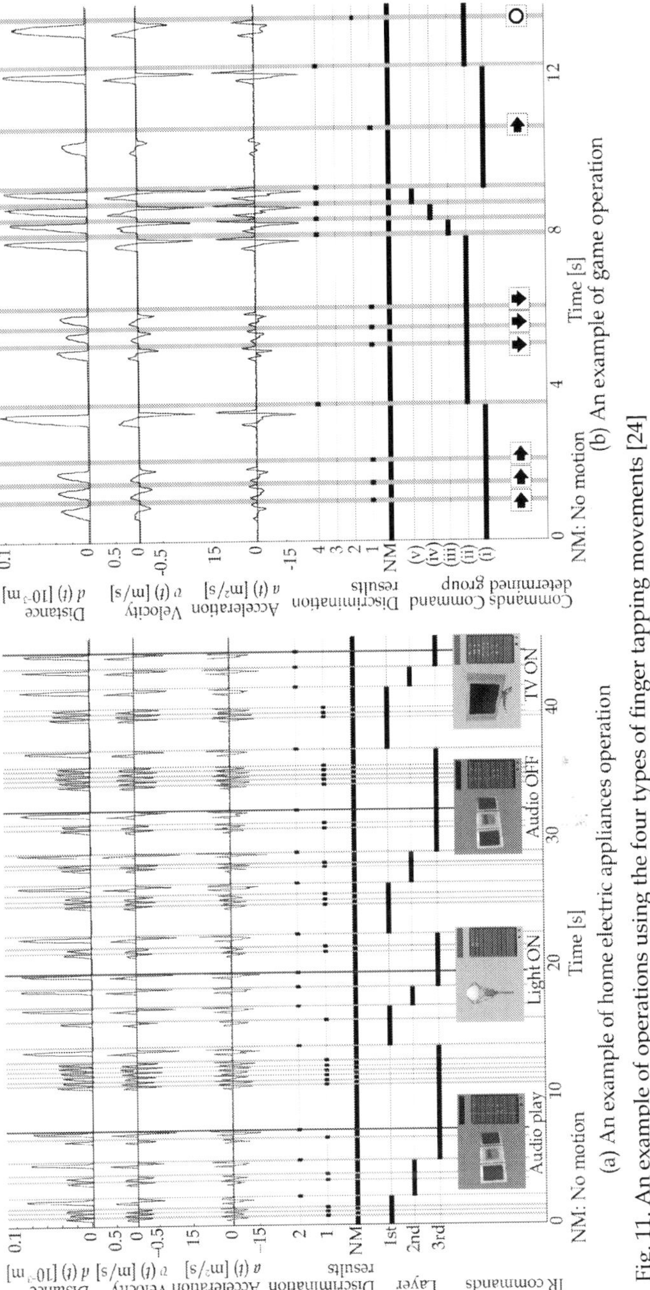

Fig. 11. An example of operations using the four types of finger tapping movements [24]

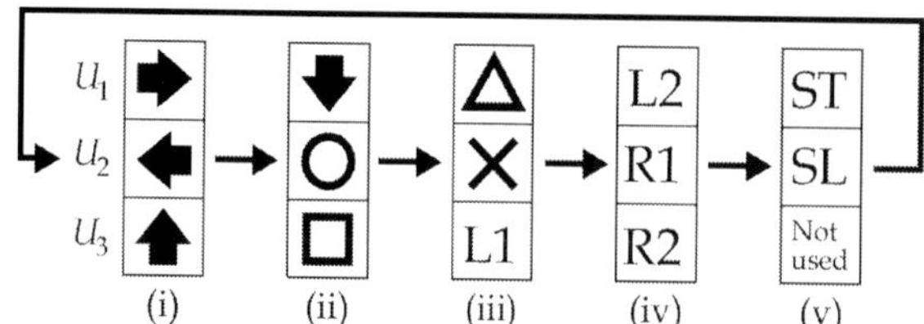

Fig. 12. The command groups in the operation experiments [24]

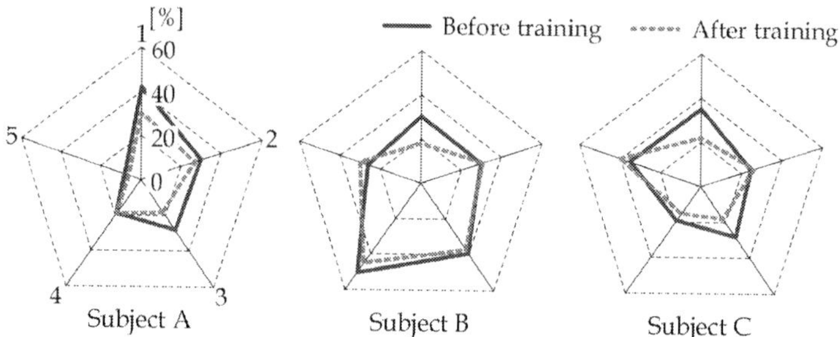

1 : CV of maximum amplitude   4 : CV of finger tapping interval
2 : CV of maximum opening velocity   5 : CV of zero-crossing number of acceleration
3 : CV of maximum closing velocity   CV : Coefficient of variation

Fig. 13. Experimental results of training with each subject [24]

5. Conclusion

A movement evaluation and training system of finger tapping movements has been explained in this Chapter. The system involves the computation of ten evaluation indices measured from finger movements using magnetic sensors, and enables operation of game machines and domestic appliances for rehabilitation training.
The results obtained in the experiments using the prototype developed are summarized below.

- The average and coefficient of variance (CV) of the tapping interval (x_4, x_5) and the average zero-crossing occurrences of acceleration (x_{10}) in normal elderly subjects and those of Parkinson's disease patients differ significantly at the 5% level, and the other indices differ significantly at the 1% level.
- The system was able to discriminate finger tapping movements voluntarily conducted by the subjects with high accuracy. The average discrimination rate was 98.56 $\pm$ 1.15 [%] with all subjects.
- The subjects were able to operate the domestic appliances and game machine as instructed, and the subjects' finger tapping movements can be then evaluated in real time.
- In the case of finger movement training, the coefficient of variance in the features of each finger tap was reduced in comparison to before game-operation training.

Our future research will involve improving the evaluation indices in order to enable diagnosis of the severity of the disease, as well as investigating the effects of aging with an increased number of subjects. We also plan to investigate the effects of training for patients with motor function impairment such as cerebrovascular disease using the proposed interface with an increased number of subjects, and to discuss adjusting the complexity of control tasks in domestic appliances and game machines for effective training.

Publications concerning this Chapter are listed in the bibliography [23],[24].

6. Acknowledgements

This study was supported in part by a Grant-in-Aid for JSPS Fellows (19·9510) from the Japan Society for the Promotion of Science.

7. References

Statistics and Information Department, Minister's Secretariat, Ministry of Health, Labour and Welfare: Patient survey, http://www.mhlw.go.jp/toukei/saikin/hw/kanja/ 05/index.html (in Japanese)

Parkinson's Disease Socity. The number of patients with Parkinson's disease, http://www.parkinsons.org.uk/about-parkinsons/whatisparkinsons/how-many-people-have-parkinson.aspx

Fahn, S.; Elton, RL.; Members of The UPDRS Development Committee. (1987) Unified Parkinson's Disease Rating Scale, In: S. Fahn, CD. Marsden, DB. Calne, M. Goldstein, Recent Developments in Parkinson's Disease, Macmillan Health Care Information, vol. 2, pp. 153–304

Holmes, G. (1917). The symptoms of acute cerebellar injuries due to gunshot injuries, *Brain*, vol. 40, no. 4, pp. 461–535

Goetz, CG.; Stebbins, GT.; Chumura, TA.; Fahn, S.; Klawans, HL.; Marsden, CD. (1995). Teaching tape for the motor section of the unified Parkinson's disease rating scale, *Movement Disorders*, vol. 10, no. 3, pp. 263–266

Shimoyama, I.; Hinokuma, K.; Ninchoji, T.; Uemura, K. (1983). Microcomputer analysis of finger tapping as a measure of cerebellar dysfunction, *Neurologia Medico Chirurgica*, vol. 23, no. 6, pp. 437–440

Konczak, J.; Ackermann, H.; Hertrich, I.; Spieker, S.; Dichgans, J. (1997). Control of repetitive lip and finger movements in parkinson's disease, *Movement Disorders*, vol. 12, no. 5, pp. 665–676

Agostino, R.; Curra, A.; Giovannelli, M.; Modugno, N.; Manfredi, M.; Berardelli, A. (2003). Impairment of individual finger movements in Parkinson's disease, *Movement Disorders*, vol. 18, no. 5, pp. 560-565

Okuno, R.; Yokoe, M.; Akazawa, K.; Abe, K.; Sakoda, S. (2006) Finger taps acceleration measurement system for quantitative diagnosis of Parkinson's disease, *Proceedings of the 2006 IEEE International Conference of the Engineering in Medicine and Biology Society*, pp. 6623–6626

Okuno, R.; Yokoe, M.; Fukawa, K.; Sakoda S.; Akazawa, K. (2007). Measurement system of finger-tapping contact force for quantitative diagnosis of Parkinson's disease, *Proc. 2007 IEEE International Conference of the Engineering in Medicine and Biology Society*, pp. 1354-1357

Kandori, A.; Yokoe, M.; Sakoda, S.; Abe, K.; Miyashita, T.; Oe, H.; Naritomi, H.; Ogata, K.; Tsukada, K. (2004). Quantitative magnetic detection of finger movements in parients with Parkinson's disease, *Neuroscience Research*, vol. 49, no. 2, pp. 253–260

Shima, K.; Kan, E.; Tsuji, Toshio; Tsuji, Tokuo; Kandori, A.; Miyashita, T.; Yokoe, M.; Sakoda, S. (2007). A new calibration method of magnetic sensors for measurement of human finger tapping movements, *Transactions of the Society of Instrument and Control Engineers*, vol. 43, no. 9, pp. 821-828 (in Japanese)

Thaut, M.H.; McIntosh, G.C.; Rice, R.R. (1997). Rhythmic facilitation of gait training in hemiparetic stroke rehabilitation, *Journal of Neurological Sciences*, vol. 151, pp. 207–212

Enzensberger, W.; Oberlander, U.; Stecker K. (1997). Metronomtherapie bei Parkinson-Patienten, *Der Nervenarzt*, vol. 68, pp. 972–977

Del Olmo, M.F.; Arias, P.; Furio, M.C.; Pozo, M.A.; Cudeiro J. (2006). Evaluation of the effect of training using auditory stimulation on rhythmic movement in Parkinsonian patients—a combined motor and [18F]-FDG PET study, *Parkinsonism and Related Disorders*, vol. 12, pp. 155–164

Barea, R.; Boquete, L.; Mazo M.; Lopez, E. (2002). System for Assisted Mobility using Eye Movements based on Electrooculography," *IEEE Trans. on Neural Systems and Rehabilitation Engineering*, vol. 10, no. 4, pp. 209–218

Tanaka, K.; Matsunaga, K.; Wang, H. O. (2005). Electroencephalogram-Based Control of an Electric Wheelchair," *IEEE Trans. on Robotics*, vol. 21, no. 4, pp. 762–766

Shima, K.; Eguchi, R.; Shiba, K.; Tsuji, T. (2005). CHRIS: Cybernetic Human-Robot Interface Systems, *Proceedings of 36th International Symposium on Robotics*, WE1C3

Shima, K.; Okamoto, M.; Bu, N.; Tsuji, T. (2006). Novel Human Interface for Game Control Using voluntarily Generated Biological Signals, *Journal of Robotics and Mechatronics*, vol. 18, no. 5, pp. 626–633

Fukuda, O.; Tsuji, T.; Kaneko M.; Otsuka, A. (2003). A Human-Assisting Manipulator Teleoperated by EMG Signals and Arm Motions, *IEEE Trans. on Robotics and Automation*, vol. 19, no. 2, pp. 210–222

Usui, S.; Amidror, I. (1982). Digital Low-Pass Differentiation for Biological Signal Processing, *IEEE Trans. on Biomedical Engineering*, vol. BME-29, no. 10, pp. 686–693

Tsuji, T.; Fukuda, O.; Ichinobe, H.; Kaneko, M. (1999). A Log-Linearized Gaussian Mixture Network and Its Application to EEG Pattern Classification, *IEEE Trans. on Systems, Man, and Cybernetics-Part C: Applications and Reviews*, vol. 29, no. 1, pp. 60–72

Shima, K.; Tsuji, T.; Kan, E.; Kandori, A.; Yokoe, M.; Sakoda S. (2008). Measurement and Evaluation of Finger Tapping Movements Using Magnetic Sensors, *Proceedings of the 30th Annual International Conference of the IEEE Engineering in Medicine and Biology Society*, pp. 5628–5631

Shima, K.; Tsuji, T.; Kandori, A.; Yokoe, M.; Sakoda S. (2008). A Tapping Interface for Finger Movement Training Using Magnetic Sensors, *Proceedings of the 2008 IEEE International Conference on Systems, Man and Cybernetics (SMC 2008)*, pp. 2597–2602

21

Ambulatory monitoring of the cardiovascular system: the role of Pulse Wave Velocity

Josep Solà[1], Stefano F. Rimoldi[2] and Yves Allemann[2]
[1]CSEM – Centre Suisse d'Electronique et de Microtechnique
Switzerland
[2]Swiss Cardiovascular Center Bern, University Hospital
Switzerland

1. Introduction

Currently the leading cause of mortality in western countries, cardiovascular diseases (CVD) are largely responsible for the ever increasing costs of healthcare systems. During the last decade it was believed that the best trade-off between quality and costs of a healthcare system would pass through the promotion of healthy lifestyles, the early diagnosis of CVD, and the implantation of home-based rehabilitation programs. Hence, the development of novel healthcare structures will irremediably require the availability of techniques allowing the monitoring of patients' health status at their homes. Unfortunately, the ambulatory monitoring of the cardiovascular vital parameters has not evolved as required to reach this aim.

To be exploitable in the long term, ambulatory monitors must of course provide reliable vital information, but even more important, they must be comfortable and inconspicuous: whoever has experimented wearing an ambulatory blood pressure monitor (ABPM) for 24 hours understands what cumbersomeness means. Surprisingly, even if intermittent and obtrusive, ABPM prevails nowadays as the single available method to assess a vascular-related index at home. Hence, a clear demand to biomedical engineers arises: healthcare actors and patients require the development of new monitoring techniques allowing the non-invasive, unobtrusive, automatic and continuous assessment of the cardiac and vascular health status. Concerning cardiac health status, the ambulatory measurement of the electrical and mechanical activities of the heart is already possible by the joint analysis of the electrocardiogram, the phonocardiogram and the impedancecardiogram. But surprisingly, little has been proposed so far for the ambulatory monitoring of vascular-related parameters.

Because several studies have recently highlighted the important role that arterial stiffness plays in the development of CVD, and since central stiffness has been shown to be the best independent predictor of both cardiovascular and all-cause mortality, one might suggest stiffness to be the missing vascular-related parameter in ambulatory cardiovascular monitoring. However, the only available technique for measuring arterial stiffness non-invasively so far is the so-called Pulse Wave Velocity (PWV). In this chapter we will see that the state of the art in PWV assessment is not compatible with the requirements of ambulatory monitoring. The goal of our work is thus to examine the limitations of the current techniques, and to explore the introduction of new approaches that might allow PWV to be established as the new gold-standard of vascular health in ambulatory monitoring.

This chapter is organized as follows: in Section 2 we introduce the phenomenon of pulse propagation through the arterial tree. In section 3 we provide a large review on the clinical relevance of aortic stiffness and its surrogate, PWV. In Section 4 we perform an updated analysis of the currently existing techniques available for the non-invasive assessment of PWV. Section 5 describes a novel approach to the measurement of PWV based on a non-obtrusive and unsupervised beat-to-beat detection of pressure pulses at the sternum. Finally, Section 6 reviews the historic and current trends on the use of PWV as a non-obtrusive surrogate for arterial blood pressure.

2. The genesis and propagation of pressure pulses in the arterial tree

In cardiovascular research and clinical practice, PWV refers to the velocity of a pressure pulse that propagates through the arterial tree. In particular, we are interested in those pressure pulses generated during left ventricular ejection: at the opening of the aortic valve, the sudden rise of aortic pressure is absorbed by the elastic aorta walls. Subsequently a pulse wave naturally propagates along the aorta exchanging energy between the aortic wall and the aortic blood flow (Figure 1). At each arterial bifurcation, a fraction of the energy is transmitted to the following arteries, while a portion is reflected backwards. Note that one can easily palpate the arrival of arterial pressure pulses at any superficial artery, such as the temporal, carotid or radial artery: already in the year 1500, traditional chinese medicine performed clinical diagnosis by palpating the arrival of pressure pulses at the radial artery (King et al., 2002). But why do clinicians nowadays get interested on the velocity of such pulses, and especially in the aorta? The reason is that the velocity of propagation of aortic pressure pulses depends on the elastic and geometric properties of the aortic wall. We will show later that while arterial stiffness is difficult to measure non-invasively, PWV is nowadays available *in vivo* to clinicians. Hence, the PWV parameter is an easily-accessible potential surrogate for the constitutive properties of the arterial walls.

In order to provide a better understanding of the biomechanics of pulse propagation, we describe here the commonly accepted model of pulse propagation: the Moens-Korteweg equation. For a complete derivation of the model see (Nichols & O'Rouke, 2005). This model assumes an artery to be a straight circular tube with thin elastic walls, and assumes it being filled with an inviscid, homogeneous and incompressible fluid. Under these hypotheses the velocity of a pressure pulse propagating through the arterial wall is predicted to be:

$$PWV^2 = Eh \; / \; d\rho \tag{1}$$

where E stands for the elasticity of the wall (Young's modulus), h for its thickness, D for its diameter and ρ corresponds to the density of the fluid. Even if this model is only a rough approximation of reality, it provides an intuitive insight on the propagation phenomenon in arteries and, in particular, it predicts that, the stiffer the artery (increased E), the faster a pressure pulse will propagate through it. Therefore, for large elastic arteries such the aorta where the thickness to diameter ratio (h / D) is almost invariable, PWV is expected to carry relevant information related to arterial stiffness.

3. Clinical relevance of Pulse Wave Velocity as a marker of arterial stiffness

We already demonstrated that, from a biomechanical point of view, the velocity of propagation of pressure pulses in large arteries is a surrogate indicator of arterial stiffness. Due to the recent commercialization of semi-automatic devices performing routine measurements of PWV, numerous studies investigating the clinical relevance of arterial stiffness have been conducted during the last decade (Asmar, 1999). In this section we review the most prominent conclusions of these studies. An additional review is given by (Mitchel, 2009).

Cardiovascular disease is the leading cause of morbidity and mortality in western countries and is associated with changes in the arterial structure and function. In particular, arterial stiffening has a central role in the development of such diseases. Nowadays, aortic PWV is considered the gold standard for the assessment of arterial stiffness and is one of the most robust parameters for the prediction of cardiovascular events. Because the structure of the arterial wall differs between the central (elastic) and the peripheral (muscular) arteries, several PWV values are encountered along the arterial tree, with increasing stiffness when moving to the periphery. Because carotid-to-femoral PWV is considered as the standard measurement of aortic arterial stiffness, we will refer to it as simply PWV. In the following we review the most important factors influencing PWV, then we justify the need for a reliable PWV monitoring: on one hand we analyse the pathophysiological consequences of increased arterial stiffness and, on the other hand we highlight the clinical relevance of PWV as an independent marker of cardiovascular risk.

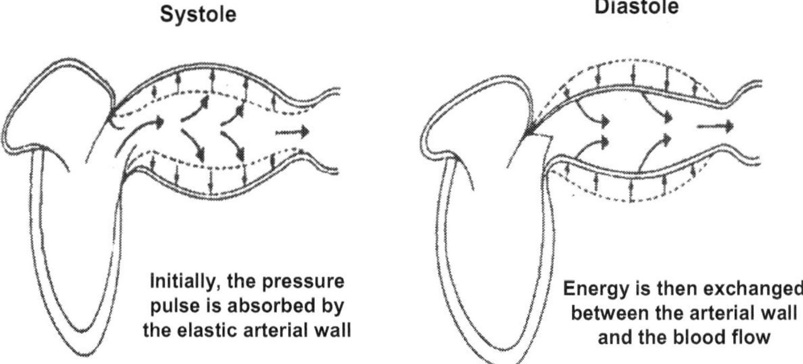

Fig. 1. Genesis of pressure pulses: after the opening of the aortic valve the pulse propagates through the aorta exchanging energy between the aortic wall and the blood flow. Adapted with permission from (Laurent & Cockcroft, 2008).

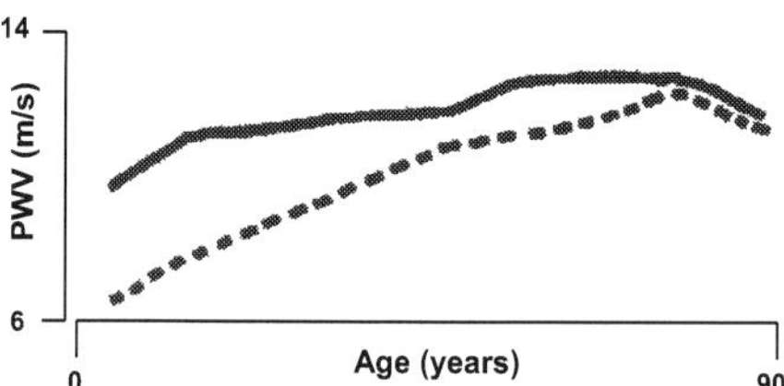

Fig. 2. The dependency of PWV with age for central elastic arteries (dashed line) and peripheral muscular arteries (continuous line). Adapted from (Avolio et al., 1985).

Major determinants of PWV under normal conditions

Before elucidating the role that PWV plays in the generation and diagnosis of pathological situations, it is necessary to understand which are its determinant factors under normal conditions. It is currently accepted that the four major determinants of PWV are age, blood pressure, gender and heart rate.

Age affects the wall proprieties of central elastic arteries (aorta, carotid, iliac) in a different manner than in muscular arteries (brachial, radial, femoral, popliteal). With increasing age the pulsatile strain breaks the elastic fibers, which are replaced by collagen (Faber & Oller-Hou, 1952). These changes in the arterial structure lead to increased arterial stiffness, and consequently to increased central PWV (Figure 2). On the other hand, there is only little alteration of distensibility of the muscular, *i.e.*, distal, arteries with age (Avolio, 1983; Avolio, 1985; Nichols et al., 2008). This fact supports the use of generalized transfer functions to calculate the central aortic pressure wave from the radial pressure wave in adults of all ages, as will be described in Section 4 (Nichols, 2005).

Arterial blood pressure is also a major determinant of PWV. Increased blood pressure is associated with increased arterial stiffness and vice versa. Ejection of blood into the aorta generates a pressure wave that travels along the whole arterial vascular tree. A reflected wave that travels backwards to the ascending aorta is principally generated in the small peripheral resistance arterioles. With increasing arterial stiffness both the forward and the reflected waves propagate more rapidly along the vessels. Consequently, instead of reaching back the aorta during the diastole, the reflected pulse wave reaches it during the systole. This results in an increase of aortic pressure during systole and reduced pressure during diastole, thus leading to an increase of the so-called Pulsatile Pressure (PP) parameter (Figure 3). Asmar (Asmar et al., 2005) studied large untreated populations of normotensive and hypertensive subjects and found that the two major determinants of PWV were age and systolic blood pressure in both groups. This result confirms the close interdependence between systolic blood pressure and arterial stiffness.

Concerning gender, studies in children revealed no gender difference in PWV, whereas in young and middle age, healthy adult men displayed higher PWV values compared to women (London et al., 1995; Sonesson et al., 1993). Indeed premenopausal women show lower carotid-radial PWV values than age-matched men, but carotid-femoral PWV is found to be similar. Once women become postmenopausal, PWV values become similar to those of age-matched men (London, 1995).

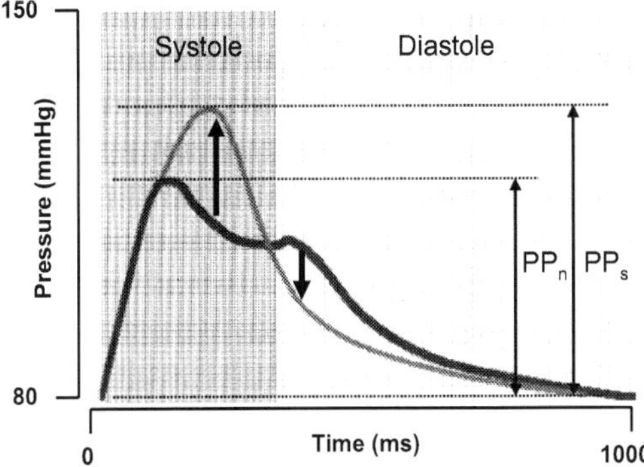

Fig. 3. Consequences of increased arterial stiffness on central blood pressure: increase of systolic and decrease of diastolic central pressures. Pulsatile Pressure is defined as the difference of both pressure amplitudes. PP_n stands for PP under normal conditions and PP_s stands for PP under stiff conditions.

Heart rate is related to PWV through two independent mechanisms. Firstly, heart rate influences PWV because of the frequency-dependant viscoelasticity of the arterial wall: if heart rate increases, the time allowed to the vessels to distend is reduced, resulting in an increased rigidity of the arterial wall. Hence, increasing rate is associated with increasing arterial stiffness. In a recent study, (Benetos et al., 2002) showed that particularly in hypertensive patients increased heart rate was one of the major determinants of accelerated progression of arterial stiffness. Secondly, heart rate is related to PWV through the influence of the sympathetic nervous system: sympathetic activation is associated with increased stiffness of the arteries (Boutouyrie et al., 1994) due to an increase in heart rate, blood pressure and smooth muscle cells tonus.

Why keep arterial stiffness under control?

Up to this point we simply outlined that increased arterial stiffness appears to be normally associated to factors such as aging and blood pressure, among others. As natural as it seems, one might then wonder, why do we need to keep arterial stiffness under controlled (low) values? We will answer this question backwards: what would happen if we did not do so? In other words, we are interested in understanding the pathophysiological consequences of increased arterial stiffness.

Firstly we describe the role of arterial stiffness in the development of endothelial dysfunction. Endothelial dysfunction is the first step in the development of atherosclerosis and plays a central role in the clinical emergence and progression of atherosclerotic vascular disease (Figure 4). The endothelium plays not only an important role in atherogenesis but also in the functional regulation of arterial compliance since endothelial cells release a number of vasoactive mediators such as the vasodilatator nitric oxide (NO) and the vasoconstrictor endothelin. The complex interplay between endothelial function and arterial stiffness leads to a vicious cycle of events, as illustrated in Figure 4 (Dart & Kingwell, 2001).

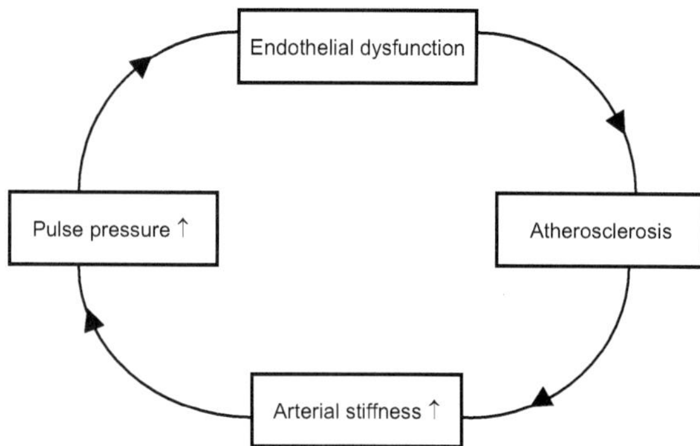

Fig. 4. Vicious circle of events resulting from endothelial dysfunction and augmented arterial stiffness.

Increased arterial stiffness is also an important determinant of myocardium and coronary perfusions. In Figure 3 we already described the mechanism through which increasing arterial stiffness leads to augmented central PP, *i.e.,* the difference between systolic and diastolic aortic pressures. The increase in central systolic pressure is thus associated with an increased afterload, which if persistent, promotes the development of left ventricular (LV) hypertrophy, an independent cardiovascular risk factor (Bouthier et al., 1985; Toprak et al., 2009). Conversely, the decrease in central diastolic pressure compromises myocardial blood supply, particularly in patients with coronary artery stenosis. However, the increased LV-mass induced by the augmented afterload will require an increased oxygen supply. Therefore, a mismatch between oxygen demand and supply may occur, leading to myocardial ischemia, LV diastolic and later systolic dysfunction. The full mechanism is illustrated in Figure 5.

Finally, the widening of central PP induced by increasing arterial stiffness may affect the vascular bed of several end-organs, particularly of brain and kidney. Because both organs are continually and passively perfused at high-volume flow throughout systole and diastole, and because their vascular resistance is very low, pulsations of pressure and flow are directly transmitted to the relatively unprotected vascular bed. By contrast, other organs if exposed to increased PP may protect themselves by vasoconstriction (O'Rourke & Safar, 2005). This unique situation predisposes the brain and kidney to earlier micro- and macrovascular injuries (Laurent et al, 2003; Henskens et al, 2008; Fesler et al., 2007).

Relevance of PWV in clinical conditions
We already described the factors that modify arterial stiffness in normal conditions. We also reviewed the consequences of an increase of arterial stiffness to endothelial function, coronary perfusion and possible damages to heart muscle, brain and kidneys. We are interested in reviewing now the broad uses of PWV as an independent cardiovascular risk factor and its interaction with the others classical risk factors such as arterial hypertension, diabetes mellitus, and dyslipidemia. The independent predictive value of PWV for cardiovascular and all-cause mortality is finally underlined.

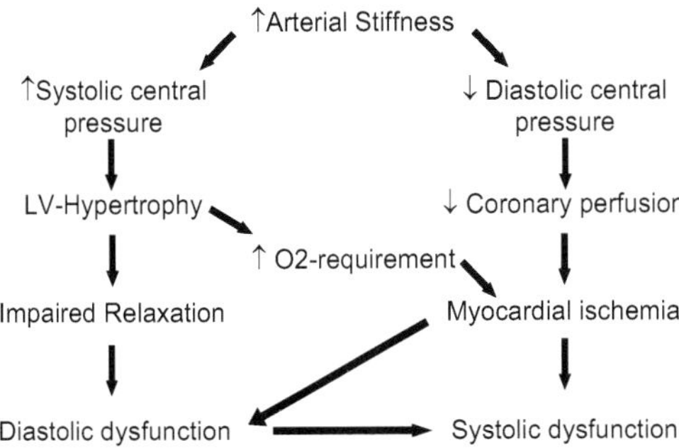

Fig. 5. Effects of increased arterial stiffness on the myocardium and its function.

Structural arterial abnormalities are already observed at an early stage of hypertension. Changes in the structure of the arterial wall, particularly of the matrix and the three-dimensional organization of the smooth muscle cells, have an important impact in determining arterial stiffness. Studies of white-coat hypertension (Glen et al., 1996) and borderline hypertension (Girerd et al, 1989) showed higher values of PWV compared to controls. Moreover, for a similar blood pressure, PWV was higher in patients than in controls, suggesting that the increased PWV was not only due to the elevated blood pressure but also to some structural changes of the arterial wall. As already mentioned, increased arterial stiffness leads to increased central systolic blood pressure, augmented afterload and ultimately left ventricular hypertrophy (Figure 5), which is itself a major cardiovascular risk factor (Bouthier et al., 1985; Lorell et al., 2000). Arterial stiffness and its associated augmented PWV is now recognized as an independent marker of cardiovascular risk (Willum-Hansen et al, 2006; Laurent et al., 2001) especially in hypertensive patients (Mancia et al., 2007).

Diabetes mellitus is one of the major cardiovascular risk factors and has been associated with premature atherosclerosis. There are numerous studies showing that both patients suffering from type 1 diabetes (van Ittersum et al., 2004) and type 2 diabetes (Cruickshank et al., 2002; Schram et al., 2004) have an increased arterial stiffness compared to controls. The increase in arterial stiffening in patients with type 1 and type 2 diabetes mellitus is evident even before clinical micro- and macrovascular complications occur (Giannattasio et al, 1999; Ravikumar et al., 2002), being already present at the stage of impaired glucose tolerance (Henry et al., 2003). Moreover, as in hypertensive patients, increased aortic PWV is identified as an independent predictor of mortality in diabetics (Cruickshank et al., 2002). The increase in arterial stiffness in patients suffering from diabetes mellitus is multifactorial (Creafer et al., 2003) and is associated with structural (Airaksinen et al., 1993) (extracellular matrix), functional (endothelium dysfunction) and metabolic (increased oxidative stress, decreased nitric oxide bioavailability) alterations. The most important mechanism seems to be the glycation of the extracellular matrix with the formation of advanced glycation end-products (AGEs): hyperglycemia favors AGEs formation which is responsible for the altered collagen content of the arterial wall (Airaksinen et al., 1993). A new class of drugs called "AGE breakers" is able to decrease the numbers of collagen cross-links and improve arterial stiffness in both diabetic rats (Wolffenbuttel et al., 1998) and humans (Kass et al., 2001).

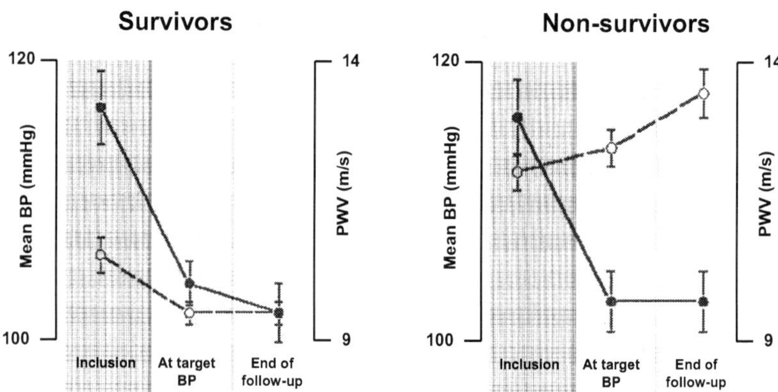

Fig. 6. Changes in mean BP (solid circles) and aortic PWV (open circles) of patients with end-stage renal disease for survivors and non-survivors: despite achievement of target BP non-survivors showed no improvement or even an increase in PWV, demonstrating on the one hand the presence of a pressure-independent component of PWV, and on the other hand, the relevance of PWV as an independent predictor for mortality. Adapted from (Guerin et al., 2001).

The association between lipids and arterial stiffness has been studied since the seventies, but the results are so far controversial. In patients suffering from coronary artery disease (CAD), an association between increased arterial stiffness and higher LDL has been proved (Cameron et al., 1995). On the other hand, in the general population the results regarding the relationship between LDL and arterial stiffness are controversial and some studies have reported a lack of association between total cholesterol and arterial stiffness (Dart et al., 2004).

Acute smoking is associated with increased arterial stiffness in healthy individuals and several patients subgroups, including normotensive, hypertensive and CAD. Studies on the chronic effects of smoking demonstrated contradictory results. However, the largest studies showed that chronic cigarette smoking was associated with increased PWV both in normotensive and hypertensive subjects (Liang et al., 2001; Jatoi et al., 2007).

Arterial hypertension and arterial stiffness induce the same end-organ damages such as coronary artery disease (CAD), cerebrovascular disease (CVD), peripheral artery disease (PAD) and chronic kidney disease (CKD) (Mancia et al., 2002). Many studies showed an association between increased PWV and the severity of CAD (Hirai et al., 1989; Giannattasio et al., 2007), CVD (Laurent et al., 2003; Henskens et al., 2008; Mattace-Raso et al., 2006), PAD (van Popele et al., 2001) and CKD (London et al., 1996; Shinohara et al., 2004).

Beyond its predictive value of morbidity, aortic stiffness appears to be relevant because of its independent predictive value for all-cause and cardiovascular mortality, in patients with arterial hypertension (Laurent et al., 2001), with type-2 diabetes (Cruickshank et al., 2002), with CKD (Blacher et al., 1999), older age (Mattace-Raso et al, 2006; Mcaume et al., 2001; Sutton-Tyrrell et al., 2005) and even in the general population (Willum-Hansen et al., 2006). Figure 6 demonstrates PWV to be a blood-pressure-independent cardiovascular risk factor for patients with end-stage renal disease.

Hence, if it is nowadays accepted (Nilsson et al., 2009) that arterial stiffness and PWV may be regarded as a "global" risk factor reflecting the vascular damage provoked by the different classical risk factors and time, how can we explain its limited use in clinical practice? The main reason seems to be its difficulty to measure. While blood pressure and heart rate are at present easily automatically measured, reliable PWV measurements still require complex recent equipments and, even worse, they require the continuous presence of a skilled well-trained operator.

4. Measuring aortic Pulse Wave Velocity *in vivo*

In the preceding sections we pointed out the need of including a vascular-related parameter into ambulatory monitoring, and we highlighted the clinical relevance of PWV as a surrogate measurement of arterial stiffness. In this section we analyse the strategies and devices that have been so far developed to measure PWV *in vivo*. Although in some cases these techniques rely on rather simplistic physiologic and anatomic approximations, their commercialization has triggered the interest in the diagnostic and prognostic uses of PWV (Boutouyrie et. al., 2009). For the sake of clearness, Table 1 summarizes the different approaches described in this section.

In general, given an arterial segment of length D, we define its PWV as:

$$PWV = D\ /\ PTT \tag{2}$$

where PTT is the so-called Pulse Transit Time, *i.e.*, the time that a pressure pulse will require to travel through the whole segment. Formally PTT is defined as:

$$PTT = PAT_d - PAT_p \tag{3}$$

where PAT_p corresponds to the arrival time of the pressure pulse at the proximal (closer to the heart) extremity of the artery, and PAT_d corresponds to the arrival time of the pressure pulse at its distal (distant to the heart) extremity.

In particular, concerning the aorta, we define PWV as the average velocity of a systolic pressure pulse travelling from the aortic valve (proximal point) to the iliac bifurcation (distal point), as Figure 7 illustrates. Note that this definition concerns the propagation of the pulse through anatomically rather different aortic segments, namely the ascending aorta, the aortic arch and the descending aorta. Accordingly, we re-define aortic PWV as:

$$PWV = (D_{asc} + D_{arch} + D_{desc})/\ PTT_a \tag{4}$$

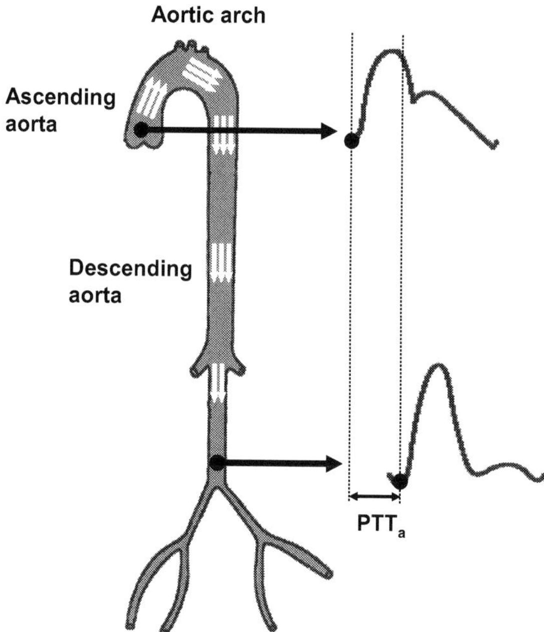

Fig. 7. Aortic PWV is defined as the average velocity of a pressure pulse when travelling from the aortic valve, through the aortic arc until it reaches the iliac bifurcation.

Hence, the *in vivo* determination of aortic PWV is a two-step problem: first one need to detect the arrival times of a pressure pulse at both the ascending aorta and the iliac bifurcation, and secondly one needs to precisely measure the distance travelled by the pulses.

A first group of aortic PWV measurement methods corresponds to those approaches that measure transit times in the aorta in a straight-forward fashion, that is, without relying in any model-based consideration. Because the aorta is not easily accessible by neither optical nor mechanical means, the strategy is to detect the arrival of a pressure pulse at two substitute arterial sites, remaining as close as possible to the aorta (Asmar et al., 1995). Starting from the aorta and moving to the periphery, the first arteries that are accessible are the common carotid arteries (at each side of the neck) and the common femoral arteries (at the upper part of both thighs, near the pelvis). This family of devices assumes thus the carotid-to-femoral transit time to be the best surrogate of the aortic transit time. Currently four commercial automatic devices based on this assumption are available: the Complior (Artech Medical, Paris, France), the Vicorder (Skidmore Medical, Bristol, UK), the SphygmoCor (AtCor Medical, New South Wales, Australia), and the PulsePen (DiaTecne, Milano, Italy). While Complior simultaneously records the arrival of a pressure pulse at the carotid and femoral arteries by means of two pressure sensors (Figure 8), Sphygmocor and PulsePen require performing the two measurements sequentially by means of a single handheld tonometer. A simultaneously recorded ECG supports the post-processing of the data obtained from both measurements (Figure 9). It has been suggested that because measurements are not performed on the same systolic pressure pulses, the SphygmoCor might introduce artifactual PTT variability (Rajzer et al., 2008). Unfortunately, there is so far no consensus on whether the transit times obtained by Complior and SphygmoCor display significant differences (Millasseau et al., 2005; Rajzer et al., 2008). Concerning the estimation of the travelled distance D, each manufacturer provides different and inconsistent recommendations on how to derive D from superficial morphological measurements with a tape (Rajzer et al., 2008). Regrettably Complior, SphygmoCor and PulsePen require the constant presence of a skilled operator who manually localizes the carotid and femoral arteries and holds the pressure sensors during the examination.

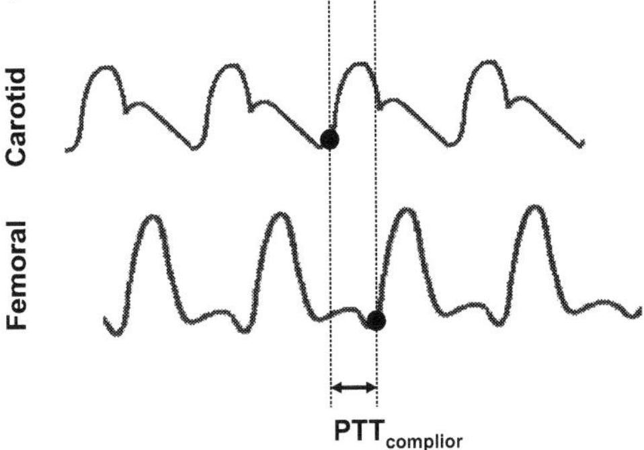

Fig. 8. Pulse transit time (PTT) as measured by Complior. The arrival time of a pressure pulse is simultaneously detected on the carotid and femoral artery. Complior implements as well a correlation-based PTT estimation.

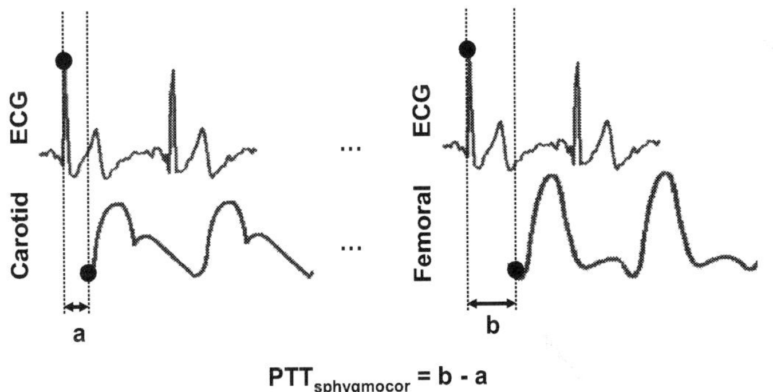

Fig. 9. Pulse transit time (PTT) as measured by SphysgmoCor. The delay between the R-Wave on the ECG and the arrival time of a pressure pulse is sequentially measured on the carotid and the femoral arteries. Both measurements are further combined to obtain a single PTT value.

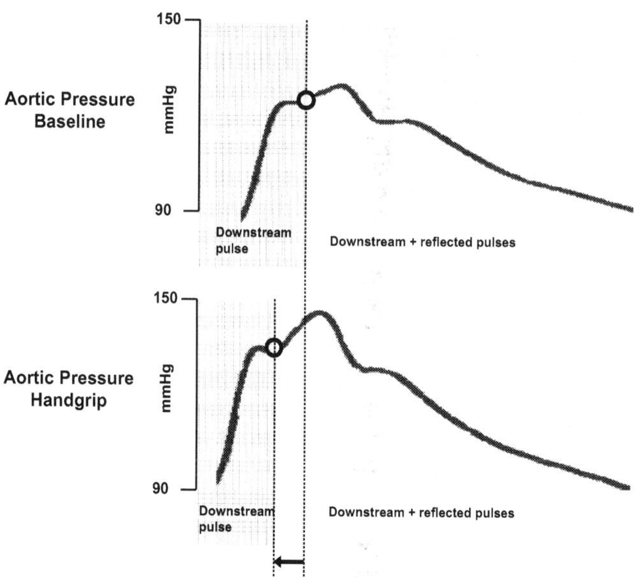

Fig. 10. Time to reflection (Tr) is defined as the arrival time of a pressure pulse that has been reflected in the arterial tree and travels back towards the heart. This example illustrates an important shortening of Tr for a male adult when performing a handgrip effort. During the sustained handgrip, mean arterial pressure is augmented, increasing the stiffness of the aorta and thus aortic PWV. Consequently, the reflected pulse reaches the aortic valve prematurely: Tr is shifted to the left in the bottom pressure pulse.

A second group of devices estimate aortic transit time based on wave reflection theory (Segers et al., 2009). It is generally accepted (Westerhof et al., 2005) that any discontinuity on the arterial tree encountered by a pressure pulse traveling from the heart to the periphery (downstream) will create a reflected wave on the opposite direction (upstream). Main reflection sites in humans are high-resistance arterioles and major arterial branching points. In particular, the iliac bifurcation at the distal extremity of the descending aorta has empirically been shown to be a main source of pulse reflections (Latham et a., 1985). Consequently, a pulse pressure generated at the aortic valve is expected to propagate downstream through the aorta, to reflect at the iliac bifurcation and to propagate upstream towards the heart, reaching its initial point after Tr seconds (Figure 10). Commonly depicted as Time to Reflection, Tr is related to the aortic length (D) and the aortic pulse wave velocity as:

$$Tr = 2\,D/\,PWV \qquad (5)$$

Even though the concept of a unique and discrete reflection point in the arterial tree is not widely accepted and is currently the source of fervent discussions (Nichols, 2009), PWV values derived from the time to reflection method have been shown to be at least positively correlated to PWV measured by Complior, r=0.69 (Baulmann et al., 2008) and r=0.36 (Rajzer et al., 2008).

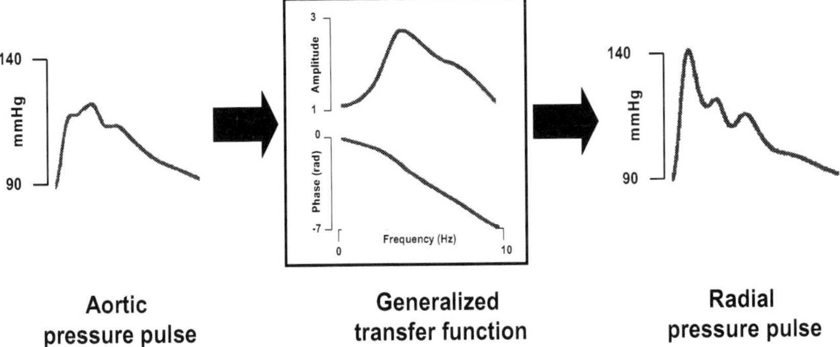

Fig. 11. Example of aortic pressure pulse, radial pressure pulse and the generalized transfer function that relates them. Adapted from (Chen et al., 1997).

Obviously a main issue is how to record aortic pressure pulses non-invasively (Hirata et al., 2006). Two approaches have been proposed so far. A first device, Arteriograph (TensioMed, Budapest, Hungary), records a sequence of pressure pulses at the upper arm by inflating a brachial cuff above systolic pressure, typically 35 mmHg. The brachial pressure waveform is then simply assumed to be a surrogate of the aortic one. Regardless of its manifest lack of methodological formalism, Arteriograph is so far the unique fully automatic and unsupervised commercial available device. Similarly, some recent studies aim at analyzing pressure pulses recorded at the finger to obtain similar results (Millasseau et al., 2006). A second device, SphygmoCor (AtCor Medical, New South Wales, Australia), records pressure pulses at the radial artery by a hand-held tonometer and then estimates an associated aortic pressure pulse by applying a generalized transfer function. In brief, the generalized transfer function approach relies on a series of empirical studies conducted during the 90s in which it was proven that the relationship between aortic and radial pressure pulses is consistent among subjects and unaffected even by aging and drug action (O'Rourke, 2009). Consequently, transfer functions provide a method for universally estimating aortic pressure pulses from radial artery measurements in a non-invasive fashion. Figure 11 illustrates the modulus and phase of the widely accepted aortic-to-radial general transfer function (Chen, et al. 1997). Large population studies (Gallagher et al., 2004) and numerical models of the arterial tree (Karamanoglu et al., 1995) have shown that the generalized transfer function is indeed consistently unchanged for frequencies below 5 Hz.

A third group of approaches comprises those developments based on the R-wave-gated pulse transit time. In brief, this technique exploits the strength of the ECG signal on the human body, and assumes its R-wave to trigger the genesis of pressure pulses in the aorta, at time $T_{R\text{-wave}}$. Then, by detecting the arrival time of a pressure pulse on a distal location (PAT_d) one calculates:

$$PTT_{R\text{-wave}} = PAT_d - T_{R\text{-wave}} \tag{6}$$

Unfortunately the physiological hypothesis relating $PTT_{R\text{-}wave}$ to PWV neglects the effects of cardiac isovolumetric contraction: indeed, after the onset of the ventricle depolarization (R-Wave in the ECG) left ventricles start contracting while the aortic valve remains closed. It is only when the left ventricle pressure exceeds the aortic one, that the aortic valve opens and generates the aortic pressure pulse. The introduced delay is commonly known as Pre-Ejection Period (PEP) and depends on physiological variables such as cardiac preload, central arterial pressure, and cardiac contractibility (Li & Belz, 1993). Hence, $PTT_{R\text{-}wave}$ is to be corrected for the delay introduced by PEP as proposed in (Payne et al., 2006):

$$PTT'_{R\text{-}wave} = PAT_d - (T_{R\text{-}wave} + PEP) \tag{7}$$

Several strategies to assess PEP non-invasively are nowadays available, mainly based on the joint analysis of the ECG (Berntson et al., 2004) and either an impedance cardiogram or a phono-cardiogram (Lababidi et al., 1970; DeMarzo & Lang, 1996; Ahlström 2008). Nevertheless, even obviating the PEP correction, $PTT_{R\text{-}wave}$ has been shown to be correlated with PWV (r=0.37) (Abassade & Baudouy, 2002) and systolic blood pressure (r=0.64) (Payne et al. 2006). Concerning the distal detection of the pressure pulse arrival time (PAT_d), different approaches have been proposed so far. We describe here the most relevant ones. Novacor (Cedex, France) commercializes an ambulatory method to monitor PWV based on a fully automatic auscultatory approach: the so-called Qkd index. Qkd is defined as the time interval between the R-Wave on the ECG and the second Korotkoff sound detected on an inflated brachial cuff. The device is currently being used to evaluate long-term evolution of systemic sclerosis in large population studies (Constans et al., 2007). A different technology, photo-plethysmography, is probably the approach that has given rise to the largest number of research developments and studies in the field (Naschitz et al., 2005). Being non-obtrusive and cheap, this technology consists in illuminating a human perfused tissue with an infra-red light source and to analyse the changes in absorption due to arterial pulsatility (Allen, 2007). Each time a pressure pulse reaches the illuminated region, the absorption of light is increased due to a redistribution of volumes in the arterial and capillary beds. The analysis of temporal series of light absorption then allows the detection of the arrival of the pressure pulse. Regrettably, to obtain reliable photo-plethysmographic signals is not a simple task and, so far, only those body locations displaying very rich capillary beds have been exploited: namely the finger tips or phalanxes (Smith et al., 1999; Fung et al. 2004; Schwartz, 2004; Muehlsteff et al., 2006, Banet, 2009), the toes (Sharwood-smith et al., 2006; Nitzan et al., 2001) and the ear lobe (Franchi et al, 1996). Undoubtedly, the listed locations correspond to the classical placement of probes for pulse oximetry, or SpO2, in clinical practice (Webster, 1997). It is to be highlighted that recent studies have investigated the feasibility of performing pulse oximetry at innovative regions such as the sternum (Vetter et al., 2009). To reduce the cumbersomeness of measuring ECG has also been the aim of recent researches: a capacitively-coupled ECG mounted on a chair has been recently proposed to monitor $PTT_{R\text{-}wave}$ in computer users (Kim et al., 2006).

Finally, an emerging non-invasive technique remains to be cited, although its implantation in ambulatory monitoring seems nowadays unfeasible: the phase-contrast MR imaging (PCMRI) (Lotz et al., 2002). PCMRI opens the possibility to perform local measurements of PWV for any given segment of the aorta, by simply defining two regions of interest on the image: a proximal and a distal region. By analysing the evolution of the regional blood flow velocity in each region, one determines the arrival times (PTT_p and PTT_d) of the pressure pulse. Because the distance between both aortic regions (D) can now be precisely measured, this approach is expected to provide highly accurate regional aortic PWV measurements. PCMRI was already introduced in the 90s (Mohiaddin et al., 1989), but the recent advances in MRI capturing rates seem to be encouraging the apparition of new studies (Boese et al., 2000; Gang et al., 2004; Laffon et al., 2004; Giri et al., 2007; Butlin et al., 2008). Fitting in the same category, some studies have been published on the assessment of PAT_d by means of ultrasound Doppler probes (Baguet et al. 2003; Meinders et al., 2001; Jiang et al., 2008).

Note that we have intentionally skipped from our analysis some works that have been performed on the tracking of pressure pulses artificially induced to the arterial wall by mechanical oscillators (Nichols & O'Rourke, 2005). Similarly, we have excluded those works based on the analysis of pressure-diameter and flow-diameter measurements (Westerhof et al., 2005).

Segments of the arterial tree	Method	Measurements of PTT and *D*	AMB	COM
	Carotid to Femoral PTT (simultaneous)	PTT is measured by two pressure sensors placed over the carotid and femoral arteries. *D* is estimated from superficial morphologic measurements.	No	Complior Vicorder
	Carotid to Femoral PTT (sequential)	PTT is measured by a single pressure sensor placed sequentially over the carotid and femoral arteries. ECG is used for synchronization purposes. *D* is estimated from superficial morphologic measurements.	No	SpyhgmoCor PulsePen
	Time to reflection, from brachial pressure pulse	PTT is measured by extracting Tr from the brachial pressure pulse recorded by a brachial obtrusive cuff. *D* is estimated from superficial morphologic measurements.	Yes	Arteriograph
	Time to reflection, from radial pressure pulse (generalized transfer function)	The aortic pressure pulse is estimated by applying a generalized transfer function to a radial pressure pulse recorded by a handheld tonometer. PTT is measured from the associated Tr. D is estimated from superficial morphologic measurements.	No	SphygmoCor

	ECG to brachial pulse transfer time	PTT is approximated as the delay between the R-Wave at the ECG, and the arrival of the pressure pulse at the brachial artery, recorded by a brachial obtrusive cuff. D is estimated from superficial morphologic measurements	Yes	NovaCor
	ViSi	PTT is approximated as the delay between the R-Wave at the ECG, and the arrival of the pressure pulse at the digital artery, recorded by photo-plethysmography. D is estimated from superficial morphologic measurements	Yes	-
	MR Imaging of aortic blood flow	PTT is measured by detecting the arrival of the pressure pulse at two or more different aortic sites, associated to different regions of interest in the PCMR images. D is accurately determined from the images.	No	-
	Sequential Doppler measurements of aortic blood flow	PTT is measured by detecting the arrival of the pressure pulse at two or more different aortic sites, by performing ECG-gated Doppler measurements. D is estimated from superficial morphologic measurements	No	-

Table 1. Summary of most relevant approaches to measure aortic PWV. Detailed descriptions are available on the text. PTT stands for Pulse Transit Time, D for distance, AMB for ambulatory compatibility, and COMM for commercial devices.

Determination of Pulse Arrival Times

Up to this point we assumed that detecting the arrival time of a pressure pulse at a certain aortic site was an obivous operation. Yet, clinical experience has shown that this is not the case: given a pressure pulse recorded either by tonometry, photo-plethysmography or any other measurement technique, it is not straight-forward to objectively define its Pulse Arrival Time, or PAT (Chiu et al., 1991; Solà et al., 2009). In the past, originally based on the analysis of pressure pulses obtained from cardiac catheterization, PAT was proposed to be estimated by identifying a collection of characteristic points (Chiu et al., 1991). Simply stated, a characteristic point is a typical feature that is expected to be found in any pressure pulse waveform. In particular one is interested in those features describing the position of the wavefront of a pulse. The justification is rather simple: on one hand the wavefront is the most patent representative feature of the arrival time of a pulse (Chiu et al., 1991), and on the other hand it is expected to be free of deformations created by reflected waves, thus maintaining its identity while propagating through the arterial tree. Conversely, any other feature of the pressure pulse waveform cannot be assigned an identity in a straight-forward manner (Westerhof et al., 2005).

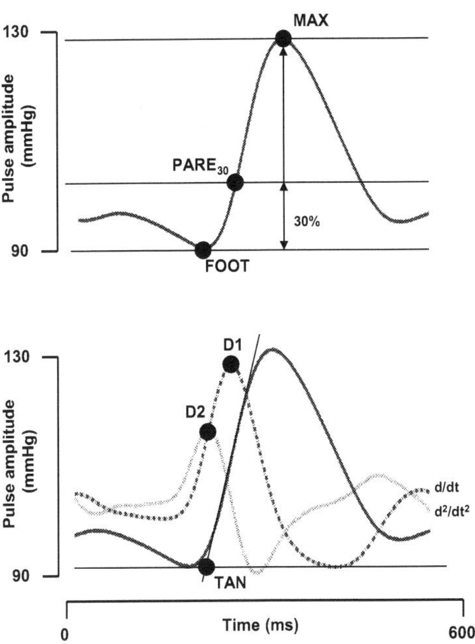

Fig. 12. Characteristic points encountered on a pressure pulse (bold curve) according to state-of-the-art definitions. Time zero corresponds to the R-Wave of a simultaneously recorded ECG.

Hence, the state-of-the-art extraction of characteristic points relies on the morphologic analysis of the wavefront of pressure pulses. The analysis is commonly based on empirically-determined rules, as illustrated in Figure 12. For the sake of completeness, we briefly describe them: the foot of a pressure pulse (FOOT) is defined as the last minimum of the pressure waveform before the beginning of its upstroke. In (Chiu et al., 1991) an iterative threshold-and-slope technique to robustly detect FOOT was proposed. The partial amplitude on the rising edge of the pulse (PARE) is defined as the location at which the pressure pulse reaches a certain percentage of its foot-to-peak amplitude. The maximum of the pressure pulse (MAX) is defined as the time at which the pressure pulse reaches it maximum amplitude. The maximum of the first derivative (D1) is defined as the location of the steepest rise of the pressure pulse. The first derivative is commonly computed using the central difference algorithm in order to reduce noise influences (Mathews & Fink, 2004). The maximum of the second derivative (D2) is defined as the location of the maximum inflection point of the pressure pulse at its anacrotic phase. Finally, the intersecting tangent (TAN) is defined as the intersection of a tangent line to the steepest segment of the upstroke, and a tangent line to the foot of the pressure pulse. Nowadays TAN is the characteristic point commonly implemented in commercial devices such as SphygmoCor.

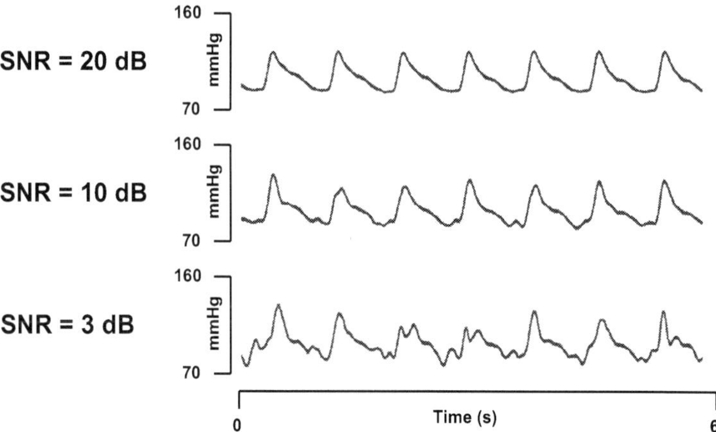

Fig. 13. Six seconds of simulated photo-plethysmographic signals, corresponding to different signal-to-noise scenarios. Noise model according to (Hayes & Smith, 1998).

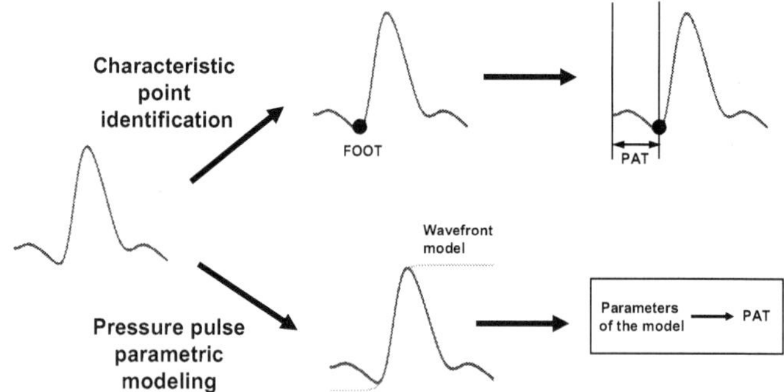

Fig. 14. Given a pressure pulse, the state-of-the-art strategy consists on determining its Pulse Arrival Time (PAT) by identifying a characteristic point on its waveform. The novel parametric approach consists in modeling the whole pulse wavefront, and to extract from this model a PAT-related index. While highly correlated (r=0.99), the robustness to noise is five times higher.

Unfortunately, when targeting ambulatory applications, one must consider that the recording of pressure pulses is severely affected by measurement and artefact noises, with signal to noise ratios (SNR) reaching values below 10dB. In order to illustrate the influence of such noises on the waveform analysis of pressure pulses, Figure 13 displays a series of simulated photo-plethysmographic recordings to which noises of different amplitudes have been introduced (Hayes & Smith, 1998). Unquestionably, the straight-forward identification of state-of-the-art characteristic points under such noisy conditions leads to erratic and unrepeatable results (Solà et al., 2009).

A common strategy to reduce the influence of noise in the determination of PAT is the pre-processing of the raw recorded data. Commercial PWV devices mostly rely on the so-called ensemble averaging approach (Hurtwitz et al. 1990), that is, by assuming the source of pressure pulses (*i.e.* the heart) to be statistically independent from the source of noise, the averaging of N consecutive pressure pulses is expected to increase the signal-to-noise ratio by a factor of $\sqrt{N}$. However, the main drawback of such an approach is that while increasing N, one eliminates any information concerning short-term cardiovascular regulation: by instance, the Complior device requires averaging at least 10 heart cycles, blurring thus any respiration-related information contained into PWV. To overcome the smoothing effects of ensemble averaging some authors have explored the use of innovative pre-processing strategies based either on ICA denoising (Foo, 2008), neighbor PCA denoising (Xu et al., 2009), sub-band frequency decomposition (Okada et al., 1986), or ECG-assisted projection on local principal frequency components (Vetter et al., 2009). The main limitation is that, in order to preserve information on the original arrival time, any pre-processing operator applied to the raw pressure pulse signals must by designed to control any source of (phase) distortions.

According to this principle we have recently proposed a novel PAT estimation approach (Solà et al., 2009): instead of initially de-noising the raw pressure pulse, we design a robust PAT detector that minimizes the need of pre-processing, and thus works on a real beat-to-beat basis (Figure 14). The so-called parametric PAT estimation relies on the analysis of the whole wavefront of the pressure pulse, rather than searching for a punctual feature on it. The approach consists on initially fitting a parametric model to the pressure pulse wavefront and then on obtaining arrival time information from the parameters of the model. The correlation analysis performed on more than 200 hours of photo-plethysmographic data has shown that the new parametric approach highly correlates with the state-of-the-art characteristic points D1 (r=0.99) and TAN (r=0.96) when hyperbolic models were used. Concerning the robustness to noise, the parametric approach has been shown to improve the temporal resolution of PAT estimations by at least a five-fold factor (Solà et al., 2009).

5. Towards the ambulatory monitoring of Pulse Wave Velocity

The review of existing technologies in Table 1 highlights the current lack of approaches allowing the ambulatory non-obtrusive monitoring of aortic PWV. So far, the only commercial devices that might be considered as being ambulatory-compatible rely on the use of brachial cuffs, and hence require a pneumatic inflation each time a measurement is to be performed (Arteriograph and NovaCor). Other devices (Complior, SphygmoCor and PulsePen) are limited to clinical uses because they require the supervision of a well-trained operator. Moreover in ambulatory scenarios one must additionally consider the important role of hydrostatic pressure: while in supine position variations of hydrostatic pressure through the arterial tree are negligible, at standing or sitting positions the pressure gradient from the iliac bifurcation to the aortic arch can reach values of almost 60 mmHg, *i.e.* about 75 mmHg par meter of altitude difference (Westerhof et al., 2005). Therefore, because PWV is affected by blood pressure to a high degree, changes in patient position would severely affect PWV measurements in setups such as Complior, SphygmoCor or PulsePen. Although a few methods for compensating for punctual hydrostatic pressure changes have been proposed in the past in the field of ambulatory blood pressure monitoring (Hiroyuki Ota & Kenji Taniguchi, 1998; Mccombie et al., 2006), these cannot be applied to PWV for two reasons. Firstly, because contrary to blood pressure, PWV is not a point measurement but a distributed one, depicting propagation properties of a whole segment of the arterial tree. Secondly, because there is no one-to-one relationship between pressure and PWV changes, different unknown factors playing important roles as depicted by the Moens-Korteweg model in Equation 1.

In conclusion, there is a lack of methods that provide aortic PWV measurements automatically, continuously and in a non-obtrusive way, while remaining unaffected by changes in body position. A novel approach fulfilling these requirements is currently under investigation at CSEM, based on the continuous measurement of transit times of a pressure pulse when travelling from the Aortic Valve to the Sternum, the so-called av2sPTT. We describe now the benefits of introducing such an approach in ambulatory monitoring.

From a metrological perspective, the av2sPTT parameter is prone to be assessed continuously and non-obtrusively, a possible measurement setup being a textile harness mounted on the thorax. In particular we are working on a harness that integrates two dry ECG electrodes, a phono-cardiograph and a multi-channel photo-plethysmograph. While the joint analysis of the ECG and the phono-cardiogram provides information on the opening of the aortic valve (Alhstrom, 2008), the ECG-supported processing of the multi-channel photo-plethysmograph provides information on the arrival of the pressure pulse at the sternum (Vetter et al., 2009). Hence, PTT values are obtained through Equation 7. Note that for assessing av2sPTT none of the implemented sensing technologies requires the inflation of any cuff, and thus the approach remains fully non-obtrusive.

From a physiological perspective, the clinical relevance of the av2sPTT parameter is supported by a simple anatomical model of the arterial tree (Figure 15). In Table 2 we have detailed the arterial segments through which a pulse pressure propagates before reaching the sternum, together with the expected delays introduced at each segment. Typical PWV values have been obtained from (Nichols & O'Rourke, 2005) and (Acar et al., 1991). According to the model, the timing information contained into the av2sPTT parameter is expected to be 85% related to large vessels (aortic and carotid) and only 15% related to conduit arteries (internal thoracic artery). In other words, the arrival time of a pressure pulse at the sternum is mainly expected to be determined by the propagation through large vessels, and only minimally affected by secondary muscular arteries.

The simple anatomical model in Table 2 foresees that the av2sPTT parameter should be a good surrogate for arterial PTT, the incidence of central elastic arteries in the total measured PTT being of 85%. The statistical consistence of such an approach has not been validated yet, and it is currently under investigation: the results of a validation study will be published in the future.

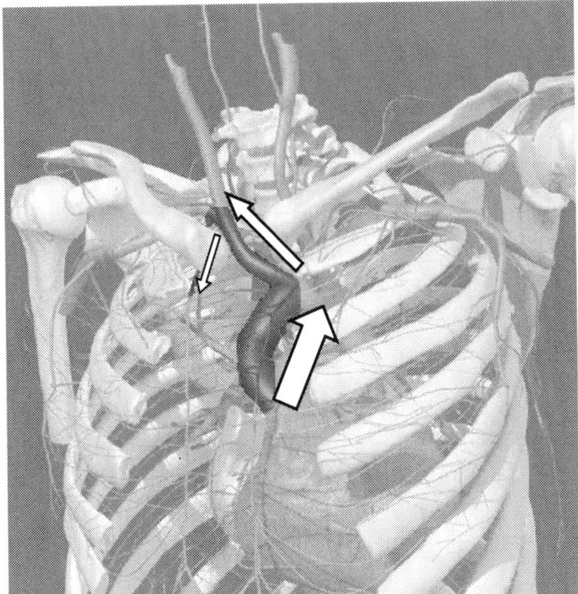

Fig. 15. 3D model of arterial segments involved in the measurement of av2sPTT: the pressure pulse propagates through the ascending aorta, the aortic arch, the brachiocephalic trunk and the internal thoracic artery. 3D model courtesy and copyright from Primal Pictures Ltd.

Ascending aorta and aortic arch	4.8 m/s	7 cm	15 ms
Brachiocephalic trunk	5.1 m/s	10 cm	20 ms
Internal thoracic artery (mammary)	8.5 m/s	5 cm	6 ms

Table 2. Propagation delays for the different arterial segments involved in the av2sPTT parameter.

In the following, we illustrate the potential use of the av2sPTT parameter as a method for the unsupervised continuous non-obtrusive monitoring of aortic PWV. The experiment consisted in sixty minutes of continuous recording on a healthy male subject on whom we simultaneously assessed the av2sPTT parameter and a carotid-to-radial PTT, obtained by a Complior device (Artech Medical, Paris, France). Beat-to-beat blood pressure was measured as well by a PortaPres device (FMS, Amsterdam, The Netherlands). During the experiment, three types of stresses were induced to the subject aiming at increasing his aortic stiffness, and thus to decrease the measured PTT values. The stresses were, by chronological order: an arithmetic task stress, a sustained handgrip test and a cold stress test. Finally, the influence of muscular arteries on the av2sPTT parameter was tested by the oral administration of 250µg isosorbid-dinitrate (UCB-Pharma, Bulle, Switzerland). Isosorbid-dinitrate is expected to create a dilatation of conduit arteries, and thus to augment av2sPTT because of the propagation through the internal thoracic artery. As depicted in Figure 16, av2sPTT was successfully decreased by all three stresses, in accordance with the Complior measurements. As one would expect (Payne et al., 2006), the decrease of PTT coincided with a marked increase of blood pressure. After administrating isosorbid-dinitrate, both Complior and av2sPTT detected an increase of PTT even if systolic blood pressure remained unchanged. Overall, a correlation coefficient of r=0.89 was encountered between the n=9 Complior measurements and the synchronous av2sPTT estimations. Although this experiment confirmed the hypothesis underlying the av2sPTT measurement principle, larger populations are required to validate the approach.

In conclusion, a novel method of assessing aortic PWV has been proposed that can be measured continuously (beat-by-beat), automatically (*i.e.* unsupervised) and non-obtrusively, thus paving the way towards the ambulatory measurement of PWV. Even more, since the measurement site is located at the sternum, perturbations due to hydrostatic pressure changes at different body positions have been minimized. Although high correlation with aortic PWV has been demonstrated from a theoretical perspective, statistically consistent data on the reliability of the approach is still missing.

6. Pulse Wave Velocity as a surrogate of mean arterial pressure

During the last 20 years a lot has been written on the use of PWV as a surrogate of arterial blood pressure (BP). The current lack of non-obtrusive devices for measuring BP has probably awakened the interest on this particular use of the PWV parameter. Yet, no commercial device has so far been released on the market. We present here the basics of this approach and we analyse the obstacles that researches are currently facing.

Historically, the dependency of PWV with respect to blood pressure was already observed in 1905 by Frank (Frank, 1905), although the underlying mechanism was not fully understood until half a century later (Hughes et al., 1979). We already described that PWV depends on arterial stiffness, and we introduced a mathematical model for this relationship: the Moens-Korteweg equation (Equation 1). Accordingly, the greater the stiffness of an artery, the faster a pressure pulse will propagate through it. Assume now that we increase the transmural pressure of the arterial wall, for instance by increasing systemic blood pressure. Because of the elastic properties of the wall, the artery will increase in diameter and decrease in thickness, while becoming stiffer. Additionally, at a certain point the recruitment of collagen fibers will start and will enhance the stiffness in a highly non-linear way (Nichols & O'Rourke, 2005). Hence, the stiffness of the arterial wall will depict a strong dependence to its transmural pressure. Putting now the two puzzle pieces together, we conclude that an increase of blood pressure will raise arterial stiffness and thus, increase PWV. Unfortunately, the relationship blood pressure - arterial stiffness - PWV is not unique, and several other parameters play important roles, as illustrated by Figure 17.

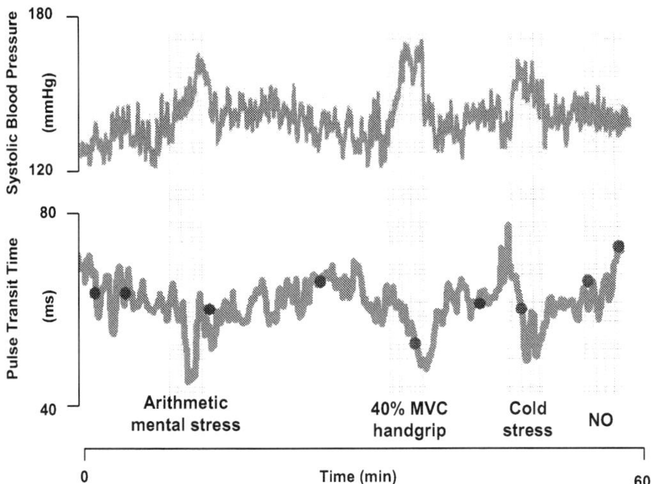

Fig. 16. Example of sixty minutes of non-invasive cardiovascular monitoring performed on a healthy male subject. The upper figure plots the evolution of systolic blood pressure as recorded by PortaPres. The lower figure shows continuous av2sPTT measurements (bold line) and simultaneous Carotid-to-Radial Complior measurements (black dots). Aortic Pulse Transit Time was altered during the experiment through different stress tasks.

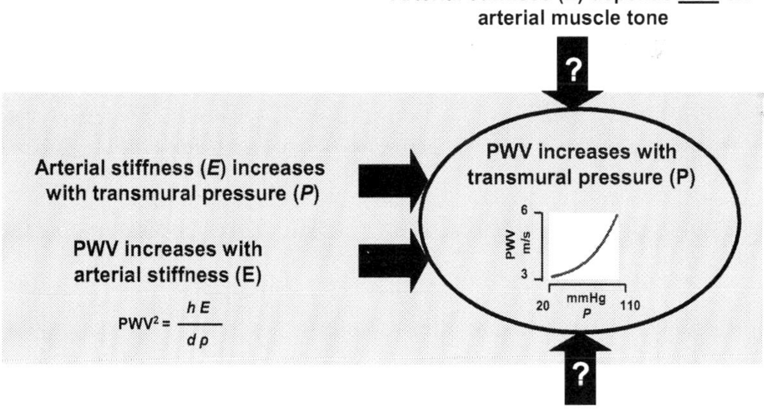

Fig. 17. Under controlled situations, increasing the transmural pressure (P) of an artery increases its stiffness (E), and consequently augments its PWV. Unfortunately other factors such as arterial muscular tonus and geometric modifications influence PWV as well.

A prominent study published in 2006 analyzed the dependency of PTT with respect to blood pressure for 12 subjects to whom vasoactive drugs were administered (Payne et al., 2006). The goal of the experiment was to quantify how the predictive capacities of PTT were degraded by drug alterations of arterial stiffness. All subjects and all drug conditions confounded, Payne still found that PTT was correlated with Diastolic Blood Pressure (DBP) with r=0.64. However, when "speaking in mmHg" this correlation appeared to be insufficient. Assuming that one would generate a calibration function for each subject in order to use PTT measurements to predict DBP, one would obtain a BP measurement device classed as "grade D" according to the British Society of Hypertension (BSH) (O'Brien et al., 2001), the cumulative percentage of readings falling within 5 mmHg, 10 mmHg and 15 mmH of actual DBP values being 44%, 66% and 73% respectively. Consequently, following the BSH directives, a PTT-based blood pressure monitor should not be recommended.

Nevertheless, the dependency of PWV versus blood pressure has still been shown to be sufficiently dominant to be statistically exploitable under standard conditions (Poon & Zhang, 2005; Meigas et al., 2006; Foo et al., 2006). In this sense, and especially because of the expected clinical and commercial impact of a non-obtrusive BP monitor, promising research works and developments have been released in the past years. We now review the most relevant ones.

A good illustrative development of the state-of-the-art is that of (Chen et al., 2000): assuming that the factors that may interfere with the relationship blood pressure - PWV have slow time dynamics, *i.e.* slower than actual blood pressure changes, Chen investigated the use of a hybrid BP monitor: while a brachial oscillometric cuff regularly inflated to perform reference BP measurements, continuous PTT measurements were performed through a non-obtrusive ECG-fingertip approach. Chen then proposed to use the PTT series to interpolate the BP intermittent readings, beat-by-beat. Such a setup still demanded the use of brachial cuffs, but was a first step towards the non-obtrusive beat-to-beat BP monitoring. With this setup, Chen analyzed 42 hours of data on 20 subjects and obtained BSH cumulative percentages of 38.8%, 97.8% and 99.4%. Note that Chen did not account for PEP changes in his measurements, and that therefore, his results might have been improved.

Hence, PWV-based methods rely nowadays on the mapping of measured PTT values (in ms) to estimated BP values (in mmHg) through some initial or intermittent calibrations performed by oscillometric brachial cuffs (Steptoe et al., 1976). Several different calibration strategies and techniques have been described so far, mainly based on the use of neural networks (Barschdorff et al., 2000), linear regressions (Park et al., 2005; Kim et al., 2007; Poon & Zhang, 2008), model-based functions (Chen et al. 2003; Yan & Zhang, 2007) or hydrostatic-induced changes (McCombie et al., 2007).

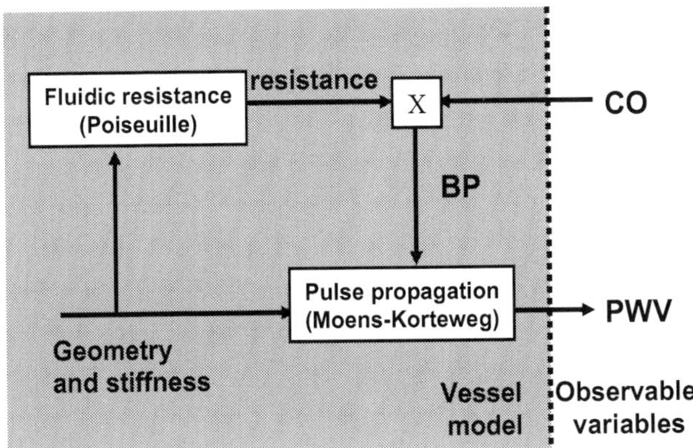

Fig. 18. When estimating BP from PWV measurements, we suggest accounting for changes of arterial geometry and stiffness in order to reduce the frequency of calibrations (Sola et al., 2008). The proposed model requires introducing Cardiac Output (CO) as an additional parameter.

In 2008 we proposed a novel approach aiming at reducing the frequency of these calibrations (Sola et al., 2008). Assuming that the major source of calibration modifications are the changes of diameter and stiffness of conduit arteries (Madero, et al., 2003), we proposed a technique that compensates for these changes without necessitating additional calibrations. In order to do so, the technique requires the continuous measurement of both PWV and Cardiac Output (CO), and assumes a Moens-Korteweg-like model of pulse wave propagation together with a Poiseuille's model of fluidic resistance (Figure 18). The most likely BP value is then computed by solving:

$$BP = \mathrm{argmin}_{BP}\, d\,(PWV_m, PWV_p(CO, BP)\,) \qquad (8)$$

that is, by finding the BP value that makes the measured PWV_m to be as close as possible to the PWV_p predicted by the model (given BP and CO). A distance metric (d) between two series of PWV measurements needs to be previously defined. Although the approach has been shown to reliably provide BP measurements even during induced vasoconstriction (Sola et al., 2008), its consistency in large population studies remains to be demonstrated.

In conclusion, the use of PWV as a surrogate for blood pressure appears to be justified under controlled conditions, that is, when the effects of vasomotion can be neglected. Unfortunately, the ambulatory monitoring of PWV currently passes through the detection of pressure pulses at distal sites such as the radial artery, or the fingertip. Because such measurement setups involve the propagation of pressure pulses through conduit arteries, the effects of vasomotion are, at least, unfavorable. The ideal solution would pass through the monitoring of PWV of proximal arteries only. However, as we demonstrated, there is currently no available technology capable of providing ambulatory very-proximal (*i.e.* aortic) PWV measures. The development of novel technologies as the herein presented aortic valve-to-sternum PTT (Figure 15) might provide great chances for the implantation of PWV into the field of portable BP monitoring.

7. Conclusion and outlook

The continuous ambulatory monitoring of cardiac and vascular functions is a clear requirement for the deployment of the new generation of healthcare structures. Unfortunately, there is so far no technology available for the non-obtrusive measurement of vascular-related health status. The recent spread of automatic devices for the measurement of aortic PWV has promoted numerous research studies on the clinical uses of PWV. Widely accepted as a surrogate for arterial stiffness, PWV appears to be an independent global marker of vascular damage risk. In this chapter we reviewed the major clinical findings and we analyzed the developed technologies. The results suggest that PWV could be promoted as a candidate to fill in the gap of vascular-related health indexes. However, the state-of-the-art in PWV measurement is currently inappropriate for the ambulatory monitoring of arterial stiffness. Therefore, we propose a novel aortic PWV measurement approach that can be integrated into a chest belt and that fulfils the requirements of continuity (beat-by-beat) and non-obtrusiveness. The strategy relies on measuring the transit time of pressure pulses from the opening of the aortic valve to their arrival at the sternum capillaries. In contrast with existing techniques, the new approach does not require the presence of skilled operators, and is expected to minimize the influences of hydrostatic pressure interferences due to postural changes.

Independently of the actual measurement approach, aortic PWV might in the near future play a central role in the diagnosis and follow up of cardiovascular diseases. It is in this context that the coordinated work of biomedical engineers and clinicians will determine to which extent PWV will be able to penetrate into clinical and medical practice.

8. References

Abassade, P. & Baudouy, Y. (2002). Relationship between arterial distensibility and left ventricular function in the timing of Korotkoff sounds (QkD internal). An ambulatory pressure monitoring and echocardiographic study. *American Journal of Hypertension,* 15, 4, (2002) 67A

Acar, C.; Jebara, V. A.; Portoghèse, M.; Fontaliran, F.; Dervanian, P.; Chachques, J. C., Meininger, V. & Carpentier, A. (1991). Comparative anatomy and histology of the radial artery and the internal thoracic artery. *Surg Radiol Anat,* 13, (1991) 283-288

Ahlström, C. (2008). *Nonlinear Phonocardiographic Signal Processing,* Linköpings Universitet, 978-91-7393-947-8, Linköping, Sweden

Airaksinen, K.E.; Salmela, P.I.; Linnaluoto, M.K.; Ikaheimo, M.J.; Ahola, K & Ryhanen, L.J. (1993) Diminished arterial elasticity in diabetes: association with fluorescent advanced glycosylation end products in collagen. *Cardiovasc Res,* 27 (1993) 942-945

Allen, J. (2007). Photoplethysmography and its application in clinical physiological measurement. *Physiol Meas,* 28, (2007) R1-R39

Asmar, R. (1999). *Arterial Stiffness and Pulse Wave Velocity. Clinical Applications,* ELSEVIER, 2-84299-148-6

Asmar, R.; Beneros, A.; Topouchian, J.; Laurent, P.; Pannier, B. Brisac, A.; Target, R. & Levy, B. (1995). Assessment of Arterial Distensibiliy by Automatic Pulse Wave Velocity Measurement. *Hypertension,* 26, 3, (1995) 485-490

Avolio, A.P.; Deng, F. Q.; Li, W. Q. et al. (1985) Effects of aging on arterial distensibility in populations with high and low prevalence of hypertension: comparison between urban and rural communities in China. *Circulation*, 71 (1985) 202-210

Avolio, AP; Chen, SG; Wang, R.P.; Zhang, C.L.; Li, M.F. & O'Rourke, M.F. (1983) Effects of aging on changing arterial compliance and left ventricular load in a northern Chinese urban community. *Circulation*, 68, (1983) 50-58

Baguet, J.; Kingwell, B. A.; Dart, A. L; Shaw, J.; et al. (2003). Analysis of the regional pulse wave velocity by Doppler: methodology and reproducibility. *J Human Hypertension*, 17, (2003) 407-412

Banet, M. (2009) ViSi: Body-Worn System for Monitoring Continuous, Non-Invasive Blood Pressure cNIBP. *Proceedings of DARPA Workshop on Continuous, Non-Invasive Monitoring of Blood Pressure (CNIMBP)*, 2009, Coronado

Barschdorff, D.; Erig, M. & Trowitzsch E. (2000). Noninvasive continuous blood pressure determination, *Proceedings XVI IMEKO World Congress*, 2000, Wien

Baulmann, J.; Schillings, U.; Rickert, S.; Uen, S.; Düsing, R.; Cziraki, R.; Illyes, M. & Mengden, T. (2008). A new oscillometric method for assessment of arterial stiffness: comparison with tonometric and piezo-electronic methods. *Journal of Hypertension*, 26, 3, (2008) 523-528

Benetos, A.; Adamopoulos, C.; Bureau, J. M. et al. (2002) Determinants of accelerated progression of arterial stiffness in normotensive subjects and in treated hypertensive subjects over a 6-year period. *Circulation*, 105 (2002) 1202-1207

Berntson, G. G.; Lozano, D. L., Chen Y. J. & Cacioppo J. T. (2004). Where to Q in PEP. *Psychophysiology*, 41, 2, (2004) 333-337

Blacher, J.; Guerin, A.P.; Pannier, B.; Marchais, S.J.; Safar, M.E. & London, G.M. (1999) Impact of aortic stiffness on survival in end-stage renal disease. *Circulation* 99 (1999) 2434-2439

Boese, J. M.; Bock, M.; Bahner, M. L.; Albers, J. & Schad, L. R. (2000) In vivo Validation of Aortic Compliance Estimation by MR Pulse Wave Velocity Measurement, *Proc. Intl. Soc. Mag. Reson. Med.*, 8 (2000) 357

Bouthier, J.D.; De Luca, N.; Safar, M.E. & Simon, A.C. (1985) Cardiac hypertrophy and arterial distensibility in essential hypertension. *Am Heart J*, 109 (1985) 1345-52.

Boutouyrie, P.; Briet, M.; Collin, C.; Vermeersch, S. & Pannier, B. (2009). Assessment of pulse wave velocity. *Artery Research*, 3, (2009) 3-8

Boutouyrie, P.; Lacolley, P.; Girerd, X.; Beck, L.; Safar, M. & Laurent S. (1994) Sympathetic activation decreases medium-sized arterial compliance in humans. *Am J Physiol*, 267 (1994) H1368-H1376

Butlin, M.; Hickson, S.; Graves, M. J.; McEniery, C. M; et al. (2008). Determining pulse wave velocity using MRI: a comparison and repeatability of results using seven transit time algorithms. *Artery Research*, 2, 3, (2008) 99

Cameron, J.D.; Jennings, G.L. & Dart, A.M. (1995) The relationship between arterial compliance, age, blood pressure and serum lipid levels. *J Hypertens*, 13 (1995) 1718-1723

Chen, C. H.; Nevo, E.; Fetics, B.; Pak, P. H.; Yin, F. C.; Maughan, W. L. & Kass, D. A.(1997). Estimation of central aortic pressure waveform by mathematical transformation of radial tonometry pressure. Validation of generalized transfer function. *Circulation*, 95, 7, (1997) 1827-1836

Chen, W.; Kobayashi, T.; Ichikawa, S.; Takeuchi, Y. & Togawa, T. (2000). Continuous estimation of systolic blood pressure using the pulse arrival time and intermittent calibration. *Medical & Biological Engineering & Computing,* 38, (2000) 569-574

Chen, Y.; Li, L.; Hershler, C. & Dill, R. P. (2003). Continuous non-invasive blood pressure monitoring method and apparatus. *US Patent 6,599,251,* July 2003

Chiu, Y. C.; Arand, P. W.; Shroff, S. G.; Feldman, T. Et al. (1991). Determination of pulse wave velocities with computerized algorithms. *Am Heart J,* 121, 5, (1991) 1460-1470

Constans, J.; Germain, C.; Gossec; P. Taillard, J. et al. (2007). Arterial stiffness predicts severe progression in systemic sclerosis: the ERAMS study. *J Hypertension,* 25, (2007) 1900-1906

Creager, M.A.; Luscher, T.F.; Cosentino, F. & Beckman, J.A. (2003) Diabetes and vascular disease: pathophysiology, clinical consequences, and medical therapy: Part I. *Circulation,* 108 (2003) 1527-32

Cruickshank, K.; Riste, L.; Anderson, S.G.; Wright, J.S.; Dunn, G. & Gosling, R.G. (2002) Aortic pulse-wave velocity and its relationship to mortality in diabetes and glucose intolerance: an integrated index of vascular function? *Circulation,* 106 (2002) 2085-90

Dart, A.M. & Kingwell, B. A. (2001) Pulse pressure--a review of mechanisms and clinical relevance. *J Am Coll Cardiol,* 37 (2001) 975-984

Dart, A.M.; Gatzka, C.D.; Cameron, J.D., et al. (2004) Large artery stiffness is not related to plasma cholesterol in older subjects with hypertension. *Arterioscler Thromb Vasc Bio,* 24 (2004) 962-968

DeMarzo, A. P. & Lang, R. M. (1996). A new algorithm for improved detection of aortic valve opening by impedance cardiography. *Computers in Cardiology,* 8, 11, (1996) 373-376

Faber M. & Oller-Hou G. (1952). The human aorta. V. Collagen and elastin in the normal and hypertensive aorta. *Acta Pathol Microbiol Scand,* 31, (1952) 377-82.

Fesler, P.; Safar, M.E.; du Cailar, G.; Ribstein, J. & Mimran, A. (2007) Pulse pressure is an independent determinant of renal function decline during treatment of essential hypertension. *J Hypertens ,* 25 (2007) 1915-1920

Foo, J. Y. A. (2008). Use of Independent Component Analysis to Reduce Motion Artifact in Pulse Transit Time Measurement. *Signal Processing Letters,* 15 , (2008) 124-126

Foo, J. Y. A.; Lim, C. S. & Wang, P. (2006). Evaluation of blood pressure changes using vascular transit time. *Physiol. Meas.,* 17 , (2006) 685-694

Franchi, D.; Bedini, R.; Manfredini, F.; Berti, S.; Palagi, G.; Ghione, S. & Ripoly, A. (1996). Blood pressure evaluation based on arterial pulse wave velocity. *Computers in Cardiology,* 8, 11, (1996) 397-400

Frank, O. (1905) Der Puls in den arterien, *Zeitschrift für Biologie,* 45 (1905) 441-553

Fung, P.; Dumont, G.; Ries, C.; Mott, C. & Ansermino, M. (2004). Continuous Noninvasive Blood Pressure Measurement by Pulse Transit Time, *Proceedings of the 26th Annual International Conference of the IEEE EMBS,* pp. 738-741, 0-7803-8439-3, San Francisco, September 2004, IEEE

Gallagher, D.; Adji, A. & O'Rourke, M. F. (2004). Validation of the transfer function technique for generating central from peripheral upper limb pressure waveform. *Am J Hypertens,* 17, 11, (2004) 1059-1067

Gang, G.; Mark, P.; Cockshott, P., Foster, J., et al. (2004). Measurement of Pulse Wave Velocity using Magnetic Resonance Imaging, *Proceedings of the 26th Annual International Conference of the IEEE EMBS*, pp. 3684-3687, 0-7803-8439-3, San Francisco, September 2004, IEEE

Giannattasio, C.; Capra, A.; Facchetti, R. et al. (2007) Relationship between arterial distensibility and coronary atherosclerosis in angina patients. *J Hypertens*, 25 (2007) 593-598.

Giannattasio, C.; Failla, M.; Piperno, A. et al. (1999) Early impairment of large artery structure and function in type I diabetes mellitus. *Diabetologia*, 42 (1999) 987-994

Girerd, X.; Chanudet, X.; Larroque, P.; Clement, R.; Laloux, B. &, Safar, M. (1989) Early arterial modifications in young patients with borderline hypertension. *J Hypertens Suppl*, 7 (1989) S45-S47.

Giri, S.S.; Ding, Y.; Nishikima, Y.; Pedraza-Toscano, et al. (2007). Automated and Accurate Measurement of Aortic Pulse Wave Velocity Using Magnetic Resonance Imaging. *Computuers in Cardiology*, 34, (2007) 661-664

Glen, S.K.; Elliott, H.L.; Curzio, J.L.; Lees, K.R. & Reid J.L. (1996) White-coat hypertension as a cause of cardiovascular dysfunction. *Lancet*, 348 (1996) 654-657

Guerin, A. P.; Blacher, J.; Pannier, B.; Marchais, S. J.; Safar, M. E. & London, G. (2001). Impact of Aortic Stiffness Attenuation on Survival of Patients in End-Stage Renal Failure. *Circulation*, 103, (2001) 987-992

Hayes, M. J. & Smith, P. R. (1998). Artifact reduction in photoplethysmogrpahy. *Applied Optics*, 37, 31, (1998) 7437-7446

Henry, R.M.; Kostense, P.J.; Spijkerman, A.M. et al. (2003) Arterial stiffness increases with deteriorating glucose tolerance status: the Hoorn Study. *Circulation* 107 (2003) 2089-95

Henskens, L.H.; Kroon, A.A.; van Oostenbrugge, R.J., et al. (2008) Increased aortic pulse wave velocity is associated with silent cerebral small-vessel disease in hypertensive patients. *Hypertension*, 52 (2008) 1120-1126

Hirai, T.; Sasayama, S.; Kawasaki, T. & Yagi, S. (1989) Stiffness of systemic arteries in patients with myocardial infarction. A noninvasive method to predict severity of coronary atherosclerosis. *Circulation*, 80 (1989) 78-86

Hirata, K.; Kawakami, M. & O'Rourke M. F. (2006) Pulse Wave Analysis and Pulse Wave Velocity – A review of Blood Pressure Interpretatoin 100 Years After Korotkov, *Circ J*, 70 (2006) 1231-1239

Hiroyuki Ota, H.; Kenji Taniguchi, K.; (1998). Electronic blood pressure meter with posture detector. *US Patent 5,778,879*, July 1998

Hughes, D. J.; Babbs, C. F.; Geddes, L. A. & Bourland, J. D. (1979) Measurement of Young's Modulus of Elasticity of the Canine Aorta with Ultrasound, *Ultrasonic Imaging*, 1 (1979) 356-367

Hurtwitz, B. E.; Shyu, L. Y.; Reddy, S P.; Shneiderman, N. & Nagel, J. II (1990). Coherent ensemble averaging techniques for impedance cardiography, *Proceedings of Third Annual IEEE Symposium on Computer-Based medical Systems*, 2009

Jatoi, N.A.; Jerrard-Dunne, P.; Feely, J. & Mahmud, A. (2007) Impact of smoking and smoking cessation on arterial stiffness and aortic wave reflection in hypertension. *Hypertension*, 49 (2007) 981-5

Jiang, B.; Liu, B.; McNeill, K. L. & Chowienczyk, P. J. (2008) Measurement of Pulse Wave Velocity Using Pulse Wave Doppler Ultrasound: Comparison with Arterial Tonometry, *Ultrasound in Med. & Biol.*, 34, 3 (2008) 509-512

Karamanoglu, M; Gallegher, D. E.; Avolio, A. P. & O'Rourke, M. F. (1995). Pressure wave propagation in a multibranched model of the human upper limb. *Am J Physiol*, 269, 4, (1995) H1363-1369

Kass, D.A.; Shapiro, E.P.; Kawaguchi, M. et al. (2002) Improved arterial compliance by a novel advanced glycation end-product crosslink breaker. *Circulation*, 104 (2002) 1464-1470

Kim, J. S.; Kim, K. K.; Lim Y. G. & Park K. S. (2007) Two unconstrained methods for blood pressure monitoring in a ubiquitous home healthcare, *Proceedings of the Fifth International Conference Biomedical Engineering*, pp. 293-296, 978-0-88986-648-5, Innsbruck, February 2007

Kim, J.; Park, J.; Kim, K.; Chee, Y.; Lim, Y. & Park, K. (2006). Development of a Nonintrusive Blood Pressure System for Somputer Users. *Telemedicine and e-Health*, 13, 1, (2006) 57-64

King, E.; Cobbin, D.; Walsh, S. & Ryan, D. (2002). The Reliable Measurement of Radial Pulse Characteristics. *Acupuncture in Medicine*, 20, 4, (2002) 150-159

Lababidi, Z.; Ehmke, D. A.; Durnin, R. E.; Leaverton, P. E. & Lauer, R. M. (1970). The First Derivative Thoracic Impedance Cardiogram. *Circulation*, 41, (1970) 651-658

Laffon, E.; Marthan, R.; Mantaudon, M.; Latrabe, V.; Laurent F. & Ducassou, D. (2005) Feasibility of aortic pulse pressure and pressure wave velocity MRI measurement in young adults, *J. Magn. Reson. Imaging*, 21, 1 (2005) 53-58

Latham, R.D.; Westerhof, N.; Sipkema, P. et al. (1985). Regional wave travel and reflections along the human aorta: a study with six simultaneous micromonometric pressures. *Circulation*, 72, 3, (1985) 1257-1269

Laurent, S. & Cockroft, J. (2008). *Central aortic blood pressure*, Elsevier, 978-2-84299-943-8

Laurent, S.; Boutouyrie, P.; Asmar, R. et al. (2001) Aortic stiffness is an independent predictor of all-cause and cardiovascular mortality in hypertensive patients. *Hypertension*, 37 (2001) 1236-41

Laurent, S.; Katsahian, S.; Fassot, C. et al. (2003) Aortic stiffness is an independent predictor of fatal stroke in essential hypertension. *Stroke*, 34 (2003) 1203-1206

Li, Q. & Belz, G. G. (1993). Systolic time intervals in clinical pharmacology. *Eur J Clin Pharmacol*, 44, (1993) 415-421

Liang, Y.L.; Shiel, L.M.; Teede, H. et al. (2001) Effects of Blood Pressure, Smoking, and Their Interaction on Carotid Artery Structure and Function. *Hypertension*, 37 (2001) 6-11

London, G.M.; Guerin, A.P.; Marchais, S.J. et al. (1996) Cardiac and arterial interactions in end-stage renal disease. *Kidney Int*, 50 (1996) 600-8

London, G.M.; Guerin, A.P.; Pannier, B.; Marchais, S.J. & Stimpel, M. (1995) Influence of sex on arterial hemodynamics and blood pressure. Role of body height. *Hypertension* ,26 (1995) 514-519

Lorell, B.H. & Carabello, B.A. (2000) Left ventricular hypertrophy: pathogenesis, detection, and prognosis. *Circulation*, 102 (2000) 470-9

Lotz, J.; Meier, C.; Leppert, A. & Galanski, M. (2002). Cardiovascular flow measurement with phase-contrast MR imaging: basic facts and implementation. *Radiographics*, 22, 3, (2002) 651-671

Madero, R.; Lawrence, H. & Sai, K. (2003). Continuous, non-invasive technique for measuring blood pressure using impedance plethysmography. *European Patent Office, EP 1 344 4891 A1,* February 2003

Mancia, G.; De Backer, G.; Dominiczak, A. et al. (2007) Guidelines for the Management of Arterial Hypertension: The Task Force for the Management of Arterial Hypertension of the European Society of Hypertension (ESH) and of the European Society of Cardiology (ESC). *J Hypertens,* 25 (2007) 1105-1187

Mathews, J. H & Fink, K. D. (1998). *Numerical Methods Using MATLAB,* Prentice Hall, 978-0132700429

Mattace-Raso, F.U.; van der Cammen, T.J.; Hofman, A., et al. (2006) Arterial stiffness and risk of coronary heart disease and stroke: the Rotterdam Study. *Circulation,* 113 (2006) 657-663

McCombie, D. B.; Reisner, A. T. & Asada, H. H. (2006). Adaptive blood pressure estimation from wearable PPG sensors using peripheral pulse wave velocity measurement and multi-channel blind identification of local artery dynamics, *Proceedings of the 28th Annual International Conference of the IEEE EMBS,* pp. 3521-3524, 1-4244-0033-3, New York City, September 2006, IEEE

McCombie, D. B.; Shaltis, P. A.; Reisner, A. T. & Asada, H. H. (2007). Adaptive hydrostatic blood pressure calibration: Development of a wearable, autonomous pulse wave velocity blood pressure monitor, *Proceedings of the 29th Annual International Conference of the IEEE EMBS,* pp. 370-373, 1-4244-0788-5, Lyon, August 2007, IEEE

Meaume, S.; Benetos, A.; Henry, O.F.; Rudnichi, A. & Safar, M.E. (2001) Aortic pulse wave velocity predicts cardiovascular mortality in subjects >70 years of age. *Arterioscler Thromb Vasc Biol,* 21 (2001) 2046-2050

Meigas, K.; Lass, J.; Karai, D.; Kattai, R. & Kaik, J. (2006). Pulse Wave Velocity in Continuous Blood Pressure Measurements, *Proceedings of the Worls Congress on Medical Physics and Biomedical Engineering,* pp. 626-629, 978-3-540-36839-7, Seoul, September 2006, Springer

Meinders, J. M.; Kornet, L.; Brands, P.J. & Hoeks, A. P. (2001) Assessment of local pulse wave velocity in arteries using 2D distension waveforms, *Ultrason Imaging,* 23, 4 (2001) 199-215

Millasseau, S. C.; Ritter, J. M.; Takazawa, K. & Chowienczyk, P. J. (2006). Contour analysis of the photoplethysmographic pulse measured at the finger. *Journal of Hypertension,* 24, 8, (2006) 1149-1456

Millasseau, S. C.; Stewart, A. D.; Patel, S. J.; Redwood, S. R. & Chowienczyk, P. J. (2005). Evaluation of carotid-femoral pulse wave velocity: influence of timing algorithm and heart rate. *Hypertension,* 45, 2, (2005) 222-226

Mitchell, G. F. (2009) Arterial stiffness and wave reflection: Biomarkers of cardiovascular risk, *Artery Research,* 2 (2009) 56-64

Mohiaddin, R. H.; Longmore, D. B. (1989). MRI studies of atherosclerotic vascular disease: structural evaluation and physiological meaurements. *Bristisch Medical Bulletin,* 45, (1989) 968-990

Muehlsteff, J.; Aubert, X. L. & Schuett, M. (2006). Cuffless Estimation of Systolic Blood Pressure for Short Effort Bicycle Tests: The Prominent Role of the Pre-Ejection Period, *Proceedings of the 28th Annual International Conference of the IEEE EMBS,* pp. 5088-5092, 1-4244-0033-3, New York City, September 2006, IEEE

Naschitz, J. E.; Bezobchuk, S.; Mussafia-Priselac, R.; Sundick, S.; et al.(2004). Pulse transit time by R-wave-gated infrared photoplethysmography: review of the literature and personal experience. *J Clin Monit Comput,* 18, 5-6, (2004) 333-342

Nichols W.W. (2005) Clinical measurement of arterial stiffness obtained from noninvasive pressure waveforms. *Am J Hypertens,* 18 (2005) 3S-10S

Nichols, W. W. & O'Rourke, M. F (2005). *McDonald's blood flow in arteries,* Hodder Arnold, 0 340 80941 8

Nichols, W. W. (2009). Aortic Pulse Wave Velocity, Reflection Site Distance, and Augmentation Index. *Hypertension,* 53, 1, (2009) e9

Nichols, W. W.; Denardo, S. J.; Wilkinson, I. B.; McEniery, C. M.; Cockroft, J. & O'Rourke, M. F. (2008) Effects of Arterial Stiffness, Pulse Wave Velocity, and Wave Reflections on the Central Aortic Pressure Waveform, *J Clin Hyoertens,* 10 (2008) 295-303

Nilsson, P. M.; Boutouyrie, P. & Laurent, S. (2009) Vascular Aging : A Tale of EVA and ADAM in Cardiovascular Risk Assessment and Prevention, *Hypertension,* 54 (2009) 3-10

Nitzan, M.; Khanokh, B. & Slovik, Y. (2002). The difference in pulse transit time to the toe and finger measured by photoplethysmography. *Phyiol Meas,* 23, (2002) 85-93

O'Brien, E.; Waeber, B.; Parati, G.; Staessen, J. & Myers M. G. (2001) Blood pressure measuring devices: recommendations of the European Society of Hypertension. *BMJ,* 322 (2001) 531-536

O'Rourke M. F. (2009). Time domain analysis of the arterial pulse in clinical medicine. *Med Biol Eng Comp,* 47, 2, (2009) 119-129

Okada, M.; Kimura, S. & Okada, M. (1986) Estimation of arterial pulse wave velocities in the frequency domain: method and clinical considerations, *Medical & Biological Engineering & Computing,* 24, 3 (1986) 255-260

O'Rourke, M.F. & Safar, M.E. (2005) Relationship between aortic stiffening and microvascular disease in brain and kidney: cause and logic of therapy. *Hypertension,* 46 (2005) 200-204

Park E. K.; Cho B. H.; Park, S. H.; Lee, J. Y.; Lee, J. S.; Kim, I. Y. & Kim S. I (2005). Continuous measurement of systolic blood pressure using the PTT and other parameters, *Proceedings of the 27th Annual International Conference of the IEEE EMBS,* pp. 3555-3558, 0-7803-8740-6, Shanghai, September 2005, IEEE

Payne, R. A.; Symeonides, C. N.; Webb, D. J. & Maxwell, S. R. (2006). Pulse transit time measured from the ECG: an unreliable marker of beat-to-beat blood pressure. *J Appl Physiol,* 100, 1, (2006) 136-141

Poon, C. C. Y. & Zhang Y. T. (2005). Cuff-less and Noninvasive Measurement of Arterial Blood Pressure by Pulse Transit Time, *Proceedings of the 27th Annual International Conference of the IEEE EMBS,* pp. 5877-5880, 0-7803-8740-6, Shanghai, September 2005, IEEE

Poon, C. Y. & Zhang, Y. T. (2008). The Beat-toBeat Relationship between Pulse Transit time and Systolic Blood Pressure, *Proceedings of the 5th International Conference on Information Technology and Application in Biomedicine,* pp. 342-343, 978-1-4244-2255-5, Shenzhen, May 2008, IEEE

Rajzer, M.; Wojciechowska, W.; Klocek, M.; Palka, I.; Brzozowska, B. & Kawecka-Jaszcz, K. (2008). Comparison of aortic pulse wave velocity measured by three techniques: Complior, SphygmoCor and Arteriograph. *Journal of Hypertension,* 26, 10, (2008) 2001-2007

Ravikumar, R.; Deepa, R.; Shanthirani, C. & Mohan, V. (2002) Comparison of carotid intima-media thickness, arterial stiffness, and brachial artery flow mediated dilatation in diabetic and nondiabetic subjects (The Chennai Urban Population Study [CUPS-9]). *Am J Cardiol,* 90 (2002) 702-7

Schram, M.T.; Henry, R.M.; van Dijk, R.A. et al. (2004) Increased central artery stiffness in impaired glucose metabolism and type 2 diabetes: the Hoorn Study. *Hypertension,* 43 (2004) 176-81

Schwartz, D. J. (2005). The pulse transit time arousal index in obstructive sleep apnea before and CPAP. *Sleep Medicine,* 6, (2005) 199-2003

Segers, P.; Kips, J.; Trachet, B.; Swillens, A.; Vermeersch, S.; Mahieu, D.; Rietzschel, E.; Buyzere, M. D. & Bortel, L. V. (2009) Limitations and pitfalls of non-invasive measurement of arterial pressure wave reflections and pulse wave velocity, *Artery Research,* 3, 2 (2009) 79-88

Sharwood-Smith, G.; Bruce, J. & Drummond, G. (2005). Assessment of pulse transit time to indicate cardiovascular changes during obstetric spinal anaestheisa. *Br J Anaesthesia,* 96, 1, (2006) 100-105

Shinohara, K.; Shoji, T.; Tsujimoto, Y. et al. (1999) Arterial stiffness in predialysis patients with uremia. *Kidney Int,* 65 (1999) 936-43

Smith, R. P.; Argod, J.; Pépin, J. & Lévy, A. (1999). Pulse transit time: an appraisal of potential clinical applications. *Thorax,* 54, (1999) 452-457

Solà, J.; Chételat, O. & Luprano, J. (2008) Continuous Monitoring of Coordinated Cardiovascular Responses, *Proceedings of the 30th Annual International Conference of the IEEE EMBS,* pp. 1423-1426, 978-1-4244-1814-5, Vancouver, August 2008, IEEE

Solà, J.; Vetter, R.; Renevey P.; Chételat, O.; Sartori, C. & Rimoldi, S. F. (2009) Parametric estimation of Pulse Arrival Time: a robust approach to Pulse Wave Velocity, *Physiol. Meas.,* 30 (2009) 603-615

Sonesson, B.; Hansen, F.; Stale, H. & Lanne, T. (1993) Compliance and diameter in the human abdominal aorta--the influence of age and sex. *Eur J Vasc Surg,* 7 (1993) 690-697.

Steptoe, A.; Smulyan, H. & Gribbin B. (1976) Pulse Wave Velocity and Blood Pressure Change: Calibration and Applications. *Psychophysiology,* 13, 5 (1976) 488-493.

Sutton-Tyrrell, K.; Najjar, S.S.; Boudreau, R.M. et al. (2005) Elevated aortic pulse wave velocity, a marker of arterial stiffness, predicts cardiovascular events in well-functioning older adults. *Circulation,* 111 (2005) 3384-90

Toprak, A.; Reddy, J.; Chen, W.; Srinivasan, S. & Berenson, G. (2009) Relation of pulse pressure and arterial stiffness to concentric left ventricular hypertrophy in young men (from the Bogalusa Heart Study). *Am J Cardiol,* 103 (2009) 978-984.

van Ittersum, F.J.; Schram, M.T.;, van der Heijden-Spek, J.J. et al. (2004) Autonomic nervous function, arterial stiffness and blood pressure in patients with Type I diabetes mellitus and normal urinary albumin excretion. *J Hum Hypertens,* 18 (2004) 761-8

van Popele, N.M.; Grobbee, D.E.; Bots, M.L. et al. (2001) Association between arterial stiffness and atherosclerosis: the Rotterdam Study. *Stroke,* 32 (2001) 454-460

Vetter, R.; Rossini, L.; Ridolfi, A.; Solà, J.; Chételat, O.; Correvon, M. & Krauss, J. (2009). Frequency domain SpO2 estimation based on multichannel photoplethysmographic measurements at the sternum, to appear in *Proceedings of Medical Physics and Biomedical Engineering World Congress,* Munich, September 2009

Webster, J. G. (1997). *Design of pulse oximeters,* CRC Press, 978-0-750-30467-2

Westerhof, N.; Stergiopulos, N. & Noble, M. (2005). *Snapshots of Hemodynamics,* Springer, 978-0-387-23345-1

Willum-Hansen, T.; Staessen, J.A.; Torp-Pedersen, C. et al. (2006) Prognostic value of aortic pulse wave velocity as index of arterial stiffness in the general population. *Circulation,* 113 (2006) 664-670

Wolffenbuttel B.H.; Boulanger, C.M.; Crijns, F.R., et al. (1998) Breakers of advanced glycation end products restore large artery properties in experimental diabetes. *Proc Natl Acad Sci USA,*95 (1998) 4630-4634

Xu, P.; Bergsneider, M. & Hu, X. (2009) Pulse onset detection using neighbor pulse-based signal enhancement, *Medical Engineering & Physics,* 31 (2009) 337-345

Yan, Y. S. & Zhang, Y. T. (2007). A Novel Calibration Method for Noninvasive Blood Pressure Measurement Using Pulse Transit Time, *Proceedings of the 4th IEEE-EMBS International Summer School and Symposium on Medical Devices and Biosensors,* Cambridge, August 2007

22

Biomagnetic Measurements for Assessment of Fetal Neuromaturation and Well-Being

Audrius Brazdeikis[1] and Nikhil S. Padhye[2]
[1]Department of Physics and Texas Center for Superconductivity, University of Houston
[2]The University of Texas Health Science Center at Houston
U. S. A.

1. Introduction

There has been an explosion of knowledge about the human genome and the complex interplay between the genome and environment that shapes the development of the central nervous system. The development of new quantitative measures that reliably capture early function of the central nervous system is fundamental to assessing the development of the human fetus. Fetal magnetocardiography (fMCG) is a recording of the spatiotemporal magnetic fields created by the fetal cardiac electrical activity that is regulated by the developing central nervous system. It is measured non-invasively by the use of superconducting quantum interference device (SQUID), the most sensitive and stable detector of magnetic flux currently available. The SQUID sensor provides unmatched sensitivity and temporal resolution used for detection of the electromagnetic field perturbation associated with the neuronal currents in the brain, fetal cardiac activity, and the nuclear spin magnetization in ultra-low field nuclear magnetic resonance spectroscopy or in magnetic resonance imaging.

Biomagnetic fMCG measurements remain predisposed to interferences both internal and external to the subject's body, low signal-to-noise ratio, and sensitivity to fetal movements. Successful implementation of the fMCG requires advanced biomagnetometer systems, which usually include arrays of SQUID sensors with automated signal acquisition and control electronics. Specialized software tools are required for signal processing, noise suppression, and artifact removal. In this chapter, we will describe the current status of fMCG applications relevant to their present scientific, technological, and clinical challenges, focusing on fundamental technological breakthroughs in the corresponding fields. Section 2 is devoted to a discussion of SQUID sensor technology, flux transformers, and noise reduction methods. Technological challenges and biomagnetic models that are specific to fetal biomagnetic measurements are described in Section 3.

Considerations in regard to signal processing of fMCG signals and separation of maternal and fetal signals are addressed in Section 4. In contrast to obstetric ultrasound, fMCG permits direct evaluation of the electrophysiological properties of the fetal heart, providing information for assessing fetal arrhythmia, prolonged QT-syndrome, and fetal cardiac wave morphology. In addition, fMCG has the precision to accurately quantify beat-to-beat variability such that small, rapid fetal heart rate oscillations associated with respiratory sinus arrhythmia can be detected, quantified, and analyzed to provide a measure of autonomic nervous system control and fetal well-being. Unlike electrocardiography, which is hampered by changing electrical conductance of the fetal-abdominal body during the course of pregnancy, fMCG permits successful recordings from an early stage in the pregnancy. In Section 5, a recent application of fMCG in an unshielded clinical setting is presented that compares spectral and complexity characteristics of heart rate variability in fetuses and in prematurely born neonates of the same age.

2. Superconducting Sensor Technologies for Weak Magnetic Field Detection

SQUIDs make use of several physical phenomena including flux-conservation, flux-quantization, and the Josephson effect (Tinkham, 1996). In fact, a SQUID is a superconducting ring, interrupted with one or two weak links called Josephson junctions, which govern the flow of a zero voltage supercurrent. These weak links alter the compensation of the external field by the circulating persistent current, thus making it possible to exploit flux-quantization for measurements of the magnetic fields. Flux-quantization is a unique characteristic of superconductors that provides superconducting sensors with a stability that is possessed by no other magnetic field sensing device. The dc SQUID is generally operated in a finite voltage regime and is effectively a flux-to-voltage transducer characterized by the transfer function which has a periodic sinusoidal function of applied flux with a period equal to one flux quantum Φ_0 ($\Phi_0 \equiv h/2e \approx 2.07\times10^{-15}$ Wb).

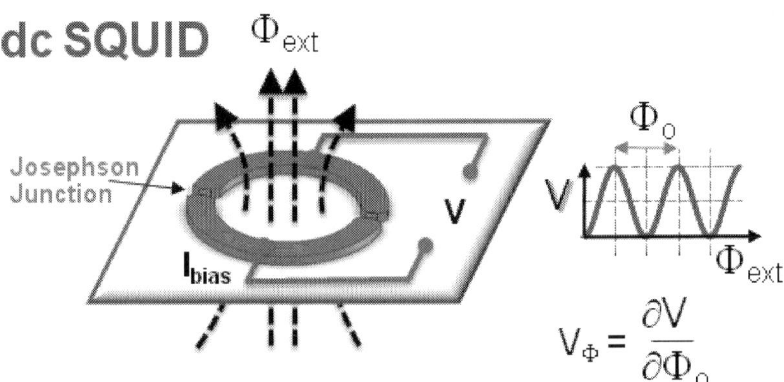

Fig. 1. A schematic illustration of a dc SQUID and its readout characteristic (V - Φ_{ext}). A small change in external magnetic field will produce a change in the readout voltage.

The maximum supercurrent I_0 through two parallel Josephson junctions in the superconducting ring is modulated periodically by the flux enclosed. When SQUID is biased with a current I_{bias} slightly higher than I_0, voltage is developed across the junctions. When magnetic flux threading the superconducting ring Φ_{ext} is changed, the voltage V across the SQUID oscillates with period of one Φ_0 as shown in Fig. 1. Any small changes in an external magnetic flux Φ_{ext} coupled to the SQUID e.g. due to time varying biomagnetic fields will produce large change in the readout voltage $\delta V = V_\Phi \delta \Phi_{ext}$ where V_Φ is the transfer function. The nonlinear SQUID output can be linearized by using flux-locked loop (FLL) electronics (Drung & Mück, 2004).

The magnetic field resolution of SQUID sensors is given by their noise performance that is characterized in terms of energy sensitivity, which for dc SQUIDs reach unsurpassed values of 10^{-32} J/Hz. In the frequency range of interest for biomagnetic measurements (dc $-$ 100 Hz) noise of commercial SQUID biomagnetometer is typically about 5 fT rms Hz$^{-1/2}$ (5 fT = 5×10^{-15} T), in part due to magnetic noise generated by electrically conductive radiation-shields of cryogenic dewars (Neonen et al., 1996).

The principal reason for choosing a SQUID sensor for weak magnetic signal detection is because of the tremendous sensitivity in its theoretical and actual performance (e.g. Weinstock, 1996; Weinstock, 2000). The SQUID-based biomagnetic instruments (biomagnetometers) offer the unique combination of sensitivity, wide dynamic range, and frequency response. Measurement of weak magnetic fields generated by nearby biomagnetic sources such as a fetal heart is affected by ambient noise from distant sources, both internal and external to the subject body. Sources of external ambient noise include electrical equipment and instruments connected to the power grid, and various moving magnetic objects such as machinery, cars, and elevators to mention a few. Internal noise sources of biomagnetic origin that are specific to fMCG include the bioelectrical activity of the maternal heart, muscles, gastro-intestinal system, and uterine contractions, especially when close to term. Other specific problems include fetal activity (fetal kicks and movements), maternal breathing moments, and pulsations associated with blood flow (Mosher et al., 1997).

One of the most effective means to reduce the noise detected by a SQUID is through the use of a superconducting flux transformer. All leads of the flux transformer are superconducting, resulting in the total flux linking the SQUID and the coils to be quantized, and therefore stable in time. Any change in the field in the proximity of the pickup coil will modify the total flux in the system, resulting in a change in the persistent current, which in turn will generate an equal but opposite compensating flux such that the total flux trapped is unchanged. This flux change is detected by a SQUID typically placed in a small superconducting (shielded) enclosure far from the measured fields.

The flux transformer coils can have diverse configurations that vary from a single-loop magnetometer to a multi-loop gradiometer as illustrated in Fig. 2. In a single-loop configuration, the flux transformer forms a magnetometer that is sensitive to the normal field component (perpendicular to the plane of the loop). Such a magnetometer is also sensitive to a majority of distant noise sources. A distant noise source is one that is roughly at a distance r of 2 meters or more, as the magnetic field from dipolar sources coupled to a magnetometer falls off as $1/r^3$. The output of two loops can be subtracted, effectively forming a first-gradient field sensor, also referred to as a first-order gradiometer.

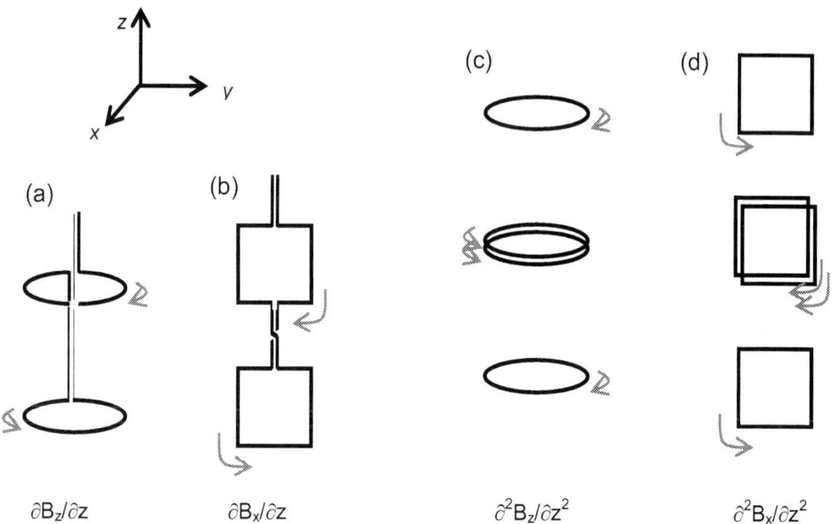

Fig. 2. A schematic illustration of various flux transformer gradiometer configurations: (a,b) first-order gradiometers, (c,d) second-order gradiometers; (b) and (d) show planar configurations.

In most situations, flux transformer output consists of measured biomagnetic signals and ambient noise, and digital filtering methods fail to separate these. The gradiometers, on the other hand, exploit the fact that the gradient of the magnetic field falls off with increasing distance much more rapidly than the uniform field itself. The n-th order field gradient falls off as $1/r^{3+n}$. Thus, gradiometers have a significantly higher sensitivity to nearby sources than distant ones, effectively behaving as spatial high-pass filters that suppress noise from distant sources (Vrba, 1996; Vrba, 2000). An axial gradiometer (Fig. 2a and Fig. 2c) consists of a set of subtracting (wound in the opposite direction) pick-up coils that measure either first- or second-order spatial derivatives $\partial B_z/\partial z$ or $\partial^2 B_z/\partial z^2$ (B_z is the z-component of the magnetic field). A planar gradiometer measures either first- or second-order spatial derivatives $\partial B_x/\partial z$ or $\partial^2 B_x/\partial z^2$, as shown in Fig. 2b and Fig. 2d.

An alternative approach is to subtract the output signals from two or more gradiometers either electronically or with software to form an electronic (Koch et al., 1993) or a higher-order synthetic gradiometer (Vrba & Robinson, 2001). Practical gradiometers are characterized by their imbalance (Fagaly, 2006) or unwanted sensitivity to uniform field components and lower-order gradient terms (for second- and higher-order gradiometers). Achieving high gradiometer balance is rather difficult and requires very precise fabrication methods and time-consuming post-assembly balancing using superconducting trim tabs or trim coils. An electronic gradiometer balancing using a reference array of three or more element vector/tensor sensors greatly improves noise rejection by several orders of magnitude (Williamson et al., 1985; Matlashov et al., 1989) — all very important for unshielded clinical operation. An axial third-order gradiometer, consisting of two symmetric second-order gradiometers can also be used for improved noise rejection over a wide range of environmental noise conditions (Uzunbajakau et al., 2005).

Other hardware approaches to reduce noise at the location of the sensitive measurements include use of various passive and active shielding methods (Fagaly, 2006). The AC and DC magnetic interferences can be shielded using passive shielding enclosures that employ single- or multi-layer shields of special high permeability and conducting materials. Active shielding strategies employ passive shields together with magnetic field compensation systems, which include separate feedback circuits and sensors that measure the magnetic field and the field gradients. Biomagnetic signals remain predisposed to large interferences, low SNR, and require specialized signal processing tools for noise suppression and artifact removal. Digital signal processing (filtering, averaging) methods and advanced mathematical algorithms that explore linear and nonlinear techniques to reduce noise and various signal artifacts are widely used (Sternickel & Braginski, 2006). Statistical signal processing techniques (Comani et al., 2004; Hild et al., 2007a; de Araujo et al., 2005; Hild et al., 2007b) such as Independent Component Analysis (ICA) or Blind Source Separation (BSS) are especially useful for extracting fetal MCG data from noisy biomagnetic recordings.

In recent years, development of SQUID instrumentation for acquisition of fetal magnetocardiograms in unshielded environments has become technically feasible (Stolz et al., 2003; Brisinda et al., 2005). Properly designed second-order gradiometers enable detection of weak fetal cardiac signals with signal amplitudes less than 5 pT peak-to-peak in unshielded hospital settings (Brazdeikis et al., 2007).

3. Factors Affecting the SNR of the Fetal Magnetocardiographic Recordings

The successful extraction of reliable information such as FHRV from noisy fMCG recordings depends on several factors, including the fetal gestational age and fetal behavioral state. Other factors that also have impact on the signal-to-noise ratio (SNR) are the fetal presentation, placenta location, and maternal bladder volume. As the fetus develops, the fetal myocardium volume increases rapidly from about 20 mm to 40 mm (longitudinal axis) during its gestation from 20 to 30 weeks (Chang et al., 1997). Considering fetal myocardium volume as an equivalent current dipole Q inside a spherically symmetric conductor (feto-abdominal body), the increase in active myocardium volume is reflected in increased Q, and consequently on the measured magnetic fields (Sarvas, 1987). Kandori et al. (1999a; 1999b) suggested the practical relationship between the strength of an equivalent current dipole Q and gestational age GA as: $Q = 18\,GA - 295$ [nAm].

The fetal abdominal depth (source-sensor separation distance) or FAD is a significant factor when estimating the SNR. Based on obstetric ultrasound measurements from 215 pregnant women, Osei & Faulkner (1999) estimated that the FAD changes with GA as FAD = 0.15 GA + 5.01 [cm]. During weeks 20 to 40, the FAD increases nearly linearly on average from about 80 mm to 110 mm. The increase in Q during the same period however is more rapid. There is a consistent improvement in the total SNR as fetal gestational age increases (Fig. 3).

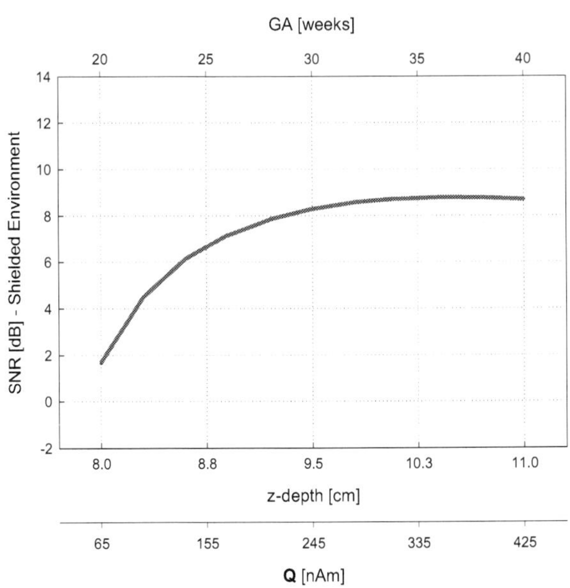

Fig. 3. The monotonic increase in the SNR plotted against the gestational age GA (upper x-axis) in shielded environment. The fetal abdominal depth (z-depth) and equivalent current dipole Q values (lower x-axes) added for illustration purposes. The biomagnetic model uses an axial second-order-gradiometer pickup, $\partial^2 B_z / \partial z^2$, with a baseline of 70 mm. The flux transformer is assumed to be electronically balanced to $C_B = 10^{-3}$ (Vázquez-Flores, 2007).

Clinical investigations of fetal heart rate patterns over gestation may be hindered by fetal behavioral state transitions and fetal movements. These behavioral states are distinct and discontinuous modes of autonomic nervous system (ANS) activity. Strong and systematic fetal heart rate changes are accompanied by increased fetal trunk and fetal respiratory movements clearly visible in fMCG recordings (Zhao & Wakai, 2002; Wakai, 2004). Prolonged heart rate accelerations or decelerations may be associated with directed fetal activity and movement, while irregular heart rate patterns on short timescales may be related to fetal breathing movements (van Leeuwen et al., 2007). Furthermore, fetal activity (fetal kicks and movements) may produce artifacts seen as variation in signal baseline and amplitude, and require reliable techniques to assess fetal gross movements using multichannel SQUID systems (van Leeuwen et al., 2009).

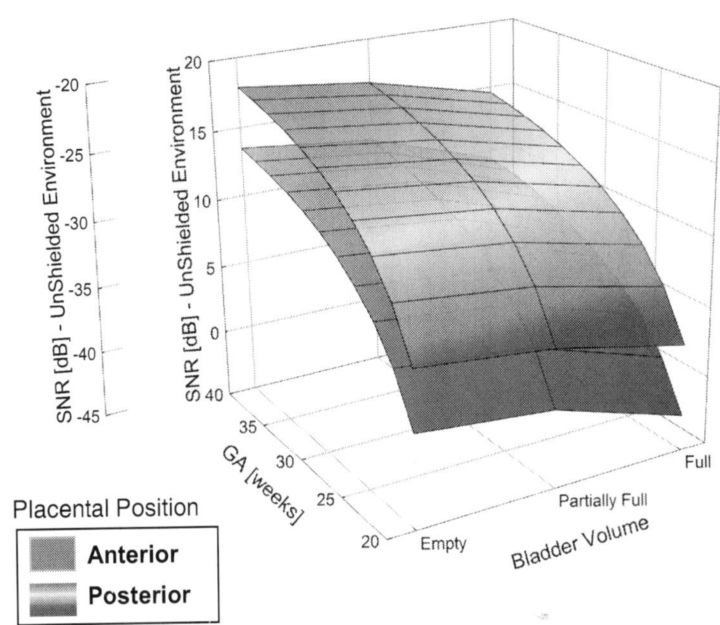

Fig. 4. The SNR calculated as a function of GA and maternal urinary bladder volumes (empty, partially full and full) for posterior and anterior placental positions. Vertical (SNR) axes are shown for shielded and unshielded environments (Vázquez-Flores, 2007).

Ultrasound examination of gravid abdomens (Osei & Faulkner, 1999) also reveals that the mean FAD is affected by the placenta location and maternal bladder volume. The fetal distance from the anterior surface of a gravid abdomen is shorter for posterior but longer for anterior placental position. When the placenta is located on the anterior uterine wall, the FAD increases by an average of 16 mm. Furthermore, the size of the maternal urinary bladder (full, partially full or empty) also has an effect on the fetal depth and consequently on the SNR. The fetal distance from the anterior surface of a gravid abdomen is shorter for empty bladder but longer for full maternal bladder. When the maternal bladder is full, the FAD increases by an average of 11 mm. Figure 4 shows calculated SNR in shielded and unshielded environments plotted as a function of fetal gestational age and maternal urinary bladder size for anterior and posterior placental positions. The SNR varies by as much as 4 dB depending on whether the maternal bladder is full or fully distended. In addition, simulation results show a 5 dB variation in the SNR between posterior and anterior placental positions. The biomagnetic model used for SNR calculations was based on an axial second-order-gradiometer pickup, $\partial^2 B_z / \partial z^2$, with a baseline of 70 mm. The flux transformer was assumed to be electronically balanced to $C_B = 10^{-3}$ (Vázquez-Flores, 2007).

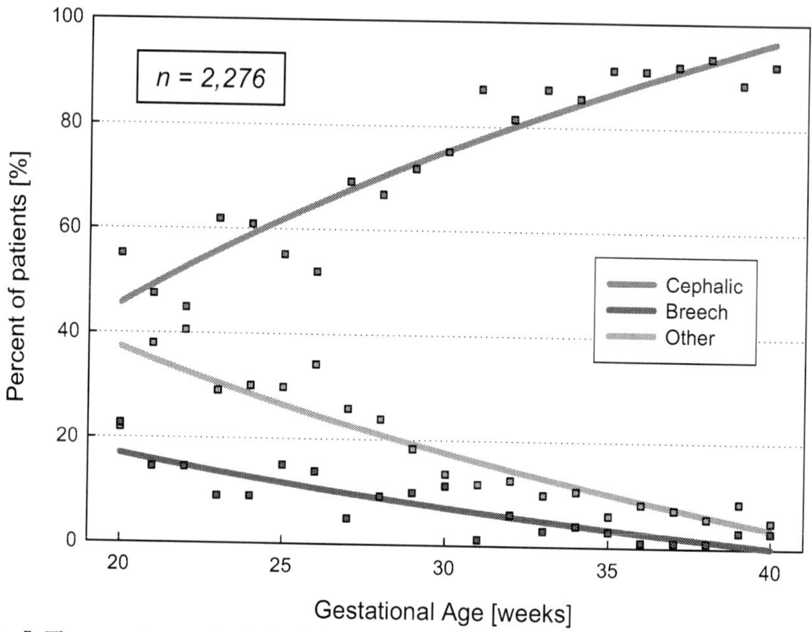

Fig. 5. The prevalence of principal classes of fetal presentation along gestation, as observed in 2,276 subjects by Scheer and Nubar (1976).

Another significant factor affecting fMCG waveform morphology and the SNR is fetal presentation. Fetal presentations are categorized into three principal classes: cephalic, breech, and transverse. Scheer and Nubar (1976) made an exhaustive study of 2,276 pregnant women in which they classified their respective babies into one of the principal presentations. The observed prevalence of fetal presentations in the longitudinal study is summarized in Fig. 5. There is limited published information about the SNR variation and changes in fMCG waveform morphology for various fetal presentations (Horigome et al. 2006). Although the incidence of cephalic presentation increases with increasing gestational age, the non-cephalic presentation is a common occurrence in early pregnancy when the fetus is highly mobile within a relatively large volume of amniotic fluid. Figure 6 illustrates rather large changes occurring in magnetic field distribution (B_z component) above a gravid abdomen (GA = 40 weeks) calculated for cephalic presentation and various axial rotations of fetal body

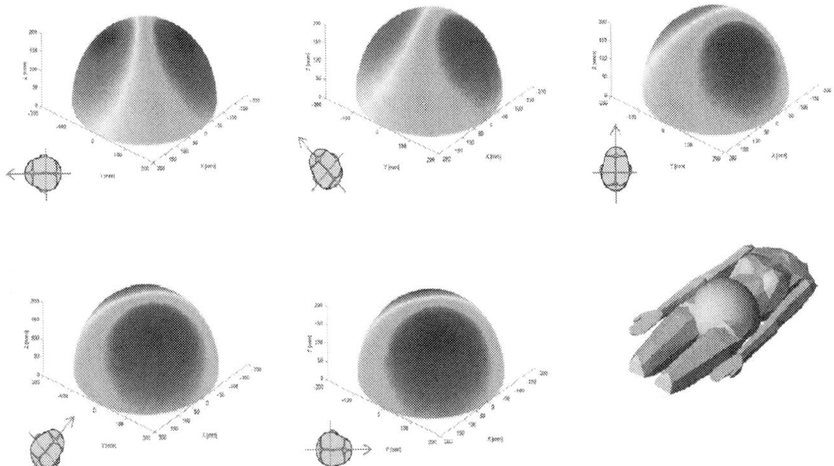

Fig. 6. Magnetic field (normal component) distribution above a gravid abdomen (GA=40 weeks) for a cephalic presentation for various fetal body rotations. Biomagnetic modeling data show that up to 30% signal amplitude variation is possible due to fetal body rotation (Vázquez-Flores, 2007).

4. Biomagnetic Signal Processing and QRS Detection

The beat-to-beat changes in fetal heart rate may be masked by incorrect signal processing and QRS detection procedures. Although a wide diversity of QRS detection schemes for electrocardiographic signals have been developed (Köhler et al., 2002; Friesen et al., 1990), automatic QRS techniques specific to fetal magnetocardiograhic signals are rare. A modified Pan-Tompkins QRS detection algorithm has been successfully implemented for automatic QRS detection in normal pregnancies of gestational ages 26–35 weeks (Brazdeikis et al., 2004). The general Pan-Tompkins QRS detection scheme (Pan & Tompkins, 1985) consists of a band-pass filtering stage, a derivative, squaring and windowing stage, and peak detection and classification stage that matches results from the two previous stages, as illustrated in Fig. 7. Quantitative analysis of fMCG showed excellent QRS detection performance with signal pre-processing and parameter tuning.

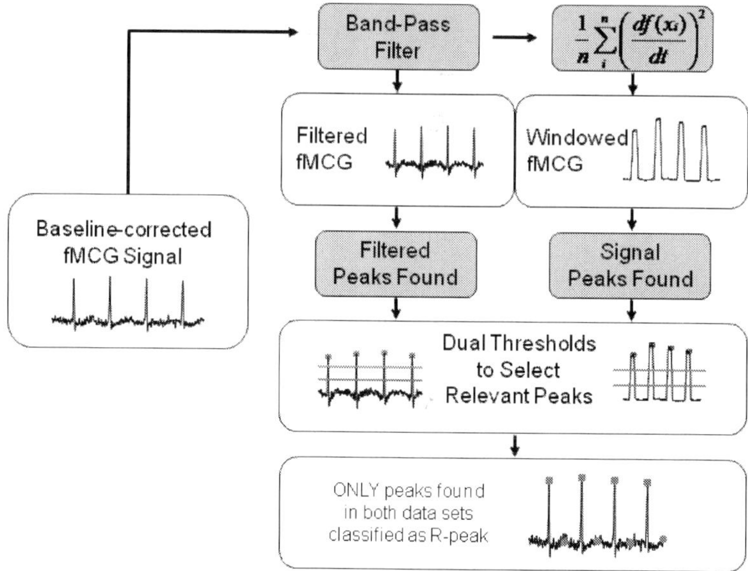

Fig. 7. The general Pan-Tompkins QRS detection scheme adapted for fetal magnetocardiographic signals (Brazdeikis et al., 2004).

When recording fMCG with a second-order gradiometer, the interference from the maternal heart is almost completely absent due to strong spatial high-pass filtering effect. Any remaining maternal MCG signals can be reliably removed by following the cross-correlation procedure illustrated in Fig. 8. In the first step, a classical Pan-Tompkins algorithm was used to extract the maternal RR time series using a reference ECG signal. In the second step, QRS complexes were selectively averaged using a template based on the extracted RR time series. In the final step, the averaged QRS complex was subtracted from the original biomagnetic signal at each location of the maternal QRS, thereby effectively suppressing maternal MCG.

5. Application of Fetal Magnetocardiography in a Clinical Study

The application presented in this section utilized clinical data that were collected during two studies of heart rate variability (HRV) at the Texas Medical Center. HRV provides a measure of autonomic nervous system balance, making it possible to gauge maturation of the autonomic nervous system.

In the first study, SQUID technology was used to record magnetocardiograms of fetuses who were 26−35 weeks gestational age. While fMCG recordings are typically done in magnetically shielded environments, the data collected in this study provided evidence that it was possible to obtain fMCG signal in various unshielded hospital settings (Padhye et al., 2004; Verklan et al., 2006; Padhye et al., 2006; Brazdeikis et al., 2007; Padhye et al., 2008). The fMCG signal had sufficiently high signal-to-noise ratio to permit the automated detection of QRS complexes in the fetal magnetocardiograms.

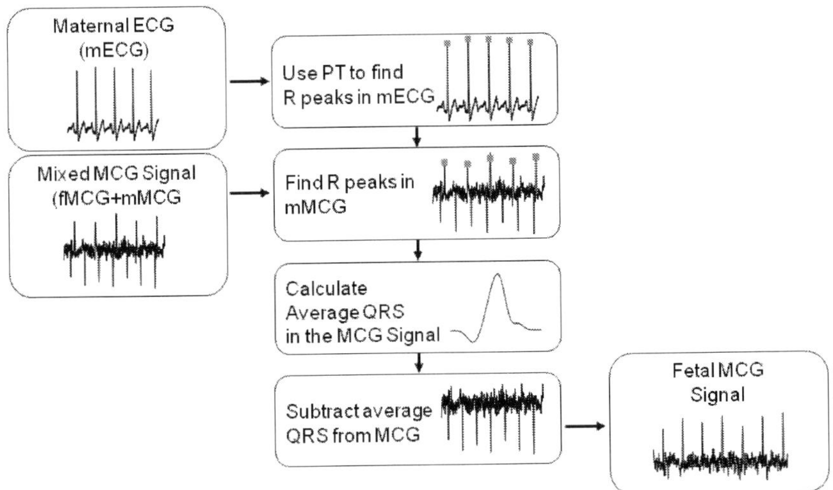

Fig. 8. The Pan-Tompkins QRS detection scheme adapted for removing any interfering maternal signals from fetal magnetocardiograms.

In the second study, electrocardiograms were recorded from prematurely born neonates of 24 to 36 weeks PMA in a neonatal intensive care unit (NICU). The first few minutes of baseline measurements were obtained while the infants were either asleep or lying quietly. The neonates were followed longitudinally and spectral powers of HRV in two frequency bands during the baseline observations were observed to increase as infants matured (Khattak et al., 2007). The increase in HRV is a reflection of the maturing autonomic nervous system. HRV is studied in high and low frequency bands in order to separate the effects of parasympathetic and sympathetic branches of the autonomic nervous system. The question of interest was to compare differences in characteristics of HRV between the fetuses and neonates at closely matched PMA.

HRV was explored in two spectral bands for both fetuses and neonates and modeled statistically to account for the growth of HRV with advancing PMA. Complexity of HRV was studied with multiscale entropy (Costa et al., 2002), which is a measure of irregularity of the fetal and neonatal RR-series. Multiscale entropy is the sample entropy (Richman & Moorman, 2000) at different timescales of the RR-series, with each scale representing a coarse-graining of the series by that factor. The sample entropy is an inverse logarithmic measure of the likelihood that pairs of observations that match would continue to match at the next observation. Lowered levels of multiscale entropy have been found to be an indicator of fetal distress (Hanqing et al., 2006; Ferrario et al., 2006). Van Leeuwen et al. (1999) reported a closely related quantity, approximate entropy, in fetuses ranging from 16 to 40 weeks and found an increasing trend with age of the fetus. In adult HRV, multiscale entropy has been used successfully to distinguish between beat-to-beat series of normal hearts and those with congestive heart failure and atrial fibrillation (Costa et al., 2002).

Fractal properties of the RR-series include self-similarity, a property by virtue of which the series appears similar when viewed on different timescales. Self-similarity was quantified for fetal and neonatal RR-series by means of detrended fluctuation analysis (Peng et al., 1994; Goldberger et al., 2000). The presence of log-linear scaling of fluctuations with box sizes provided evidence of self-similar behavior. Two scaling regions were generally present among the fetuses as well as neonates. The scaling in the region with smallest box sizes is closely related to the asymptotic spectral exponent.

5.1 Data Collection

Fetal magnetocardiograms were collected at the MSI Center at the Memorial Hermann Hospital in the Texas Medical Center. Seventeen fMCG recordings were obtained from six fetuses with PMA $\geq$ 26 weeks. Two fetuses were studied on more than one occasion and the rest were one-time observations. All but one of the recordings were in pairs of consecutive data collection sessions in magnetically shielded and unshielded environments.

As discussed in Section 3, the magnetic signals are largely unaffected by tissue density or conductance variation but fall rapidly with the distance away from the source. This property was used advantageously to filter out interferences arising from the maternal heart, muscle noise, and distant environmental noise sources. A 9-channel SQUID biomagnetometer was employed with second-order gradiometer pick-up coils (see Section 2) that effectively suppressed noise from distant sources while enabling the detection of signals from near sources that generally have stronger gradients at the location of the detector (Brazdeikis et al., 2003). After careful placement of the sensor array over the gravid abdomen it was possible to record fetal magnetocardiograms at several spatial locations largely unaffected by the maternal signal.

Neonatal electrocardiograms were obtained at Children's Memorial Hermann Hospital NICU during the course of a prospective cohort study following 35 very low birth weight (<1500 grams) infants over several weeks after admission to the NICU. The neonates ranged from 23 to 38 weeks GA with an entry criterion that required GA at birth <30 weeks. A subset was selected of 33 recordings from 13 infants that were relatively healthy and did not require mechanical ventilation. The subset included in the analysis ranged from 24 to 36 weeks GA. Electrocardiograms were recorded from study infants while they were resting for approximately 10 minutes before a blood draw procedure. At the outset, infants were relaxed, eyes were generally closed, and movements were limited to startles and jaw jerks. The Institutional Review Board approved all studies.

5.2 Measures of HRV

The fMCG signal was digitized at 1 kHz in each of 9 SQUID channels and signal from the best channel was selected for further analysis. High-frequency noise, baseline drifts, artifacts, and occasionally maternal-MCG were removed using standard techniques of biomagnetic signal processing (see Section 4). The neonatal electrocardiograph signal was similarly digitized at 1 kHz. The RR-series for HRV analysis was obtained from either type of signal after implementing a QRS detector using a modified Pan-Tompkins algorithm that was outlined in Section 4.

The RR-series for each neonatal data set spanned 1000 beats that were part of the baseline recordings, while the full lengths of the fetal RR-series (average of 690 beats per series) were utilized. Far outliers were removed using interquartile range boxes with asymmetric tolerance factors of 3 and 6 on the lower and upper side, respectively, to accommodate strong, natural variability. On average, 0.27% of data points were deemed far outliers in any data set, while most sets were not affected by far outliers at all.

Since heartbeats are not equispaced in time, the Lomb periodogram (Lomb, 1976) was computed after removing slow trends with a cubic polynomial filter. The Lomb algorithm has some advantages in accuracy of computing the power spectrum for non-uniformly spaced data points over using the fast Fourier transform on an interpolated uniform grid (Laguna & Moody, 1998; Chang et al., 2001). Spectra were computed on all available segments of RR-series with 192 beats in each segment and skipping forward by 96 beats. Segments had to satisfy a stationarity test that was implemented with the Kolmogorov-Smirnov test of differences between distributions on sub-segments (Shiavi, 1999). For inclusion, a segment also had to satisfy the condition that the average Nyquist frequency exceed 1.0 Hz, which was the upper limit of our high-frequency band. The band powers were averaged across all segments that passed the criteria. The resulting power spectrum was integrated in the low-frequency (LF) band from 0.05 to 0.25 Hz and in the high-frequency (HF) band from 0.25 to 1.00 Hz, and band powers were expressed in decibel units with respect to a reference level of 0.02 ms^2.

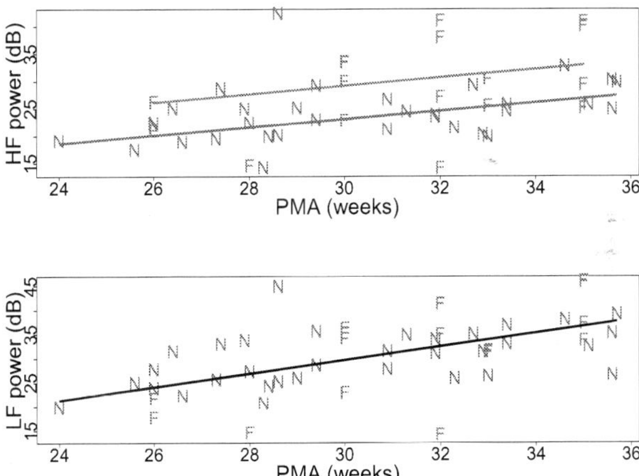

Fig. 9. Top panel depicts growth of HF power with post-menstrual age, differentiated between fetal and neonatal groups. Bottom panel depicts growth of LF power with post-menstrual age. Blue triangles represent fetal observations and red circles are neonatal observations. The lines are model predictions; in the top panel the upper and lower lines are for fetuses and neonates, respectively.

At any given scale, the sample entropy was computed for pair-wise matching with tolerance set at 20% of the standard deviation (Richman & Moorman, 2000). The RR-series was considered to be a point process for the computation of entropy. A self-similar series must necessarily be nonstationary. In first-order detrended fluctuation analysis, the signal at any time is transformed into a signal that has been integrated up to that time instant, ensuring nonstationarity. Fluctuations around linear trends are then computed for varying box sizes. If the resulting logarithm of fluctuations varies linearly with the logarithm of box size, there is evidence of self-similarity. The self-similarity parameter a represents the slope of the linear relationship. It is closely related to the asymptotic spectral exponent and to the Hurst exponent. The slopes of log-linear scaling regions of fluctuations were estimated from regression models. Continuously sliding windows were used in order to minimize estimation error. Since it is important to have precision in the timescales or box sizes in the computation of a, the RR-series was uniformly resampled on a grid with 400 ms spacing between points. The grid spacing corresponds closely to the average RR interval for the sample.

5.3 Results

Statistical models were constructed for HF and LF band powers to estimate age related changes and differences between fetal and neonatal HRV with adjustment for age. Robust regression technique was used in order to minimize impact of any large residuals on the model parameters (Yohai et al., 1991). All statistical significances were tested at the 95% confidence level. The HF power increased 0.75 ±0.29 dB per week in both groups, however the level of HF power was 6.08 ±2.11 dB higher in the fetuses than in the neonates (Fig. 9). The expected value of fetal HF power at 30 weeks PMA was 29.16 ±1.80 dB. The LF power increased 1.40 ±0.27 dB per week in fetuses and neonates, but there was neither a significant difference in the LF power levels nor in the rates of growth between the two groups. The expected value of fetal as well as neonatal LF power at 30 weeks PMA was 29.62 ±0.87 dB.

The expectation value of the mean RR-interval at 30 weeks PMA was 406.7 ±8.6 ms for a fetus and 13.0 ±3.3 ms lower for a neonate. The mean RR-interval increased by 9.2 ±3.0 ms per week for the fetal group, whereas it declined slightly for the neonates over the age range of the study. The mean heart rate is inversely related to the mean RR-interval.

Estimates of multiscale entropy are progressively less reliable at higher scales. The constraint of series length capped the highest scale at 7. Sample entropy was higher in the fetuses at all scales, as shown in Fig. 10. Statistical models showed differences of $0.24 - 0.30$, with mean difference of 0.28. Age-dependent changes in the entropy were not detected at any scale. There was no apparent effect of the magnetic environment, shielded or unshielded, on the shape of the multiscale entropy curves, suggesting that fMCG recordings obtained in unshielded settings are suitable for FHRV studies. The multiscale entropy of a 26 week old fetus showed high entropy at scale 1 and dropped thereafter. This is similar to the relationship of entropy to scale in adults with atrial fibrillation (Costa et al., 2002). The relationship of entropy to scale is reversed in the fetuses 30 weeks GA or older, and resembles that of normal adults (Fig. 11).

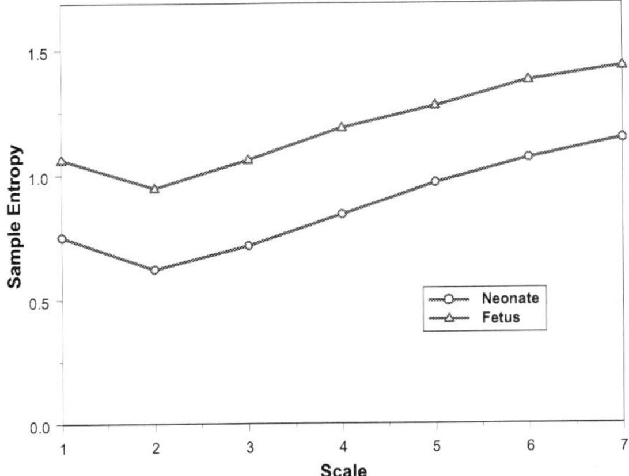

Fig. 10. Average fetal and neonatal entropy vs. scale of RR-series.

Fluctuations scaled linearly with box size on a log-log plot in both fetuses and neonates, indicating the presence of self-similar behavior of the RR-series (Fig. 12). There were typically 2 regions of linear scaling, one at box sizes below 25 (corresponds to timescales below 10 s) and a region with reduced slope of scaling at box sizes between 50 and 100 (corresponding to timescales between 20 and 40 s). This is in agreement with findings from studies of other fractal properties of fetal HRV (Felgueiras et al., 1998; Kikuchi et al., 2005). Spectral exponents were estimated from the scaling exponent at the fast timescales. The spectral exponent β represents the asymptotic slope of the power spectrum $(1/f^\beta)$. The exponent ranged between 1.3 and 2.6, with a tendency for neonates to exhibit a level that was nearly constant in the age range of the study, while the younger fetuses had a tendency toward lower spectral exponents. The middle 50% of all exponents were distributed in a narrow band around 2.0, from 1.9 to 2.1.

5.4 Implications

Cardiovascular variance in the HF band is closely related to respiration largely due to the shared control mechanism of the vagus nerve that is part of the parasympathetic nervous system. The decreased level of HRV in neonates in the HF band suggests that the sympathetic/parasympathetic balance of their autonomic nervous system is distinct from that of fetuses at identical post-menstrual ages. It is hypothesized that the physiological stresses of prematurity suppress the activity of the parasympathetic nervous system. Even the healthy "feeder-grower" premature neonate is encumbered with independent respiration and additional metabolic tasks that the fetus is not required to perform. It may be that growth of many systems, including the nervous system, becomes secondary to processes necessary for survival.

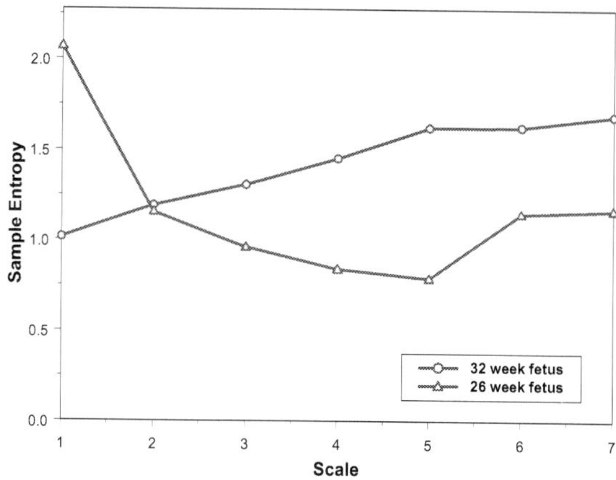

Fig. 11. Multiscale entropy of the heart rate variability of a 26-week fetus and a 32-week fetus show a reversal of relationship between entropy and scale.

The increasing trend of HRV in HF and LF bands in both fetuses and neonates reflects the maturation of parasympathetic and sympathetic nervous systems. The absence of a significant difference in the LF variance between neonates and fetuses suggests that the sympathetic fight-or-flight response is equally well-developed in the two groups.

Entropy of fetal RR-series was higher than the entropy of neonatal RR-series at all scales, which suggests that fetal HRV is more complex and non-repeating than its neonatal counterpart of the same PMA. We investigated the possibility of systematic bias in estimation of entropy due to greater length of the neonatal RR-series, and concluded that stability of estimation was sufficient to discount this possibility. Given the paradigm in the science of complex systems that higher levels of complexity are associated with healthier physiological systems (Goldberger et al., 2002), this may be another indicator that fetal HRV is in a more healthy state than HRV of the prematurely born neonate.

Two regions of scaling were present in the RR-series fluctuations, and there was no discernible difference of scaling regions between fetuses and neonates. Spectral exponents for neonates and fetuses were distributed around the value 2.0, which corresponds to the spectral exponent of a normal diffusion process. This represents a lower level of complexity compared to HRV in healthy adults that exhibits spectral exponents closer to 1 (Yamamoto & Hughson, 1994). The observed tendencies were for the neonates to have a higher spectral exponent that was steady, while the exponent increased in fetuses with advancing age. However, robust statistical models could not establish the increasing trend in fetuses at the 95% confidence level. Age-related changes in the scaling exponent were not detected in a larger study of fetal HRV (Lange et al., 2005) suggesting that relative constancy of the spectral exponent may be a property that is shared by fetuses and prematurely born neonates.

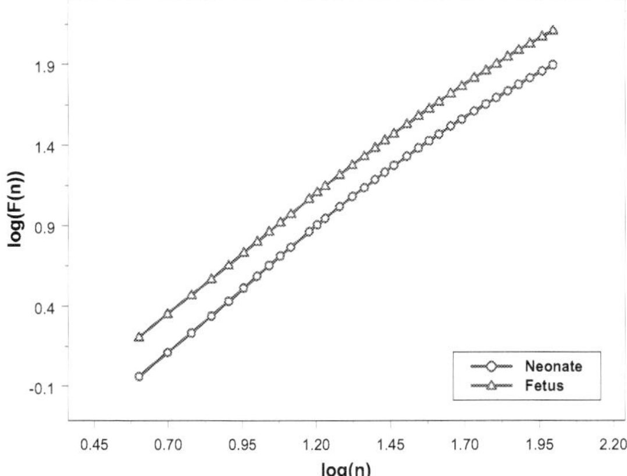

Fig. 12. Fluctuations vs. box size on a log-log scale shows linear relationship below timescale of 10 seconds. Curves represent averages over groups of neonates and fetuses.

The relationship of entropy to scale reversed in observations of fetuses at 26 weeks and 30 weeks gestational age, which may be indicative of a critical stage of maturation in the autonomic nervous system that controls their heart rate variability. This pilot study is limited by the sample size. More data is required, especially for fetuses younger than 30 weeks gestational age, before a more confident conclusion can be drawn. Spectral as well as complexity measures were computed from recordings in the unshielded environment that did not differ appreciably from corresponding measures computed from recordings in magnetically shielded rooms.

6. Conclusion

Fetal magnetocardiography offers direct evaluation of the electrophysiological properties of the fetal heart from an early stage of fetal development. It offers potentially more accurate examination of beat-to-beat intervals than does fetal ultrasound or fetal ECG. At present its wide clinical adoption is limited since it requires expensive magnetically shielded rooms. Recent successes in recording fetal magnetocardiograms with relatively small systems outside the shielded environment are a promising development. Application of the technical and computational tools was illustrated in a clinical study that compared spectral and complexity properties of heart rate variability in fetuses and age-matched, prematurely born neonates. Future work in fetal magnetocardiography is likely to focus on development of technology that is affordable for wide clinical deployment at the bedside and that is supported by diagnostics of fetal neuromaturation and stress based on measures of heart rate variability.

7. References

Brazdeikis, A.; Xue, Y. Y. & Chu, C. W. (2003). Non-invasive assessment of the heart function in unshielded clinical environment by SQUID gradiometry. *IEEE Trans. Appl. Supercond.*, 13, pp 385-388

Brazdeikis, A.; Guzeldere, A. K.; Padhye, N. S. & Verklan, M. T. (2004). Evaluation of the performance of a QRS detector for extracting the heart interbeat RR time series from fetal magnetocardiography recordings, *Proc. 26th Ann. Intl. Conf. IEEE Eng. in Med. and Biol. Soc.*, pp. 369–372, San Francisco, CA, USA

Brazdeikis, A.; Vázquez-Flores, G. J.; Tan, I. C.; Padhye, N. S. & Verklan, M. T. (2007). Acquisition of fetal magnetocardiograms in an unshielded hospital setting. *IEEE Transactions on Applied Superconductivity*, 17, 2, pp. 823-826

Brisinda, D.; Comani, S.; Meloni, A. M.; Alleva, G.; Mantini, D. & Fenici, R. (2005). Multichannel mapping of fetal magnetocardiogram in an unshielded hospital setting. *Prenatal Diagnosis*, 25, pp. 376-382

Chang, F. M.; Hsu, K. F.; Ko, H. C.; Yao, B. L.; Chang, C. H.; Yu, C. H.; Liang, R. I. & Chen, H. Y. (1997). Fetal heart volume assessment by three-dimensional ultrasound. *Ultrasound. Obstet. Gynecol.*, 9, pp. 42-48

Chang, K. L.; Monahan, K. J.; Griffin, M. P.; Lake, D. & Moorman, J. R. (2001). Comparison and clinical application of frequency domain methods in analysis of neonatal heart rate time series. *Ann. Biomed. Eng.*, 29, pp. 764-774

Comani, S.; Mantini, D.; Alleva, G.; Di Luzio, S. & Romani, G. L. (2004). Fetal magnetocardiographic mapping using independent component analysis. *Physiol. Meas.*, 25, 6, pp. 1459–1472

Costa, M.; Goldberger, A. L. & Peng, C. K. (2002). Multiscale entropy analysis of complex physiologic time series. *Phys. Rev. Lett.*, 89, 068102

De Araujo, D. B.; Barros, A. K.; Estombelo-Montesco, C.; Zhao, H.; da Silva Filho, A. C.; Baffa, O.; Wakai, R.; Ohnishi, N. (2005). Fetal source extraction from magnetocardiographic recordings by dependent component analysis. *Phys. Med. Biol.*, 50, 19, pp. 4457-4464

Drung, D. & Mück, M. (2004). SQUID electronics, In: *The SQUID Handbook*, Clarke, J. & Braginski, A. I. (Eds.), pp. 127-170, Wiley-VCH

Fagaly, R. L. (2006). Superconducting quantum interference device instruments and applications. *Rev. Sci. Instrum.*, 77, 101101-45

Felgueiras, C. S.; de Sa´ Marques, J. P.; Bernardes, J. & Gama, S. (1998). Classification of foetal heart rate sequences based on fractal features. *Med. Biol. Eng. Comput.*, 36, pp. 197–201

Ferrario, M.; Signorini, M. G.; Magenes, G. & Cerutti, S. (2006). Comparison of entropy-based regularity estimators: Application to the fetal heart rate signal for the identification of fetal distress. *IEEE Transactions on Biomedical Engineering*, 53, pp. 119-125

Friesen, G. M.; Jannett, T. C.; Jadallah, M. A.; Yates, S. L.; Quint, S. R. & Nagle, H. T. (1990). A comparison of the noise sensitivity of nine QRS detection algorithms. *IEEE Trans. Biomed. Eng.*, 37, pp. 85–98

Goldberger, A. L.; Amaral, L. A. N.; Glass, L.; Hausdorff, J. M.; Ivanov, P. C.; Mark, R. G.; Mietus, J. E.; Moody, G. B.; Peng, C. K. & Stanley, H. E. (2000). PhysioBank, PhysioToolkit, and PhysioNet: Components of a new research resource for complex physiologic signals. *Circulation*, 101, 23, pp. e215-e220 [Circulation Electronic Pages; http://circ.ahajournals.org/cgi/content/full/101/23/e215]

Goldberger, A. L.; Peng, C. K. & Lipsitz, L. A. (2002). What is physiologic complexity and how does it change with aging and disease? *Neurobiol. Aging*, 23, pp. 23-26

Hanqing, C.; Lake, D. E.; Ferguson, J. E.; Chisholm, C. A.; Griffin, M. P. & Moorman, J. R. (2006). Toward quantitative fetal heart rate monitoring. *IEEE Transactions on Biomedical Engineering*, 53, pp. 111-118

Hild, K. E.; Alleva, G.; Nagarajan, S. & Comani, S. (2007a). Performance comparison of six independent components analysis algorithms for fetal signal extraction from real fMCG data. *Phys. Med. Biol.*, 52, pp. 449-462

Hild, K. E.; Attias, H. T.; Comani, S. & Nagarajan, S. S. (2007b). Fetal cardiac signal extraction from magnetocardiographic data using a probabilistic algorithm. *Signal Proc.*, 87, pp. 1993–2004

Horigome, H.; Ogata, K.; Kandori, A.; Miyashita, T.; Takahashi-Igari, M.; Chen, Y. J.; Hamada, H. & Tsukada, K. (2006). Standardization of the PQRST waveform and analysis of arrhythmias in the fetus using vector magnetocardiography. *Pediatr. Res.*, 59, pp. 121-125

Kandori, A.; Miyashita, T.; Tsukada, K.; Horigome, H.; Asaka, M.; Shigemitsu, S.; Takahashi, M. I.; Terada, Y. & Mitsui, T. (1999a). Sensitivity of foetal magnetocardiograms versus gestation week. *Med. Biol. Eng. Comput.*, 37, pp. 545-548

Kandori, A.; Miyashita, T.; Tsukada, K.; Horigome, H.; Asaka, M.; Shigemitsu, S.; Takahashi, M.; Terada, Y.; Mitsui, T. & Chiba, Y. (1999b). A vector fetal magnetocardiogram system with high sensitivity. *Rev. Sci. Instrum.*, 70, pp. 4702-4705

Khattak, A. Z.; Padhye, N. S.; Williams, A. L.; Lasky, R. E.; Moya, F. R. & Verklan, M. T. (2007). Longitudinal assessment of heart rate variability in very low birth weight infants during their NICU stay. *Early Hum. Dev.*, 83, pp. 361-366

Kikuchi, A.; Unno, N.; Horikoshi, T.; Shimizu, T.; Kozuma, S. & Taketani, Y. (2005). Changes in fractal features of fetal heart rate during pregnancy. *Early Hum. Dev.*, 81, pp. 655-661

Köhler, B.-U.; Hennig, C. & Orglmeister, R. (2002). The principles of software QRS detection. *IEEE Eng. Med. Biol. Mag.*, 21, pp. 42–57

Koch, R. H.; Rozen, J. R.; Sun, J. Z. & Gallagher, W. J. (1993). Three SQUID gradiometer. *Appl. Phys. Lett.*, 63, pp. 403–405

Laguna, P. & Moody, G. B. (1998). Power spectral density of unevenly sampled data by least-square analysis: Performance and application to heart rate signals. *IEEE Trans. Biomed. Eng.*, 45, pp. 698-715

Lange, S.; Van Leeuwen, P.; Geue, D.; Cysarz, D. & Grönemeyer, D. (2005). Application of DFA in fetal heart rate variability. *Biomedizinsiche Technik*, 50, suppl. 1, pp. 1481-1482

Lomb, N. R. (1976). Least-squares frequency analysis of unequally spaced data. *Astrophys. and Space Sci.*, 39, pp. 447-462

Matlashov, A.; Zhuravlev, Y.; Lipovich, A.; Alexandrov, A.; Mazaev, E.; Slobodchikov, V. & Washiewski, O. (1989). Electronic noise suppression in multi-channel neuromagnetic system, In: *Advances in Biomagnetism*, Williamson, S. J.; Hoke, M.; Stroink, G. & Kotani, M. (Eds.), pp. 7725–7728, Plenum Press, New York

Mosher, J. C.; Flynn, E. R.; Quinn, A.; Weir, A.; Shahani, U.; Bain, R. J. P.; Maas, P. & Donaldson, G. B. (1997). Fetal magnetocardiography: methods for rapid data reduction. *Rev. Sci. Instrum.*, 68, pp. 1587-1595

Neonen, J.; Montonen, J. & Katila, T. (1996). Thermal noise in biogmagnetic measurements. *Rev. Sci. Instrum.*, 67, pp. 2397-2405

Osei, E. K. & Faulkner, K. (1999). Fetal position and size data for dose estimation. *Br. J. Radiol.*, 72, pp. 363-370

Padhye, N. S.; Brazdeikis, A. & Verklan, M. T. (2004). Monitoring fetal development with magnetocardiography, *Proc. 26th Ann. Intl. Conf. IEEE Eng. in Med. and Biol. Soc.*, pp. 3609–3610, San Francisco, CA, USA

Padhye, N. S.; Brazdeikis, A. & Verklan, M. T. (2006). Change in complexity of fetal heart rate variability, *Proc. 28th Ann. Intl Conf. IEEE Eng. in Med. and Biol. Soc.*, pp. 1796–1798, New York City, NY, USA

Padhye, N. S.; Verklan, M. T.; Brazdeikis, A.; Williams, A. L.; Khattak, A. Z. & Lasky, R. E. (2008). A comparison of fetal and neonatal heart rate variability at similar post-menstrual ages, *Proc. 30th Ann. Intl Conf. IEEE Eng. in Med. and Biol. Soc.*, pp. 2801–2804, Vancouver, BC, Canada

Pan J. & Tompkins, W. J. (1985). A real-time QRS detection algorithm. *IEEE Trans. Biomed. Eng.*, 32, pp. 230-236

Peng, C. K.; Buldyrev, S. V.; Havlin, S.; Simons, M.; Stanley, H. E. & Goldberger, A. L. (1994). Mosaic organization of DNA nucleotides. *Phys. Rev. E*, 49, pp. 1685-1689

Richman, J. S. & Moorman, J. R. (2000). Physiologic time series analysis using approximate entropy and sample entropy. *Am. J. Physiol.*, 278, pp. 2039-2049

Sarvas, J. (1987). Basic mathematical and electromagnetic concepts of the biomagnetic inverse problem. *Phys. Med. Biol.*, 32, pp. 11-22

Scheer, K. & Nubar, J. (1976). Variation of fetal presentation with gestational age. *Am. J. Obstet. Gynecol.*, 125, pp. 269-270

Shiavi, R. (1999). *Introduction to applied statistical signal analysis*, 2nd ed., Academic Press, San Diego

Sternickel, K. & Braginski, A. I. (2006). Biomagnetism using SQUIDs: status and perspectives. *Supercond. Sci. Technol.*, 19, pp. S160-S171

Stolz, R.; Bondarenko, N.; Zakosarenko, V.; Schulz, M. & Meyer, H. G. (2003). Integrated gradiometer-SQUID system for fetal magneto-cardiography without magnetic shielding. *Superconductivity Science Technologies*, 16, pp. 1523-1527

Tinkham, M. (1996). *Introduction to Superconductivity*, McGraw-Hill, New York

Uzunbajakau, S. A.; Rijpma, A. P.; ter Brake, H. J. M. & Peters, M. J. (2005). Optimization of a third-order gradiometer for operation in unshielded environments. *IEEE Trans. Appl. Supercond.*, 15, pp. 3879-3885

Van Leeuwen, P.; Lange, S.; Bettermann, H.; Grönemeyer, D. & Hatzmann, W. (1999). Fetal heart rate variability and complexity in the course of pregnancy. *Early Hum. Dev.*, 54, pp. 259-269

Van Leeuwen, P.; Cysarz, D.; Lange, S. & Geue, D. (2007). Quantification of fetal heart rate regularity using symbolic dynamics. *Chaos*, 17, 015119-9

Van Leeuwen, P.; Geue, D.; Lange, S. & Groenemeyer, D. (2009). Analysis of fetal movement based on magnetocardiographically determined fetal actograms and fetal heart rate accelerations, In: *ECIFMBE 2008, IFMBE Proceedings Vol. 22*, Vander Sloten, J.; Verdonck, P.; Nyssen, M. & Haueisen, J. (Eds.), pp. 1386-1389, Springer, Berlin

Vázquez-Flores, G. J. (2007). A realistic biomagnetic model for optimized acquisition of fetal magnetocardiograms in unshielded clinical settings, Thesis, University of Houston

Verklan, M. T.; Padhye, N. S. & Brazdeikis, A. (2006). Analysis of fetal heart rate variability obtained by magnetocardiography. *J. Perinat. Neonat. Nurs.*, 20, pp. 343-348

Vrba, J. (1996). SQUID gradiometers in real environments, In: *SQUID Sensors: Fundamentals, Fabrication and Applications*, Weinstock, H. (Ed.), pp. 117-178, Kluwer Academic Publishers, Dordrecht

Vrba, J. (2000). Multichannel SQUID biomagnetic systems, In: *Applications of Superconductivity*, Weinstock, H. (Ed.), pp. 61-138, Kluwer Academic Publishers, Dordrecht

Vrba, J. & Robinson, S. E. (2001). Signal processing in magnetoencephalography. *Methods*, 25, pp. 249-271

Wakai, R. T. (2004). Assessment of fetal neurodevelopment via fetal magnetocardiography. *Experimental Neurology*, 190, Suppl. 1, pp. S65-S71

Weinstock, H. (1996). *SQUID Sensors: Fundamentals, Fabrication and Applications*, Kluwer Academic Publishers, Dordrecht

Weinstock, H. (2000). *Applications of Superconductivity*, Kluwer Academic Publishers, Dordrecht

Williamson, S. J.; Pellizone, M.; Okada, Y.; Kaufman, L.; Crum, D. B. & Marsden, J. R. (1985). Five channel SQUID installation for unshielded neuromagnetic measurements, In: *Biomagnetism: Applications and Theory*, Weinberg, H.; Stroink, G. & Katila T. (Eds.), pp. 46-51, Pergamon Press, New York

Yamamoto, Y. & Hughson, R. L. (1994). On the fractal nature of heart rate variability in humans: effects of data length and beta-adrenergic blockade. *Am. J. Physiol.*, 266, pp. R40-R49

Yohai, V.; Stahel, W. A. & Zamar, R. H. (1991). A procedure for robust estimation and inference in linear regression, In: *Directions in Robust Statistics and Diagnostics, Part II*, Stahel W. A. & Weisberg, S. W. (Eds.), Springer-Verlag, Berlin

Zhao, H. & Wakai, R. T. (2002). Simultaneity of foetal heart rate acceleration and foetal trunk movement determined by foetal magnetocardiogram actocardiography. *Phys. Med. Biol.*, 47, pp. 839-846

23

Optical Spectroscopy on Fungal Diagnosis

Renato E. de Araujo, Diego J. Rativa, Marco A. B. Rodrigues
Department of Electronic and Systems, Federal University of Pernambuco
Brazil

Armando Marsden, Luiz G. Souza Filho
Department of Mycology and Tropical Medicine, Federal University of Pernambuco
Brazil

1. Introduction

Occurring globally, most fungi are undetectable to naked eye, living for the most part in soil, dead matter, as well as symbionts of plants, animals, or other fungi. Fungal infections are of important concern in several patients submitted to treatment with prolonged antibiotic therapy, immunosuppressive drugs, corticosteroids, degenerative diseases, diabetes, neoplasias, blood dyscrasias, endocrinopathies and other debilitating conditions as transplanted patients. In the most of cases, a rapid diagnostic and treatment is therefore critical (Davies, 1988).

In dermatological mycology, diagnostics modalities available are histopathology, direct microscopic examination of clinical specimen, culture and serology. Visual examination of skin, nail and hair samples for detect the presence of fungi is an essential step to confirm the clinical diagnosis of cutaneous fungus infection. Normally, the identification of fungi is done mainly by morphological *in vivo* studies based on visual macroscopic and microscopic aspects. Therefore, visual inspection requires a lot of training.

Characteristics of an organism's growth on culture media, such as colony size, color, and shape, provide clues to species identification. The prolonged incubation time is a major limitation of fungal cultures as a diagnostic tool. Biochemical and molecular biology techniques such as serology are also used for that purpose (Rippon, 1999; De Hoog et al., 2001). In particular, the serology test for detection of fungal antibodies take about 2 to 3 weeks, and it is of limited value especially in immunocompromised patients in whom production of antibodies is impaired. Multiple test techniques can be highly accurate but may require several days to yield results, creating delay in diagnosis, which may even culminate in a fatal outcome.

Here we exploit the autofluorescence spectroscopy of fungi as a tool to identify microbial infections. Different types of light source were used to excite endogenous fungal fluorochromes and a simple mathematical method was developed to identify specific features of the emission spectrum of six fungal species.

2. Fungal autofluorescence

Fluorescence consists of the electromagnetic radiation emitted by a material, especially of visible light, after absorption of incident radiation and persisting only as long as the stimulating radiation is continued. A number of cellular constituents fluoresce when excited directly or excited by energy transfer from another constituent, this fluorescence is called autofluorescence (Prasad, 2003). In the most of cases, excitation can be obtained by use of near ultraviolet (UV) light, with wavelength (λ) going from 320 to 400 nm (Prasad, 2003; Richards-Kortum & Sevick-Muraca, 1996). After the absorption of UV light by a fluorochrome, radiation of longer wavelength (visible light) is emitted.

The autofluorescence spectroscopic technique is a simple and quick procedure that can be exploited on fungal detection from *in vivo* diagnosis of dermatophytic infection to *in vitro* tissue or incubation on culture media by immunofluorescent techniques (Mustakallio & Korhonen, 1966; Asawanonda & Charles, 1999).

The first use of fluorescence by UV excitation in dermatology was reported in 1925 (Margarot & Deveze, 1925), with the detection of fungal infection on hair. At the present time UV light in dermatology is used predominantly in diagnostic areas involving pigmentary disorders, cutaneous infections, and the porphyrias (Asawanonda & Charles, 1999). Moreover, UV light can be very helpful establishing the extent of infection by *Malassezia furfur*, which presents a yellowish autofluorescence (Mustakallio & Korhonen, 1966). Blue-green fluorescence can be observed in *Microsporum audouinii* and *Microsporum canis* infections (Asawanonda & Charles, 1999). *Microsporum distortum* and *Microsporum ferrugineum* also present a greenish fluorescence. A faint blue color is emitted by *Trichophyton schoenleinii* and a dull yellow is seen in *Microsporum gypseum* fluorescence (Asawanonda & Charles, 1999). *In vitro* studies indicate that the chromophores pteridine is one of the chemical substances responsible for the fluorescence of *M. canis* and *M. gypseum* (Wolf, 1957; Chattaway & Barlow, 1958; Wolf, 1958). It was also showed the tryptophan dependence on the fluorochrome synthesis of *Malassezia* yeasts (Mayser et al., 2004; Mayser et al., 2002).

The advantages and limitations of UV light on fungal diagnosis are already known (Asawanonda & Charles, 1999). The emission spectrum overlap of different fungi can make them indistinguishable by a visual inspection of fluorescence. Moreover, some species of fungi do not contain fluorescent chemicals and therefore not all the fungi infections can be detected by visual analyses of their autofluorescence. To overcome this limitation nonspecific fluorochrome stains, such as Calcofluor White (λ~440nm) and Blancophor (λ~470nm) that binds to cellulose and chitin in cell walls of fungi, can be used to detect without ambiguity fungal elements in dermatological assays (in vitro) (Harrington & Hageage 1991).

3. UV Light Sources

In dermatology, the long-wave ultraviolet (UV) light source, known as Wood's lamp, has become an invaluable tool for diagnostic procedure. Wood's lamp was invented in 1903 by Robert W. Wood (1868–1955) (Wood, 1919). Wood's lamp is a high-pressure mercury fluorescent lamp that emits a broad band spectrum, with wavelength going from 320 to 400 nm, with a peak at 365 nm. In fluorescent lamps, mercury atoms are excited through collisions with electrons and ions. When the atoms return to their original energy level, they emit photons. The output intensity of a Wood's lamp is typically of few mW/cm^2.

For medical purposes, light on the UV region of the electromagnetic spectrum can be obtained with optoeletronics devices rather than Wood's lamp. A light-emitting diode (LED) is a semiconductor device that generates light when an electric current passes through it. LEDs are completely solid-state technology, making them extremely durable. On other hand, vibration or shock easily breaks the fragile glass tubing of a fluorescent lamp. In addition to being robust and efficient producers of light, LEDs are compact, low voltage and low power consuming devices, suitable to be used in small equipments. Moreover, it is possible to find LEDs in a wide range of colors, extending from ultraviolet (350 nm) to the far-infrared (1500 nm) region of the electromagnetic spectrum.

Ultraviolet light can also be obtained by the use of medical LASER systems, as excimer LASER (XeCl, XeF) and by infrared pulse LASERS (exploring the generation of second and third harmonic). The number of LASERS in medical clinics has rapidly increased in the last two decades, turning LASER therapy and diagnostic more accessible.

4. Autofluorescence spectroscopy

This section is devoted to describe the possibility of applying different UV light sources on the identification of fungi by optical spectroscopy.

Here six species of filamentous fungi were used: Five dermatophytes (*Microsporum gypseum, Microsporum canis, Trichophyton schoenleinii, Trichophyton rubrum, Epidermophyton floccosum*) and one *hyalohyphomycetes* (*Fusarium solani*). Theses fungi are recognized as emergent pathogens in the Northeast of Brazil. All of the samples studied were isolated from patients with dermatomycoses (superficial mycoses) attended in the medical mycology laboratory at the Federal University of Pernambuco. The biological materials were cultivated on Petri dishes with a Sabouraud Dextrose Agar (SDA) medium containing chloranphenicol (0.05 g/L). After isolation and identification (by microscopic and macroscopic morphological analysis) of the fungi, the samples were placed in glass tubes with SDA without antibiotic and preserved at room temperature (25ºC).

Four different light sources were explored in the experiment: 4 Watts UV fluorescent lamp (Wood's lamp) from Toshiba (BLUE FL4BLB) and from XELUX (G5), UV LEDs from Roithner LASER (UVLED365-10), and the third harmonic from a Nd:YAG nanosecond pulsed laser (Continuum/ Surelte). The light sources spectra are presented on figure 1. All light sources radiates on the UV-A region of the electromagnetic spectrum. The bandwidth and the peak wavelength of the light sources used were respectively 43 and 353nm for the Toshiba lamp, 18 and 375nm for the Xelux lamp, 19 and 363nm for the Roithner LED. The bandwidth of the UV LASER light at 352 nm was 3.5nm.

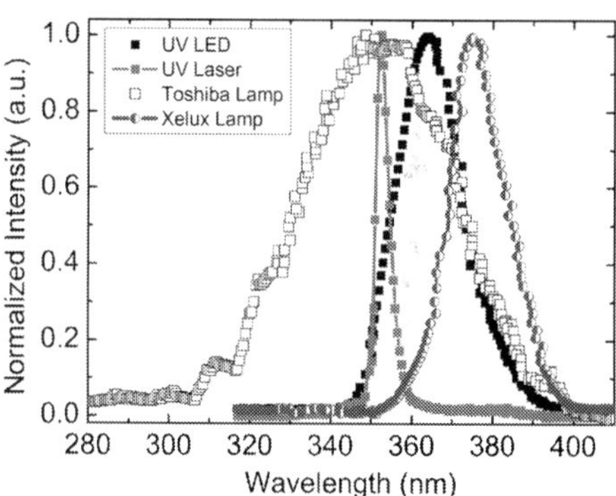

Fig. 1. Light sources emission spectra

In our experimental setup for fungal autofluorescence spectroscopy, the excitation UV light was focused on the sample. To keep the UV intensity with about the same value ($5mW/cm^2$) for all light sources, neutral density filters were used. The fungal autofluorescence light was collected by a lens system and sent to a spectrometer (SPEX/Minimate). A color filter (Corning 3-73) was placed at the entrance of the spectrometer to ensure that the excitation light would not reach the photomultiplier. A GaAs photomultiplier (RCA Electronic Device) was used to convert the collected light to an electrical signal. The signal was digitalized by a lock-in amplifier (SR530 Stanford Research) and sent to a computer, where it was stored and analyzed. The spectrum resolution of the experimental system was 0.5 nm. The experimental setup scheme is shown in Figure 2.

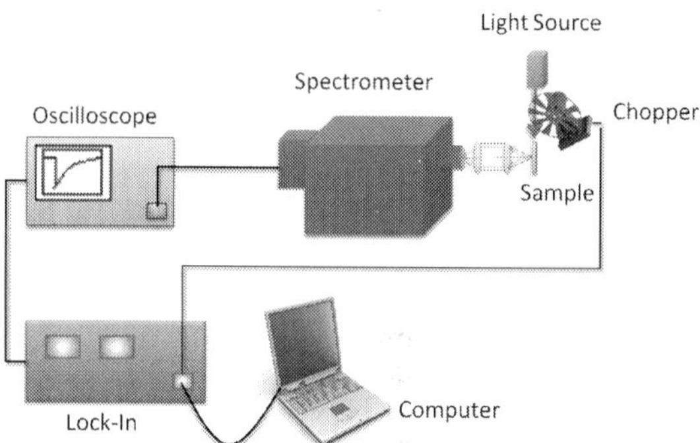

Fig. 2. Scheme of the experimental setup used.

For all fungi, the first fluorescence measurements were taken seven days after inoculation, and repeated 14 and 21 days later. In all experiments, all samples were investigated applying different light sources (UV Lamp, LED, and LASER). The excitation light power was monitored to ensure similar excitation conditions. Two set of attempts were performed one month apart. Spectroscopic analysis of isolated growth medium fluorescence was also performed.

5. Spectroscopic results and analysis

All samples studied fluoresced. Figure 3 shows the fluorescence of *F. solani*, *T. rubrum* and *T. schoenleinii*, *M. gypseum*, *M. canis* and *E. floccosum* excited with the UV LED 21 days after inoculation. An increase of the fluorescence intensity at the 21st day was noticed for several fungi. Spectroscopic results show (Figure 4) that fluorescence emissions induced by UV Lamps (Toshiba and Xelux) are quite similar from the ones obtained with UV LED (Figure 3). It can be observed on Figure 3 and 4 that the *T. rubrum* has a fluorescence spectrum very distinct from the other microorganisms.

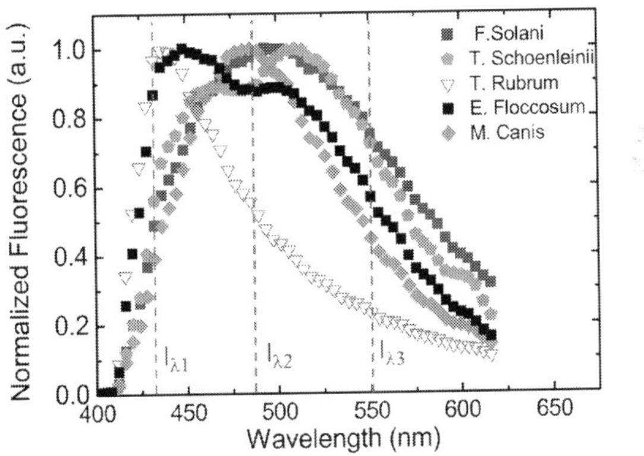

Fig. 3. Fungal emission after UV LED excitation (21 days after inoculation).

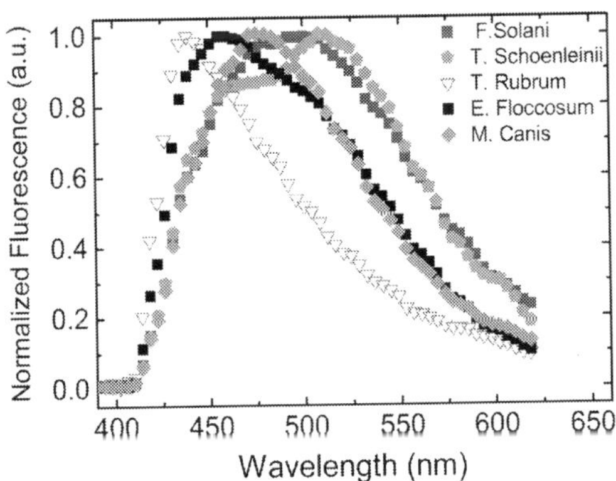

Fig. 4. Fungal emission after UV lamp excitation (21 days after inoculation).

The closeness of the peak emission wavelength and the spectrum shape of all samples, other than the *T. rubrum*, make it hard to distinguish fungi by a visual analysis of their autofluorescence. Although a careful spectroscopic analysis of the fluorescence shows distinct features on the detected emissions. Difference between fungi fluorescence spectra can be better perceived by analyzing the emission intensity at specific wavelength. Table 1 presents the values of a relative intensity defined as $(I_{\lambda 1}\text{-}I_{\lambda 2}\text{-}I_{\lambda 3})/(I_{\lambda 1}+I_{\lambda 2}+I_{\lambda 3})$, where $I_{\lambda 1}$, $I_{\lambda 2}$ and $I_{\lambda 3}$ are respectively the intensity of the fluorescence at 430, 485 and 550 nm, obtain in Fig. 3.

--------	$(I_{\lambda 1}\text{-}I_{\lambda 2}\text{-}I_{\lambda 3})/(I_{\lambda 1}+I_{\lambda 2}+I_{\lambda 3})$	
Fungi	**1° experiment**	**2° experiment**
T. rubrum	1.25 ± 0.05	1. 25 ± 0.05
F. solani	-4.15 ± 0.05	-4.20 ± 0.05
T. schoenleinii	-3.50 ± 0.05	-3.50 ± 0.05
M. canis	-7.50 ± 0.05	-7.55 ± 0.05
E. floccosum	-1.60 ± 0.05	-1.60 ± 0.05

Table 1. Fungal fluorescence spectral characteristics (LED excitation).

Fungal emission spectra obtained using the narrow band UV LASER excitation source is presented in Figure 5. UV LASER induced fluorescence present three peaks, resulting from specific energy decaying channels. The graphics in Figure 5 are normalized at 460 nm, to better show the spectra distinctions. Relative intensities of the peaks (417, 460 and 505 nm) can be explored to identify the studied fungi. Table 2 presents values of a relative intensity defined as $(I_{\lambda 1}\text{-}I_{\lambda 2})/(I_{\lambda 1}+I_{\lambda 2})$, where $I_{\lambda 1}$ and $I_{\lambda 2}$ are respectively the intensity of the fluorescence at 417 and 505nm, obtain by Fig. 5. The results in Table 2 indicate that a spectroscopic analysis of UV LASER induced fluorescence can be explored on the identification of fungi.

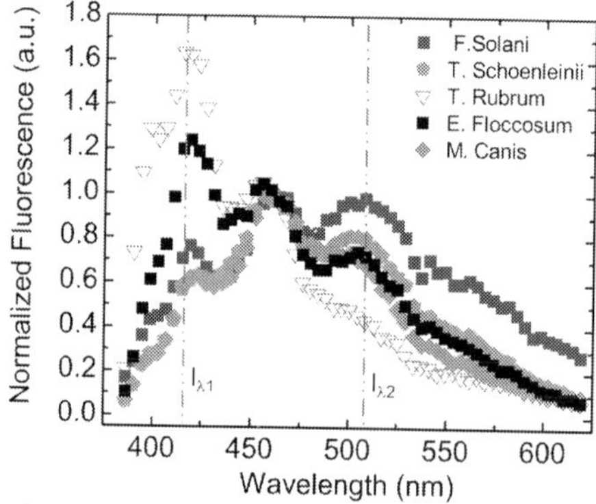

Fig. 5. Fungal emission after UV LASER excitation (21 days after inoculation).

--------	$(I_{\lambda 1}-I_{\lambda 2})/(I_{\lambda 1}+I_{\lambda 2})$	
Fungi	**1° experiment**	**2° experiment**
T. rubrum	0.55	0.54
F. solani	-0.09	-0.13
T. schoenleinii	-0.13	-013
M. canis	-0.10	-0.08
E. floccosum	0.28	0.26

Table 2. Fungal fluorescence spectral characteristics (LASER excitation)

6. Conclusion

Here it was demonstrated that optical spectroscopy can be exploit as a tool for fungal diagnosis. We observed distinct features on fungal emission. Although it is impossible do distinguish several microorganisms only by a visual analysis of their fluorescence. A careful spectroscopic analysis of fungal autofluorescence is required on the on the identification of microbial infections.

By exciting fungal fluorochromes with a broadband UV light source (LED and Lamp), we showed that a multiple wavelength (430, 485 and 550 nm) analysis of their autofluorescence spectrum can differentiate several fungi species. It has been proposed before a device for fungal diagnosis base on the analysis of the relative intensity of two specific wavelengths (Rativa, 2008). Here a better method for fungal identification is presented, based on the evaluation of three spectra regions of the fluorescent emission. We believe that a more refine mathematical model should be explored on a bigger group of fungi species. For that we are currently working with the Kolmogorov-Smirnov method on the fungal autofluorescence spectrum.

Here we also showed that UV narrow band light source (LASER) can lead to special features on the fluorescent spectrum. In that case a dual-wavelength analysis can be use to distinguish all the six fungal species studied. Although UV LASERS are still too expensive to be used for fungal diagnosis, their prices are constantly decreasing over the past decade. In the near feature UV LASER can be an important tool for dermatological diagnosis.

7. References

Asawanonda, P. & Charles, T.R. Wood's light in dermatology. *Int J Dermatol*, 38 (1999) 801-807.

Davies, S. F. Diagnosis of pulmonary fungal infections. *Semin Respir Infect*; 3, (1988) 162-171.

De Hoog, G. S.; Guarro, J.; Gene, J. & Figueras, M. J. (2001) *Atlas of Clinical Fungi*. 2nd ed., American Society Microbiology, Washington.

Chattaway, F. W. and Barlow, A. J. E. Fluorescent substances produced by Dermatophytes. *Nature*, 4604 (1958) 281-282.

Harrington, B. J. & Hageage, G. J. Jr. Calcofluor white: Tips for improving its use. *Clin Microbiol Newslett*, 13 (1991) 3–5.

Mayser, P.; Schäfer, U.; Krämer, H. J.; Irlinger, B. & Steglich, W. Pityriacitrin – a ultraviolet-absorbing indole alkaloid from the yeast Malassezia furfur. *Arch Dermatol Res*; 94 (2002) 131– 134.

Mayser, P.; Tows, A.; Kramer, H. J. & Weiss, R. Further characterization of pigment-producing Malassezia strains. *Mycoses*, 47 (2004) 34–39.

Margarot, J. & Deveze, P. Aspect de quelques dermatoses lumiere ultraparaviolette. *Bull Soc Sci Med Biol Montpellier*, 6 (1925) 375-378.

Monod, M.; Jaccoud, S.; Stirnimann, R.; Anex, R.; Villa, F.; Balmer, S. & Panizzon, R. Economical Microscope Configuration for Direct Mycological Examination with Fluorescence in Dermatology. *Dermatology*, 201 (2000) 246-248.

Mustakallio, K. & Korhonen, P. Monochromatic ultraviolet photography in dermatology. *J. Investig. Derm.*, 47 (1966) 351-356.

Prasad, P. N. (2003) *Introduction to Biophotonics*, 1st ed. Wiley-Interscience, New York.

Rativa, D. J.; Gomes, A. S. L.; Benedetti, M. A.; Souza Filho, L. G.; Marsden, A. & de Araujo, R. E. (2008) Optical spectroscopy on in vitro fungal diagnosis, *Proceedings of 30th Annual International EMBS Conference*, pp. 4871 – 4874, Vancouver, Aug. 2008, IEEE, Vancouver.

Richards-Kortum, R. & Sevick-Muraca, E. Quantitative Optical Spectroscopy for Tissue Diagnosis. *Annu. Rev. Phys. Chem.*, 47 (1996) 555–606.

Rippon, J. W. (1988) *Medical Mycology: The Pathogenic Fungi and the Pathogenic Actinomycetes*. 3rd ed. W B Saunders Co. Philadelphia

Wolf, F. T. Chemical nature of the fluorescent pigment produced in Microsporum-infected hair. *Nature*, 4591 (1957) 180-181.

Wolf, F. T. Fluorescent Pigment of Microsporum. *Nature*, 182 (1958) 475-476.

Wood, R. W. Secret communications concerning light rays. *J. of Physiol*; 5e serie: t IX (1919).

24

Real-Time Raman Spectroscopy for Noninvasive *in vivo* Skin Analysis and Diagnosis

Jianhua Zhao, Harvey Lui, David I. McLean and Haishan Zeng
*Laboratory for Advanced Medical Photonics and Photomedicine Institute,
Department of Dermatology and Skin Science,
University of British Columbia & Vancouver Coastal Health Research Institute
Cancer Imaging Department, British Columbia Cancer Research Center,
Vancouver, Canada*

1. Introduction

Human skin has been the object of numerous investigations involving noninvasive optical techniques including infrared (IR) spectroscopy and Raman spectroscopy (Zeng *et al.* 1995; Zeng *et al.* 2008; Kollias *et al.* 2002; Richards-Kortum *et al.* 1996; Mahadevan-Jansen *et al.* 1996; Hanlon *et al.* 2000). IR and Raman spectroscopy are complimentary techniques. Both techniques probe the vibrational properties of molecules according to different underlying physical principles. For example, IR spectroscopy is based on the absorption properties of the sample where the signal intensity follows the Beer's Law, while Raman spectroscopy relies on detecting photons that are scattered inelastically by the sample. The intensity of the Raman shift is directly proportional to molecular concentration. The differences in underlying mechanisms confer certain advantages for each method. The instrument for IR spectroscopy is simpler, but the spectra are strongly affected by water absorption in the IR region. The instrumentation for Raman spectroscopy is more complicated than for IR because the Raman signal is extremely weak, but its intensity is proportional to the concentration and independent of the sample thickness. Comparing these two techniques, Raman spectroscopy is more useful for *in vivo* applications. Since its introduction by Williams *et al.* for skin research, Raman spectroscopy has gained increasing popularity (Williams *et al.* 1992; Barry *et al.* 1992). Gniadecka *et al* studied human skin, hair and nail *in vitro* and the signatures of cutaneous Raman spectra have been well documented (Gniadecka *et al.* 1997; Gniadecka *et al.* 1998; Gniadecka *et al.* 2003; Gniadecka *et al.* 2004; Edwards *et al.* 1995). Caspers *et al* reported the Raman properties of different skin layers using *in vivo* confocal microscopy (Caspers *et al.* 1998; Caspers *et al.* 2001; Caspers *et al.* 2003). Raman spectroscopy has also been used to study dysplasia and cancer in a variety of human tissues, including skin (Huang *et al.* 2001a; Huang *et al.* 2005; Huang *et al.* 2006; Gniadecka *et al.* 1997; Gniadecka *et al.* 2004; Lieber *et al.* 2008a; Lieber *et al.* 2008b; Nijssen *et al.* 2002). Because the probability of Raman scattering is exceedingly low it has heretofore been characterized by weak signals or relatively long acquisition times on the order of several seconds to minutes (Barry *et al.* 1992; Williams *et al.* 1992; Edwards *et al.* 1995; Chrit *et al.* 2005; Gniadecka *et al.* 1997; Gniadecka *et al.* 1998; Gniadecka *et al.* 2003; Gniadecka *et al.* 2004; Shim *et al.* 1997; Nijssen *et al.* 2002). These factors have limited its clinical application in medicine.

The key to implementing Raman in a clinical setting is an integrated system that can provide real-time spectral acquisition and analysis. We are the first to demonstrate the feasibility of real-time *in vivo* Raman spectroscopy for practical clinical applications to the skin by reducing the integration time to less than one second (Huang *et al.* 2001a). Schut *et al.* also reported real-time *in vivo* Raman spectra of the finger, arm, nail, tooth, and tongue using a commercially available probe in combination with software post-processing (Schut *et al.* 2002). Motz *et al* reported a real-time Raman system for studying *in vivo* atherosclerosis (Motz *et al.* 2005a). In this chapter, we detail the design aspects of an integrated real-time Raman spectroscopy system for evaluating the skin. The system includes an image aberration correction feature for full-chip vertical hardware binning, and a software module for real-time data processing. Good signal-to-noise ratio (SNR) Raman spectra can be acquired within one second. This technique can be easily extended to other medical research fields such as lung, cervix or colon cancer diagnosis.

2. Raman Instrumentation

A real-time NIR Raman system is shown schematically in Fig. 1. It consists of five components: light source, light delivery, Raman probe, signal delivery, and signal detection (spectrometer). For real-time Raman spectroscopy, specific design features must be incorporated into each of these components.

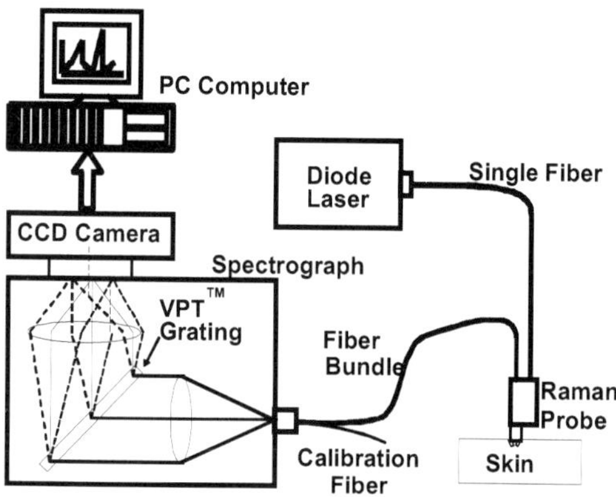

Fig. 1. Block diagrams of the integrated real-time Raman spectrometer system for skin evaluation and diagnosis (Adopted from figure 1a in Zhao *et al.* 2008a with permission).

2.1. Light source

The light sources used in Raman spectroscopy are mainly lasers because of their higher power output and narrower bandwidth. The choice of wavelength for Raman measurement depends on the specific application. For biologic tissue, a NIR laser is commonly used because of its deep penetration depth (700-1100 μm is regarded as the optical window of biological tissues) and the lower level of tissue autofluorescence under NIR excitation. For example, 632 nm, 690 nm, 785 nm, 810nm, 830 nm, and 1064 nm lasers have been reported in *in vivo* and *in vitro* Raman spectroscopy of human tissues (Short *et al.* 2006; Gniadecka *et al.* 1998; Huang *et al.* 2001a; Zhao *et al.* 2008a; Caspers *et al.* 1998; Caspers *et al.* 2001; Caspers *et al.* 2003). Shorter wavelengths are usually used for *ex vivo* thin tissue samples. Both pulsed and continuous-wave lasers are used in Raman spectroscopy. Pulsed lasers are mainly used in time-resolved Raman measurement or time-gated Raman spectroscopy to separate fluorescence from Raman scattering (Morris *et al.* 2005). Ultra-short pulsed lasers can be used in coherent anti-stokes Raman spectroscopy (CARS) (Cheng *et al.* 2004). For conventional Raman spectroscopy, continuous-wave lasers are used most commonly. The critical requirements for the laser source are its intensity and wavelength stability. Solid-state and diode lasers are popular choices for their portability. Our real-time Raman system initially used an external-cavity stabilized diode laser (785 nm, 300 mW, Model 8530, SDL, San Jose, CA) that was subsequently replaced by a solid-state diode laser (785 nm, 350 mW, Model BRM-785-0.35-100-0.22-SMA, B&W Tek Inc., Newark, DE, USA).

2.2. Light delivery

Optical fibers are most commonly used for light delivery in medical applications. The main considerations for choosing optical fibers are numerical aperture, core diameter, core material and its transmission properties. Single mode or polarization-maintaining fibers are rarely used for light delivery in Raman measurement because it is difficult to couple the laser beam into the small core (several microns) of these fibers. Multi-mode 100 – 200 μm core diameter fibers are commonly used. The choice of the numerical apertures (0.22 or 0.37) depends on the collection capability (numerical aperture matching) of the laser system and the lens system. The transmission properties depend on the core and cladding materials. High-OH fibers have high UV and visible wavelength transmission, while low-OH fibers are preferred for NIR and IR wavelength range. Raman signals may arise from the fiber's core material itself and contaminate the tissue signals. Puppels *et al.* studied the Raman properties of a number of commercially-available optical fibers (Santos *et al.* 2005). Choosing the right optical fiber is therefore important for *in vivo* Raman spectroscopy. Our system uses a 200-μm core-diameter low-OH single fiber for laser beam delivery because of its high NIR transmission.

2.3. Raman probe design

Of all the components in biomedical Raman systems, the Raman probe varies significantly according to the specific applications. For endoscopy, Raman probe is entirely composed of fibers because of size limitations. The amount of light delivered to the sample is limited by the thermal hazards. The design of a fiber-based Raman probe is driven by the need to maximize light collection. Because there are huge background signals originating from the laser source, the delivery fibers and other optical components, inline band-pass or long-pass filters are usually deposited onto the fiber tips to reduce noise, as with the lung (Short *et al.* 2008) and the gastrointestinal (Huang *et al.* 2009) probes. For other applications where size is less critical, specialized lens-and-filter based illumination and collection probes have been designed, such as the graded-indexed GRIN lenses probe (Myrick *et al.* 1990), the compound parabolic concentrator probe (Berger *et al.* 1997), the cervical Raman probe (Mahadevan-Jansen *et al.* 1996) and the ball lens Raman probe (Motz *et al.* 2005b).

The optical layout of our skin Raman probe is schematically shown in figure 2. It is designed to maximize the collection efficiency of the tissue Raman scattering and reduce the interference of the backscattered laser light, fiber fluorescence, and silica Raman signals. It consists of two arms: a 1.27 cm (0.5-inch) diameter illumination arm and a 2.54 cm (1-inch) diameter signal collection arm. In the illumination arm, the laser beam illuminates a 3.5 mm spot on the skin surface at a $40°$ degree incident angle after having passed through a collimating lens, a band pass filter (785 ± 2.5 nm; Model HQ785/5x, Chroma, Rockingham, VT), and a focusing lens. The band-pass filter can effectively reject Raman scattering and fluorescence that may arise from within the delivery fiber. The laser intensity is controlled so that the surface skin irradiance is 1.56 W/cm^2, which is lower than the ANSI maximum permissible exposure (MPE) limit of 1.63 W/cm^2 for a 785-nm laser beam (ANSI Standard Z136.1-1993, American National Standards Institute, Washington, DC) (Huang *et al.* 2001a).

The collection arm has a double-lens (FPX11685/102, JML, Rochester, NY) configuration, with the first lens for signal collection and beam collimation and the second lens for focusing the signal to the fiber bundle. Both lenses have a diameter of 25.4 mm with 90% of clear aperture and an effective focal length of 50 mm, which matches the numerical aperture (N.A.) of the fiber for good throughput. The focal point of the collection lens overlaps the focal point of the illumination lens on the illumination arm. The diameter of the fiber bundle determines the measurement size (1.3 mm on skin surface). In between the two collection lenses lies a high transmission interference 785 nm long pass (LP) filter (LP01-785RU-25, Semrock, Rochester, NY). Because the rejection by the interference LP filter depends on the incident beam angle, two 17.7 mm-aperture windows are used before the LP filter to reject stray light. This arrangement more effectively rejects the laser line and allows us to record Raman shifts down to 500 cm^{-1} for *in vivo* skin tissue.

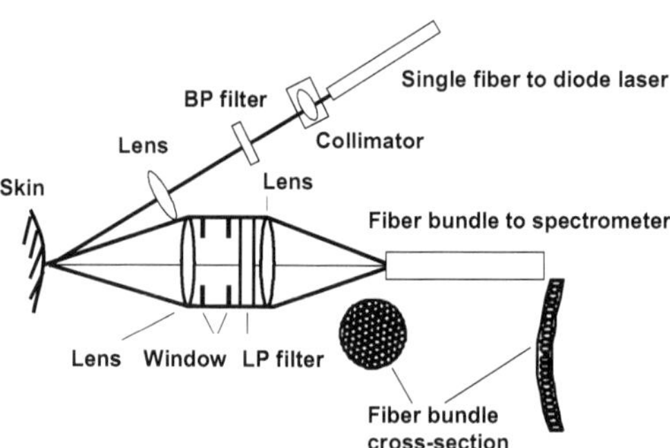

Fig. 2. Block diagrams of the specially designed skin Raman probe. See details in text (Adopted from figure 1b in Zhao *et al.* 2008a with permission).

2.4. Signal delivery

The raw signal, which is composed of Raman scattering and the tissue autofluorescence background, is collected by the probe and transmitted to the spectrometer detection system through a fiber bundle. The fiber bundle is composed of 58 low-OH fibers (100-µm core-diameter). The number of fibers is determined by the height of the CCD detectors (6.9 mm). The distal end of the fiber bundle that connects the Raman probe is packed into a 1.3-mm diameter circular area, which also defines the measurement spot size at the skin surface.

The proximal end of the fiber bundle that is coupled to the spectrograph has a patented design that substantially improves the signal to noise ratio (S/N) of the Raman system (Zeng 2002) and is discussed in detail below under the signal detection section.

2.5. Signal detection

The detection system is equipped with an NIR-optimized back-illumination deep-depletion CCD array (LN/CCD-1024EHRB, Princeton Instruments, Trenton, NJ) and a transmissive imaging spectrograph (HoloSpec-f/2.2-NIR, Kaiser, Ann Arbor, MI) with a volume phase technology based holographic grating (HSG-785-LF, Kaiser, Ann Arbor, MI). The CCD has a 16 bit dynamic range and is liquid nitrogen-cooled to -120°C. The f-number of the spectrograph (f = 2.2) matches the numerical aperture (N.A. = 0.22) of the fiber, so the throughput is much better than that of a traditional f/4 Czerny-Turner spectrographs (Owen *et al.* 1995).

Conventionally the spectrograph is equipped with a straight slit, whose image is well known to be parabolic through a plane grating (HoloSpec, VPT System Operations Manual, Kaiser Optical System, Ann Arbor, MI, 1994). The parabolic shape arises from the fact that rays from different positions along the length of the slit are incident on the grating at varying degrees of obliqueness. For spectrographs with short focal lengths, this obliqueness causes significant distortion that can affect the performance of the detector. For example, the horizontal displacement of a spectral line of our system is shown graphically in figure 3 (Huang *et al.* 2001a), with the displacement rounded to pixels (dashed lines). The maximum horizontal displacement is 5 pixels (135 µm). The solid line is a linear regression-fitted parabolic curve described by $x = 1.1904{\times}10^{-5}\, y^2 - 1.9455{\times}10^{-4}\, y - 0.98613$, where x is the horizontal displacement at a vertical position, y. This image aberration causes two problems for hardware binning of CCD detectors: (1) It decreases the spectral resolution and (2) it decreases the S/N ratio. It also causes problems in wavelength calibration. The manufacturer (Kaiser) of the HoloSpec spectrograph suggested a combination of hardware and software binning in which the neighboring pixels along the dashed vertical line are hardware binned, then shifted to the appropriate number of pixels and summing them up with software. As shown in figure 3, there are 11 such hardware-binning groups. Another simple method is a complete software binning procedure, in which the whole image is acquired first and then all the pixels along the curve are added up together using software. However, the improvement of S/N ratio using software binning or combined hardware-software binning is limited because the binning only improves the S/N ratio by as much as the square root of the number of pixels binned together. For signal levels that are readout-noise limited, i.e., weak Raman signal measurements, hardware binning is preferred because it improves the S/N ratio linearly with the number of pixels grouped together. We proposed a simple novel solution for full-chip hardware binning by eliminating this image

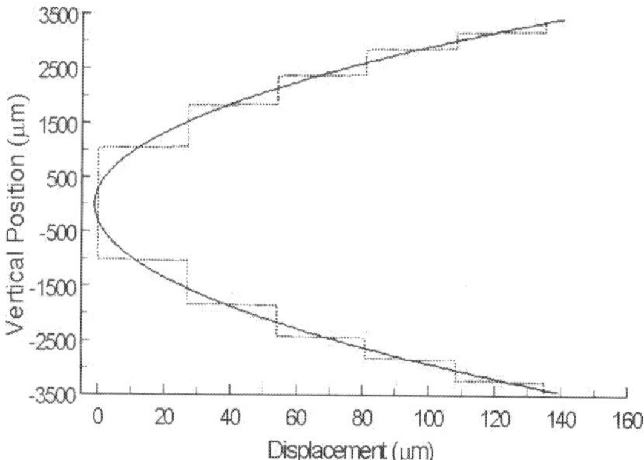

Fig. 3. Graphic representation of the curve observed in horizontal displacement rounded to pixels (dashed lines). The solid curve is a linear-regression-fitted parabolic line (Adopted from figure 3 in Huang *et al.* 2001a with permission).

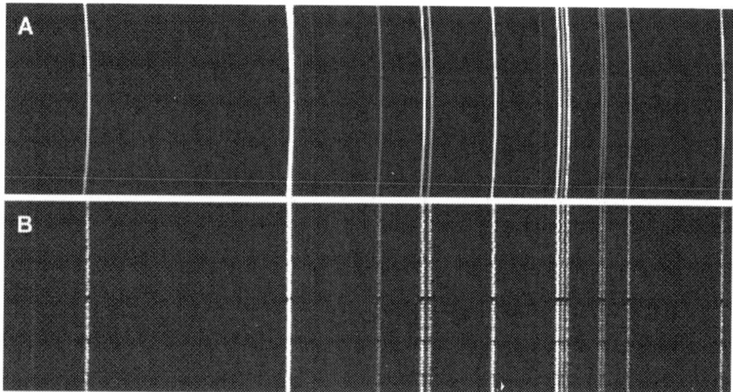

Fig. 4. (a) Mercury-argon lamp image of a 100-μm slit on the CCD through the HoloSpec spectrograph, demonstrating the image aberration. (b) CCD image of 58 fibers aligned along a parabolic line at the entrance of the spectrograph, demonstrating that the image aberration has been corrected (Adopted from figure 2 in Huang *et al.* 2001a with permission).

aberration. As shown in Fig. 2, the 58 fibers of the fiber bundle are aligned at the spectrograph end along a curve formed by the horizontal displacement, but in the reverse orientation. Figure 4a shows the image aberration of a 100-μm slit through the spectrograph in our uncorrected system when it is illuminated by a mercury argon lamp. Figure 4b shows a CCD image of the fiber bundle illuminated by a mercury argon lamp after image aberration correction. The center fiber (dark spot) is used for calibration so that the image of the fibers is symmetrical along the centerline of the CCD detectors. With this specific fiber arrangement the spectral lines are substantially straighter, which enables image-aberration and full-chip hardware binning along the entire CCD vertical line (256 pixels) without losing resolution and reducing the S/N ratio. The S/N ratio improvement that we achieve with our system is 3.3 times that of the combined hardware and software binning procedure, and 16 times that of the complete software binning (Huang *et al.* 2001a). The spectral resolution of the system with 100-um fiber is 8 cm^{-1}.

3. Software Implementation

The real-time Raman control and data acquisition & analysis system are implemented with Labview (National Instruments, Austin, TX drivers from R Cubed Software, Lawrenceville, NJ) (Zhao *et al.* 2008a). A flow chart of the software implementation is shown in figure 5. The estimate of time cost for each step is marked in millisecond. There are three key steps: system initialization, real-time data acquisition, and real-time data processing.

3.1. Raman system initialization

Before clinical measurement, a number of system calibrations are necessary. These calibrations include wavelength calibration, system spectral response calibration, intensity calibration and CCD dark-noise subtraction. The CCD dark-noise is first measured before each measurement and sequentially subtracted immediately after the CCD readout. Wavelength calibration can be performed using cyclohexane, acetone and barium sulfate, in combination with an Hg-Ar lamp. In our system, 10 major peaks that span the whole wavelength range are used for wavelength calibration. A fifth-order polynomial fitting is used to correlate the CCD pixels with the wavelengths. Because system configuration does not change during the Raman measurement, wavelength calibration can be implemented before the measurement. The spectral response calibration is critical to correct the optical transfer function, which varies from system to system. It is performed using an NIST (National Institute of Standards and Technology) traceable tungsten calibration lamp. The ratios of the known spectral irradiance of the lamp to the measured spectra yield the spectral response correction factors. System-independent spectra are then obtained from the measured spectrum through multiplication by the spectral response correction factors. To facilitate intensity calibration, a NIST traceable reflectance standard disk (SRS-99-020, Labsphere, New Hampshire, USA) was used, which showed stable Raman peaks at 726.56 cm^{-1} and 1379.06 cm^{-1}. The Raman spectrum of the standard disk was measured before each experiment, and then used to correct the intensity variations of the laser beam. The laser output can also be monitored directly for laser intensity correction.

The program starts with system initialization, including the above wavelength calibration, spectral response calibration, intensity calibration and CCD dark-noise subtraction. It also loads all databases or files needed for PCA and LDA analysis as well as the reference Raman spectra for biochemical composition analysis. Other steps are also included such as those necessary for the real time measurement and archiving, setting specific regions of interest (ROI) of the CCD detector, data auto-saving, patient information, and comments etc.

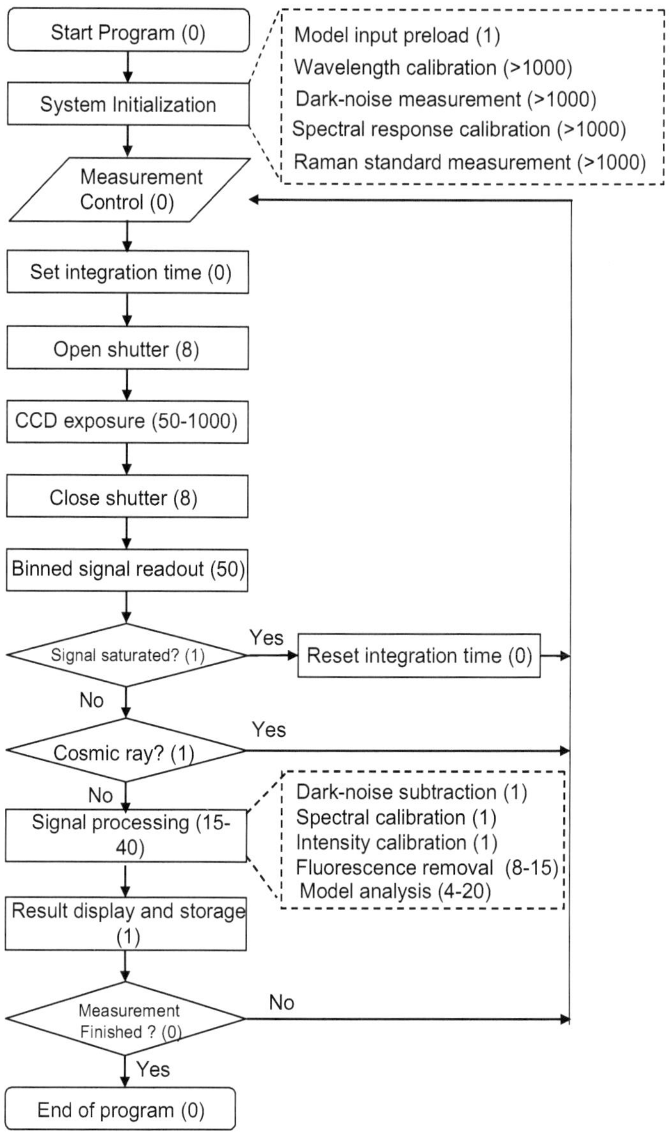

Fig 5. Flow chart of the real-time Raman system. It shows all the necessary steps for processing Raman spectra. The numbers in parentheses are estimates in millisecond (ms) required for each module (Adopted from figure 4 in Zhao *et al.* 2008a with permission).

3.2. Raman data acquisition

After initialization, the system is ready for real-time measurements. Measurements are started via a control signal that can be triggered from the keyboard, hand switch, foot switch, or a signal generated by the program itself. There are two shutters in the system, which essentially have identical response times. One internal shutter lies in the front of the CCD camera to prevent over-exposure or exposure during the readout process. The other lies in the path of laser output to prevent any effect on the skin before measurement, such as photobleaching of tissue autofluorescence (Zeng *et al.* 1998). Both shutters are synchronized to open after the control signal is triggered and then close after a pre-set exposure time. The raw signal (including tissue Raman and autofluorescence background) is read out after the shutter closure.

Both Raman and fluorescence intensities vary according to subject and site within the same subject; for example pigmented lesions exhibit relatively higher NIR autofluorescence (Huang *et al.* 2006; Han *et al.* 2009). The initial choice of integration time may not be optimal. Therefore, signal saturation control is necessary for real-time systems. Signal saturation control can be implemented by reducing the laser intensity as in the atherosclerosis Raman system (Motz *et al.* 2005a), or by reducing the integration time. For our skin Raman measurement, signal saturation control was implemented by reducing the integration time with close to 100% accuracy. Basically we compare the signal with the dynamic range of the CCD detector before background subtraction (i.e. 65535 for a 16-bit dynamic range). To account for noise, any five successive values (except near laser line) of the spectrum beyond the dynamic range will indicate that saturation has occurred. The saturated spectra are then discarded and the data acquisition procedures are repeated automatically with a lower exposure time. The initial integration time is usually set to be equal to or less than 1 second. Experiments show that half of the initial integration time can always suffice for preventing saturation.

Another issue for real-time measurement is cosmic rays, which are detected by the Raman system at an average rate of 1-5% per one-second exposure time. To our knowledge automatic cosmic ray rejection has not yet been incorporated into real-time biomedical Raman systems. Our algorithm for cosmic ray rejection is based on the striking differences between the peak bandwidths of biological tissue Raman peaks which are usually a few tens of pixels, and those of cosmic rays which are usually limited to a couple of pixels. Our algorithm compares each data point with its adjacent 5 points on both sides to determine whether a cosmic ray is present. A sharp peak with bandwidth of only 1-2 pixels will define a cosmic ray signal and prompt the system to repeat the measurement automatically until a cosmic ray-free Raman signal is obtained. For measurements with longer integration times, cosmic rays are unavoidable, and thus, an alternative would be to remove the cosmic ray through software.

3.3. Raman data processing

Real-time data processing includes CCD dark-noise subtraction, spectral response calibration, intensity calibration, fluorescence background removal, and data modeling and analysis (i.e. GLS fitting, PCA, LDA etc). The CCD dark-noise is first subtracted from the cosmic ray-free raw signal before further analysis. After dark-noise subtraction, the spectral response of the system is also corrected using a standard tungsten-halogen lamp, which was loaded during the system initialization. The laser intensity variation is also corrected. All signals are then scaled to an equivalent integration time of 1 second.

The most important step in real-time Raman spectroscopy is the rejection of NIR autofluorescence background that is superimposed on the Raman signal. The most commonly used method in biomedical Raman measurement is single polynomial curve-fitting (Mahadevan-Jansen *et al.* 1996). As discussed, the major weakness of polynomial fitting is its dependence on the spectral range and the choice of polynomial order (Zhao *et al.* 2007). Lieber *et al* proposed an iterative modified polynomial method to improve the fluorescence background removal (Lieber *et al.* 2003). Recently we proposed the Vancouver Raman Algorithm, which combines peak-removal with a modified polynomial fitting method. This method substantially improves the fluorescence background removal, particularly for spectra with high noise or intense Raman peaks. The advantages of the Vancouver Raman Algorithm are that it not only reduces the computation time, but also suppresses the artificial peaks on both ends of the spectra that may be introduced by other polynomial methods. The algorithm is less dependent on the choice of the polynomial order as well (Zhao *et al.* 2007). A copy of the algorithm for noncommercial use can be downloaded from http://www.bccrc.ca/ci/people_hzeng.html.

A detailed diagram of the Vancouver Raman Algorithm can be found in the reference by Zhao et al. (Zhao *et al.* 2007). It starts from a single polynomial fitting $P(v)$ using the raw Raman signal $O(v)$, followed by calculation of its residual $R(v)$ and its standard deviation DEV, where v is the Raman shift in cm^{-1}. The quantity of DEV is considered an approximation of the noise level. In order to construct data for the next round of fitting, we compared the original data with the sum of the fitted function and the value of its DEV, defined as SUM. The data set is reconstructed following the rule that if a data point is smaller than its corresponding SUM, it is kept; otherwise it is replaced by its corresponding SUM. Setting DEV=0, is equivalent to Lieber's method (Lieber *et al.* 2003), but applying our rule provides a means for taking into account the noise effect and avoiding artificial peaks that may arise from noise and from both ends of the spectra. In order to minimize the distortion of the polynomial fitting by major Raman signals, the major peaks are identified and are removed from the subsequent rounds of fitting. Peak removal is limited to the first few iterations to prevent unnecessary excessive data rejection. The iterative polynomial fitting procedure is terminated when further iterations cannot significantly improve the fitting, determined by $|(DEV_i - DEV_{i-1})/DEV_i| < 5\%$. As with many iterative computation methods, the percentage can be empirically adjusted by the user according to the problem involved and computation time allowed. However, we recommend it be fixed in the whole process for a given clinical study. The final polynomial fit is regarded as the fluorescence background. The final Raman spectra are derived from the raw spectra by subtracting the final polynomial fit function.

An example of the Vancouver Raman Algorithm and the final Raman spectra is shown in Fig. 6. It is the spectra obtained from solid phase urocanic acid (Sigma Aldrich, USA), which exhibits multiple intense Raman peaks. For comparison purpose, the results for single

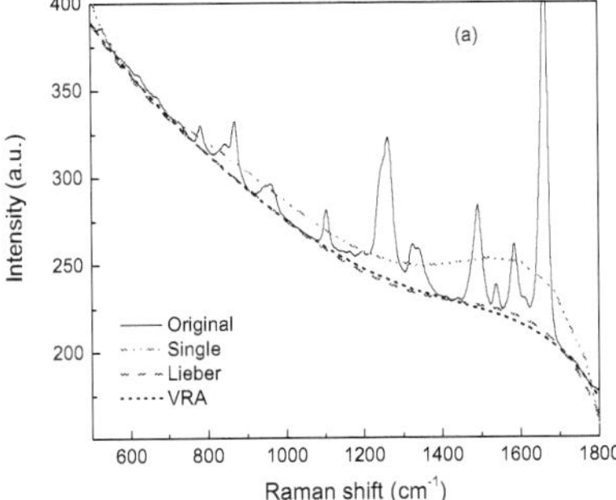
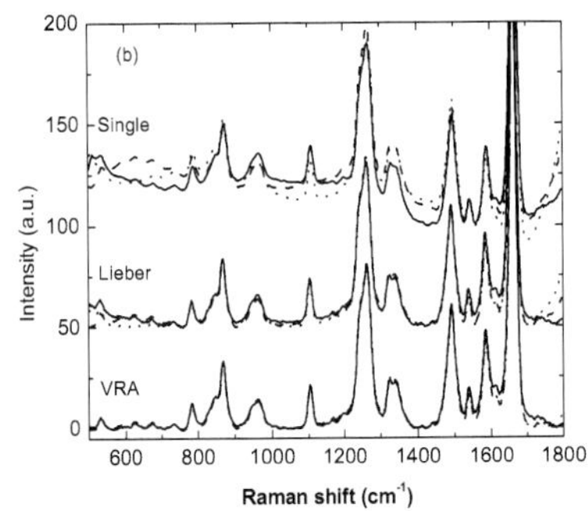

Fig. 6. (a) Raw Raman spectra and the fitted fluorescence background using a fifth order single polynomial (Single), Lieber's modified polynomial (Lieber) and the Vancouver Raman Algorithm (VRA). (b) The final Raman spectra obtained from the three methods with the choice of the fourth-, fifth- and sixth-order polynomial fitting. The sample is solid phase urocanic acid, obtained from Sigma Aldrich, USA without further processing (Adopted from figures 6a and 7 in Zhao *et al.* 2007 with permission).

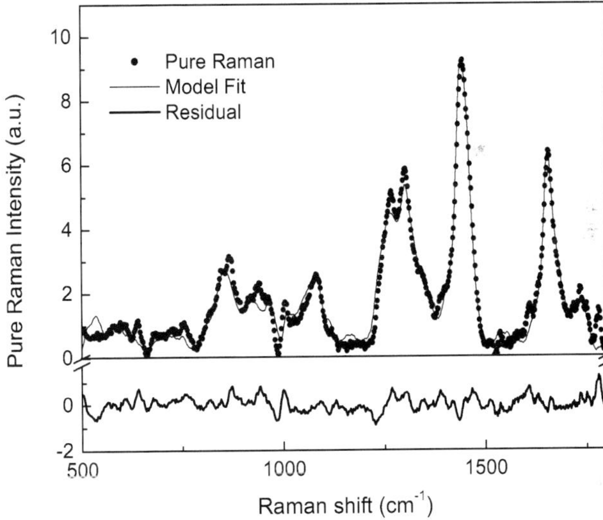

Fig. 7. Modeling of Raman spectra of an Asian volunteer (volar forearm skin) with integration time of 1 second, showing the "pure" Raman spectrum, the general least square fitting, and the fitting residuals for a 5-component reference model (see text) (Adopted from figure 5c in Zhao *et al.* 2008a with permission).

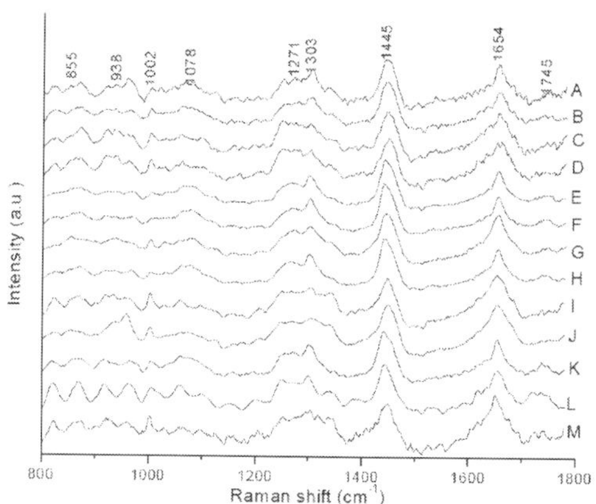

Fig. 8. *In vivo* skin Raman spectra obtained from different skin locations of a healthy volunteer. (A) forehead, (B) cheek, (C) chest, (D) abdomen, (E) volar side of the forearm, (F) surface of the forearm, (G) palm of the hand, (H) dorsal hand, (I) fingertip, (J) fingernail, (K) leg, (L) dorsal foot; (M) sole of the foot (Adopted from figure 2 in Huang *et al.* 2001b with permission).

Peak position (cm⁻¹)	Protein Assignment	Lipid Assignment	Others
822 (w)	δ(CCH) aliphatic		
855 (mw)	δ(CCH) aromatic, olefinic		polysaccharide
880 (mw, sh)	ρ(CH₃)		
936 (mw)	ρ(CH₃) terminal, ν(CC) proline, valine		
1002 (mw)	ν(CC) phenyl ring		
1031 (mw)	ν(CC) skeletal		
1065 (mw, sh)		νₐₛ(CC) skeletal	
1080 (ms)		ν(CC) skeletal	ν(CC), νₛ(PO₂), nucleic acid
1128 (mw, sh)		νₛ(CC) skeletal	
1269 (s, sh)	ν(CN), δ(NH), amide III		
1303 (s, sh)		δ(CH2) twisting, wagging	
1445 (vs)	δ(CH₂), δ(CH₃)	δ(CH₂) scissoring	
1655 (s)	ν(C=O) amide I		
1745 (m)		ν(C=O)	

Table 1. Summary of major Raman bands identified in skin. w: weak, m: medium, s: strong, v: very, sh: shoulder; ν: stretching mode, νₛ: symmetric stretching mode, νₐₛ: asymmetric stretching mode, ρ: rocking mode, δ: bending mode (Adopted from table 1 in Huang *et al.* 2001b with permission).

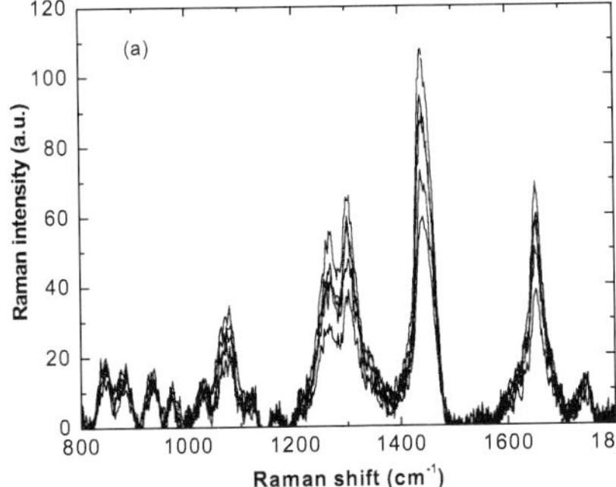
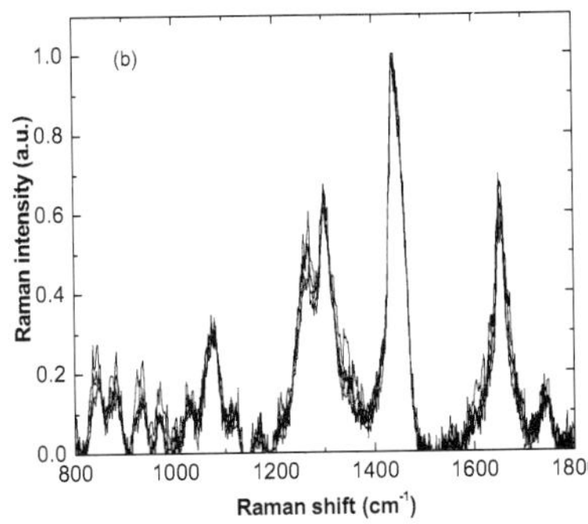

Fig. 9. Sample spectra of human volar forearm skin of 5 subjects showing that the absolute spectra are dramatically different, whereas the normalized spectra have very little variation. (a) absolute Raman spectra, and (b) normalized Raman spectra (Adopted from figure 3 in Zhao *et al.* 2008b with permission).

polynomial fitting and modified polynomial fitting are also presented. Figure 6a is the raw spectra and the fitted fluorescence background of the three methods with the fifth-order polynomial fitting. Note how the intense peak at 1664 cm⁻¹ heavily biases the single polynomial fitting. Neither single polynomial fitting method nor Lieber's method generates satisfactory results. Because the peak regions are removed in the Vancouver Raman Algorithm, the bias of the major peaks is minimized. Potential artifacts at both the upper and lower spectral boundary regions are also prevented. Fig. 6b shows the final Raman spectra of the solid phase urocanic acid sample after the fluorescence background removal using the above three methods with the choice of the fourth- (solid line), fifth- (dashed line) and sixth-order (dotted line) polynomial fittings. No method was found to be totally independent of the polynomial order. The Raman spectra from the single polynomial fitting differ significantly for different orders. Lieber's method substantially reduces the variability amongst the choices of orders. The Vancouver Raman Algorithm is the most indifferent with respect to the choice of polynomial order.

Both the Raman spectra and the fluorescence background can be further analyzed. For example, combining the Raman and fluorescence has been shown to improve the sensitivity and specificity of tumor detection (Huang *et al.* 2005). Data analysis models can include reference spectra of morphological and chemical components for general least square fitting, or tissue-specific diagnostic algorithms. Figure 7 shows the Raman spectra, the model fits, and the residuals. In this particular model, the reference Raman spectra of oleic acid, palmitic acid, collagen I, keratin and hemoglobin standard are used. The reference Raman spectra are measured directly from the commercially obtained samples (Sigma Aldrich, St. Luis, MO) without any further processing. The results demonstrated that the skin Raman spectra can be modeled based on these separate components.

4. Applications

The integrated real-time skin Raman system can provide the final Raman spectra in real-time. Its usefulness for *in vivo* skin assessment and skin diseases diagnosis is currently under investigation in our laboratory, and some preliminary results are summarized below.

4.1. *In vivo* Raman spectra of normal skin

We have measured *in vivo* Raman spectra of normal skin on 25 different body sites of 30 healthy volunteers (15 female, 15 male; 17 Caucasian and 13 Asian, average age of 37 years old) (Zhao *et al.* 2008b). Before each measurement, the skin was cleaned with a single wipe of tissue saturated in 70% isopropyl alcohol. The *in vivo* Raman spectra of the skin from different skin regions of the body are shown in Fig. 8. Prominent spectral features in the range of 800-1800 cm^{-1} are the major vibrational bands around 1745, 1655, 1445, 1301, 1269, 1080, 1002, 938, and 855 cm^{-1}. The vibrational assignments for the major skin Raman bands are summarized in Table 1. The strongest band is located at 1445 cm^{-1}, and is assigned to the CH_2 deformations of proteins and lipids. The 1655 cm^{-1} and 1269 cm^{-1} bands are assigned to protein vibrational modes involving in amide I and amide III. The strong band centered at 1301 cm^{-1} is assigned to a twisting deformation of the CH_2 methylene groups of intracellular lipid. The region from 1000 to 1150 cm^{-1} contains information on the hydrocarbon chain. Peaks at 1128 and 1062 cm^{-1} are consistent with C-C stretching modes, while the peak at 1080 cm^{-1} is due to a random conformation vibrational mode. The 1002 cm^{-1} peak, assigned to the phenylalanine breathing mode, is seen in nearly all skin sites, particularly in nail and palm skin.

Distinct Raman peaks in the 800–1800cm^{-1} range can be discerned clearly from various skin sites of the body. We found that within the same subject, skin Raman signals vary significantly according to body sites (Fig. 8). The absolute skin Raman signals for a given body site are also significantly different between subjects, but the normalized Raman spectra (normalized to the strongest peak at 1445 cm^{-1}) have relatively minimal differences as shown in Fig. 9. This may provide unique advantage in skin disease diagnosis. The ratio of the 1655 to 1445 cm^{-1} differs by body site. It shows that keratin-abundant skin sites such as finger-tip and palm regions have the highest mean value (1.023-1.051), and the earlobe the lowest (0.702) (Huang *et al.* 2001b). This means that the lipid/protein compositions are not uniform throughout the body, and this body-site differences need to be factored into skin Raman assessment and disease diagnosis.

4.2. Raman spectra of *in vivo* melanin

Melanin is one of the most ubiquitous and biologically important natural pigments. It is largely responsible for the color of skin, hair, and eyes. Functionally, melanin can act as a sunscreen, scavenge active chemical species, and produce active radicals that can damage DNA. Melanin can be divided into two main classes: a black-to-dark-brown insoluble eumelanin found in black hair and retina of the eye, and a yellow-to-reddish-brown alkali soluble pheomelanin found in red hair and red feathers. Because of its biological importance, particularly its role in skin, melanin has been extensively studied using a wide variety of techniques including mass spectrometry, x-ray diffraction, nuclear magnetic resonance, and scanning tunneling microscopy. Although eumelanin is currently believed to be a heteropolymer, its chemical structure and biological functions are still subject to debate. Optical measurement is a standard tool for *in vivo* melanin detection and measurement. At the present time, *in vivo* optical measurements of melanin are largely based on its absorption properties. However, melanin has no distinctive absorption peaks to distinguish itself from other cutaneous chromophores such as oxy- and deoxy-hemoglobin, which makes it very difficult to quantify *in vivo*. Raman studies on synthetic melanin and persulfate oxidized tyrosine were carried out by Panina *et al.* (Panina *et al.* 1998) and Cooper *et al.* (Cooper *et al.* 1987). Because the extremely low quantum efficiency of Raman excitation, *in vivo* Raman measurement of melanin has been difficult. We successfully measured for the first the *in vivo* Raman spectra of human skin melanin using the real-time Raman system. Under 785 nm excitation, we have observed two intense and one weak Raman bands from *in vivo* skin and hair as well as from synthetic and natural eumelanins. The three Raman bands are around 1368, 1572 and 1742 cm^{-1}, with subtle differences for different conditions (Huang *et al.* 2004).

In vivo Raman spectra of cutaneous melanin obtained under 785-nm laser excitation are shown in Fig. 10, including dark forearm skin of a volunteer of African descent, a benign compound pigmented nevus, a malignant melanoma, and a normal skin site adjacent to the malignant melanoma. The Raman spectra of normal white skin, dark skin and pigmented lesions are different. Dark skin and pigmented lesions show three intense melanin Raman bands. These three bands can serve as a spectral signature for eumelanin and can potentially be used for noninvasive *in situ* clinical analysis and diagnosis.

4.3. *In vivo* Raman spectra of skin diseases

In vitro Raman spectra of skin diseases and skin cancers have been reported (Gniadecka *et al.* 1997; Gniadecka *et al.* 2003; Gniadecka *et al.* 2004). It was found that for *in vitro* studies, a sensitivity of 85% and a specificity of 99% could be achieved for diagnosis of melanoma (Gniadecka *et al.* 2004). Case studies of *in vivo* Raman spectroscopy of skin cancers are also reported (Huang *et al.* 2001a; Zeng *et al.* 2008; Caspers *et al.* 1998; Caspers *et al.* 2001; Caspers *et al.* 2003; Chrit *et al.* 2005; Gniadecka *et al.* 1997; Gniadecka *et al.* 2003; Gniadecka *et al.* 2004; Lieber *et al.* 2008a; Lieber *et al.* 2008b). Currently we are conducting a large-scale clinical study of skin cancers and skin diseases in order to evaluate the utility of Raman spectroscopy for noninvasive skin cancer detection. We have conducted an intermediate data analysis of 289 cases, of which 24 cases were basal cell carcinoma, 49 cases of squamous cell carcinoma, 37 cases of malignant melanoma, 24 cases of actinic keratosis, 53 cases of seborrheic keratosis, 32 cases of atypical nevus, 22 cases of compound nevus, 25 cases of intradermal nevus, and 23 junctional nevus (Zhao *et al.* 2008c). The normalized mean Raman spectra for different skin cancers and benign skin lesions are shown in Fig. 11. All of them are normalized to the strongest 1445 cm^{-1} peak. Differences in molecular signatures for different skin cancers and skin diseases are apparent. We used partial least squares (PLS) regression of the measured Raman spectra to derive the biochemical constituents in each lesion, and then used linear discriminant analysis (LDA) to classify the skin diseases. Our preliminary results showed that malignant melanoma can be differentiated from other pigmented benign lesions with a diagnostic sensitivity of 97% and specificity of 78%, while precancerous and cancerous lesions can be differentiated from benign lesions with a sensitivity of 91% and specificity of 75%, based on leave-one-out cross-validation (LOO-CV).

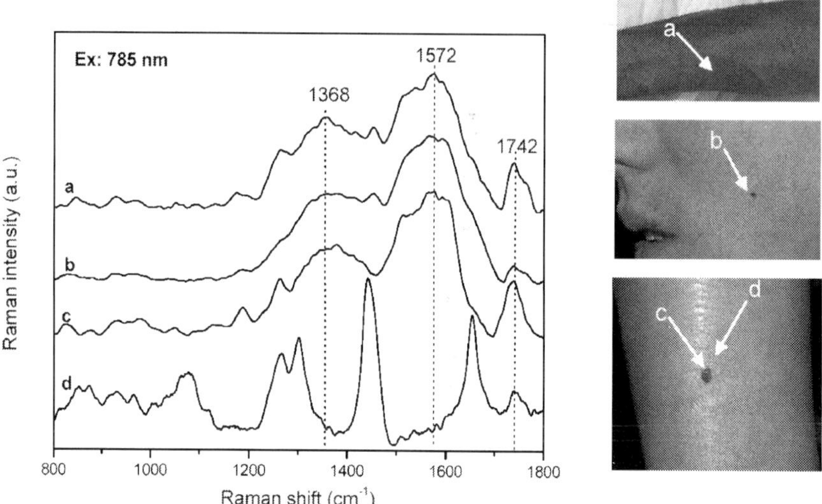

Fig. 10. *In vivo* Raman spectra of cutaneous melanin obtained under 785-nm laser excitation from: (a) volar forearm skin of a volunteer of African descent, (b) benign compound pigmented nevus, (c) malignant melanoma, and (d) normal skin site adjacent to the malignant melanoma. Also shown at the right side are clinical pictures of the corresponding skin sites for *in vivo* Raman measurements (Adopted from figure 7 in Huang *et al.* 2004 with permission).

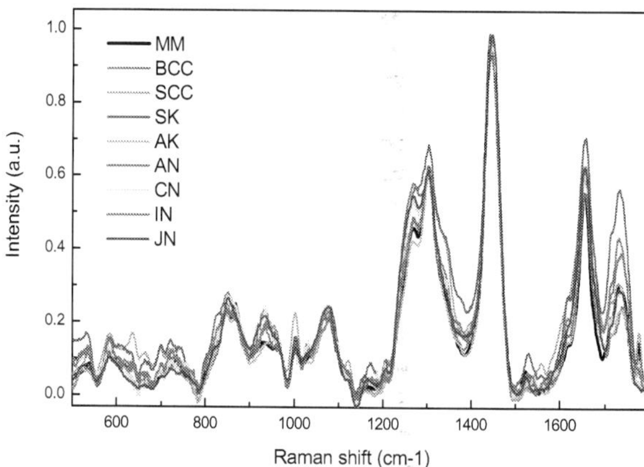

Fig. 11. Normalized Raman spectra of skin cancers and benign skin diseases, including melanoma (MM), basal cell carcinoma (BCC), squamous cell carcinoma (SCC), seborrheic keratosis (SK), actinic keratosis (AK), atypical nevus (AN), compound nevus (CN), intrademal nevus (IN) and junctional nevus (JN) (Adopted from figure 2 in Zhao *et al.* 2008c with permission).

5. Conclusions and future directions

We have developed an integrated real-time Raman spectroscopy system for *in vivo* skin evaluation and skin disease diagnosis. The device includes hardware instrumentation and software implementation. The skin Raman probe maximizes Raman signal collection and minimizes back scattered laser light. It can easily access most body sites. The aberration of the spectrograph image was corrected and the CCD full-chip vertical hardware binning was implemented. Real-time data acquisition and analysis include CCD dark-noise subtraction, wavelength calibration, spectral response calibration, intensity calibration, signal saturation detection and fixing, cosmic ray rejection, fluorescence background removal, and data model analysis. The *in vivo* clinical results validated the utility of the system for potential clinical applications for skin disease diagnosis. Although designed initially for examining the skin, this system can serve as a platform for *in vivo* Raman analysis of tissues from other organs.

We also presented a few examples of real-time *in vivo* Raman spectroscopy for skin. Many potential applications of Raman spectroscopy in skin research remain to be explored. Near future directions include: (1) further clinical trial of real-time Raman spectroscopy as an method for skin cancer and skin disease diagnosis; (2) real-time clinical Raman spectra database management and analysis; (3) Real-time Raman spectroscopy as a method in monitoring cutaneous drugs delivery; (4) Real-time Raman spectroscopy as a method in studying wound healing process; (5) Combination of Raman spectroscopy with confocal microscopy for depth resolved analysis (Wang *et al.* 2009); and (6) Combination of Raman spectroscopy with other imaging methodologies.

6. Acknowledgements

This work is supported by the Canadian Cancer Society, the Canadian Dermatology Foundation, the Canadian Institutes of Health Research, the VGH & UBC Hospital Foundation In It for Life Fund, and the BC Hydro Employees Community Services Fund. We would like to acknowledgment the contributions of our previous group members: Dr. Zhiwei Huang, Dr. Iltefat Hamzavi, Dr. Abdulmajeed Alajlan, Dr. Hana Alkhayat, Dr. Ahmad Al Robaee, and Miss Michelle Zeng. We also thank Mr. Wei Zhang for his technical assistance, and Dr. Michael Chen and Dr. Michael Short for their help.

7. References

Barry B., Edwards H. & Williams A. (1992). Fourier transform Raman and infrared vibrational study of human skin: assignment of spectral bands. *J. Raman Spectrosc.* 23, 641-645, ISSN 0377-0486.

Berger A., Itzkan I. & Feld M. (1997). Feasibility of measuring blood glucose concentration by near-infrared Raman spectroscopy. *Spectrochimica Acta Part A* 53A, 287-292, ISSN 1386-1425.

Caspers P., Lucassen G., Wolthuis R., Bruining H. & Puppels G. (1998). *In vitro* and *in vivo* Raman spectroscopy of human skin. *Biospectroscopy* 4, S31-S39, ISSN 1075-4261.

Caspers P., Lucassen G., Carter E., Bruining H. & Puppels G. (2001). *In vivo* confocal Raman Microspectroscopy of the skin: noninvaisve determination of molecular concentration profiles. *J. Invest. Dermatol.* 116, 434-442, ISSN 0022-202X.

Caspers P., Lucassen G. & Puppels G. (2003). Combined *in vivo* confocal Raman spectroscopy and confocal microscopy of human skin. *Biophys. J.* 85, 572-580, ISSN 0006-3495.

Cheng J. & Xie X. (2004). Coherent anti-Storkes Raman scattering microscopy: instrumentation, theory and applications. *J. Phys. Chem.* B 108, 827-840, ISSN 1520-6106.

Chrit L., Hadjur C., Morel S., Sockalingum G., Lebourdon G., Leroy F. & Manfait M. (2005). *In vivo* chemical investigation of human skin using a confocal Raman fiber optic microprobe. *J. Biomed. Opt.* 10, 44007, ISSN 1083-3668.

Cooper T., Bolton D., Schuschereba S. & Schmeisser E. (1987). Luminescence and Raman spectroscopic characterization of tyrosine oxidized by oersulfate. *Appl. Spectrosc.* 41, 661-667, ISSN 0003-7028.

Edwards H., Williams A. & Barry B. (1995). Potential applications of FT-Raman spectroscopy for dermatological diagnostics. *J. Mol. Struct.* 347, 379-388, ISSN 0166-1280.

Gniadecka M., Wulf H., Mortensen N., Nielsen O. & Christensen D. (1997). Diagnosis of basal cell carcinoma by Raman spectroscopy. *J. Raman Spectrosc.* 28, 125-129, ISSN 0377-0486.

Gniadecka M., Nielsen O., Christensen D. & Wulf H. (1998). Structure of water, proteins, and lipids in intact human skin, hair, and nail. *J. Invest. Dermatol.* 110, 393-398, ISSN 0022-202X.

Gniadecka M., Nielsen O. & Wulf H. (2003). Water content and structure in malignant and benign skin tumours. *J. Mol. Struct.*, 661-662, 405-410, ISSN 0166-1280.

Gniadecka M., Philipsen P., Sigurdsson S., Wessel S., Nielsen O., Christensen D., Hercogova J., Rossen K., Thomsen H., Gniadecki R., Hansen L. & Wulf H. (2004). Melanoma diagnosis by Raman spectroscopy and neural networks: structure alterations in proteins and lipids in intact cancer tissue. *J. Invest. Dermatol.* 122: 443-449, ISSN 0022-202X.

Han X., Lui H., McLean D. & Zeng H. (2009). Near-infrared autofluorescence imaging of cutaneous melanins and human skin *in vivo*. *J. Biomed. Opt.* 14: 024017, ISSN 1083-3668.

Hanlon E., Manoharan R., Koo T., Shafer K., Motz J., Fitzmaurice M., Kramer J., Itzkan I., Dasari R. & Feld M. (2000). Prospects for *in vivo* Raman spectroscopy. *Phys. Med. Biol.* 45: R1-R59, ISSN 0031-9155.

Huang Z., Zeng H., Hamzavi I., McLean D. & Lui H. (2001a). Rapid near-infrared Raman spectroscopy system for real-time *in vivo* skin measurements. *Opt. Lett.* 26: 1782-1784, ISSN 0146-9592.

Huang Z., Zeng H., Hamzavi I., McLean D. & Lui H. (2001b). Evaluation of variations of biomolecular constituents in human skin *in vivo* by near-infrared Raman spectroscopy. *Proceedings of SPIE*, vol. 4597, pp. 109-114.

Huang Z., Lui H., Chen X., Alajlan A., McLean D. & Zeng H. (2004). Raman spectroscopy of *in vivo* cutaneous melanin. *J. Biomed. Opt.* 9, 1198-1205, ISSN 1083-3668.

Huang Z., Lui H., McLean D., Mladen K. & Zeng H. (2005). Raman spectroscopy in combination with background near-infrared autofluorescence enhances the *in vivo* assessment of malignant tissues. *Photochem. Phobiol.* 81, 1219-26, ISSN 0031-8655.

Huang Z., Zeng H., Hamzavi I., Alajlan A., Tan E., McLean D. & Lui H. (2006). Cutaneous melanin exhibits fluorescence emission under near-infrared light excitation. *J. Biomed. Opt.* 11, 034010, ISSN 0146-9592.

Huang Z., Teh S., Zheng W., Mo J., Lin K., Shao X., Ho K., Teh M. & Yeoh K. (2009). Integrated Raman spectroscopy and trimodal wide-field imaging techniques for real-time *in vivo* tissue Raman measurements at endoscopy. *Opt. Lett.* 34, 758-760, ISSN 0146-9692.

Kollias N. & Stamatas G. (2002). Optical non-invasive approaches to diagnosis of skin diseases. *J. Invest. Dermatol. Symposium Proceedings* 7, 64-75.

Lieber C. & Mahadevan-Jansen A. (2003). Automated method for subtraction of fluorescence from biological Raman spectra. *Appl. Spectrosc.* 57, 1363-1367, ISSN 0003-7028.

Lieber C., Majumder S., Billheimer D., Ellis D. & Mahadevan-Jansen A. (2008a). Raman microspectroscopy for skin cancer detection *in vitro*. *J. Biomed. Opt.* 13, 024013, ISSN 1083-3668.

Lieber C., Majumder S., Ellis D., Billheimer D. & Mahadevan-Jansen A. (2008b). *In vivo* nonmelanoma skin cancer diagnosis using Raman microspectroscopy. *Lasers in Surgery and Medicine* 40: 461-467, ISSN 0196-8092.

Mahadevan-Jansen A. & Richards-Kortum R. (1996). Raman spectroscopy for the detection of cancers and precancers. *J. Biomed. Opt.* 1, 31-70, ISSN 1083-3668.

Morris M., Matousek P., Towrie M., Parker A., Goodship A. & Draper E. (2005). Kerr-gated time-resolved Raman spectroscopy of equine cortical bone tissue. *J. Biomed. Opt.* 10, 14014, ISSN 1083-3668.

Motz J., Gandhi S., Scepanovic O., Haka A., Kramer J., Dasari R. & Feld M. (2005a). Real-time Raman system for *in vivo* disease diagnosis. *J. Biomed. Opt.* 10, 031113, ISSN 1083-3668.

Motz J., Hunter M., Galindo L., Gardecki J., Kramer J., Dasari R. & Feld M. (2005b). Optical fiber probe for biomedical Raman spectroscopy. *Appl. Opt.* 43, 542-554, ISSN 0003-6935.

Myrick M., Angels S. & Desiderio R. (1990). Comparison of some fiber optic configurations for measurements of luminescence and Raman scattering. *Appl. Opt.* 29: 1333-13444, ISSN 0003-6935.

Nijssen A., Schut T., Heule F., Caspers P., Hayes D., Neumann M. & Puppels F. (2002). Discriminating basal cell carcinoma from its surrounding tissue by Raman spectroscopy. *J. Invest. Dermatol.* 119, 64-69, ISSN 0022-202X.

Owen H., Battey D., Pelletier M. and Slater J. (1995). New spectroscopic instrument based on volume holographic optical elements. *Proceedings of SPIE*, vol. 2406, 260-267.

Panina L., Kartenko N., Kumzerov Y. and Limonov M. (1998). Comparative study of the spatial organization of biological carbon nanostructures and fullerene-related carbon. *Mol. Mater.* 11, 117-120, ISSN 1058-7276.

Richards-Kortum R. & Sevick-Muraca E. (1996). Quantative optical spectroscopy for tissue diagnosis. *Annu. Rev. Phys. Chem.* 47: 555-606, ISSN 0066-426X.

Santos L., Wolthuis R., Koljenovic S., Almeida R. and Puppels F. (2005). Fiberoptic probes for *in vivo* Raman spectroscopy in the high-wavenumber region. *Anal. Chem.* 77, 6747-6752, ISSN 0003-2700.

Schut T., Wolthuis R., Caspers P. & Puppels G. (2002). Real-time tissue characterization on the basis of *in vivo* Raman spectra. *J. Raman Spectrosc.* 33: 580-585, ISSN 0377-0486.

Shim M. & Wilson B. (1997). Development of an *in vivo* Raman spectroscopic system for diagnostic applications. *J. Raman Spectrosc.* 28, 131-142, ISSN 0377-0486.

Short M., Lui H., McLean D., Zeng H., Alajlan A. & Chen X. (2006). Changes in nuclei and peritumoral collagen within nodular basal cell carcinomas via confocal micro-Raman spectroscopy. *J. Biomed. Opt.* 11: 034004, ISSN 1083-3668.

Short M., Lam S., McWilliams A., Zhao J., Lui H. & Zeng H. (2008). Development and preliminary results of an endoscopic Raman probe for potential *in-vivo* diagnosis of lung cancers. *Opt. Lett.* 33: 711-713, ISSN 0146-9592.

Wang H., Huang N., Zhao J., Lui H., Korbelik M. & Zeng H. (2009). *In vivo* confocal Raman spectroscopy for skin disease diagnosis and characterization - preliminary results from mouse tumor models. *Proceedings of SPIE,* vol. 7161, 716108.

Williams A., Edwards H. & Barry B. (1992). Fourier transform Raman spectroscopy: a novel application for examing human stratum corneum. *Int. J. Pharm.* 81, R11-R14, ISSN 0378-5173.

Zeng H., MacAulay C., McLean D. & Palcic B. (1995). Spectroscopic and microscopic characteristics of human skin autofluorescence emission. *Photochem. Phobiol.* 61: 639-645, ISSN 0031-8655.

Zeng H., MacAulay C., McLean D., Palcic B. & Lui H. (1998). The dynamics of laser-induced changes in human skin autofluorescence - experimental measurements and theoretical modeling. *Photochem. Phobiol.* 68: 227-236, ISSN 0031-8655.

Zeng H. (2002). Apparatus and methods relating to high speed Raman spectroscopy. United States Patent #: 6486948.

Zeng H., Zhao J., Short M., McLean D., Lam S., McWilliams A. & Lui H. (2008). Raman spectroscopy for *in vivo* tissue analysis and diagnosis, from instrument development to clinical applications. *J. Innovative Optical Health Sciences,* 1, 95-106, ISSN 1793-5458.

Zhao J., Lui H., McLean D. & Zeng H. (2007). Automated Autofluorescence Background Subtraction Algorithm for Biomedical Raman Spectroscopy. *Appl. Spectrosc.* 61, 1225-1232, ISSN 0003-7028.

Zhao J., Lui H., McLean D. & Zeng H. (2008a). Integrated real-time Raman system for clinical *in vivo* skin analysis. *Skin Res. and Tech.* 14, 484-492, ISSN 0909-752X.

Zhao J., Huang Z., Zeng H., McLean D. & Lui H. (2008b). Quantitative analysis of skin chemicals using rapid near-infrared Raman spectroscopy. *Proceedings of SPIE,* vol. 6842, 684209.

Zhao J., Lui H., McLean D. & Zeng H. (2008c). Real-time Raman spectroscopy for non-invasive skin cancer detection - preliminary results. *Proceedings of the 30th Annual International Conference of the IEEE Engineering in Medicine and Biology Society,* pp. 3107-3109, ISBN 978-1-4244-1815-2, Vancouver, British Columbia, Canada, August 20-24, 2008.

25

Design and Implementation of Leading Eigenvector Generator for On-chip Principal Component Analysis Spike Sorting System

Tung-Chien Chen[1,2], Kuanfu Chen[2], Wentai Liu[2] and Liang-Gee Chen[1]
[1.] *Graduate Institute of Electronic Engineering, National Taiwan University*
Taiwan
[2.] *Electrical Engineering Department, University of California, Santa Cruz*
USA

1. Introduction

On-chip implementation of neural signal processing along with the recording circuitry can significantly reduce the data bandwidth, and is a key to enable the wireless neural recording system with a large amount of electrodes (Zumsteg et al., 2005). Without such data processing, large amount of data need to be transferred to a host computer, and typically a cable is required. In this case, patients and test subjects are restrained from free movement, which impedes the progress in fundamental neuroscience research and the advance in closed-loop neural prosthetic devices.

Several approaches to achieve the bandwidth reduction have been investigated. One example is to transmit the encoded version of the whole neural waveform by using either lossless or lossy compression algorithms. In Oweiss et al., 2003, a 30-fold data reduction is demonstrated by using wavelet transformation and variable length coding algorithms. However, more data reduction is still desired. Another approach is to detect the spike events with threshold methods, and transmit either the binary event streams or the time stamps of the detected events (Olsson & Wise, 2005, Harrison, 2003). The compression performance increases to more than 100-fold data reduction. However, the significant loss of information limits the ability of classification and sorting of the individual neuron signal sources.

A promising approach to achieve the bandwidth reduction is to extract spike features immediately after spike detection on the implant site (Oweiss et al., 1977, Letelier & Weber, 2000, Hulata et al., 2002). Only the event times and some additional features about classification are transmitted after the signal processing. This approach achieves a similar data reduction as the threshold method does while preserving the capability for the neuron-to-neuron discrimination. The principal component analysis (PCA) (Zumsteg et al., 2005, Oweiss et al., 1977) and wavelet transformation (Letelier & Weber, 2000, Hulata et al., 2002) are currently the most widely used tools in this approach.

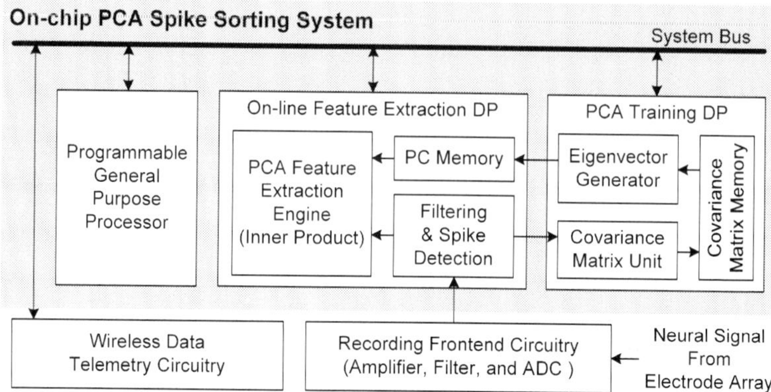

Fig. 1. The proposed on-chip system for a PCA-based spike sorting. The system has several heterogeneous processors with application specific functionalities reflecting the needs of spike sorting. Dedicated processors (DPs) are designed to accelerate the computationally intensive spike sorting algorithm. A programmable general purpose processor (GPP) is embedded for the system controlling and scheduling.

There are many architectures (Andra et al., 2002, Huang et al., 2004, Kamboh et al., 2007) that have been designed for wavelet transformation. However, there have not been seen a demonstration of prototype chip propose to achieve for wavelet-based spike sorting. In this paper, we propose to achieve the first hardware prototype in the form of an integrated circuit for PCA-based approach.

For PCA-based spike sorting, the PCA algorithm finds an optimal linear transformation which reduces d-dimensional spike waveform to h-dimensional feature scores (d>>h) in such a way that the information is maximally preserved in terms of minimum mean squared error. Note that d is the sample number of spike waveforms while the h is the desired number of principal components (PCs). In general, the spike waveforms with similar feature scores are corresponding to the same firing neuron. After the dimension reduction, the classification algorithm such as K-means (Kanungo et al., 2002, Ding & He, 2004)} or Mean-shift (Comaniciu & Meer, 2002) can be more effectively applied to sort the spikes into clusters corresponding to the different firing neurons.

The PCA feature extraction has two major phases---the parameter training phase and the on-line processing phase. In the parameter training phase, the algorithm collects the detected spikes, constructs the covariance matrix, and then calculating the corresponding eigenvectors. The major characteristic vectors, the PCs that can optimally differentiate neurons in a least square error term, are the first few eigenvectors with largest eigenvalues. In the on-line processing phase, the feature scores are extracted by projecting the detected spike waveforms on the PCs that are calculated in the training phase. The operation of inner product between the extracted spikes and the trained PCs is required for the vector projection. Note that the trained parameters may need to be updated through the periodic re-training in order to reflect the environment perturbations for long-duration experiments (Shenoy et al., 2006).

Fig. 1 shows the proposed on-chip PCA-based spike sorting system. The system has several heterogeneous processors with application specific functionalities reflecting the needs of spike sorting. The operations on raw neural data such as noise filtering, spike detection and feature extraction require the most computation. Dedicated processors (DPs) are used to accelerate these computationally intensive tasks, utilizing customized parallel architectures and memory hierarchies. The PCA training DP collects the detected spike events and then calculates the co-variance matrix and the corresponding eigenvectors. After the training, the leading eigenvectors are transmitted to the on-line feature extraction DP and stored in the PC memory. The feature extraction DP then generates the feature scores of the following detected spike events by projecting them on the leading eigenvectors. Apart from DPs, a programmable general purpose processor (GPP) is embedded for the system controlling and scheduling. The GPP can also provide some flexibility in the algorithm development.

In realizing this on-chip PCA-based spike sorting system, the most challenging problem is to design a hardware unit to calculate leading eigenvectors. There are many algorithms to calculate eigenvectors from a covariance matrix (Golub et al., 1996, Roweis, 1998, Schilling & Harris, 2000, Sirovich, 1987), but most of them can hardly be mapped into an efficient VLSI architecture. The most well-known algorithm is the Cyclic Jacobi's method (Golub et al., 1996) based on eigenvalue decomposition (EVD). It generates all eigenvalues and eigenvectors after diagonalizing the symmetric covariance matrix. However, EVD has high computational complexity. The architecture design for matrix diagonalization is very complicated and will be expensive in silicon area. Expectation maximizing (EM) (Roweis, 1998) is proposed for PCA with less computation complexity compared to EVD method. However, it requires matrix inverse operation in both the E-step and M-step for each of the iteration, and the matrix inverse operation also cannot be efficiently implemented. Furthermore, EM algorithm may not converge to a global optimal and a good initial setup is required. The power method (Schilling & Harris, 2000) is another less computationally expensive method but can compute only the most leading eigenvector. Another snap-shot algorithm (Sirovich, 1987) also requires matrix inversion and is not hardware-friendly. Note that very small silicon area and power consumption are usually required by the implantable hardware in order to avoid neural tissue damage.

In this chapter, based on a computationally fast and hardware friendly algorithm (Sharma & Paliwal, 2007), the first VLSI architecture to calculate the leading eigenvectors is proposed for the on-chip PCA-based spike sorting system. The reminder of this paper is organized as follows. In section 2, the algorithm is introduced and then validated for the spike sorting through software simulations. In section 3, the low power and low area VLSI architecture is proposed with a flipped structure and adaptive level shifting method. Section 4 presents the implementation and fabrication results and Section 5 concludes this work.

2. Iterative Eigenvector Distilling Algorithm

In this section, a computationally fast and hardware friendly algorithm to find the desired number of leading eigenvectors is introduced. We will go through the algorithm first and then summarize the advantages of the algorithm in terms of hardware implementation. Finally, neural data are used in the software simulation to validate the algorithm for PCA-based spike sorting. For the detailed mathematic proof of the algorithm, please refer to (Sharma & Paliwal, 2007). To facilitate the description, we name this algorithm iterative eigenvector distilling algorithm.

---

1. Choose h, the number of eigenvectors required to estimate,
   Choose r, the iteration number of eigenvector distilling,
   Compute covariance matrix Σ_{cov}, and set p and q to 1.
2. Initialize eigenvector φ_p up, e.g. randomly.
3. Do the eigenvector distilling process :
$$\varphi_p = \Sigma_{cov}\, \varphi_p$$
4. Do the Gram $-$ Schmidt orthogonalization process :
$$\varphi_p = \varphi_p - \sum_{j=1}^{p-1} \left(\varphi_p^T \varphi_j\right) \varphi_j$$
5. Normalize up φ_p by dividing it by its norm :
$$\varphi_p = \varphi_p / \left\| \varphi_p \right\|$$
6. Increase counter q = q + 1 and go to step 3 until q equals r.
7. Increase counter p = p + 1 and go to step 2 until p equals h.

Table 1. Fast PCA algorithm based on the iterative eigenvector distilling algorithm.

2.1 Algorithm Description

Table 1 depicts the fast PCA algorithm based on the iterative eigenvector distilling algorithm. "h" is the required number of the PCs. "r" is the algorithm iteration number, and "Σ_{cov}" is the covariance matrix calculated from the detected spike waveforms. In the beginning, the eigenvectors, "ϕ_p", are initialized randomly. Afterwards, the leading eigenvectors of the covariance matrix are calculated one by one in a reducing order of dominance. The calculation of each eigenvector has r iterations and each of the iterations has two procedures---the eigenvector distilling process and the orthogonal process.

The key of this algorithm is to intensify the major component on the initial eigenvector through continuously multiplying the initial eigenvector with the covariance matrix. This procedure is called the eigenvector distilling process. The most PC can be simply derived after several iterations of this distilling process. For the remaining h-1 PCs, the orthogonal process is required. In order to continuously intensify the pth PC on the initial eigenvector, the previously measured p-1 components are removed from the intermediate results of "ϕ_p" by the orthogonal process after every iteration of distilling process. Note that the Gram-Schmidt method is used in our orthogonal process.

This algorithm has several advantages in terms of hardware implementation. The first one is the simple math operation. This algorithm is free from eigenvalue decomposition. The matrix diagonalization, symmetric rotation, and matrix inverse are not required. Second, the algorithm exactly meets the requirement without calculating the eigenvalues as well as the remainder minor eigenvectors. This fact combined with the simple operation results in the low computation complexity. Third, the algorithm can globally converge in a few iterations without the need for any specific initial setting. Also, the algorithm has a very regular procedure. As a result, the presented algorithm is computationally efficient and hardware friendly, and is a good starting point for VLSI implementation.

2.2 Simulation Results

We realized the iterative eigenvector distilling algorithm in Matlab, and used the neural data download from Quian Quiroga to validate the algorithm for PCA-based spike sorting. The "eig" function, a standard Matlab function to generate the eigenvectors, is used as our benchmark (Anderson et al., 1999). Note that the nonlinear energy operation (NEO) algorithm (Kim & Kim, 2000) is adopted as our spike detection method. After spike detection, the detected spike waveforms are aligned horizontally and vertically according to their peaks and 8/12 samples are used before/after the peak to represent each spike waveform. Fig. 2 illustrates the mean squared error between the benchmark and the iterative eigenvector distilling algorithm with different iterations. According to the simulation results, the eigenvector usually converges within five iterations when its eigenvalue is much larger than the eigenvalue of the previous eigenvector. Otherwise, it takes around 10 to 15 iterations for the convergence.

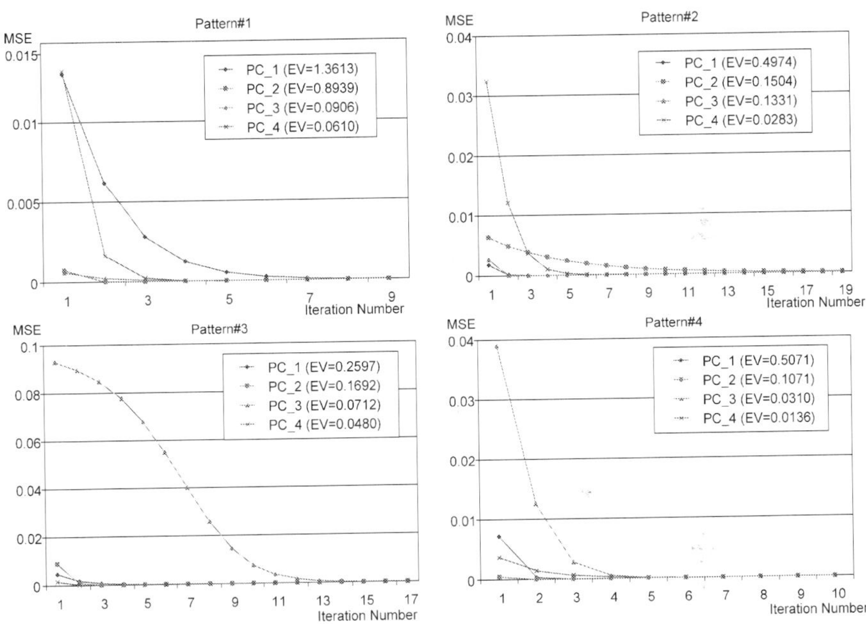

Fig. 2. Mean squared error (MSE) between the benchmark and the iterative eigenvector distilling algorithm of different iterations. EV and PC in the figures denote the abbreviation of eigenvalue and principal component. According to the simulation results, the eigenvector converges within five iterations when its eigenvalue is much larger than the eigenvalue of the previous eigenvector. Otherwise, it takes around 10 to 15 iterations for the convergence. The test patterns are downloaded from Quian Quiroga. Pattern #1 to #4 are C_Easy1_noise005, C_Easy2_noise005, C_Difficult1_noise005, and C_Difficult2_noise005.

3. Architecture Design

In this section, based on the iterative eigenvector distilling algorithm, two techniques are proposed to enable the efficient VLSI implementation. A flipped structure is used to save the power and silicon area by discarding the division and square root operations in the orthogonalization process. The adaptive level shifting scheme is applied to achieve the highest accuracy in a fixed-point processing system with only a small bit-width. Finally, the architecture as well as the corresponding processing schedule is designed for the modified iterative eigenvector distilling algorithm.

$$
\begin{aligned}
&for(p = 1 : 4) \\
&\{ \quad \varphi_p = [\ 1, \quad 1, \quad ..... \quad 1, \ ]^T) \\
&\quad\quad for(i = 1 : 10) \\
&\quad\quad\quad \{ \quad \varphi_p = \Sigma_{cov}\cdot\varphi_p \\
&\quad\quad\quad\quad for(j = 1 : p-1) \\
&\quad\quad\quad\quad\quad \{ \quad \varphi_p = \varphi_p - (\varphi_p^T \varphi_j)\,\varphi_j \quad \} \\
&\quad\quad\quad\quad \varphi_p = \varphi_p / \|\varphi_p\| \quad \} \}
\end{aligned}
$$

Fig. 3. The pseudo-code of the original iterative eigenvector distilling algorithm. The $\Sigma_{\_cov}$ is the covariance matrix of the spike waveforms, and the ϕ is the demanded eigenvector. Suppose the demanded number of leading PCs is four, and the iteration number for each PC is ten.

3.1 Flipped Structure

In order to clearly explain the proposed techniques, we represent the original iterative eigenvector distilling algorithm in a pseudo code format shown in Fig. 3. The "$\Sigma_{\_cov}$" is the covariance matrix of the spike waveforms, and the "ϕ" is the demanded eigenvector. Suppose that four leading PCs are required, and the iteration number for each PC is ten. In the original algorithm, four kinds of math operations are required---addition, multiplication, division, and square root. Generally speaking, division and square root hardware units require much more silicon area and consume much more power compared with multipliers and adders. In order to optimize the power consumption and silicon area, the flipped structure is proposed to discard these hardware-expensive operations.

First, we discard the normalization process of $\varphi_p = \varphi_p / \|\varphi_p\|$, and change the orthogonal process to $\varphi_p = \varphi_p - (\varphi_p^T\varphi_j / \|\varphi_j\|)\,(\varphi_j / \|\varphi_j\|)$. Then, we multiply the whole equation by $\|\varphi_j\|^2$. Since $\|\varphi_j\|^2 = \varphi_j^T\varphi_j$, the orthogonal process finally becomes $\varphi_p = (\varphi_j^T\varphi_j)\,\varphi_p - (\varphi_p^T\varphi_j)\,\varphi_j$. In this way, the norm of the previously calculated PC is flipped to the dividend part in the orthogonal process. The division and square root operations are thus replaced by addition and multiplication. The silicon area and power consumption are thus saved by means of reusing the uncomplicated processing units of the adders and the multipliers.

3.2 Adaptive Level Shifting Scheme

After the flipped structure, the φ can be easily represented in a fixed-point integer number during the processing. It should be advantageous since the fixed-point integer DSP system is very friendly in terms of VLSI implementation. However, the dynamic range of φ increases rapidly during the iterations. For example, suppose the input covariance matrix is a 32x32 matrix, and each entry has 16-bit precision. The dynamic range of φ is increased by 16+5 bits for every eigenvector distilling process. If the current dynamic range of φ_j is n bits, the dynamic range of φ_p is increased by (2xn+5) bits for each orthogonal process. After several iterations, the final dynamic range become prohibitively large, which impedes a low area and low power implementation.

Quantization and saturation to a pre-defined bit-level is a general solution to deal with this problem in a fixed point DSP system. When the level of the processed signal can be well predicted, this method can usually result in a good trade-off between the hardware cost and signal accuracy. However, the variation of neural signals is very large for different living individual, system setup and applications. The signal level cannot be well predicted from such high dynamic range during the iterations. Another solution is to represent all intermediary data in floating point numbers and use a floating point DSP system for calculating. The floating point system can efficiently use the full range of the limited bit-width to represent as much information as possible. However, the floating point DSP system is very complicated and not cost-efficient in terms of area per bit and power per bit.

An adaptive level shifting scheme is proposed to optimize the hardware in terms of processing accuracy per hardware cost. The idea is to use the floating point concept in a fixed point DSP system. It is realized by dynamically increasing the quantization level according to the signal level until the limited bit-width can completely represent the quantized signals for each processing step. Fig. 4 (a) shows the pseudo code of the proposed flipped structure combining with the proposed adaptive level shifting scheme. After the eigenvector distilling process and the orthogonalization process, the level check and shift procedure is applied to adaptively compress the dynamic range according to the current level. The level check and shift procedure is shown in Fig. 4 (b). "bw" is the pre-defined bit-width of the system outputs of the final eigenvectors. During the level check and shift procedure, φ_p is continuously rounded by 2 until it can be completely represented in "bw" bits.

$$
\begin{aligned}
&for(p = 1:4)\\
&\quad \{ \quad \varphi_p = [\ 1, \quad 1, \quad ...., \quad 1, \ ]\\
&\quad\quad for(i = 1:10)\\
&\quad\quad\quad \{ \quad \varphi_p = \Sigma_{cov}\varphi_p\\
&\quad\quad\quad\quad Level\_Check\_And\_Shift(\varphi_p)^*\\
&\quad\quad\quad\quad for(j = 1:p-1)\\
&\quad\quad\quad\quad\quad \{ \quad \varphi_p = \left(\varphi_j^T \varphi_j\right)\varphi_p - \left(\varphi_p^T \varphi_j\right)\varphi_j\\
&\quad\quad\quad\quad\quad\quad Level\_Check\_And\_Shift(\varphi_p)^* \}\}\}
\end{aligned}
$$

$$
\begin{aligned}
&{}^* Level\_Check\_And\_Shift(\varphi_p):\\
&While\left(\max(\varphi_p) \geq 2^{(bw-1)} \| \min(\varphi_p) < -2^{(bw-1)}\right)\\
&\quad \{ \quad \varphi_p = (\varphi_p + 1) >> 1 \quad \}
\end{aligned}
$$

(a)   (b)

Fig. 4. (a) The pseudo-code of the modified iterative eigenvector distilling algorithm with the flipped structure and the adaptive level shifting scheme. For the flipped structure, the normalization process is discarded, and the norm of the calculated PC, $\|\varphi_j\|$, is flipped to the dividend part in the orthogonal process. The division and square root operations are thus replaced by addition and multiplication operations. After the processing of the eigenvector distilling or the orthogonalization, the level check and shift procedure is applied to compress the dynamic range of the intermediate results according to their signal levels. (b) The level check and shift procedure. During the procedure, φ_p is continuously rounded by 2 until it can be completely represented in a pre-defined bit-width. The adaptive level shifting scheme optimizes the hardware in terms of processing accuracy per hardware cost by using the full range of the limited bit-width to represent as much information as possible. Note that the "max(*)" function extracts the largest value in the input vector while the "min(*)" function extracts the smallest value.

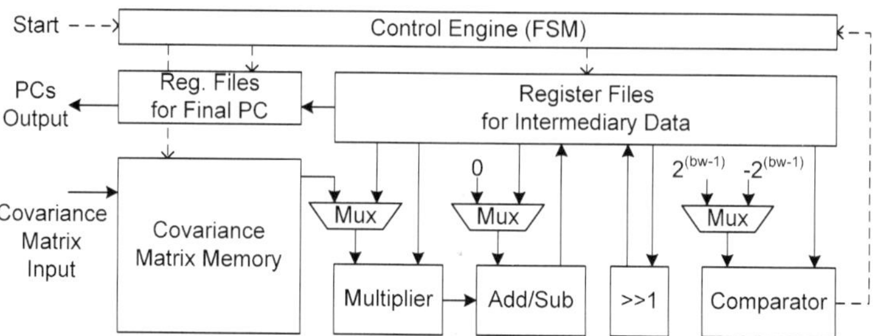

Fig. 5. The block diagram of the proposed architecture for the leading eigenvector generation. The multiplier and adder (also used as a subtractor) units are used for the eigenvector distilling process and the orthogonalization process. The right-shift and comparator units are used for the level check and shift procedure. The whole algorithm is folded into these four processing units and processed sequentially. All the intermediary data are stored in the register files. The control engine is responsible for the scheduling and resource allocation.

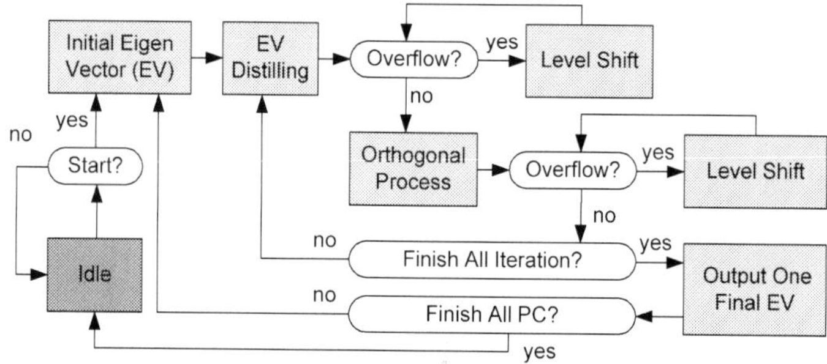

Fig. 6. The main finite state machine in the control engine. Each eigenvector distilling state takes (nxn) cycles. The orthogonal process for each pre-calculated eigenvector takes (nx4) cycles. Each overflow checking and level shift states take n cycles.

3.3 Architecture Design

Based on the modified algorithm, the block diagram of the proposed architecture for the leading eigenvector generation is shown in Fig. 5. The input is a covariance matrix of the detected spike waveforms. The outputs are several leading eigenvectors of the covariance matrix, or the PCs of the detected spike waveforms. Four major processing units are implemented. The multiplier and adder (also used as a subtractor) units form a multiply-accumulate (MAC) structure and are used for the eigenvector distilling process and the orthogonalization process. The right-shift and comparator units are used for the level check and shift procedure. The whole algorithm is folded into these four processing units and processed sequentially. All the intermediary data are stored in the register files. The control engine constructed of finite state machines (FSMs) is responsible for the scheduling and resource allocation during the processing.

After the architecture is constructed, the next step is to do the scheduling and resource allocation. Fig. 6 shows the main FSM of the control engine. Suppose each spike waveforms has n samples, and Σ_{cov} is an nxn matrix while φ is an nx1 vector. During the state of eigenvector distilling, "Σ_{cov}" and "φ_p" are input to MAC and the new "φ_p" is stored back to the register file. Because of the serial processing, every eigenvector distilling state takes nxn cycles. During the orthogonal process, "$\varphi_j^T\varphi_j$" is first computed, and two inputs of MAC are both "φ_j". Afterwards, "φ_p" and "φ_j" are input to MAC for "$\varphi_p^T\varphi_j$". Then, "$\varphi_j^T\varphi_j$" and "φ_p" are input for "$(\varphi_j^T\varphi_j)\,\varphi_p$". As the final step in the orthogonal process, the MAC is initialized with "$(\varphi_j^T\varphi_j)\,\varphi_p$". "$\varphi_p^T\varphi_j$" and "$\varphi_j$" are input with the subtraction mode. After this orthogonalization process, the "φ_j" component is removed from "φ_p". The result is also stored back to the register files. Note that the orthogonal process to remove each pre-calculated eigenvector, "φ_j", takes nx4 cycles. During the overflow checking state, "φ_p" is input to the comparator and compared with $2^{(bw-1)}$ and $-2^{(bw-1)}$. The checking result is fed back to the control engine. If an overflow occurs, the FSM will enter the level shift state, and "φ_p" is input to the right shift engine to quantize the signal by 2. This procedure will continue until the overflow checking fails. It takes n cycles to pass each overflow checking and level shift state.

Spec.: Max. Bit Width		Entire Core		Covariance Matrix Memory	Processing Units + Register Files
I/O	Internal Circuit	Area (μm^2)	Power (μW)	Area (μm^2)	Area (μm^2)
2	11	45996	93	17667	26465
4	17	70027	150	20859	47303
6	23	95054	204	25007	68182
8	29	119956	255	29154	88937
9	32	132021	282	31228	98929
10	35	145624	308	33302	110457
12	41	171074	364	37449	131760
14	47	196965	417	41597	153503
16	53	222950	469	45744	175341

Table 2. Synthesized results of different processing accuracy.

Spec.: samples per Spike Waveform		Entire Core		Covariance Memory Matrix	Processing Units + Register Files
		Area (μm^2)	Power (μW)	Area (μm^2)	Area (um^2)
16		79209	152	18135	59322
32		132021	282	31228	98929
64		255495	521	75481	178071

Table 3. Synthesized results of different sample number per spike waveform.

4. Implementation Results

In the previous section, the first VLSI architecture is designed to generate the leading eigenvectors for the PCA-based spike sorting. However, defining the hardware specifications in the spike sorting system to meet the application requirements under the minimum hardware cost is still an opened issue. In this section, we use 90 nm 1P9M process to synthesize the proposed leading eigenvector generator for various specifications. Through the simulation, the PCs generated by our verilog hardware model are compared to those generated by the standard Matlab function. Combining our hardware with the software-based classification algorithm, we also demonstrate the tradeoff between the sorting performance and the hardware cost. Finally, this eigenvector generation unit is integrated with other processors to complete a PCA-based spike sorting system and fabricated in .35 μm 2P4M process. We hope that the report in this section acts as a good reference for those who intend to define and implement a closed-loop neural prosthesis in the future.

4.1 Synthesized Results

There are four hardware parameters that can be specified in this design. The first one is the accuracy, including the bit width of input covariance matrix and the bit width of output PCs. The second one is the sample number of spike waveforms. The third and fourth are the required PC number and the iteration number for eigenvector distilling process. With a given operation frequency, the silicon area and power consumption are highly influenced by the first and second parameters, while the processing capability is influenced by the second, third, and fourth parameters. The processing capability is defined as the number of channels that can be trained in PCA algorithm within a period of time.

Table 2 reports the synthesized results of different processing accuracies. The input bit-width specifies the precision of the given covariance matrix while the output bit-width specifies the precision of the required PCs. The sample number of spike waveforms is fixed to support as large as 32 samples while the PC number and iteration number can go up to four and 128 respectively. Note that if the input/output (I/O) bit-width is n, the maximum bit-width of internal circuit is (3xn+5) which happens after the orthogonal process. The size of the on-chip static random access memory is (32x32xn) bits to store the covariance matrix. The area and power are reported in 90 nm 1P9M process at 1MHz operation frequency. When the bit width goes high, the area of covariance matrix memory, register files, and processing units increase in order to store and process more data. The hardware costs almost linearly increase in this case.

Table 3 reports the synthesized results of different sample numbers of spike waveforms. This time the I/O bit-width is fixed to 9 bits. The PC number and iteration number can still go up to 4 and 128 respectively. If the sample number of spike waveform is m, the size of the on-chip static random access memory is (mxmx9) bits. When the sample number of spike waveforms goes high, the dimensions of Σ_{cov} and φ increase. This fact increases the area of the covariance matrix memory and the register files. The area cost also linearly increases in this case.

Table 4 shows the hardware capability with different hardware parameters. The processing capability is defined as the number of channels that can be trained in PCA algorithm within one minute and the required seconds that can train 1000 channels. The number is reported for the worst case (which requires the maximum cycles for level checking and shifting) and with iteration number of 20, required PC number of 4, and 1MHz operation frequency. In the maximum specification of 64 samples per spike and 16 bits bit-width of each input spike sample and output eigenvector sample, our hardware can perform PCA parameter training for 90 channels within one minute. It requires 666 seconds to train 1000 channels.

Samples per Spike (#)	I/O Bit-width (bit)	Required Cycles for each Channel (#)	Channel Number per Minute (#)	Required Time to train 1000 Channels (sec)
64	16	666k	90	666
32	16	246k	244	246
32	9	192k	312	192
16	9	73k	822	73

Table 4. The hardware capability with different hardware parameters.

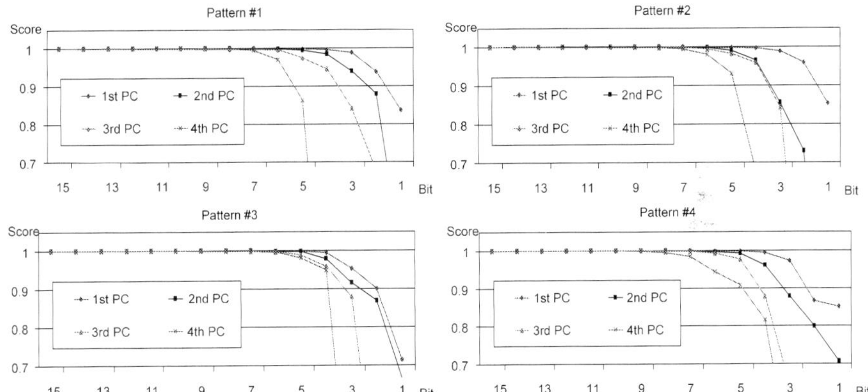

Fig. 7. The comparison between the PCs generated by the software Matlab model using floating point operations and our hardware Verilog model using fixed point operations. We use the correlation parameter as the similarity score. The simulation results show that the hardware with 9-bit precision is the cost-minimized hardware without affecting the accuracy of the output PCs.

4.2 Precision Analysis

As the synthesized results, the larger bit-width leads to the larger chip area. The precision analysis is made here in order to find the cost-minimized hardware without affecting the accuracy of the output PCs. The experimental data and the algorithm setup are the same as those used in Section 2.2. The benchmark is also the standard Matlab "eig" function. The only difference is that we use the hardware Verilog model instead of the software Matlab model to realize the leading eigenvector distilling algorithm. After the spike detection and alignment, the covariance matrix of the detected spike waveforms is calculated and quantized into n-bit precision. This n-bit fixed point covariance matrix is then fed into our hardware Verilog model. The output PCs are also n-bit fixed point number. Note that the iteration number for each PC is set to 20 in this analysis. Fig. 7 shows the comparisons between the PCs generated by the standard Matlab function and our hardware verilog models. We use the correlation function as the similarity score, and the equation is shown as follows:

$$\varphi^T{}_{Verilog}\ \varphi_{Matlab} / norm(\varphi_{Verilog}) \times norm(\varphi_{Matlab})$$

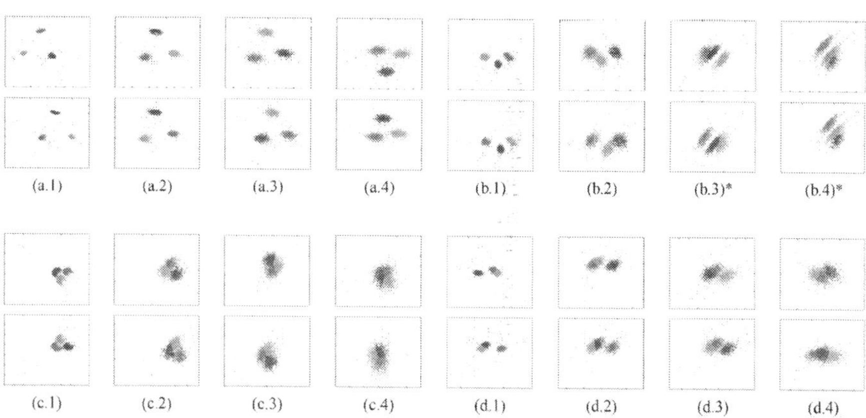

(a.1)   (a.2)   (a.3)   (a.4)   (b.1)   (b.2)   (b.3)*   (b.4)*

(c.1)   (c.2)   (c.3)   (c.4)   (d.1)   (d.2)   (d.3)   (d.4)

Fig. 8. Subjective comparison of the sorting performance with the PCs generated by our hardware Verilog model and the software Matlab model. The neural sequences #a.1~a.4, #b.1~b.4, #c.1~c.4, and #d.1~d.4 are C_Easy1_noise005~020, C_Easy2_noise005~020, C_Difficult1_noise005~020, C_Difficult2_noise005~020 from Quian Quiroga. The NEO-based spike detection, PCA-based feature extraction, and K-means classification (*watershed-based classification algorithm for b.3 and b.4) algorithms are used. For each neural sequence, the upper figure uses the software Matlab model for the eigenvector generation. 32-bit floating-point number is used to represent the input calculated covariance matrix, and the output PCs. The lower figure uses the hardware verilog model. 9-bit fixed-point precision is used instead. As the results, the PCs generated by the verilog model can achieve almost the same sorting performance compared with the Matlab model. The corresponding objective comparison is shown in Table 5.

Neural Data	a.1	a.2	a.3	a.4	b.1	b.2	b.3	b.4
Matlab (float)	98.24%	98.74%	98.34%	98.02%	98.27%	96.15%	89.02%	84.48%
Verilog (9bit)	98.24%	98.71%	98.39%	97.58%	98.15%	94.85%	90.08%	79.59%

Neural Data	c.1	c.2	c.3	c.4	d.1	d.2	d.3	d.4
Matlab (float)	96.57%	87.47%	78.03%	68.50%	93.37%	83.33%	76.81%	69.10%
Verilog (9bit)	96.87%	85.83%	78.28%	69.01%	93.33%	80.74%	75.61%	63.56%

Average: Matlab(32-bit floating point)/Verilog(9-bit fixed point) = 95.16%/94.45%

Table 5. Objective comparison of the sorting performance between the verilog and matlab models.

The simulation results show that the hardware with 9-bit precision is the cost-minimized hardware without affecting the accuracy of the output PCs.

Combined with the classification algorithm, we also demonstrate the sorting performance with the PCs generated by our hardware Verilog model, and compare it with the software Matlab model in Fig. 8. We adapt the K-means algorithm (Kanungo et al., 2002, Ding & He, 2004), the traditional classification algorithm for spike sorting, to classify most of the neural data on the PCA feature space. For data b.3 and b.4, because the K-means algorithm cannot come out with a reasonable result, another algorithm based on the watershed segmentation algorithm (Wang, 1998) is used. For each neural sequence in Fig. 8, the upper figure indicates the sorting results with the Matlab model while the lower figure is with the

Verilog model. Note that 9-bit precision is used in our final hardware. As the results, the PCs generated by the 9-bit fixed point verilog model can achieve almost the same sorting performance compared with the floating point Matlab model. The objective comparison is shown in Table 5.

In the modified eigenvector distilling algorithm, the normalization process is discarded with the proposed flipped structure. In this case, the output PCs are the orthogonal bases but not the unit vectors. That means the PCs generated by our hardware are the scaled version of the original PCs. However, our adaptive level shifting scheme uses the same bit-width to maximally represent the eigenvectors after the adaptive quantization. These orthogonal but non-orthonormal PCs will thus have similar scaling factors, and lead to almost the same classification results with the K-means algorithm as shown in Fig. 8 and Table 5.

4.3 Fabrication Results

The proposed eigenvector generator is integrated with other processors to complete the PCA-based spike sorting system shown in Fig. 1. As the first prototype chip (Chen et al., 2009), the system is fabricated in .35 µm 2P4M CMOS process for its lower cost. Figure 9 shows the chip micrograph. Table 6 describes the detailed chip specification. The chip size is 28.32 mm² with 51.1 k logic gates and 83.5 kb SRAMs. The chip is able to perform NEO-based spike detection and PCA-based feature extraction for 16 recording channels in a realtime. The power consumption is 4.11 mW with 5 volt supply voltage and 3.2MHz/400kHz operation frequency for the GPP/DPs.

Figure 10 demonstrates the functional capability of this chip. The 16-channel neural samples are input to the chip through the NI card device. The PCA training DP calculates the covariance matrix and the corresponding eigenvectors from the detected spikes. After the training, the resultant PCs are stored in the on-chip memory. This training procedure is sequentially performed channel by channel for the 16 recording channels. The embedded GPP is used to control the training and re-training schedule. After the training, the on-line 16-channel spike sorting DP uses these PCs to extract features from the following detected spikes. After the processing, the spike features and the corresponding timing information are output from the chip, recorded by the NI card device, parsed by the computer, and then displayed visually on the screen.

5. Conclusion

In this chapter, the VLSI architecture for leading eigenvector generation was designed for the on-chip PCA-based spike sorting system. The iterative eigenvector distilling algorithm is used because of its simple and regular nature. The proposed flipped structure enables the low area and low power implementation, while the adaptive level shifting scheme optimizes the accuracy and area trade-off. According to the synthesized results with specification of four PCs/channel, 32 samples/spike and 9 bits/sample, the proposed hardware can train 312 channels per minute at 1MHz operation frequency and consumes 132k µm² silicon area and 282 µW power in 90 nm process. This eigenvector generation unit is finally fabricated together with other processors in .35 µm process to complete the on-chip 16-channel PCA-based spike sorting system resulting in a 28.32 mm² chip area and 4.11 mW power consumption.

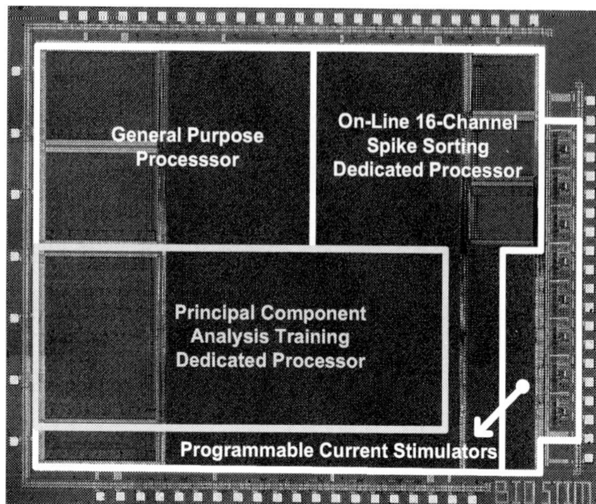

Fig. 9. Chip micrograph of the PCA-based spike sorting system. The proposed eigenvector generator is integrated with other processors to complete the PCA-based spike sorting system shown in Fig. 1. The system is fabricated in .35 μm 2P4M CMOS process.

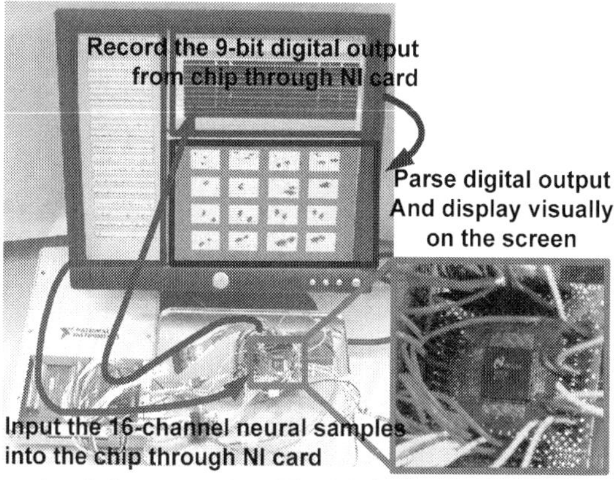

Fig. 10. Chip functional demonstration. The 16-channel neural samples are input to the chip through the NI card device. After the PCA training and the on-line feature extraction, the extracted spike features and the corresponding timing information are output from the chip, recorded by the NI card device, parsed by the computer, and then displayed visually on the screen.

Fabrication Process	0.35 μm 2P4M CMOS
Silicon Area	4.8x5.9 mm²
Logic Gate	51.1k
On-chip Memory	83.5kb
Max. Frequency	40MHz
Max. Voltage	5V
Power Consumption	4.11 mW*

*Power consumption for 16-channel PCA-based spike sorting. 3.2 MHz/400kHz frequencies are used for GPP and DPs respectively.

Table 6. Chip specifications of the PCA-based spike sorting system.

6. References

Zumsteg, Z.; Kemere, C.; Odriscoll, S.; Santhanam, G.; Ahmed, R.; Shenoy, K. & Meng, T. (2005). Power feasibility of implantable digital spike sorting circuits for neural prosthetic systems. *IEEE Transactions on Neural Systems and Rehabilitation Engineering*, Vol. 13, No. 3, pp. 272–279, 1534-4320.

Oweiss, K. G.; Anderson, D. J. & Papaefthymiou, M. M. (2003). Optimizing signal coding in neural interface system-on-a-chip modules. *Proceedings of 25th Annual Conference IEEE Engineering in Medicine and Biology Society*, Vol. 3, pp. 2216–2219, 0-7803-7789-3.

Olsson, R. H. & Wise, K. D. (2005). A three-dimensional neural recording microsystem with implantable data compression circuitry. *IEEE Journal of Solid-State Circuits*, Vol. 40, No. 12, pp. 2796–2804, 0018-9200.

Harrison, R. R. (2003). A low-power integrated cicuit for adaptive detection of action potentials in noisy signals. *Proceedings of 25th Annual Conference IEEE Engineering in Medicine and Biology Society*, Vol. 4, pp. 3325–3328, 0-7803-7789-3.

Oweiss, K. G.; Anderson, D. J. & Papaefthymiou, M. M. (1977). Multispike train analysis. *Proceedings of the IEEE*, Vol. 65, No. 5, pp. 762–773, 0018-9219.

Letelier, J. C. & Weber, P. P. (2000). Spike sorting based on discrete wavelet transform coefficients. Journal of Neuroscience Methods, Vol. 101, No. 2, pp. 93–106, 0165-0270.

Hulata, E.; Segev, R. & Ben-Jacob, E. (2002), A method for spike sorting and detection based on wavelet packets and Shannon's mutual information. Journal of Neuroscience Methods, Vol. 117, No. 1, pp. 1–12, 0165-0270.

Andra, K.; Chakrabarti, C. & Acharya, T. (2002). A VLSI architecture for liftingbased forward and inverse wavelet transform. *IEEE Transactions on Signal Processing*, Vol. 50, No. 4, pp. 966–977, 1053-587X.

Huang, C. T.; Tseng, P. C. & Chen, L. G. (2004). Flipping structure: an efficient VLSI architecture for lifting-based discrete wavelet transform. *IEEE Transactions on Signal Processing*, Vol. 52, No. 4, pp. 1080–1089, 1053-587X.

Kamboh, A. M.; Raetz, M.; Oweiss, K. G. & Mason, A. (2007). Area-power efficient VLSI implementation of multichannel SWT for data compression in implantable neuroprosthetics. *IEEE Transactions on Biomedical Circuits and Systems*, Vol. 1, No. 2, pp. 128–135, 1932-4545.

Kanungo, T.; Mount, D. M.; Netanyahu, N. S.; Piatko, C. D.; Silverman, R. & Wu, A. Y. (2002). An efficient k-means clustering algorithm: analysis and implementation. *IEEE Transactions on Pattern Analysis and Machine Intelligence*, Vol. 24, No. 7, pp. 881–892, 0162-8828.

Ding, C. & He, X. (2004). K-means clustering via principal component analysis. *Proceedings of International Conference on Machine Learning*, pp. 225–232, 1-58113-828-5, Banff, Alberta, Canada, July 2004, ACM, New York.

Comaniciu, D. & Meer, P. (2002). Mean shift: a robust approach toward feature space analysis. *IEEE Transactions on Pattern Analysis and Machine Intelligence*, Vol. 24, No. 5, pp. 603–619, 0162-8828.

Shenoy, K.; Santhanam, G.; Ryu, S.; Afshar, A.; Yu, B.; Gilja, V.; Linderman, M. Kalmar, R.; Cunningham, J.; Kemere, C.; Batista, A.; Churchland, M. & Meng, T. (2006). Increasing the performance of cortically controlled prostheses. *Proceedings 28th Annual Conference IEEE Engineering in Medicine and Biology Society*, pp. 6652–6656, 1-4244-0032-5.

Golub, G. H. & Van Loan, C. F. (1996). *Matrix Computations*. Johns Hopkins University Press, 0-8018-5414-8, Baltimore, USA.

Roweis, S. (1998). Em algorithms for PCA and SPCA. *Proceedings of the 1997 Conference on Advances in Neural Information Processing Systems*, pp. 626–632, 0-262-10076-2, Denver, Colorado, United States, 1998, MIT Press, Cambridge, MA, USA.

Schilling, R. J. & Harris, S. L. (2000). *Applied Numerical Methods for Engineers Using Matlab and C.* Brooks/Cole Publishing Company, 0-5343-7014-4, Pacific Grove, CA, USA.

Sirovich, L. (1987). Turbulence and the dynamics of coherent structures. *Quarterly of Applied Mathematics*, Vol. 45, pp. 561–571, 0033-569X.

Sharma, A. & Paliwal, K. K. (2007). Fast principal component analysis using fixed-point algorithm. *Pattern Recognition Letters*, Vol. 28, No. 10, pp. 1151–1155, 0167-8655.

Quian Quiroga, R. Simulated extracellular recordings. http://www2.le.ac.uk/departments/ engineering/research/bioengineering/neuroengineering-lab.

Anderson, E.; Bai, Z.; Bischof, C.; Blackford, S.; Demmel, J.; Dongarra, J.; Du Croz, J.; Greenbaum, A.; Hammarling, S.; McKenney, A. & Sorensen, D. (1999). *LAPACK User's Guide*, Society for Industrial and Applied Mathematics, 0-89871-447-8, Philadelphia, USA.

Kim, K. H. & Kim, S. J. (2000). Neural spike sorting under nearly 0-db signal-to-noise ratio using nonlinear energy operator and artificial neural-network classifier. *IEEE Transactions on Biomedical Engineering*, Vol. 47, No. 10, pp. 1406–1411, 0018-9294.

Wang, D. (1998). Unsupervised video segmentation based on watersheds and temporal tracking. *IEEE Transactions on Circuits System on Video Technology*, Vol. 8, No. 7, pp. 539–546, 1051-8215.

Chen, T. C.; Chen, K.; Yang, Z.; Cockerham, K. & Liu, W. (2009) A biomedical multiprocessor soc for closed-loop neuroprosthetic applications. *Proceedings of IEEE International Solid-State Circuits Conference*, Vol. 25, pp. 434–435.

26

Noise Impact in Designed Conditioning System for Energy Harvesting Units in Biomedical Applications

Aimé Lay-Ekuakille and Amerigo Trotta
University of Salento, Polytechnic of Bari
Italy

1. Introduction

The human body is subject to the same laws of physics as other objects, gaining and losing heat by conduction, convection and radiation. Conduction between bodies and/or substances in contact; convection involving the transfer of heat from a warm body to a body of air above it or inside the human body and here the blood, gases and other fluids is the medium, radiant heat transfer is a major mechanism of thermal exchange between human body and the surface surrounding environment. These three effects in most situations operate together. In human body, metabolic processes generate its own heat as well, similar to a heat-producing engine. Human body behaviour try to be in stable state therefore, it absorbs and emits energy to be in equilibrium, stimulation is applied to the body surface, this make the activity of metabolism induced to body surface. Human beings and, more generally speaking, warmblooded animals (e.g., dangerous and endangered animals, cattle, and pets), can also be a heat source, by means of a TEG (thermoelectric generator), for the devices attached to their skin. A TEG mounted in a wristwatch is an example for powering a watch using wasted human heat. Practical applications of TEGs have been carried out by different authors. In different works, the changes in a part of human body being have been studied and analyzed before and after stimulation and compared between them, then simulate the bio heat transfer mechanism using 2nd order circuit, which designed based on 1st order introduced by Guotai et al., and analyze the human thermo response. Since the human body emits energy as heat, it follows naturally to try to harness this energy. However, Carnot efficiency puts an upper limit on how well this waste heat can be recovered. This paper illustrates a specific study of the noise limited resolution of certain signal conditioning system concerning a TEG capable of powering biomedical hearing aids. In designing instrumentation system, especially for TEG, it is often necessary to be able to predict the noise limited threshold measurand, or alternately, what input measurand level will produce a given output SNR. The paper shows that, since the inner temperature of the human body is greater than the outer temperature, hence, the trunk is the area of the body where the tissue temperature has the highest value. So this is the area from which it is suitable to locate the sensing device for the sake of extraction and of subsequent conversion from thermal to electric energy. The choice of TG, for the purposes of this research, falls on

MPG-D602 device whose. The TEG "sees" the difference in terms of temperature between the hot side and the cold one, by producing, quickly, an electric power.

2. Electric energy from human body warmth

In different works, the changes, in a part of human body being, have been studied and analyzed before and after stimulation and compared between them, then simulate the bio heat transfer mechanism using 2nd order circuit, which designed based on 1st order introduced by different authors [Jiang, 2004], and analyze the human thermo response. Since the human body emits energy as heat, it follows naturally to try to harness this energy. However, Carnot efficiency puts an upper limit on how well this waste heat can be recovered. Assuming normal body temperature and a relatively low room temperature (20 °C), the Carnot efficiency is

$$\frac{T_{body} - T_{ambient}}{T_{body}} = \frac{(310K - 293K)}{310K} = 5.5\%$$

(1)

In a hot environment (27°C) the Carnot efficiency falls to

$$\frac{T_{body} - T_{ambient}}{T_{body}} = \frac{(310K - 300K)}{310K} = 3.2\%$$

(2)

This calculation provides an ideal value. Today's thermoelectric generators that might harness this energy do not approach Carnot efficiency in energy conversion. Although work on new materials and new approaches to thermoelectric [Kishi, 1999] promise to somewhat improve conversion efficiencies, today's standard thermopiles are 0.2% to 0.8% efficient for temperature differences of five to 20°C, as expected for a wearable system in temperate environments. For the sake of discussion, the theoretical Carnot limit will be used in the analysis below, hence the numbers are optimistic. Table 1 indicates that while sitting, a total of 116W of power is available. Using a Carnot engine to model the recoverable energy yields 3.7-6.4W of power. In more extreme temperature differences, higher efficiencies may be achieved, but robbing the user of heat in adverse environmental temperatures is not practical. Evaporative heat loss from humans account for 25% of their total heat dissipation (basal, non-sweating) even under the best of conditions. This "insensible perspiration" consists of water diffusing through the skin, sweat glands keeping the skin of the palms and soles pliable, and the expulsion of water-saturated air from the lungs. Thus, the maximum power available without trying to reclaim heat expended by the latent heat of vaporization drops to 2.8-4.8W.

According to mathematical viewpoint, heat diffusion in human body can be represented according to a system of eight differential equations of a structural human body model, and the human body head is the area with the highest temperature. Consequently, we exploit the head skin to locate the sensors for gathering electric energy from body temperature. We used a thin film generator named MPG-D family and specifically MPG-D602 according to the characteristics of Table 2 [micropelt].

Activity	Kilocal/hr	Watts
sleeping	70	81
lying quietly	80	93
sitting	100	116
standing at ease	110	128
conversation	110	128
eating meal	110	128
strolling	140	163
driving car	140	163
playing violin or piano	140	163
housekeeping	150	175
carpentry	230	268
hiking, 4 mph	350	407
swimming	500	582
mountain climbing	600	698
long distance run	900	1,048
sprinting	1,400	1,630

Table 1. Human energy expenditures per activities

Type	Dimension (mm)	Number of leg pairs	Thermal resistance	Electrical resistance	Substrate type	Thickness
MPG-D602	Cold side: 2.47x2.47 Hot side: 2.47x2.47	450	9.6 K/W	189Ω	Silicon	500µm

Table 2. MPG-D602 characteristics

The MPG-D is a thermoelectric power generator based on the transfer of the thermal energy through a minimum of one leg pair consisting of p-type and n-type thermoelectric material. Micropelt utilizes Bismuth (Bi), Antimony (Sb), Tellurium (Te) and Selenium (Se) compounds that have the best material properties with operating temperatures around room temperature and up to 200 °C. The produced output voltage is direct proportional with the number of leg pairs and the applied temperature difference ΔT over the element. The resulting voltage U is given by the following equation, where α is the Seebeck coefficient in µV/K (material related) that influences the output voltage (see fig 1).

$$U = N_{legpairs} . \Delta T . \alpha$$

(3)

The circuit connections of the MPG-D are illustrated in fig. 2 and the real dimensions of MPG-D602 is depicted in fig 3. The efficiency of a thermoelectric device is given by the material properties which are combined in a figure of merit F given by the following equation

$$F = \alpha^2 T \frac{\sigma}{k}$$

(4)

where T is the absolute temperature, σ is the electrical conductivity and k the thermal conductivity. As aforementioned, the most widely used material for the fabrication of thermoelectric generators operating at room temperature is BiTe, which exhibits a F of 1. PolySiGe (F=0.12) has also been used, especially for micromachined thermoelectric generators [Leonov, 2007]. Research on nanostructured materials and multilayers is ongoing worldwide in order to optimize thermoelectric properties and F values as large as 3.5 have been reported in many researches. These encouraging results may replace BiTe in the long term. Apart from improving the material properties, miniaturization using micromachining is ongoing and the main challenges of micromachined energy harvesters are known. Selected device results reported in literature [Hagelstein, 2002]. The reported power levels however cannot be directly compared, as output values are often calculated using a well-defined temperature drop across the thermopile (i.e. the temperatures of both plates have been fixed). In real applications the temperature drop across the thermopile is lower than the one between the hot plate and the ambient, and therefore the extrapolated results are too optimistic. It has been shown that the most challenging task in designing an efficient thermoelectric converter consists in maximizing this temperature drop across the thermopiles [Van Herwaarden, 1989].

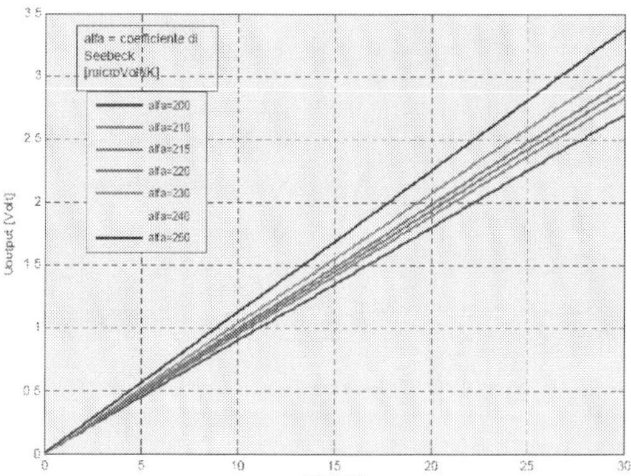

Fig. 1. MPG output in function of Seebeck coefficient

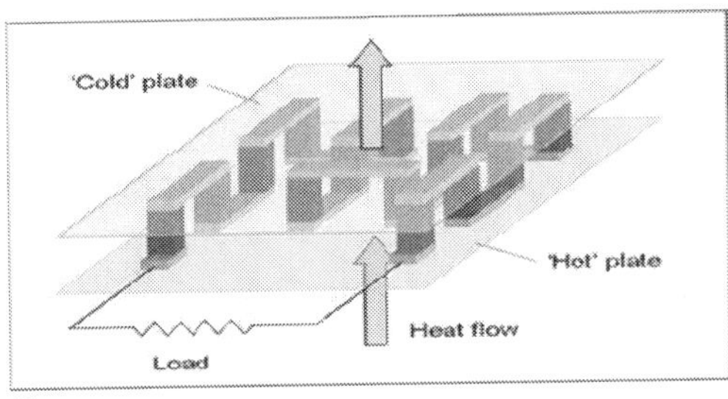

Fig. 2. Circuit connections

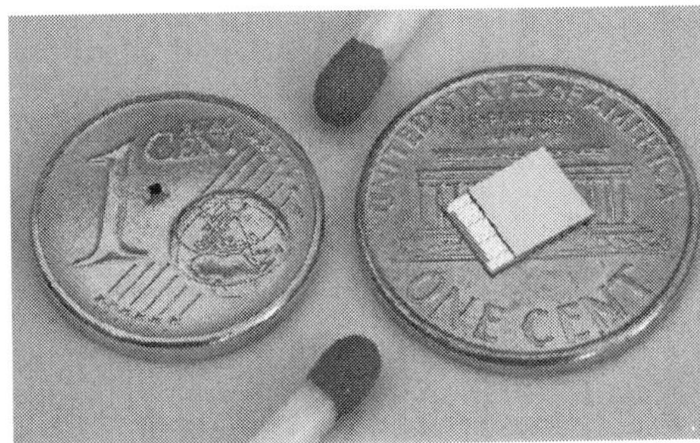

Fig. 3. MPG-D601 real dimensions

3. Conditioning system

3.1 Main Layouts and architectures

Analog conditioning signal system, in its simplest implementation, can be voltage amplification, with a change in impedance level between the conditioning amplifier's input and output. Analog signal conditioning may also involve linear filtering in the frequency domain, such as bandpass filtering to improve signal-to-noise ratio (SNR) at the amplifier's output. In the other cases, the analog input to the signal conditioning system may be processed nonlinearly. For instance, depending on the system specifications, the output of the analog signal conditioner may be proportional to the square root of the input, to the RMS value of the input, to the logarithm of the input, or to the cosine of the input, etc.., Analog signal conditioning is often accomplished by the use of operational amplifiers, as well as special instrumentation amplifiers, isolation amplifiers, analog multipliers, and dedicated nonlinear processing ICs. The output of the MPG-D must be connected to a specific conditioning circuit in order to make available the necessary voltage for hearing aids. The output voltage is an appropriate combination of single voltage released by single sensors. We illustrate two different conditioning circuits for the purposes of this research.

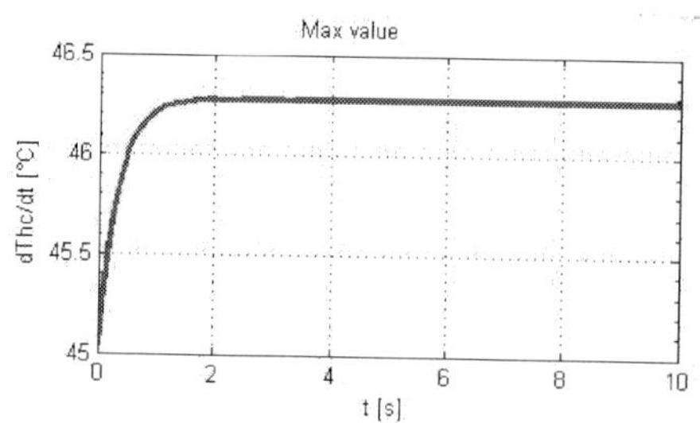

Fig. 4. Heat distribution max value within 10 s

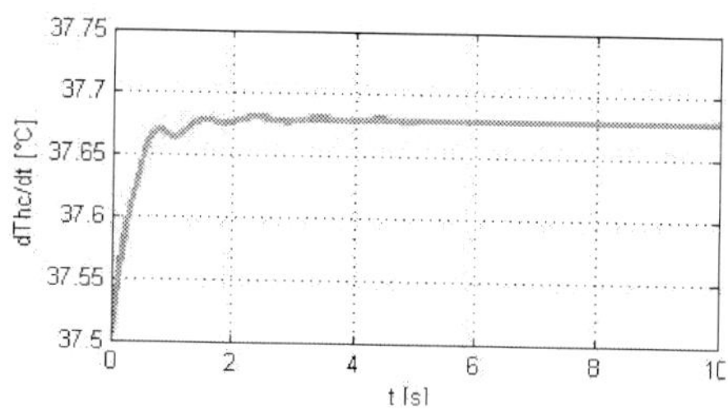

Fig. 5. Heat distribution average value within 10 s

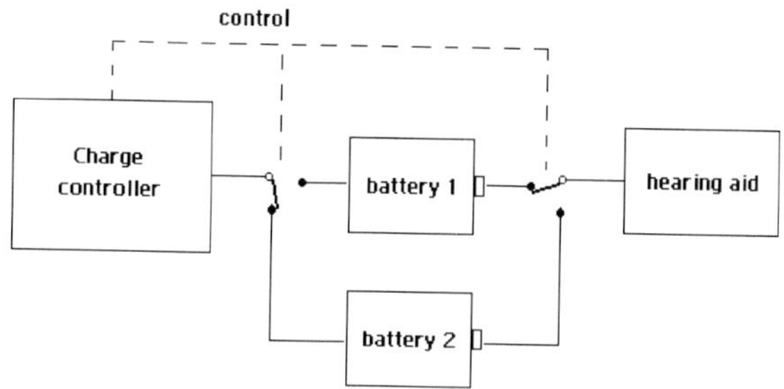

Fig. 6. Charge control architecture

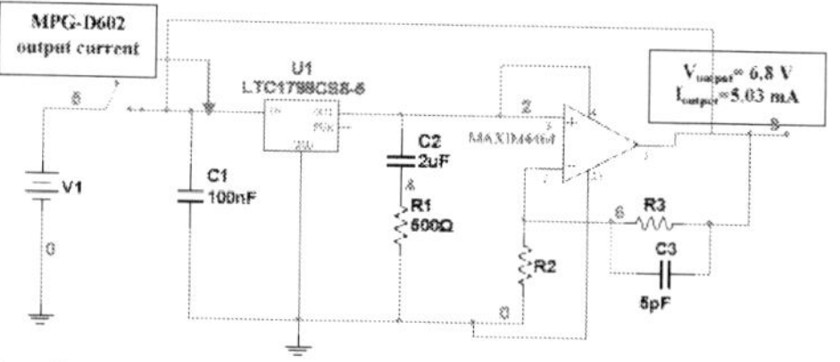

Fig. 7. Conditioning circuit

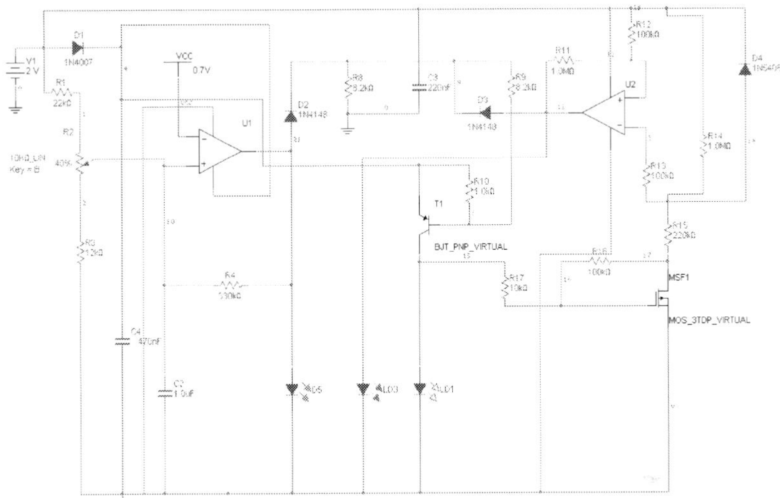

Fig. 8. Conditioning circuit including charge controller

In order to design, in a reliable way, the conditioning unit, a heat distribution for head area [Hirayama, 1998] is used as depicted in fig. 4 and fig. 5. These trends are very important for focusing the amount of heat to be converted in electric power. Since the hearing aid is, in general, supplied by a 1.4 V due to a specific battery, in order to increase the supplying reliability, an additional battery is used according to fig. 6. Hence, a conditioning unit is designed as shown in fig. 7, taking power from the sensor. A further improvement could be obtained from a charger configuration as depicted in fig. 8. In this case, three LEDs are used to simulate the operating mode of the circuit while the hearing aid is supplied.

3.2 Noise impact

The problem to be faced is the sources of noise in such signal conditioning units that can be separated into two major categories: noise from passive resistors and noise from active circuit elements such as bipolar junction transistors, field effect transistors and vacuum tubes. Noise from resistors is called *thermal or Johnson noise*. It has been observed that when dc (or average) current is passed through a resistor, the basic Johnson noise PDS (power density spectrum) is modified by the addition of a $1/f$ spectrum.

$$S_n(f) = 4kTR + AI^2/f \qquad (5)$$

where I is the average or dc component of current through the resistor, and A is a constant that depends on the material from which the resistor is constructed. An important parameter for resistors carrying average current is the crossover frequency, f_c, where the $1/f$ PDS equals the PDS of the Johnson noise. This is

$$f_c = AI^2/4kTR \qquad (6)$$

It is possible to show that the f_c, of a noisy resistor can be reduced by using a resistor of the same type, but having a higher wattage or power dissipation rating. Noise arising in JFETs, BJTs and other complex IC amplifiers is generally described by the two source input model. The total noise observed at the output of an amplifier, given that its input terminals are short circuited, is accounted for by defining an equivalent short circuited input noise voltage which replaces all internal noise sources affecting the amplifier output under short circuited input conditions [Horowitz, 1989]. The input noise voltage for many low noise, discrete transistors and IC amplifiers is specified by manufacturers.

4. Conclusion

Thermoelectric generators, for supplying autonomous biomedical devices, are necessary because they overcome battery limitations. Their conditioning units are essential to increase as great as possible the quantity of power available to feed the hearing aids. Particular attention must be paid in designing the conditioning and the charger circuits in order to lower the power consumption and the noise.

5. References

G.T Jiang, G.T.; Qu, T.T.; Zhigang S. & Zhang, X. (2004). A Circuit Simulating Method for Heat Transfer Mechanism in Human Body, *Proceedings of 26th IEEE EMBS*, pp. 5274-5276, 7803-8439-3-04, September 2004, IEEE EMBS, Piscataway.
Kishi, M.; Nemoto, H.; Hamao, T.; Yamamoto, M.; Sudou, S.; Mandai, M.; & Yamamoto S. (1999). Micro-thermoelectric modules and their application to wristwatches as an energy source, *Proceedings of 18th Int. Conf. Thermoelectrics ICT'99*, pp. 301–307, 7803-5451-6-00, Baltimore, april, 1999, ITS, Vienna.
www.micropelt.com.
Leonov, V.; Torfs, T.; Fiorini, P. & Van Hoof C. (2007). Thermoelectric Converters of Human Warmth for Self-Powered Wireless Sensor Nodes. *IEEE Sensors Journal*, Vol. 7, No 5, (may 2007) 650-657, 1530-437X.
Hagelstein, P.L. & Kucherov, Y. (2002). Enhanced figure of merit in thermal to electrical energy conversion using diode structures. *Physics Letters*, Vol. 81, No 3, (July 2002) 559–561, 0003-6951.
Van Herwaarden, A.W.; Van Duyn D.C.; Van Oudheusd, B.W. & Sarro P.M. Integrated Thermopile Sensors. Sensors and Actuators A, Vol.21-23 (1989) 621-630, 0924-4247-90.
Hirayama, H.; Kimura, T. (1998). Theoretical analysis of the human heat production system and its regulation, Proceeding of SICE '98. Proceedings of the 37th SICE Annual Conference, pp. 827-833, 1-3-98-000-0827, Yokogawa, July 1998, SICE, Tokyo
Horowitz, P. & Hill, W. (1989). Low-power design, In: *The Art of Electronics*, Horowitz & Hill, (Ed. II), 917-986, Cambridge University Press, 0-521-37095-7, Cambridge

27

A Novel Soft Actuator using Metal Hydride Materials and Its Applications in Quality-of-Life Technology

Shuichi Ino[1] and Mitsuru Sato[2]
[1]National Institute of Advanced Industrial Science and Technology
[2]Showa University
Japan

1. Introduction

Globally, social needs for daily life support systems and robots have strongly increased in an aging society with a falling birth rate. Quality-of-life technologies affect people in various settings with different needs (Cooper, 2008). To provide force and motion for rehabilitation therapy or human power assistance in quality-of-life technologies, some kinds of force devices such as electric motors, hydraulic actuators, and pneumatic actuators are used in rehabilitation apparatuses and assistive systems (Guizzo & Goldstein, 2005). It is particularly important that the force devices used for rehabilitation apparatuses or power assist systems include human-compatible softness for safety (Bicchi & Tonietti, 2004), noiselessness, and a high power-to-weight ratio.

To fulfill the above demands, we designed a novel actuator using a metal hydride (MH) alloy based on rare-earth metal compounds for a source of mechanical power. A force device using an MH alloy, which is called an MH actuator, generates a high output force, even if its size is small (Sasaki et al., 1986). The main reason is simply that the MH alloy can store a large amount of hydrogen by controlling heat energy. Moreover, the MH actuator has human-friendly flexibility and noiselessness based on a soft drive mechanism derived from the chemical reaction of metal hydrides. As you know, hydrogen is also the ideal clean energy carrier candidate because it does not have adverse effects on the environment (Sakintuna et. al., 2007).

The purpose of this chapter is threefold: (a) to outline the properties of metal hydride materials and the structure and drive mechanism of the MH actuator, (b) to describe the characteristics of a newly developed wearable MH actuator using a soft bellows made of a multilayer laminate film, which is more human-friendly than a current commercial actuator, and (c) to show some applications of the MH actuator in quality-of-life technology: a transfer aid for a wheelchair user, a continuous passive motion (CPM) machine for joint rehabilitation, and a power assist system for bed sore prevention of people with restricted mobility. Further, we describe a subsystem component to convert from hydrogen gas pressure to air pressure to facilitate safety and versatility of the MH actuator.

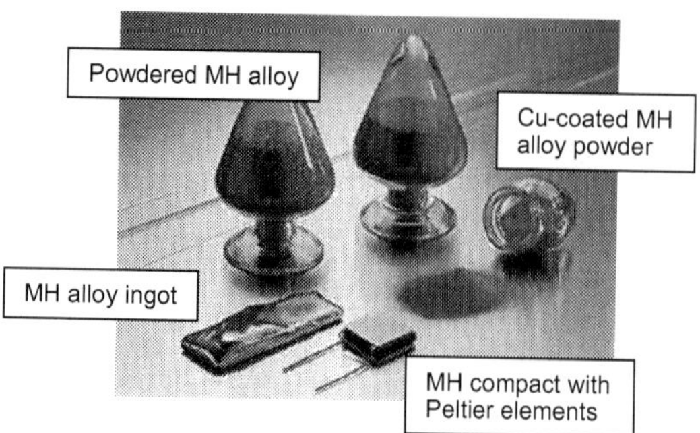

Fig. 1. Various forms of a metal hydride alloy (ingot, powder, Cu-coated powder, and compact module nipped Peltier modules) to embed in the MH actuator.

Finally, we will discuss some issues to improve the MH actuator for more suitable devices in assistive technology and rehabilitation engineering.

2. Metal Hydride Actuator

2.1 Metal Hydride Materials

MH alloys are particular materials that have the ability to store a large amount of hydrogen, about 1000 times as large as the volume of the alloy itself. The various forms of the MH alloy are shown in Fig. 1. One of the conventional metal hydride materials is Mg_2Ni, which was discovered in 1968 at Brookhaven National Laboratory, USA (Wiswall & Reilily, 1974). This is historically the first practical metal hydride material. Shortly thereafter, as it happens, $LaNi_5$ was discovered in 1970 at Philips Research Laboratories, the Netherlands (Van Mal et al., 1974). These successive discoveries became a trigger of research of various MH alloys and opened new possibilities for industrial developments.

A reversible chemical reaction between metal (M) and hydrogen gas (H_2) generates metal hydrides (MH_x) as in the following reaction formula:

$$M + \frac{x}{2}H_2 \leftrightarrow MH_x + Q \tag{1}$$

where Q is the heat of reaction, and thus, $Q > 0$ J/mol for H_2. If this reaction succeeds at a fixed temperature, then it will advance up to an equilibrium pressure, which is the plateau pressure. The PCT diagram (P: hydrogen pressure, C: hydrogen content, T: temperature) shows the basic characteristics of the MH alloy. As demonstrated in the PCT diagram in Fig. 2, changing the temperature of the MH alloy can control the plateau pressure. The MH alloy with a good hydrogen absorbing property for actuator applications has a flat and wide plateau area in the PCT diagram.

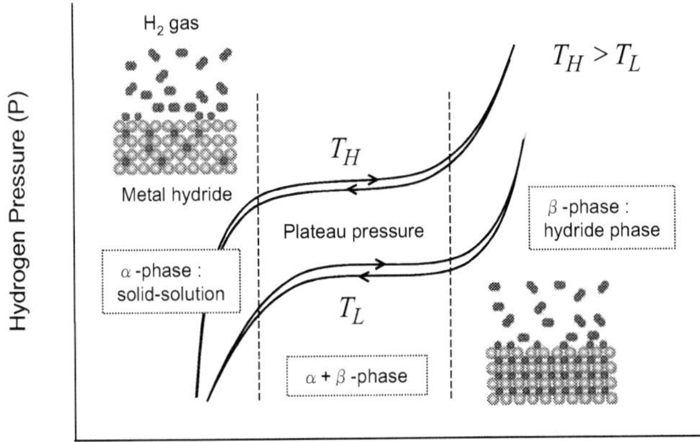

Hydrogen Content (C)

Fig. 2. Pressure-content-temperature plot (PCT diagram) of a metal hydride alloy.

Then, the hydrogen equilibrium pressure (P) is related to the changes ΔH and ΔS in enthalpy and entropy, respectively, as a function of temperature (T) by the Van't Hoff equation:

$$\log_e P = \frac{\Delta H}{R} \cdot \frac{1}{T} - \frac{\Delta S}{R} \tag{2}$$

where R is the gas constant. The PT diagram of a CaNi based alloy is shown in Fig. 3. The relationship between the hydrogen equilibrium pressure and the temperature of the CaNi₅ alloy can be partially adjusted by changing the alloy's composition with the addition of mishmetal (Mm) and aluminum (Al). Mishmetal is a common name for a mixture of unrefined rare earth elements.

Furthermore, the MH alloy is not combustible or flammable, so it is safe as a hydrogen storage material for a fuel cell in road vehicles and other mobile applications (Schlapbach & Züttel, 2001).

2.2 Fundamental Mechanism and Configuration

Not only can the MH alloy efficiently store a large amount of hydrogen gas, it also desorbs hydrogen gas by controlling its own temperature. If the reversible reaction is carried out in a hermetically closed container system, heat energy applied to the MH alloy is converted into mechanical energy via a pressure change in the container system, as shown in Fig. 4. Thus, the MH actuator functions by using the hydrogen gas pressure derived from the MH alloy through the heat energy, which is controlled by a thermoelectric Peltier device for heating and cooling force.

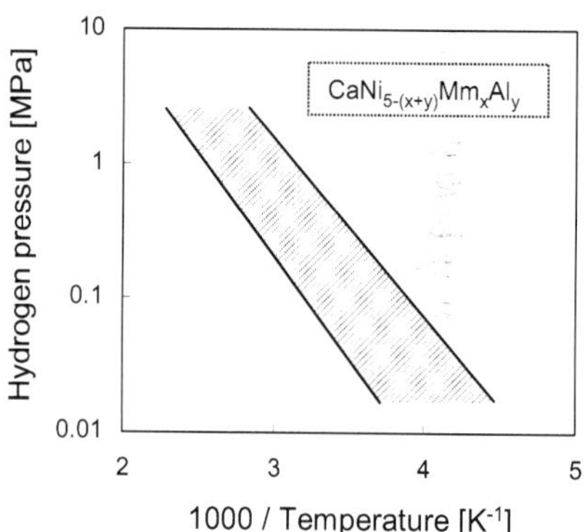

Fig. 3. Relationship between equilibrium hydrogen pressure and temperature (PT diagram) in CaNi$_5$ based MH alloys.

The MH actuator is composed of a solidified MH alloy powder, Peltier elements to electrically control the temperature of the alloy, an MH container to act as a small gas cylinder, and an end-effecter to transfer the hydrogen gas pressure into an acting force (Ino et al., 1992).

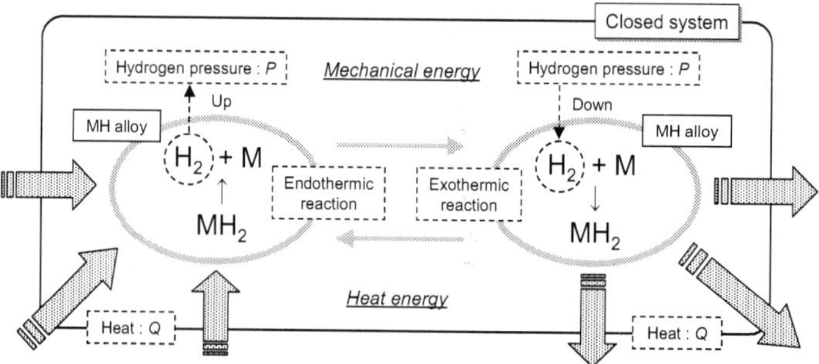

Fig. 4. Schematic illustration of actuation principles based on an energy conversion mechanism between heat, Q, and hydrogen pressure, P, in a MH actuator system.

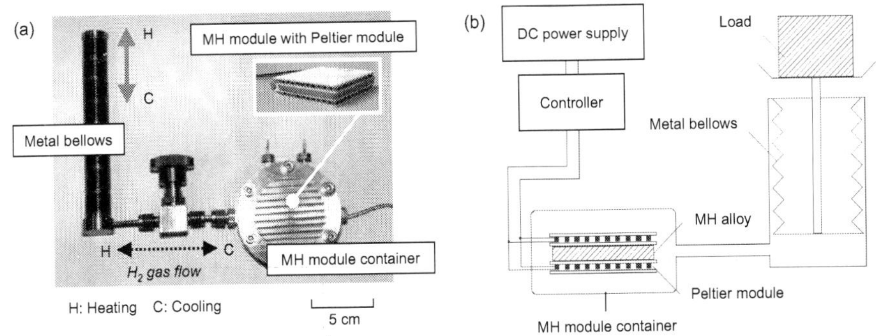

Fig. 5. Photograph of an MH actuator using a metal bellows (left) and a block diagram of an MH actuator system (right).

For example, the MH actuator shown in Fig. 5 contains six grams of an MH alloy. The maximum output force of this actuator is approximately 100 N. The power-to-weight ratio of the MH actuator is very high compared to those of traditional actuators, such as an electric motor and a hydraulic actuator (Wakisaka et al., 1997). However, the MH actuator uses the Peltier device, so it is not as energy efficient as an electric actuator. On the other hand, the heat drive mechanism of the MH actuator does not produce any noise or vibration. In addition, the reversible hydrogen absorption/desorption also has a buffering effect to act as a cushion to a human body and prevents extreme power surges or shock loads. Therefore, the MH actuator is suitable for use as a human-sized flexible actuator applied to soft and noiseless rehabilitation systems and assistive devices.

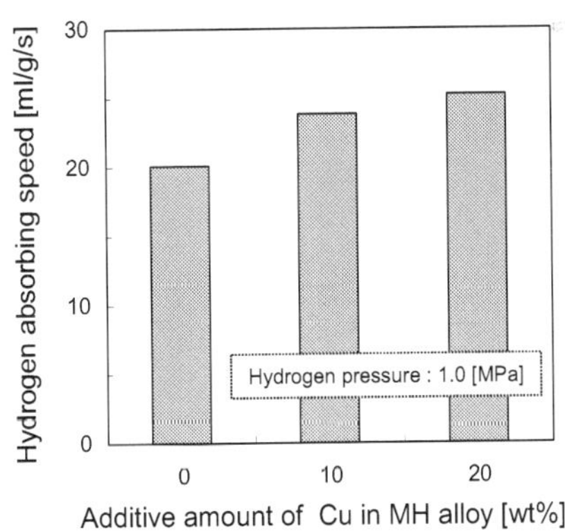

Fig. 6. Hydrogen absorbing speed versus additive amount of copper in the MH alloy powder at 1.0 MPa.

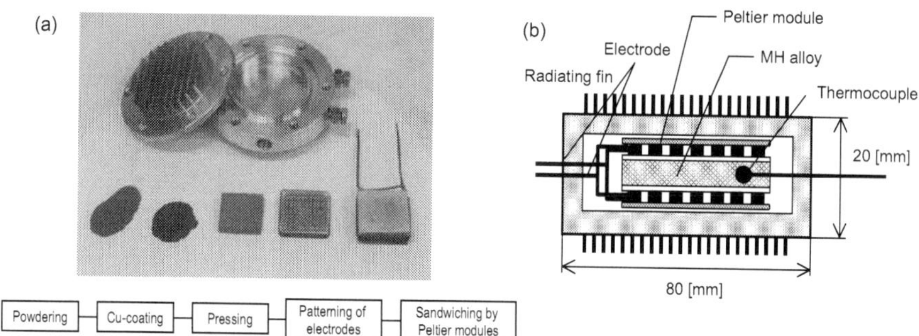

Fig. 7. Processing of the HM module components to improve heat conductivity for the acceleration of hydrogen absorbing speed of the MH alloy (left) and a cross-section of the MH module container (right).

3. Improvement on Metal Hydride Alloy

3.1 Heat Conductivity

The MH actuator has some unique properties such as a high power-to-weight ratio, lightweight, no noise, and softness. However, the speed of motion is relatively slow because the drive mechanism of the MH actuator depends on the poor heat conductivity of an activated MH alloy.

We designed the MH alloy to be powdered to improve the heat conductivity of the activated MH alloy, and this powdered MH alloy was coated with copper by chemical plating. The heat conductivity was increased about 50 times over that of only an MH alloy. As the results show in Fig. 6, the addition of Cu yields a clear increase in the hydrogen absorption speed.

From the experimental results, the powdered MH alloy was coated with a 1.0-µm-thick Cu (20 wt%). The MH alloy powder was solidified into a compact MH by pressing it to a thickness of about 3.0 mm. The heat source using a Peltier element was directly attached to the MH alloy compact to build in an integrated module. To assemble the Peltier element into this integrated module, the surface of the MH alloy compact was coated with alumina (Al_2O_3), which is an electric insulator, by plasma spraying, and the circuit pattern of the Peltier element was drawn on the alumina coating layer. These components of an MH module for the MH actuator are shown in Fig. 7 (a). The cross section of the MH module and container are illustrated in Fig. 7 (b).

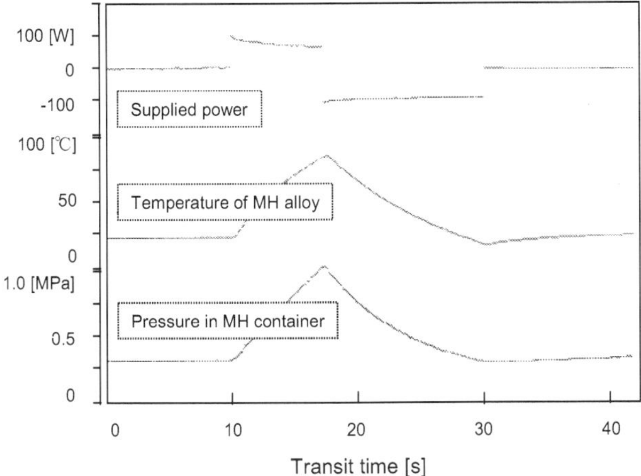

Fig. 8. Measured patterns of the pressure in the MH container and the temperature of the MH alloy with the application of a step voltage input through a DC power supply.

3.2 Motion Speed

By the improvement of the heat of conductivity of the MH module, the response speed of the MH actuator is increased, and it is potentially more useful in an actual power assist device for rehabilitation equipment.

The relationship between the temperature of the MH alloy and the pressure in the hermetically sealed container is shown in Fig. 8. The pressure rose smoothly from 0.3 to 1.0 MPa during 7.0 s. The time delay from the temperature change of the MH alloy to the pressure change of the container was about 0.1 s. Therefore, the MH actuator is sufficient for applications needing gentle motion such as joint rehabilitation or power assistance of bodily movement.

4. Design of a Soft End-Effector

4.1 Laminate Film Bellows

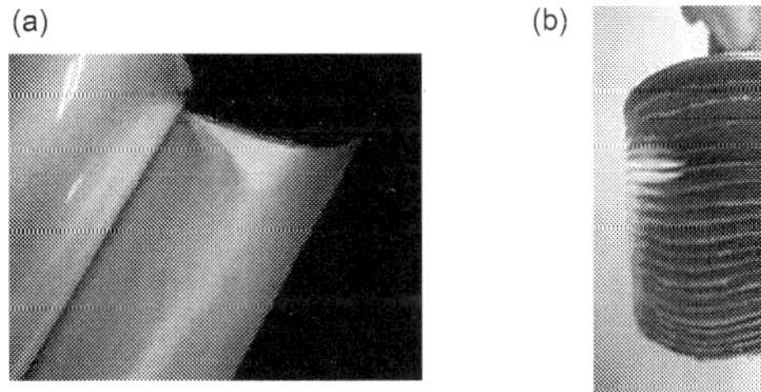

Fig. 9. Multilayer laminate film sheet (left) and a soft bellows made of the PE-Al-PET laminate film (right).

To maintain impermeability to hydrogen, a metal bellows has been used as the end-effector in conventional MH actuators. However, using stainless steel in fabricating the metal bellows has limitations in terms of weight, elongation rate, and flexibility. Rehabilitation equipment and power assist devices for human use must be light and a compatible softness with a human body. Therefore, we have attempted to develop a soft and light bellows made of non-metal materials to improve the human-friendliness of the MH actuator. The bellows of the MH actuator needs to be flexible, lightweight, and impermeable to hydrogen. However, fulfilling these conditions using only non-metal materials is very difficult. Alternatively, a polymer-metal laminate composite was selected here for a suboptimal solution (Ino et al., 2009).

The applied laminate composite is a tri-layer structure film of polyethylene (PE), aluminum (Al), and polyester (PET). The total thickness of the film is about 100 μm. The hydrogen barrier performance of the laminate film is supposed to be proportional to the thickness of the aluminum layer, but the flexibility of the film decreases as the thickness increases. These properties of the laminate film are in a trade-off relationship with the aluminum layer thickness. The aluminum layer thickness adopted in this design is 12 μm. We fabricated the laminate film bellows with a diameter of 100 mm and 20 corrugations using this laminate film, as shown in Fig. 9.

	Metal bellows	Laminate film bellows
Maxmun output [kgf]	28	28
Maxmun stroke [mm]	130	130
Weight [g]	800	35
Initial length [mm]	240	8
Withstand pressure [MPa(gauge)]	1	0.08
Section area [cm^2]	3.5	50

Table 1. Comparison between a metal bellows and a laminate film bellows in mechanical properties.

Table 1 shows a comparison between the mechanical parameters of the laminate film bellows and those of the metal bellows. The maximum force output and the maximum stroke were aligned to the same value for comparison. The weight of the laminate film bellows was 20 times lighter than that of the metal one, and the elongation range of the laminate film bellows was 30 times as large as that of the metal one. Hence, these mechanical properties of the laminate film bellows are useful to design a soft MH actuator.

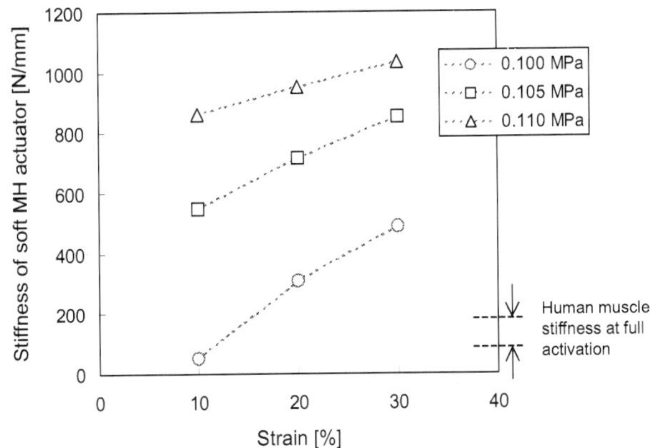

Fig. 10. Stiffness of the laminate film bellows versus applied strain changing the initial inner pressure of the MH actuator and the range of human muscle stiffness at full activation.

4.2 Hydrogen Impermeability

It is well known that a polymer-metal laminate film is a strong gas barrier to oxygen, water vapor, and other substances in the packaging industry (Schrenk & Alfrey Jr., 1969). However, data do not exist about the hydrogen impermeability of the laminate film and its adhesion area by thermo-compression bonding.

The hydrogen impermeability of the soft bellows made of the laminate film was examined by monitoring the inner pressure and displacement of the soft bellows filled with 99.99999% pure hydrogen gas. The initial inner pressure in the soft bellows was 0.02 MPa (gauge), and the water temperature of a bath to immerse the soft bellows was controlled at 20 °C.

From the experimental result, the amount of decompression of the soft bellows after 240 hours was about 0.7% of the initial inner pressure. Thus, it was clear that the laminate film bellows was capable of maintaining a hydrogen gas barrier for at least ten days.

4.3 Flex Durability

The aluminum layer of the laminate film may fracture due to metal fatigue if a bending motion is repeatedly applied for a long time period. If a fracture occurs in the laminate film, the inner pressure and stroke length of the laminate film bellows may decline rapidly. Thus, a flex durability test was performed to determine how long the laminate film bellows could continuously flex and extend.

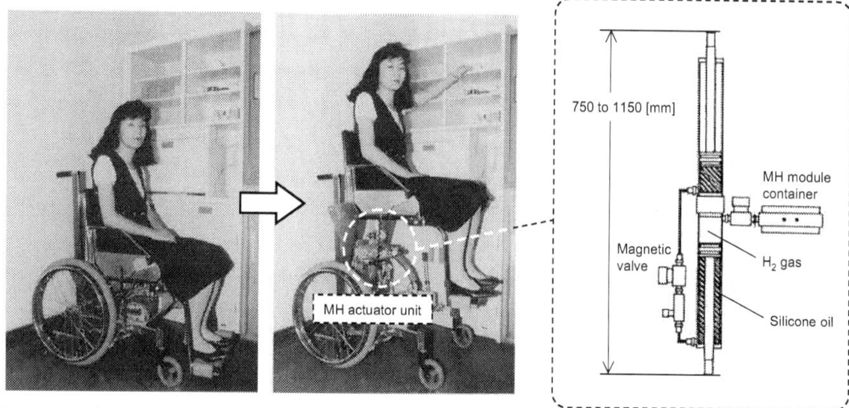

Fig. 11. Wheelchair seat lift using the MH actuator (left) and its long stroke tandem cylinder having a function that is convertible from a hydrogen gas pressure to a silicone oil one (right).

From the durability test, the laminate film did not break down by repeated motion for ten days. There was no clear change of the inner pressure and stroke length during the flex durability test, so the laminate film bellows could perform normally for more than 3,500 strokes. The number of strokes in this test should guide the assumption of a periodic replacement of this laminate film bellows, which helps maintain good hygiene.

4.4 Passive Elasticity

The passive elasticity of the soft MH actuator built in the laminate film bellows was measured by a universal tester. The relationship between the stiffness and the strain of the laminate film bellows where the parameters are the initial inner pressure ($P_0 = 0.100$, 0.105, and 0.110 MPa) of the MH actuator is shown in Fig. 10. It was found that the stiffness increased with increasing strain on the laminate film bellows, and that the rate of the stiffness change (gradient) decreased with increasing initial inner pressure of the soft MH actuator. The stiffness of the soft MH actuator with a closed valve was higher than that with an opened valve. This actuator property may be a result of hydrogen being absorbed by the MH alloy due to applying pressure from outside the bellows.

Moreover, the range of the variable stiffness of human muscle at full activation (Cook, C. S. & McDonagh, M. J. N., 1996) was included in that of the soft MH actuator, as shown in Fig. 10. Thus, the soft MH actuator may be suitable for a human power assist and rehabilitation device from the viewpoint of mechanical impedance matching and safety in passive elasticity to reduce any potential danger.

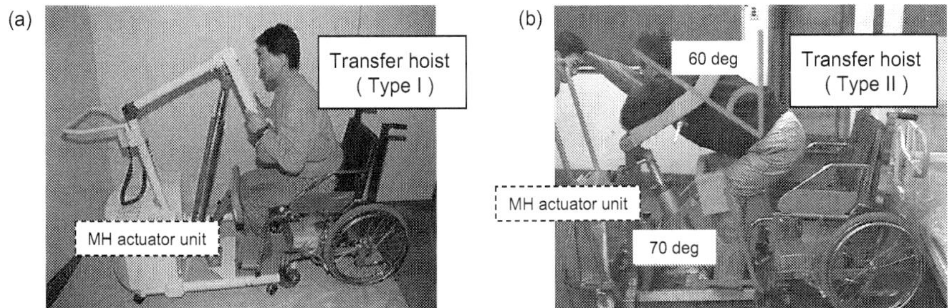

Fig. 12. Transfer hoists using a high power MH actuator unit (type I, left) and its downsized MH actuator unit with an accumulator (type II, right).

4.5 Cost-Effectiveness

The laminate bellows can be produced at very low cost compared to a metal one because a mass-produced polymer-metal laminate film is not typically expensive. Therefore, it is possible to create a disposable version of the laminate film bellows, which would satisfy the hygienic requirements of medical and rehabilitation devices.

5. Applications

5.1 Wheelchair Seat Lift

A wheelchair is a popular assistive device for persons with lower limb disability or the elderly. Recently, the wheelchair has taken significant functional advancement and many types have been developed to conform to the life style of wheelchair users. When using a wheelchair, however, some tasks meant to be performed from a standing position, such as reaching a tall shelf and cooking in the kitchen are very difficult in daily life. Thus, a wheelchair with a seat lift system using the MH actuator was developed to improve the quality of life (Wakisaka et al., 1997).

These assistive systems for human body motion need an especially long stroke displacement for lifting. Therefore, a long stroke MH actuator using a tandem piston cylinder with a solenoid valve was developed, as shown in Fig. 11. When hydrogen gas flows from the lower piston, silicone oil in the lower piston moves to the upper piston depending on the rate of flow of the hydrogen gas. By using such a drive mechanism, the stroke displacement obtained totally by an MH actuator system is doubled in comparison with an actuator drive system using only hydrogen gas. The seat height of the wheelchair can be stabilized by stopping the silicone flow via the solenoid valve.

This MH actuator, which adopts a 40-g $CaNi_5$ alloy, can produce approximately an 800 N output force and a 40 cm stroke. The lift speed was about 20 mm/s and the total weight of the seat lift equipment including the MH actuator unit and the tandem piston cylinder was about 5 kg.

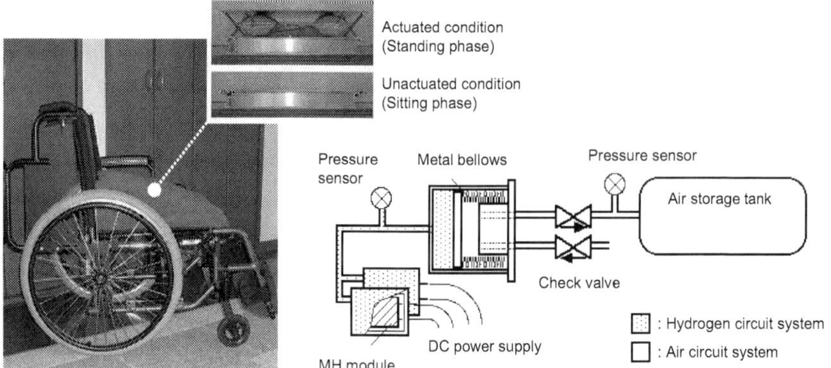

Fig. 13. Sit-to-stand assist cushion using a compact air compressor including an MH actuator unit on a wheelchair seat (left) and the schematic configuration of an MH air compressor (right).

5.2 Transfer Equipment

When people cannot stand up by themselves due to illness or injury, they need help transferring between a bed, a wheelchair, a toilet seat, a bath, etc. This transfer assistance requires a strong, safe motion. Thus, a physical and mental load exists between a patient and a helper at any time. For these reasons, we developed a transfer hoist based on an ergonomic motion analysis of transfer behavior. An MH actuator with a variable compliance function was implemented into his standing transfer hoist.

The appearance of the transfer hoist is shown in Fig. 12 (a); it has a height of 118 cm and a width of 70 cm. A kneepad, an arm pad, and a chest pad with cushioning material were built into the transfer hoist to prevent a fall with the knee flexed and to move the user's body stably and safely. These pads were designed based on the measurement of the motion analysis of elderly people (Tsuruga et al., 2001). The kneepad had a variable position mechanism using springs in consideration of changing the ankle joint angle through a transfer motion. The basic parts of the transfer hoist were a modular fashion to customize as appropriate according to the physical features of the users. We developed a double-acting MH actuator with two MH modules for the lifting mechanism of the transfer hoist. The double-acting MH actuator can control its own stiffness and position by changing the balance between the inner and outer hydrogen pressures of a metal bellows in a cylinder. This double-acting MH actuator provides a maximum lifting weight of 200 kg and a stroke of 350 mm.

The size of the transfer hoist described above is acceptable in a hospital and an assisted-living facility. However, the size is somewhat large for at home use. Thus, we redesigned a compact transfer hoist as shown in Fig. 12 (b). The MH actuator was modified to a single-acting-type mechanism using an accumulator for a reduction in size and weight. This single-acting-type MH actuator can smoothly push up and down a transfer hoist arm by use of an accumulator pressure regardless of a single MH module as well as the double-acting-type MH actuator. From this improvement, the size of the transfer hoist was a height of 80 cm and width of 45 cm, and the total weight was reduced 40% compared with the former transfer hoist (type I).

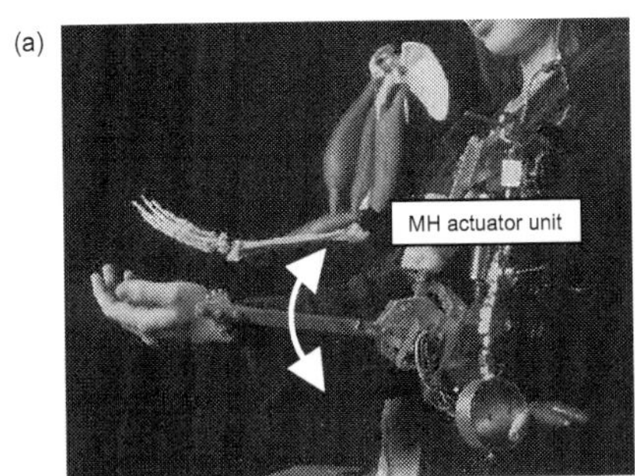

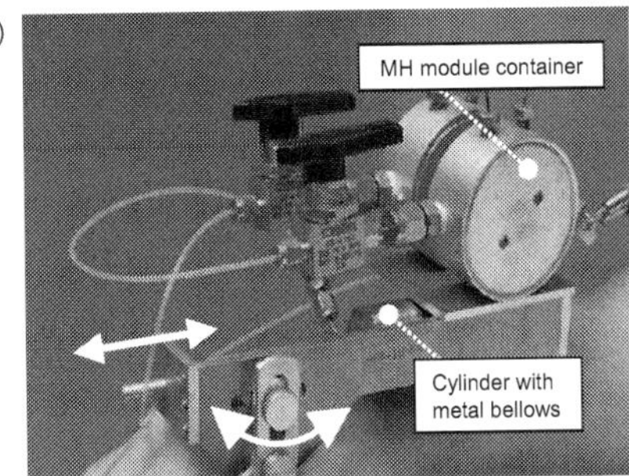

Fig. 14. Elbow CPM machine using an MH actuator unit (left) and the main components of its MH actuator unit (right).

As for the rest, our collaborative company has also developed a toilet seat lifter using an MH actuator (Wakisaka et al., 1997). This toilet seat lifter was installed in a house, which was called the Welfare Techno House in Japan (Tamura, 2006), for a case study of the well being of elderly people.

5.3 Sit-to-Stand Assist Cushion

The lifting systems of the wheelchair seat lift and the transfer hoist obviously cannot use the other assistive equipment without modification. Therefore, we have designed a portable cushion system for assisting in the sit-to-stand motion, which can easily attach to an existing wheelchair or bed (Sato et. al., 2007). The MH actuator in this cushion system was fitted with an air bag and a hydrogen-to-air pressure conversion system.

The appearance of the portable cushion system for assisting with sit-to-stand motion is shown in Fig. 13. To convert the hydrogen pressure generated by the MH module into an air pressure, a metal bellows, an air cylinder, and an accumulator were connected in series as illustrated in Fig. 13. The air cylinder and the accumulator were joined via a check valve. In other words, this system is a small and quiet air compressor using an MH actuator, what is termed an MH air compressor. The cushion part, which is applied as air bags made of laminate film sheet, comes from compressed air pressure exhausted from the accumulator to an elevating force as a stand-up support for a seated person. This cushion system contains a 12-g MH alloy. The output force is about 500 N, and the changing height of a seat is 90 mm. As the driving gas in the air bag is common air and not hydrogen, a hydrogen leakage safety concern is not an issue.

5.4 Continuous Passive Motion Machine

In the aging society, there are many needs for at-home instruments for motor rehabilitation in stroke or joint injured patients. The techniques of joint rehabilitation include manual therapy and range of motion (ROM) exercises using a continuous passive motion (CPM) machine. The therapeutic effects of these techniques were clinically clear in previous studies

(Salter et al., 1984). However, current CPM machines have some problems such as a lack of softness that inheres in human body, a bulky size for use, and noise emitted from the use of an electric motor. These problems disturb the ease and safety of use of the CPM machine at home. Hence, we have designed a compact MH actuator and prototyped a CPM device using it.

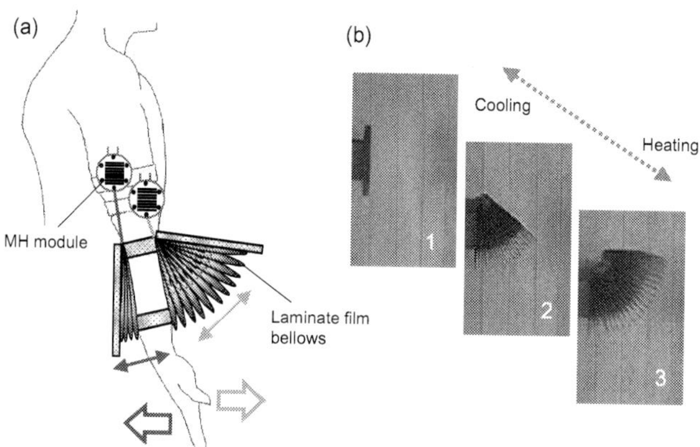

Fig. 15. Image of the elbow CPM machine using a pair of laminate film bellows and MH modules (left) and example of a motion pattern of the laminate film bellows added of an asymmetric elongation structure.

The prototyped CPM device for an elbow joint is shown in Fig. 14. The installed MH actuator contained a small metal bellows. The output torque around an elbow was about 7 Nm at maximum, which was selected based on the data obtained by the manual therapy motion of a physical therapist. The weight of this device was about 1.7 kg, and it is much lighter than that of a conventional CPM machine. The variable range of the mechanical compliance was 6.5 to 15 deg/Nm. Although this CPM machine has the potential to significantly improve joint disease, its weight and wearability are still not enough for clinical use.

In order to solve this problem, we designed a different type of CPM machine, which uses a laminate film bellows integrated into a soft MH actuator (Ino et al., 2008), as shown in Fig. 15. The antagonistic mechanism composed of two soft MH actuators allows for soft actuation of the elbow joints, and its stiffness can easily be controlled based on the sum of the inner pressure of both laminate film bellows (Sato et al., 1996).

Moreover, the range of the variable stiffness of human muscle at full activation was included in that of the MH actuator, as shown already in Fig. 10. Thus, the MH actuator using the laminate film bellows is suitable for a physical rehabilitation apparatus considering mechanical impedance matching.

By using the MH actuator, an extremely slow motion that is not available by a human hand be applied to a patient's joint, so it may allow some kind of effective exercise for early ROM rehabilitation after joint surgery, the cure of club-foot and other joint diseases.

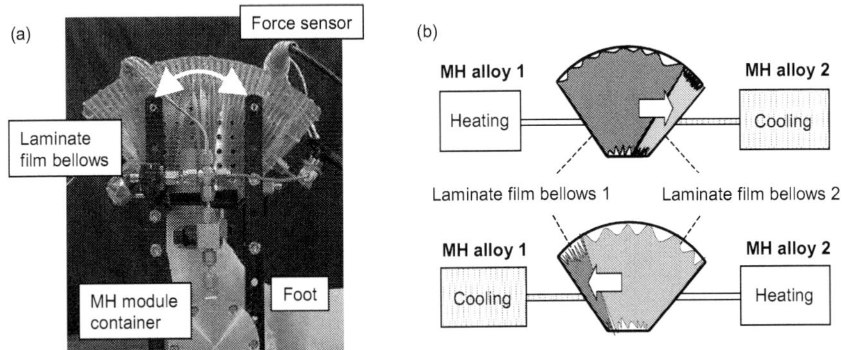

Fig. 16. Power assist system using the soft MH actuator units for toe exercises to prevent symptoms of disuse syndrome (left) and a schematic illustration of its antagonistic driving mechanism using a pair of the soft MH actuator units (right).

5.5 Power Assist Device

We have developed a bedside power assist system for toe exercises that can be configured from two of the soft MH actuators with a laminate film bellows, pressure sensors, a bipolar power supply, and a PID controller using a personal computer, as shown in Fig. 16 (a). The laminate film bellows of the soft MH actuator weighed 40 g.

A sketch of an antagonistic motion pattern of the soft MH actuators is shown in Fig. 16 (b). The extension and flexion motion of the toe joints are derived from a pair of soft bellows spreading out in a fan-like form in a plastic case. The motion of the toes in the power assist system was properly gentle and slow for joint rehabilitation. During the operation of the system, the subject's toes constantly fitted in the space between the two soft bellows.

Thus, various toe joint exercises could be easily actualized by a simple pressure control of the soft MH actuator system. In addition, we have measured the cutaneous blood flow before and during exercise to examine the preventive effect on bedsore formation by a passive motion exercise (Hosono et al., 2008). These results show a significant blood flow increase at the frequent sites of decubitus ulcers. The passive motion at toe joints using such a soft MH actuator will be useful for the prevention of disuse syndromes (Bortz, 1984).

6. Conclusion

In this chapter, we explained a novel soft actuator using an MH alloy and its applications in assistive technology and rehabilitation engineering. The MH actuator using metal hydride materials has many good human-friendly properties regarding the force-to-weight ratio, mechanical impedance, and noise-free motion, which are different from typical industrial actuators. From these unique properties and their similarity to muscle actuation styles of expansion and contraction, we think that the MH actuator is one of the most suitable force devices for applications in human motion assist systems and rehabilitation exercise systems. Additionally, by producing a much larger or smaller MH actuator by taking advantage of the uniqueness of its driving mechanism and the simplicity of its configuration, its various applications may extend in other industrial areas such as a micro-actuator for a functional endoscope, a manipulator for a submarine robot, a home elevator system, and so on.

The energy efficiency and the speed of the contraction mode of the MH actuator are the main issues to be improved when considering the increasing use of this actuator. The cause of these issues is derived from the use of a Peltier module for the temperature control of the MH alloy. Thus, technological developments on the Peltier module with supreme heat conversion efficiency or a method of high-speed heat flow control are demanded for a performance gain of the MH actuator.

In an aging society with a declining birth rate, the demand for motion assist systems and home care robots for supporting well-being in daily life will be increased from a lack of labor force supply, especially in Japan which has been faced with a super-aged society. It is important to make sure a biomedical approach is taken to developing the soft actuator considering sufficiently human physical and psychological characteristics, a thinking pattern that is different from that of a conventional industrial engineering approach. At present, a human-friendly soft actuator is strongly demanded to progress quality-of-life technologies. For a further study, we will focus on putting the soft MH actuator into practical use to serve the elderly and people with disabilities in daily life at the earliest possible date.

Acknowledgements

This work was supported in part by the Industrial Technology Research Grant Program from NEDO of Japan and the Grant-in-Aid for Scientific Research from the Japan Society for the Promotion of Science. The authors would like to thank for H. Ito, H. Kawano, M. Muro, and Y. Wakisaka of the Muroran Research Laboratory, Japan Steel Works Ltd. for outstanding technical assistance

7. References

Bicchi, A. & Tonietti, G. (2004). Fast and "soft-arm" tactics. *IEEE Robotics & Automation Magazine*, Vol. 11, No. 2, pp. 22-33

Bortz, W. M. (1984). The disuse syndrome. *Western Journal of Medicine*, Vol. 141, No. 5, pp. 691-694

Cook, C. S. & McDonagh, M. J. N. (1996). Measurement of muscle and tendon stiffness in man. *European Journal of Applied Physiology*, Vol. 72, No. 42, pp. 380-382

Cooper, R. A. (2008). Quality-of-Life Technology; A Human-Centered and Holistic Design. *IEEE Engineering in Medicine and Biology Magazine*, Vol. 27, No. 2, pp. 10-11

Guizzo, E. & Goldstein, H. (2005). The rise of the body bots. *IEEE Spectrum*, Vol. 42, No. 10, pp. 50-56

Hosono, M.; Ino, S.; Sato, M.; Yamashita, K.; Izumi, T. & Ifukube, T. (2008). Design of a Rehabilitation Device using a Metal Hydride Actuator to Assist Movement of Toe Joints, *Proceedings of the 3rd Asia International Symposium on Mechatronics*, pp. 473-476, Sapporo (Japan), August 2008

Ino, S.; Izumi, T.; Takahashi, M. & Ifukube, T. (1992). Design of an actuator for tele-existence display of position and force to human hand and elbow. *Journal of Robotics and Mechatronics*, Vol. 4, No. 1, pp. 43-48

Ino, S.; Sato, M.; Hosono, M.; Nalajima, S.; Yamashita, K.; Tanaka, T & Izumi, T. (2008). Prototype Design of a Wearable Metal Hydride Actuator Using a Soft Bellows for Motor Rehabilitation, *Proceedings of the 30th Annual International Conference of the IEEE Engineering in Medicine and Biology Society*, pp. 3451-3454, ISBN: 978-1-4244-1815-2, Vancouver (Canada), August 2008

Ino, S.; Sato, M.; Hosono, M. & Izumi, T. (2009). Development of a Soft Metal Hydride Actuator Using a Laminate Bellows for Rehabilitation Systems. *Sensors and Actuators: B. Chemical*, Vol. B-136, No. 1, pp. 86-91

Sakintuna, B.; Lamari-Darkrimb, F. & Hirscherc, M. (2007). Metal hydride materials for solid hydrogen storage: A review. *International Journal of Hydrogen Energy*, Vol. 32, pp. 1121-1140

Salter, R. B.; Hamilton, H. W.; Wedge, J. H.; Tile, M.; Torode, I. P.; O' Driscoll, S. W.; Murnaghan, J. J. & Saringer, J. H. (1984). Clinical application of basic research on continuous passive motion for disorders and injuries of synovial joints: A preliminary report of a feasibility study. *Journal of Orthopaedic Researche*, Vol. 1, No. 3, pp. 325-342

Sasaki, T.; Kawashima, T. & Aoyama, H.; Ifukube, T. & Ogawa, T. (1986). Development of an actuator by using metal hydride. *Journal of the Robotics Society of Japan*, Vol. 4, No. 2, pp. 119-122

Sato, M.; Ino, S.; Shimizu, S.; Ifukube, T.; Wakisaka, Y. & Izumi, T. (1996). Development of a compliance variable metal hydride (MH) actuator system for a robotic mobility aid for disabled persons. *Transactions of the Japan Society of Mechanical Engineers*, Vol. 62, No. 597, pp. 1912-1919

Sato, M.; Ino, S.; Yoshida, N.; Izumi, T. & Ifukube, T. (2001). Portable pneumatic actuator system using MH alloys, employed as an assistive device. *Journal of Robotics and Mechatronics*, Vol. 19, No. 6, pp. 612-618

Schlapbach, L. & Züttel, A. (2001). Hydrogen-storage materials for mobile applications. *Nature*, Vol. 414, pp. 353-358

Schrenk, W. J. & Alfrey Jr., T. (1968). Some physical properties of multilayered films. *Polymer Engineering and Science*, Vol. 9, No. 6, pp. 393-399

Tamura, T. (2006). A Smart House for Emergencies in the Elderly, In: *Smart homes and beyond*, Nugent, C. & Augusto, J. C. (Eds.), pp. 7-12, IOS Press, ISBN: 978-1-58603-623-2, Amsterdam

Tsuruga, T.; Ino, S.; Ifukube, T.; Sato, M.; Tanaka, T.; Izumi, T. & Muro, M. (2001). A basic study for a robotic transfer aid system based on human motion analysis. *Advanced Robotics*, Vol. 14, No. 7, pp. 579-595

Van Mal, H. H.; Buschow, K. H. J. & Miedema, A. R. (1974). Hydrogen absorption in LaNi5 and related compounds: experimental observations and their explanation. *Journal of Less-Common Metals*, Vol. 35, No. 1, pp. 65-76

Wakisaka, Y.; Muro, M.; Kabutomori, T.; Takeda, H.; Shimiz, S.; Ino, S. & T. Ifukube (1997). Application of hydrogen absorbing alloys to medical and rehabilitation equipment. *IEEE Transactions on Rehabilitation Engineering*, Vol. 5, No. 2, pp. 148-157

Wiswall, R. H. & Reilily, J. J. (1974). Hydrogen storage in metal hydrides. *Science*, Vol. 186, No. 4170, p. 1558

28

Methods for Characterization of Physiotherapy Ultrasonic Transducers

Mario-Ibrahín Gutiérrez, Arturo Vera and Lorenzo Leija
Electrical Engineering Department, Bioelectronics Section, CINVESTAV-IPN
Mexico City, Mexico

1. Introduction

Ultrasound (US) is an energy composed of cyclic acoustic pressures with a frequency higher than that of the upper limit of human hearing. This energy is an option to treat many diseases, from healing muscular inflammation to ablating malignant tumors. Ultrasound is an emission coming from a transducer which is chosen depending on the application. There are two main therapeutic applications of the ultrasound in medicine: low intensity ultrasound which uses unfocused transducers with acoustic intensities lower than 3 W/cm^2; and HIFU (High Intensity Focused Ultrasound) which uses focused transducers with acoustic intensities higher than 100 W/cm^2. Each application makes use of different kinds of transducers hence some standards have been established in order to characterize the equipment in accordance with the specific use. For example, in order to characterize a physiotherapy transducer (low intensity ultrasound), it is needed to determine and to validate the Effective Radiating Area (*ERA*), the Beam Non-uniformity Ratio (*BNR*) and the ultrasonic power (related to the effective acoustic intensity). The International Electrotechnical Commission (IEC) and the United States Food and Drug Administration (FDA) have established the methodology to measure all of these parameters.

A comparison of three techniques for characterization a physiotherapy ultrasonic transducer by the determination of two of the mentioned parameters, *ERA* and *BNR,* is presented in this chapter. The ultrasonic power can be measured by using a radiation force balance — a simple and accurate method that is not mentioned here because of the objective of this chapter. The techniques are based on measurements of the acoustic field which are postprocessed in order to get the characteristic parameters of the ultrasonic transducer. This chapter also includes a brief abstract of other techniques that have been used for the same objective. These techniques were not included in the comparison because of their expensiveness and the technological requirements to be implemented. The use of each technique described here depends on the necessities of the application.

2. Ultrasound in Medicine

Ultrasound has been used in medicine for many years. A wide variety of applications have been developed in order to help in diagnosis or even to treat some diseases, and all of them differ in the frequency, the kind of transducer (and therefore the kind of beam), and the acoustic intensities, among other factors. Some medical ultrasound applications that can be mentioned here are the ultrasonic imaging, the flow measurements (Doppler and Transit Time), tissue healing, bone regeneration and cancer therapy (Paliwal & Mitragotri, 2008; ter Haar, 1999; ter Haar, 2007). In this chapter, we will talk about the techniques for characterizing ultrasonic transducers used in the treatment of muscular injuries; however, general information about ultrasound in therapy is needed in order to better understand the specific necessities.

2.1 Ultrasound in Therapy

Therapeutic ultrasound is the use of ultrasonic energy in order to produce changes in tissues through its mechanical, chemical and thermal effects. Depending on the effects in the tissues and the area of application, the ultrasound therapy can have different names. In general, therapeutic ultrasound can be separated in two categories: "low" intensity ultrasound (0.125-3 W/cm^2) and "high" intensity ultrasound (more than 5 W/cm^2) (ter Haar, 1999; ter Haar, 2007). The lower intensities are used when the treatment is expected to propitiate the regeneration of tissues caused by physiological changes. In contrast, higher intensities are used when ultrasound has to produce a complete change in tissue by means of overheating (hyperthermia) or cell killing (ablation) (Feril & Kondo, 2004).

There are two main areas where the last classification is clear: physiotherapy (low intensities) and oncology (high intensities). The therapy in both areas has been called therapeutic ultrasound, but the techniques have significant differences both in the devices as in the results. In general, the effects produced by ultrasound in tissues can be divided in two types:

- *Thermal effects*, which are produced basically because of the absorption of the energy by large protein molecules commonly present in collagenous tissues. Some of these effects are the increase in blood flow, the increase in tissue extensibility, the reduction of joint stiffness, pain release, etc. (Speed, 2001).
- *Nonthermal effects*, which are produced when the therapy is delivered in a pulsed way avoiding the media heating. The first nonthermal effect reported is the "micro-massage" (ter Haar, 1999) whose effects have not been measured yet. Acoustic streaming is another effect that could have important changes in the tissues. Streaming may modify the environment and organelle distribution inside the cells, this in turn can change the concentration gradients near the membrane and therefore it modifies the diffusion of ions and molecules across it (Johns, 2002). These effects are responsible for the stimulation of the fibroblast activity, the tissue regeneration and the bone healing (Johns, 2002; Speed, 2001).

2.1.1 Oncology

Oncologic ultrasound is the therapy that uses thermal effects of ultrasound in order to ablate malignant tumors. This therapy is applied either alone or in combination with radiotherapy or chemotherapy because it has been demonstrated that the effects of these therapies are potentialized when the tumor is ultrasonically heated (Field & Bleehen, 1979). The treatment consists in heating the tumor at temperatures above 42°C, which is the maximum temperature resistance of malignant cells, but avoiding overheating healthy cells around it. Heating is applied approximately for 60 min; during this time, the temperature in the tumor must be between 42-45°C and the temperature of the healthy tissue must be lower than 41.8°C (ter Haar & Hand, 1981).

The main problem of this therapy is the accurate control of temperature in tissues because there are no appropriate methods to measure the temperature in a continuous way and in all the heated volume without damaging tissues. This is the principal reason of why this therapy has not been widely used. Methods that use ultrasound to measure the temperature non-invasively inside a tissue are being developed, but problems with the non-homogeneity of tissues and natural scatters have not been eliminated (Arthur et al., 2003; Arthur et al., 2005; Maass-Moreno & Damianou, 1996; Pernot et al., 2004; Singh et al., 1990). Thermometry by using X-rays, or MRI is another option, but these techniques are expensive (De Poorter et al., 1995; Fallone et al., 1982). It has been proposed that this problem could be avoided by heating the tissues at higher temperatures (about 60°C) so fast that the normal perfusion does not have a significant effect (ter Haar, 1999).

2.1.2 Physiotherapy

The use of ultrasound to treat muscular damage, heal bones, reduce pain, etc. has been called physiotherapy ultrasound. This therapy uses ultrasound in order to induce changes in muscular and skeletal tissues through thermal and mechanical effects. These effects can be changes in the cell permeability (Hensley & Muthuswamy, 2002) or even cellular death when the ultrasonic energy is not controlled correctly (Feril & Kondo, 2004). The desired effect is a light elevation of the temperature into the treated tissue without provoking ablation (cell killing); this phenomenon is called diathermy. This therapy is commonly confused with hyperthermia, but the main difference is that the latter is an elevation of temperature with the objective of producing changes in tissues immediately by means of the overheating. In contrast, diathermy is the phenomenon of heating a tissue in order to induce physiological changes, e.g., an increase of the blood flow rate, activation of the immunological system, changes in the cell chemical interchange among cells and the extracellular media, etc.

The therapy consists in using a transducer to produce ultrasonic waves which are directed to the treated tissue. The transducer is connected to an RF generator that produces a senoidal signal (or approximately senoidal) which has high amplitude and high frequency. The transducer acoustic impedance is relatively small compared to the acoustic impedance of the air. Should the ultrasonic energy travel from the transducer to the air, only a little part would go out and the most significant part would go backwards. This reflected energy, called reflected wave, could damage the transducer and even the RF generator. During the therapy, when the transducer is dry, there is a thin layer of air between the transducer face and the skin; this layer can produce reflected waves. Therefore, in order to avoid this problem, media with acoustic impedances between the transducer and the skin are used to improve the contact between them. The ultrasonic waves are directed to the tissues by means of either using acoustic gel between the transducer and the skin or submerging the desired part of the body in degasified water and applying the energy with the transducer submerged too. Both ways are efficient in getting a correct coupling.

3. Physiotherapy Ultrasonic Transducers

Ultrasonic transducer technology has been improved in the last 50 years. The first transducers were constructed using piezoelectric crystals as ultrasound generator elements (Christensen, 1988). Later on, piezoelectric ceramics (polarized artificially in order to produce the piezoelectric effect) were discovered and developed which allowed designers construct different configurations with many shapes, sizes, frequencies, and at higher efficiencies. New design techniques, and new materials with better properties than their predecessors have contributed to improve the piezoelectric elements (Papadakis, 1999).

The construction of a US transducer is carried out in accordance with its application. The kind of material chosen for the piezoelectric element depends on the acoustic intensity at which the device will be used. However, there is another important parameter to consider: the bandwidth. Some transducers are designed to work in a range of frequencies that allow them to keep a good amplitude either receiving US (like the hydrophones) or both emitting and receiving. Others are good just for emitting ultrasound at a specific frequency. This new consideration allows for another way of transducer classification: wideband and narrowband transducers.

Physiotherapy ultrasonic devices use narrowband transducers because they require high efficiency in the energy conversion. This kind of transducers must work in the resonance frequency to make use of their high efficiency characteristics. When continuous emission occurs through a low efficiency transducer, a great part of the energy is transformed into heat in the transducer and only a little part of the energy is emitted to the media as ultrasound. This fact is not important in some applications, but in a physiotherapeutic treatment, the transducer is in contact with the patient's skin and overheating is an undesired effect. Characterization is an excellent tool to know if a transducer is working properly at nominal values. The incorrect transducer characterization could lead to the lack of results of the treatment or even provoke some injuries to the patient. Some defects in the emission efficiency could be due to a decoupling between the generator and the transducer, so that frequency characterization should be carried out in order to know this efficiency. In this chapter, only the acoustic characterization of a physiotherapy ultrasonic transducer working at its resonant frequency of 1 MHz is shown.

3.1 Transducer Acoustic Field

When a source of ultrasound emits energy, the ultrasonic waves produced are propagated around all directions of the source. The distribution of this mechanical energy is called acoustic field. The shape of the acoustic field has a distribution of acoustic pressures in accordance with the shape of the emitter. In physiotherapy transducers, the acoustic field shape is, theoretically, cylindrical because of the proportions of the piezoelectric element, i.e., the diameter is more than ten times the wave length (Águila, 1994). The first part of the transducer acoustic field (when the last condition is true) is called near field or Fresnel zone, and the next part is called far field or Fraunhofer zone. The Fresnel zone is composed of symmetrical rings of maximum and minimum pressures along the central edge which cause a non uniformed distribution of the acoustical energy. The Fraunhofer zone is divergent and the acoustic intensity follows the inverse-square law (Seegenschmiedt, 1995):

$$I_x \approx \frac{1}{x_2}$$

(1)

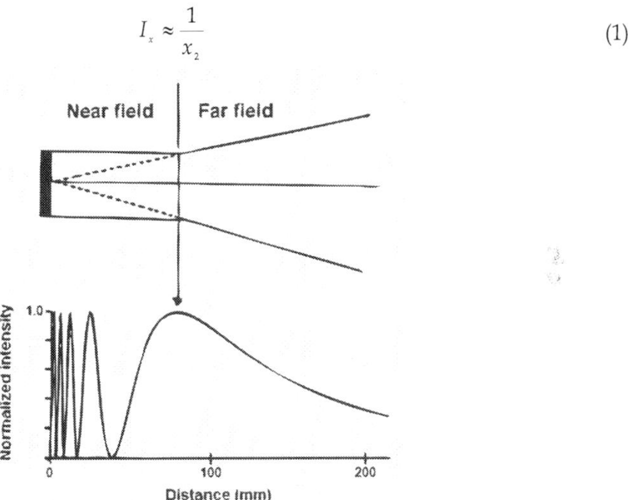

Fig. 1. *Above*, shape of the acoustic field generated by a physiotherapy ultrasonic transducer (D>10λ). *Below*, normalized acoustic intensity versus distance from the transducer (Seegenschmiedt, 1995)

The near field length ($L_{near\,field}$) is directly dependent on the diameter D and inversely proportional to the wave length (Eq. 2). The physiotherapy ultrasonic transducers have diameters bigger than the wave length and therefore they have a long near field. Because of this, when a physical therapy is being carried out, the therapeutic heating is produced inside the near field where the acoustic pressures are the result of a sum of the ones produced at different points in the piezoelectric plate. The near field of the transducer is the most important part to characterize but it is the part where the majority of the non-linearities occur.

$$L_{near\,field} = \frac{D^2}{4\lambda}$$

(2)

The divergence angle in the Fraunhofer zone is also dependent on the diameter and the wave length, and it can be calculated with Eq. 3 as follows

$$\sin \theta = 1.22 \frac{\lambda}{D}$$

(3)

3.2 Transducer Characterization

When ultrasound is used to treat a muscular problem or to heal a fractured bone, it is applied following a protocol for the specific disease. Researchers have developed many protocols to treat some diseases by using different parameters of the ultrasonic device. These parameters differ in the output intensities, time of treatment, duty cycle, and frequency, and it has been considered that all values are correct (Speed, 2001). However, there are reports about calibrating medical ultrasonic devices for therapy in which it has been found that most of them are not working within nominal values (Pye & Milford, 1994).

When a therapist uses a protocol to treat a disease and the gotten results are not sufficient, he/she is going to modify the intensities in accordance with his/her experience. This behavior adds subjectivities to a treatment that nowadays is already subjective. Results dose-response have been gotten (Lu et al., 2008; Nacitarhan et al., 2005; ter Haar, 2007) but there is not a guideline to follow in order to determine the best dose (Watson, 2008). Therapists must calculate the doses base on the results reported in some papers and they must know the characteristics of the radiation produced in order to promote the desired thermal and nonthermal effects. However, the necessity of characterization is still a problem; therefore, new techniques have been developed in order to reduce the time required to make measurements and to reduce the costs.

3.3 Characterization Parameters

There are many techniques for characterizing the emission of an ultrasonic transducer in order to get the parameters of interest. Each technique measures only one magnitude of the ultrasonic beam, but with this result and applying some mathematical calculations it is possible to obtain the others. The transducer acoustic field is composed by a superposition of many waves coming from different parts of the transducer. When the design of the piezoelectric element of the transducer was not right, the generated waves have an undesirable behavior. The parameters of interest of the transducer emission have been developed in order to determine if the transducer has this adverse performance. These parameters are described in the following part of this chapter.

3.3.1 Effective Radiating Area (*ERA*)

There have been many definitions for this parameter. One of these is given by the FDA, which defines the ERA_{FDA} as the area consisting of all points of the effective radiating surface (all points within 5 mm from the applicator face) at which the intensity is 5 percent or more of the maximum intensity at the effective radiating surface, expressed in square centimeters (FDA, 2008). Recently, a new way of measuring and of defining (Hekkenberg, 1998) *ERA* which is written in the IEC standards (ABNT, 1998; IEC, 1991) was developed. This new method consists in measuring and in registering the acoustic intensities (or the proportion in mV, mPa, etc.) in four planes parallel to the transducer face at four distances along the propagation edge z. For each measured plane, the beam cross-sectional area (A_{BCS}) is calculated. This area is defined as the minimum area in a specified plane perpendicular to the "beam alignment axis" which contains 75% of the spatial integral of the "total mean square acoustic pressure" pms_t given by:

$$pms_t = \sum_{i=1}^{N} p_i^2 \tag{4}$$

where p_i is the acoustic pressure in the ith point and N is the total number of points in the scan. After that, it is considered that the near field of the beam is linearly related to z, and hence the A_{ER} (same meaning than ERA_{FDA}, Effective Radiating Area) is calculated with a relation of the extrapolation of the calculated A_{BCS}'s at $z = 0$. The A_{ER} can be calculated with Eq. 5.

$$A_{ER} = F_{AC} A_{BCS} \tag{5}$$

and

$$F_{AC} = 2.58 - 0.0305 ka \qquad \text{for } ka \leq 40 \tag{6}$$

$$F_{AC} = 1.354 \qquad \text{for } ka > 40 \tag{7}$$

where a is the effective radio of the transducer and k is the circular wave number in cm^{-1}. In this chapter, we used the ERA_{FDA} definition. The FDA definition gives large uncertainties (more than 20%) if it is compared to the IEC definition (less than 10%). Our calculation of ERA_{FDA} cannot be extrapolated to the A_{ER} of the IEC standards because the measurements and calculations are completely different (Hekkenberg, 1998; Johns et al., 2007).

For characterizing the ultrasonic emission in solid media, there is another definition which considers the Specific Absorption Rate (SAR) given by Eq. 8. The ESHO protocols define the ERA of an applicator as the 50% SAR contour measured at a depth of 10 mm from the surface of a plane homogeneous phantom (Hand et al., 1989). This definition is needed when it is not possible to know the acoustic intensities due to the characterization technique used (Hand et al., 1989).

The SAR can be calculated with:

$$SAR = C \frac{\Delta T}{\Delta t} \approx \frac{2\mu_a I}{\rho_0} \tag{8}$$

where C is the heat capacity (J/kg·°C), ΔT is the change of the temperature (°C), Δt is the change of the time (s), μ_a is the attenuation coefficient (dB/m), I is the acoustic intensity (W/m²), and ρ_0 is the medium density (kg/m³).

3.3.2 Beam Non-uniformity Ratio (*BNR*)

This is the relation between the square of the maximum acoustic pressure (p_{max}) and the spatial mean square of the acoustic pressure (pms_t), where the spatial media is taken on the effective radiating area (ABNT, 1998; FDA, 2008; Hekkenberg, 1998). Eq. 9 indicates the process to calculate this parameter (ABNT, 1998)

$$BNR = \frac{p_{max}^2 \cdot ERA}{pms_t \cdot a_0} \tag{9}$$

where a_0 is the area per the global raster. If the transducer is for physiotherapy, BNR must be in the range of 1:6 because of the patient's security (Hekkenberg, 1998). When the value is close to 1, the transducer is safer than the case when the BNR is close to 6.

3.3.3 Penetration Depth (P_D)

It depends on the properties of the medium where the ultrasound is passing through. In this chapter, it is used to calculate the t_{max} in the IR thermography (Eq. 12), but it can also be used to determine whether the treatment has an adequate depth. By definition, the penetration depth is the distance from the transducer where the Specific Absorption Rate (SAR) magnitude is 50% of the maximum magnitude at the ERA (Hand et al., 1989).

4. Characterization Techniques

The objective of characterizing the devices is to prevent patients' injuries because of either non-uniformities of the beam, commonly called hot-spots, or an effective radiating area different to the reported one, which modifies the total power emitted. Manufacturers deliver the devices with measurements of their characteristic parameters but with high tolerance in the measurements. For example, they tell us that the value of the ERA is about 10 cm² but with a tolerance of ±20%, which means that ERA could be between 8 cm² to 12 cm²; the rest of the reported parameters have this kind of tolerance. Needless is to say that the sum of these uncertainties can result in an ineffective treatment or in injury to patients.

There are different transducer characterization techniques that can deliver accurate results. Most of these techniques were designed in order to improve a specific characteristic of the measurement. Some techniques are faster or cheaper than others, but they are not so accurate; there are some which are more accurate but they are too expensive or slow; with some of them it is possible to measure some magnitudes that with others is not possible, and vice versa. In this chapter, three techniques: C-scan with hydrophone, IR thermography, and Thermochromic Liquid Crystals (TLC) are going to be compared. A brief review of other techniques that could help in the characterization will also be included in order to have a better picture of the different solutions to this task.

4.1 C-scan

This technique consists in moving a small microprobe into the ultrasonic beam in order to measure the acoustic pressure levels punctually (Papadakis, 1999). The measurements are carried out into a tank filled with degasified water where all the elements (transducer and sensor) are immersed. The microprobe dimensions depend on the magnitude of interest, i.e., the C-scan technique can be used to measure the acoustic pressures instantly or the absorbed energy during a known interval of time. It is required that the sensor be as small as possible to get a good resolution. Also, the system for positioning the sensor must allow very small steps to prevent affecting the overall resolution. According to the literature, the sensors that have been used with this purpose are the hydrophones, the thermistors or the thermocouples (Marangopoulos et al., 1995), and even a reflecting ball as it will be explained later (Mansour, 1979).

The setup for carrying out the measurements has many common components among the variants mentioned. In general, the C-scan technique uses a tank, a base to fix the transducer, a system for positioning the sensor, an oscilloscope, an electronic card to excite the transducer, and the computer to register and process data. The tank must be made using ultrasonic absorbent material in order to avoid (or reduce) wave reflections (Selfridge, 1985). The water where the measurements are carried out must be degasified so the bubbles caused by the acoustic vibrations are eliminated thus avoiding the error in the results because of cavitation. A base with adjustable grips is required for fixing and centering the transducer. The sensor is fixed on the positioner XYZ which will move it transversally along the ultrasonic beam.

The setup of the experiment has some initial steps. At first, the transducer is fixed, and then a sequence of measurements aimed at finding the center is carried out. The sequence is composed by sweeps in each axis of the transducer transversal section in order to find the maximum acoustic pressure level which corresponds to the center of the piezoelectric plate. This procedure is repeated at different distances from the transducer until this one is completely centered which is determined when the movement of the sensor along the direction of the beam propagation occurred without losing the center at each distance (Vera et al., 2007). The measurements are started after the installation and the centering, and they are carried out in accordance with the problem necessities: characterization, data processing, modeling, etc. A system for 3D positioning is used in this technique.

4.1.1 Using a point reflector

This technique uses the same transducer to emit and receive the ultrasonic beam (Mansour, 1979); it works with the concept of pulse-echo. We have to know, initially, the sensitivity to ultrasound of the transducer to characterize at each point of the area of the transducer front face. This is because the ultrasound will arrive at the transducer and the energy will be changed to an electrical signal; the relation between the arriving ultrasonic energy and the electric signal generated is needed. The C-scan with point reflector, also called ball target (Papadakis, 1999), consists in positioning a small ball into the acoustic field by means of a positioner XYZ which will move the ball transversally along the beam. Although the transducer emits a cylindrical beam with a relatively large transversal section (approximately equals to ERA), the measured signal corresponds only to a small area just in the direction of the ball target (Fig. 2).

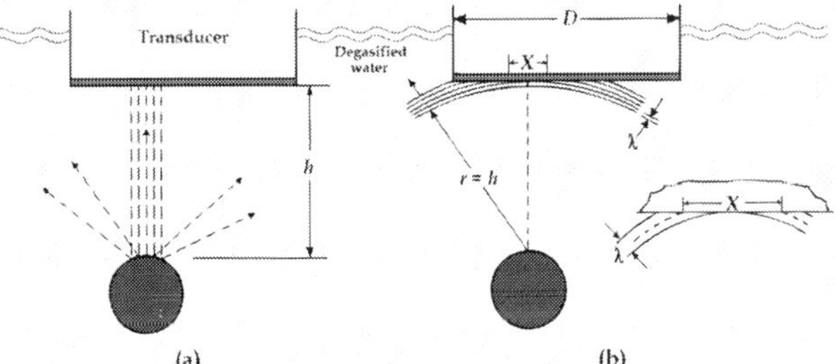

Fig. 2. C-scan with ball reflector. (a) The waves out of the pole of the ball go out of the transducer. (b) A small area above the ball performs the sampling. Destructive interference prevents the sampling of the other waves (Papadakis, 1999)

The magnitude measured represents the product of the acoustic intensity arriving at the transducer and the sensitivity of the small area above the ball of the transducer (X in Fig. 2b). When the plane wave returns to the transducer after the reflection, it is converted into a spherical wave. The measurement is taken only in the transducer area nearest to the ball because the wave arrives first at this part. Other wave segments are lost due to the cone-like reflection with a large angle (Fig. 2a). Even if some wave segments reach the transducer, waves beyond a specific radius are lost because of destructive interference (Papadakis, 1999). The wave measured, converted into voltage, is the result of the product of the acoustic pressure and the sensitivity at the point where the wave reaches the transducer. This characteristic could result in a problem because there is another unknown parameter that can influence the measurement.

4.1.2 Using a hydrophone

The most accurate technique until now, in accordance with IEC standards (Hekkenberg, 1998; IEC, 1991), is the C-scan with hydrophone, which uses a hydrophone as the sensor element of the C-scan system. This technique consists in moving a hydrophone inside the acoustic field while it registers the acoustic pressure at each point. This is a through-transmission technique which means that the ultrasonic transducer to characterize emits the energy and the hydrophone measures the signal, and no-reflection is considered. It is more acceptable to use this element as the sensor because it can register a time-dependent signal that can be used to get most of the required parameters not only used for characterization, but also for other applications. The utilization of a sensor for measuring directly the acoustic pressures, independently of the element to be characterized, eliminates unknown variables as the sensitivities required for the C-scan with ball reflector. The hydrophone sensitivity can be determined with a calibration, and the transducer gain per unit of area (if it would be required) could be determined by using the C-scan with a calibrated hydrophone.

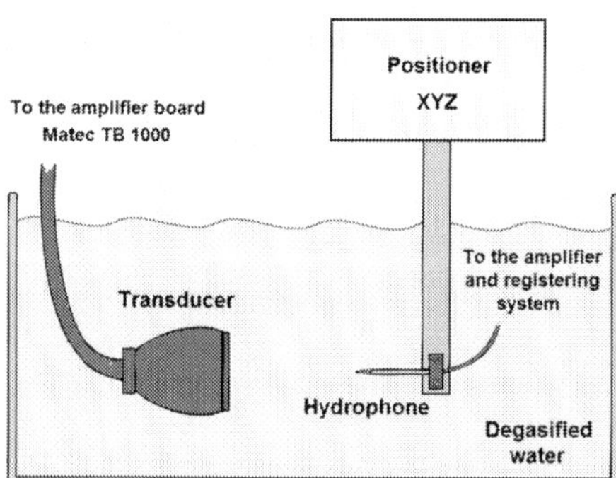

Fig. 3. Setup of C-scan with hydrophone. A more detailed diagram is shown in Fig. 10

The transducer is excited with a pulsed sinusoidal signal using either the ultrasonic equipment or a special amplifier board that produces a standard signal. The excitation signal is not continuous in order to allow the ultrasound wave to die before emitting another signal, which is required to avoid the addition of reflected waves. Therefore, a sinusoidal signal modulated by a square short pulse is used. Some parameters are required to know before applying the excitation:

Output Voltage: it is the voltage that excites the US transducer. It must be adjusted in accordance with the desired ultrasonic output power (acoustic intensity) at which the transducer is going to be characterized.

Pulse width: it is the length of the electrical square pulse that modulates the sinusoidal signal in order to excite the transducer. For example, inside an excitation with pulse width of 10 µs, there are 10 cycles of a sinusoidal signal of 1 MHz (period of 1 µs).

Repetition rate: it is the repetition period of the excitation pulses. For example, an excitation sinusoidal signal of 1 MHz modulated with a square signal of pulse width of 10 µs has a repetition rate of 13 ms because the pulse is repeated (or initiated) each 13 ms. It could be transformed into a repetition frequency which is, in this case, of $1/13e^{-3}$ Hz.

4.1.3 Using a temperature sensor

The increment of temperature in an ultrasonically irradiated medium is directly related to the acoustic intensity in the medium for a unit of time. Considering this, it is possible to use a temperature sensor as the element that registers the signal inside the acoustic field provided that the acoustic intensity is quite elevated to produce a thermal change in the medium. However, the sensor by itself is not sufficient since it must be covered by an ultrasonic absorber material which is going to be heated (Marangopoulos et al., 1995). Therefore, the temperature measured by the sensor is related to the acoustic intensity, the radiation time, and the material parameters by Eq. 10; the material parameters are the ones of the material that covers the sensor. This modality of C-scan has an overall resolution given by the size of the temperature sensor covered by the absorber material.

In contrast to the C-scans which use the above described sensors, this technique measures the energy applied during a period of time. This feature gives a relation of the measured magnitude to the applied signal which is equal to the integral of effective acoustic intensities in the media with respect to the time. The sensor cover absorbs each wave and increases its temperature as it is indicated in Eq. 10. The temperature (T) generated by the absorption of the acoustic energy for a specific time (t) is given by:

$$T = \int \frac{2\alpha I_x}{\rho C} dt \tag{10}$$

where α is the absorption coefficient of the ultrasonic energy in the medium, I_x is the acoustic intensity at a depth of x (W/cm²), ρ is the medium density (kg/m³) and C is the heat capacity of the medium (J·kg⁻¹·K⁻¹).

4.2 Schlieren technique

This technique applies the Schlieren effect, discovered by Robert Hook (Rienitz, 1975). It uses a two candle system to visualize the ultrasonic beam; the first explanation of the phenomenon in ultrasonic waves was made by Raman-Nath in 1935 (Johns et al., 2007).

Schlieren techniques make density gradients in transparent media visible based on the deflection of light that passes through it. This characterization technique consists in sending a beam of light normal to the ultrasonic beam. When the longitudinal ultrasonic beam travels through a medium, the medium local densities are changed because of the compressions and rarefactions of the beam. These changes in density modify the optical index. Hence, the light passing through the ultrasonic beam changes the direction in accordance with the acoustic intensities (Hanafy & Zanelli, 1991).

The system is composed by a source of light (emitter) which is normally a laser or an arc lamp which produces high intensity uniform light. The light has to be collimated by using a system of lenses as shown in Fig. 4. The refracted light is sensed by the camera at the other side of the emitter. The acoustic beam is covered mostly by the light beam, which allows relating the collected light intensity and the acoustic radiation pressure (Hanafy & Zanelli, 1991). The light is strobed at a fixed delay after emitting the ultrasound pulses. This does not affect the image formation at the video camera because the image appears to be static, but this permits to avoid taking the image of the ultrasound reflected wave. The ultrasound absorber does not avoid reflections; it just reduces them significantly.

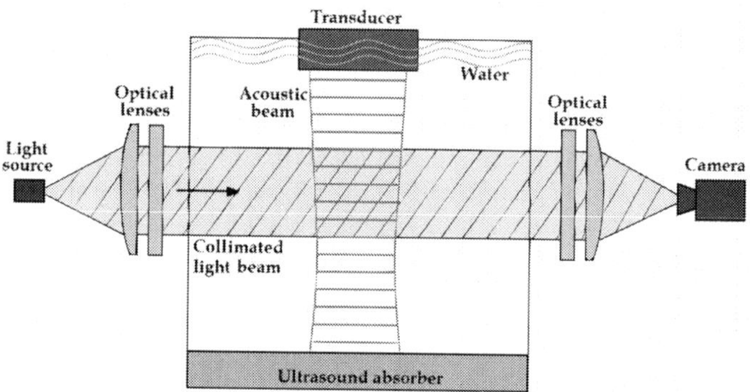

Fig. 4. Schlieren system

Optical intensity at each pixel is proportional to the acoustic intensity integrated along the line where the light passed through. This statement is true provided that

1. the acoustic wave fronts are quasi-planar and normal to the light beam, and
2. the acoustic intensity is low enough to avoid acousto-optic nonlinearities.

Both conditions are satisfied if some considerations are taken. Condition 1 is satisfied if the transducer is aligned by measuring the acoustic intensities at each point of the transversal section. Condition 2 is satisfied by adjusting the acoustic intensity in order to be sure that the changes are within 5% of linearity, which is commonly true at low acoustic intensities, less than 0.2 W/cm^2. When the system does not satisfy these conditions, the optic intensity is not linearly proportional to the acoustic intensity; hence, Schlieren system cannot be used quantitatively.

This technique is very useful because it does not affect the acoustic emission and it permits to have the acoustic beam without the previous knowledge of the shape. However, the system is expensive and it requires some critical adjustments: lense alignment, high intensity light, transparent propagation media, ultrasound low intensities, high quality optics, etc. Moreover, it is not possible to get a punctual acoustic intensity, but an acoustic intensity integrated along the optical path. Researches continue in order to find a way to eliminate these disadvantages, e.g., reducing the cost of the lamp for emitting high intensity light (Gunarathne & Szilard, 1983).

4.3 Sarvazyan technique

This method was proposed by Sarvazyan et al. in 1985. It is a simple and rapid method that consists in mapping the ultrasound fields using a white paper and an aqueous solution of methylene blue dye. The paper is an Astralux 200 µm card (Star Paper Company, Blackburn, Lancashire) that has demonstrated being suitable in characterizing the ultrasound emission at frequencies around 1 MHz. The field is directed at a sheet of paper through the blue solution during 1 minute. After this exposition time, there is a pattern of dye formed in the paper which is related to the intensity distribution of ultrasound (Watmough et al., 1990). The patterns obtained along the ultrasound beam are processed in order to get the acoustic intensities at each point in the card.

The dye diffusion is because the paper has microbubbles on the surface due to the microscopic irregularities. The size of the microbubbles depends on the paper, and because of that, it is not possible to use any kind of paper. Astralux card has microscopic holes of 3 µm of diameter which are resonant at frequencies around 1 MHz. Resonant gas bubbles are related to microstreaming of the liquid surrounding them, and this is the phenomenon that causes the increment of dye diffusion in high acoustic intensity areas (Shiran et al., 1990; Watmough et al., 1990). The resolution technique depends on the distance between the gas bubbles.

This technique has some disadvantages, e. g. the gas bubbles cause ultrasound reflections to the transducer; this can affect the radiation pattern and consequently the characterization results. Because of gas bubbles, Astralux paper is not ultrasound "transparent" and stationary waves could be formed that could even cause damages to the ultrasonic transducer. Also, it is not a reversible technique, hence the paper must be changed before the next measurement and this can result in errors because of differences in the position of the papers.

4.4 Holography with Flexible Pellicle

This technique was proposed by (Mezrich et al., 1975) to display the ultrasonic waves by using a flexible pellicle and the Michelson interferometer. The pellicle is located into the ultrasound field perpendicularly to the ultrasound propagation in order to have movement in the pellicle proportional to the acoustic intensities. As pellicle (M_2) moves, the relative phase between M_1 and M_2 varies and produces intensity changes at photodiode D. The laser beam is moved in order to scan the displacement at every point of the pellicle. The interferometer is shown in Fig. 5, and in this system, the pellicle thickness is 6 µm.

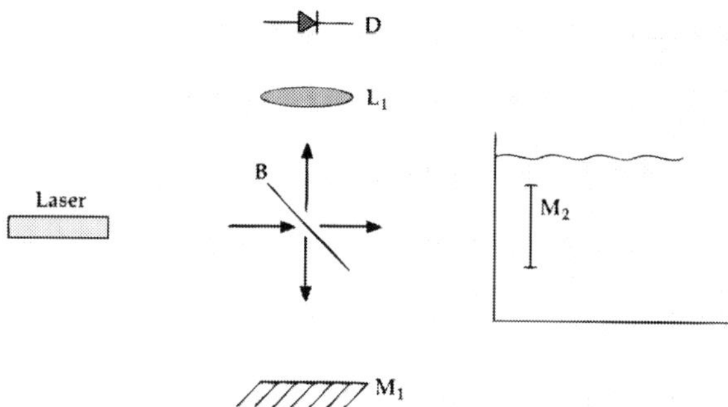

Fig. 5. Michelson interferometer used by (Mezrich et al., 1976) to detect the acoustic displacement amplitude

4.5 Optical Computerized Tomography

This technique uses a Michelson interferometer in order to visualize the ultrasonic beam based on the modified index of refraction gradient caused by the ultrasound pressures. It is similar to the Schlieren technique but it uses the Michelson interferometer to visualize the transducer beam. The light passes through the ultrasound beam and it is compared to the reference light in order to determine the optical intensity that has the information about the acoustic intensity. This method compares the light phase as well as the light intensity of each beam. The light is detected by an avalanche photodiode and the data are postprocessed in order to reconstruct the beam (Obuchi et al., 2006).

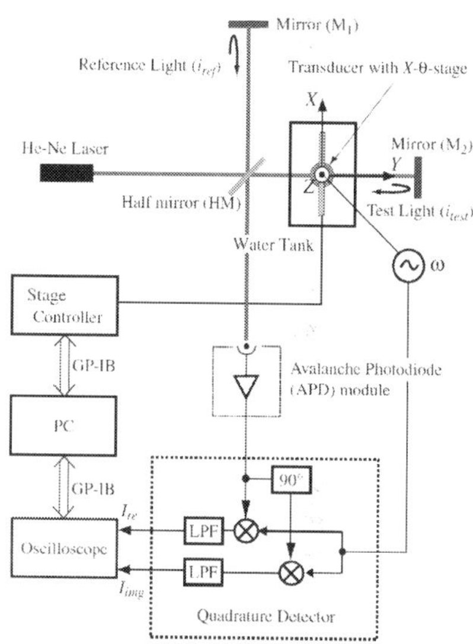

Fig. 6. Schematic diagram and experimental setup for the system proposed by (Obuchi et al., 2006)

The setup of the system for visualization of the ultrasonic beam designed by (Obuchi et al., 2006) is shown in Fig. 6. The light beam is divided in two: the reference light and the test light. When both beams are reflected by their respective mirror, they go to the avalanche photodiode which generates a signal with all the information. The signal is processed by a quadrature detector considering the driven frequency of the ultrasound transducer, ω. The optical intensity resulted is I_{out} which is given by

$$I_{out} = I_{test} + I_{ref} + 2\sqrt{I_{test}I_{ref}}\,\cos\phi(x,z,t) \tag{11}$$

where I_{test} is the test light intensity, I_{ref} is the reference light intensity and ϕ is the phase difference between these lights.

4.6 Thermography in liquids and solids

As it was described before, the increment of temperature is directly related to the acoustic intensities in a specific medium (Eq. 10). It is possible to get the characteristic parameters by measuring this temperature directly in the heating media. Next, three techniques of temperature measurement that can be used in characterization of ultrasound transducers are described.

4.6.1 Invasive Thermography

This technique consists in measuring the temperature in the irradiated solid medium (phantom) using a temperature sensor inserted in it. The sensor must not be affected by the ultrasonic radiation and it must be as small as possible in order to have a punctual measurement. The data are registered in a matrix containing all the information about the measurements and the place where they were taken with respect to the transducer. Measurements are carried out upwards using as many sensors as possible because the values are going to be processed in order to get the parameters of study. The measurement is carried out in this direction because the phantom is destroyed when the sensor is inserted; if measurements are performed in the opposite direction, this destruction can cause problems with the ultrasonic propagation. When the measurements are made starting at the bottom of the phantom, we can be sure that the propagation is correct from the transducer to the inserted sensor, and that the destroyed part is left behind. Postprocessing is required to relate the measurements to the characteristic parameters or to reconstruct the thermal field to calculate the penetration depth, the absorption (SAR), etc.

Even though this technique has some interesting advantages, the disadvantages could be even more important. This technique requires little specialized equipment and relatively simple postprocessing, and its temperature sensors (the thermocouples or the thermistors) are not affected by ultrasound. However, whichever sensor is inserted into the media will produce a hot-spot caused because the media and the sensor have different acoustic impedances. This difference causes backward wave reflections and therefore the addition of the arriving and the returning waves; this can be observed as an increment of temperature in that point. Another disadvantage is the time used for the measurements. For each line, it is required to heat the phantom while the sensors are measuring, and to wait until the phantom reaches the original temperature before taking another line.

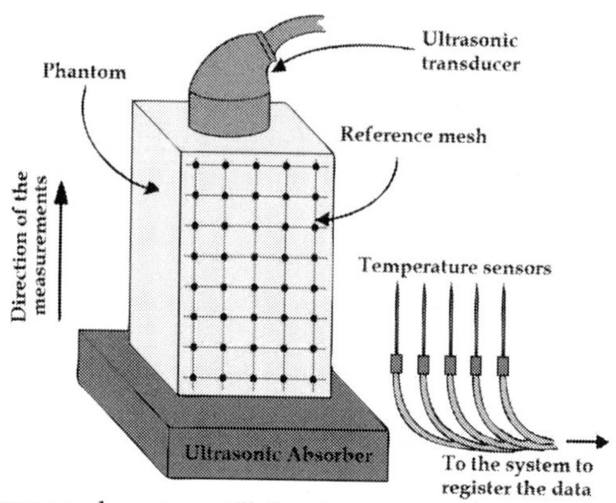

Fig. 7. Invasive Thermography setup. All the elements are fixed. The mesh is the reference for inserting the sensors. The distance between the sensors is the spatial resolution of the system

4.6.2 IR Thermography

The use of devices to capture IR images is another alternative for the characterization of the ultrasound effects (Guy, 1971). The IR radiation caused by any material depends directly on its temperature. Nowadays, there are cameras that can be used to detect the IR radiation and convert it to a thermal image related to a temperature color scale; these cameras are called IR cameras. However, for making the measurement, it is necessary to have the temperature of interest at the surface of the material. A modification of the setup proposed in 1991 for electromagnetic applicators is shown in Fig. 8 (Andreuccetti et al., 1991b). It consists in a phantom cut by the half and an IR camera that takes the picture. The phantom is heated by the US transducer during a period of time at which it is separated to make visible its internal part. The picture is taken before the complete temperature dissipation occurs. After each picture, the phantom in cooled and the transducer is moved in order to get another plane of the beam. The displacements are part of the resolution because the overall resolution is limited mainly by the IR camera and the non-homogeneities of the phantom.

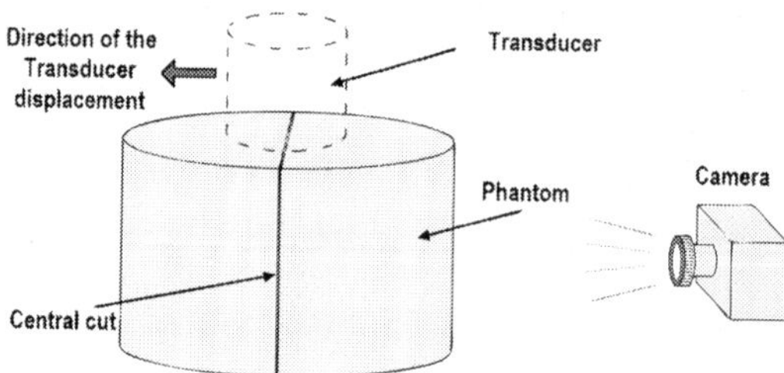

Fig. 8. IR thermography system setup. The transducer is moved after taking each picture in order to get the complete beam

Andreuccetti et al. established the maximum time to get the IR image in relation to the penetration depth; they got this empirical formula:

$$t_{max} = 13.2 P_D{}^2 \qquad (12)$$

where P_D is the penetration depth (section 3.3.3) in centimeters and t_{max} is the maximum time for taking the picture in seconds. Disadvantages of this technique are the difficulties to fix the transducer and the phantom and the difficulty in being sure that the displacement of the transducer is the desired one. Methods of registering data can solve this problem by taking some planes and rotating the transducer in order to measure another plane.

4.6.3 Thermography with Thermochromic Liquid Crystals (TLC)

This thermographic technique uses a TLC sheet to create a colored image which corresponds to the heat produced by the ultrasonic absorption in a medium. The sheets that contain TLC (sometimes called thermochromic sheets) are used as sensors and they have to be in contact with the medium heated (Gutierrez et al., 2008). The ultrasound generates heat when the media are highly absorbent; therefore, a phantom with a large absorption coefficient must be used. The technique can be applied when the characterization of the transducer emission in either liquid or solid media is required, but modifying the system setup for each situation in order to have a coherent measurement.

Thermography with TLC in solid media is made by using a setup as the one shown in Fig. 8 but by placing in the middle, where the cut is made, the TLC sheet. The heat is transmitted from the phantom to the TLC sheet which creates the thermal image. The picture is taken by using a normal camera because the image is in the visible range (Andreuccetti et al., 1991a; Andreuccetti et al., 1991b). The disadvantage of this application is that the TLC sheet has to be implemented in contact with the medium during all heating and this produces distortion of the transducer radiation pattern because of the acoustic differences between the TLC sheet and the phantom.

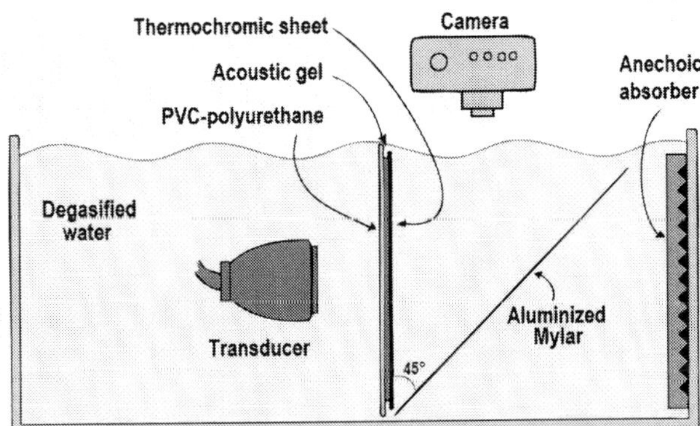

Fig. 9. Thermography with TLC setup. The color image is related to the effective acoustic intensities

The other application is in the characterization of the acoustic emission in transparent liquid media, commonly degasified water (Martin & Fernandez, 1997). In this technique, the transducer is placed inside a container as it is indicated in Fig. 9. The transducer radiates through the water in direction to the TLC sheet and the absorbing layer, which are placed perpendicular to the acoustic propagation. The ultrasound will continue beyond the layers and it will reach an absorber material at the end of the tank in order to avoid ultrasound reflections. The image is taken with a common camera through a Mylar mirror; the distributions of color obtained are related to the energy absorbed converted punctually into heat. The transducer has to be moved by a positioner along the direction of propagation in order to capture the required images along the acoustic field. Postprocessing is required in order to get the characteristic parameters or to reconstruct the complete acoustic beam.

5. Measurements

The techniques described before could be used to get characteristic parameters of an ultrasonic device. This chapter presents a comparison of the characterization results gotten with three techniques with different features: time consuming, accuracy, and kind of media where ultrasound passes through. The characterized device was a physiotherapy ultrasonic equipment Ibramed from Brazil; its principal features are shown in Table 1.

Manufacturer	Ibramed, Brazil
Model	Sonopulse
Frequency	1 or 3 MHz (+/- 10%)
ERA	3.5 cm² or 1 cm² (+/- 20%)
Output power	0.1 to 2 W/cm² (+/- 20%)
BNR	<8:1 (+/- 30%)

Table 1. Principal features of the characterized physiotherapy ultrasonic equipment

5.1 Methodology

5.1.1 C-scan with hydrophone

The C-scan used for these measurements is composed by a PZTZ44-0400 hydrophone as the sensor element. The hydrophone signal is amplified 17 dB before sending the signal to the oscilloscope, which has a 150 MHz bandwidth (TDS-340, Tektronix, USA). The transducer is excited with an amplifier/receiver board TB 1000 (Matec Instruments, USA) using the next parameters: repetition rate of 13 ms, frequency of 1.05 MHz, pulse width of 6.22 µs, and output voltage of 120 V. The generator board and the oscilloscope are synchronized and the computer registers a new value each time the oscilloscope is ready to measure, i.e., when the signal is stable. The block diagram of the C-scan system can be seen in Fig. 10.

During the characterization, the positioner XYZ and the oscilloscope are controlled by a computer with the software Scan 340 and through a GPIB interface. For these measurements, the software was configured to read transversal planes of 40 mm X 40 mm separated from the transducer by a distance that varied from 2 mm to 100 mm until completing 51 planes. These data were saved in a matrix of 40 X 40 X 51 so they could be taken in order to calculate the ultrasonic beam parameters.

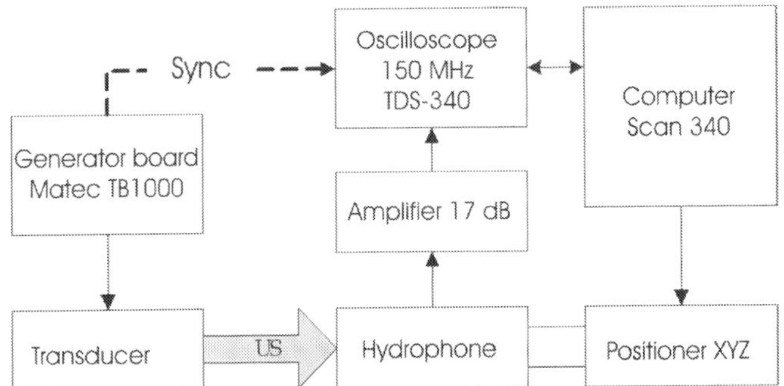

Fig. 10. Block diagram of the C-scan with hydrophone. The setup of the system is described in section 4.1.2

5.1.2 Thermochromic Liquid Crystals (TLC)

The thermochromic sheet used for the experiments (R25C5W, Hallcrest, USA) has a "red start to blue start" range of 25-30°C. The medium that absorbs the ultrasound is a sheet of PVC-polyurethane with 0.4 mm of thickness, a sound reflection coefficient in water of 0.06 (±0.01) and an attenuation coefficient of 23.5 (±1.02) dB·cm^{-1}·MHz^{-1}. All the systems are mounted in a degasified-water-filled tank as it is shown in Fig. 9. The anechoic absorber has an attenuation of 45 dB/cm at 1 MHz and 25°C (Zeqiri & Bickley, 2000). The thermal image was observed through the aluminized Mylar which is practically "transparent" for the ultrasound because of its small acoustic reflection coefficient.

The pictures were taken after 30 min of ultrasonic radiation with an acoustic intensity of 2 W/cm^2; this time was chosen because it was the moment when the stabilization of the temperature pattern took place. The transducer was moved backward the absorbing layer in steps of 2 mm starting at 2 mm from the absorbing layer until it reached 13 mm from the layer.

5.1.3 IR thermography

The temperature in a phantom of soft-tissue was obtained and a protocol to take the photographs was used. Initially, the phantom was made with a cylindrical form; then, it was cut at the middle in order to separate the two parts. After heating, the phantom was divided and a photograph was taken as fast as possible in order to avoid thermal conduction effects; before taking another thermal image, the phantom was cooled and the transducer was displaced perpendicularly to the surface where the picture had been taken in order to have images at different axial cuts of the acoustic field. The images were taken with an IR camera Mikron model TH5104. The penetration depth was measured to know the maximum time to get the image.

The phantom elaborated was agar-based with a combination of ingredients to simulate the acoustic properties of the muscle: 2.5% agar, 5% graphite, 10% glycerol and distilled water. The agar is used to solidify the resulted mixture; the graphite, to simulate the acoustic attenuation; the glycerol, to get the desired acoustic velocity; and the distilled water, to dissolve the materials. The resulted phantom had the acoustic properties shown in Table 2.

Magnitude (20°C)	Measured	Muscle
Attenuation (dB/cm)	0.807	0.5-1.3
Velocity of propagation (m/s)	1537.51	1520-1580

Table 2. Acoustic properties of the phantom compared to those of the muscle

5.2 Radiation pattern

In order to compare the results, the characteristic parameters were obtained with each technique by using the radiation pattern. Although the transducer was always the same, the radiation patterns are different because the measured magnitudes were different for each technique. However, the results can be compared because every magnitude is related to the acoustic intensity as it has been explained.

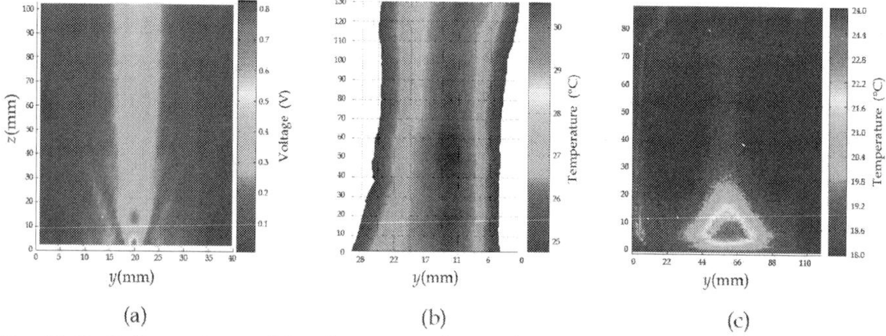

(a)   (b)   (c)

Fig. 11. Radiation pattern of the characterized transducer. (a) C-scan with hydrophone, (b) thermography with TLC, (c) IR thermography

The radiation patterns are shown in Fig. 11. The acoustic pressure distribution around the ultrasonic beam when the technique C-scan was used is shown in Fig. 11a. We can notice that the acoustic pressure magnitude represents the "free ultrasonic field" since the attenuation is negligible. This is because the medium where the ultrasound passes through was water which has an attenuation coefficient of 2.5×10^{-4} Np/cm at 1 MHz. The increments near the transducer are caused by the wave cancelations (and additions) in the near field zone.

The radiation pattern of the transducer was obtained by using the thermography with TLC; the pattern was composed by the temperatures measured, as it is shown in Fig. 11b. There was a visible effect in the inclination of the figure due to the internal inclination of the piezoelectric element with respect to the transducer face. The initial sequence to find the center (as in C-scan) was not enough because of the dependence on the system angles. The Fig. 11b shows the radiation pattern resulted from the interpolation among every image taken.

Finally, the radiation pattern of Fig. 11c was obtained using the IR thermography. This picture is completely different from the pictures showed in Fig. 11a and 11b because of the differences among the techniques. In Fig. 11a, the radiation pattern was formed with instantaneous acoustic pressures, and in Fig. 11c the magnitude measured was the quantity of the ultrasound absorbed (effective acoustic intensity was transformed into temperature). In spite of the different pattern, it is possible to calculate the characteristic parameters using this results; moreover, this is the most appropriated technique, of the three compared here, for calculating the penetration depth in the media, if it were required.

5.3 Effective Radiating Area

This was calculated using the FDA definition given above. Considering the results of the C-scan, Fig. 12a, the region with the 95% of the intensity starts at the sample 11 and ends at the sample 28. Because each sample was equal to 1 mm, we have a diameter of 17 mm, and then an ERA of 227 mm².

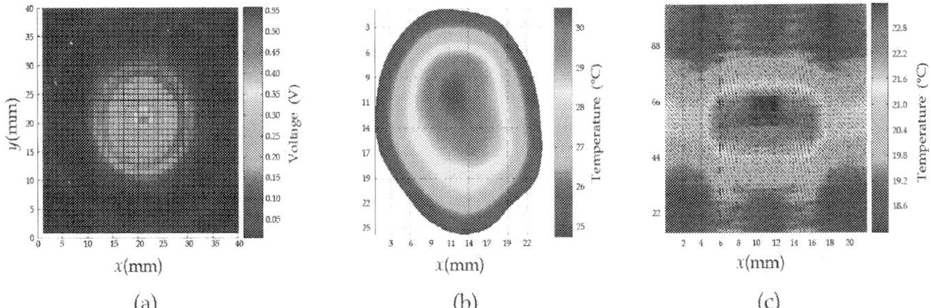

(a) (b) (c)

Fig. 12. Radiation pattern used to calculate the ERA. (a) C-scan with hydrophone, (b) thermography with TLC, (c) IR thermography

In order to calculate the ERA using the TLC, a MATLAB algorithm was used (see the Fig. 12b). This algorithm takes the color of the image, creates a relation of the color and the temperature, transforms the color image to a temperature data matrix, finds the maximum SAR, and determines the area with the 50% of the maximum SAR in order to have the ERA in agreement with the ESHO protocols (Hand et al., 1989). Same calculations were carried out to find the ERA using the measurements with the IR thermography. The results are shown in Table 3.

Technique	ERA (mm²)
C-scan with hydrophone	227
Thermography with TLC	201
IR-thermography	154

Table 3. ERA calculations using each technique. C-scan is the most accurate in accordance with the IEC standards. Thermography with TLC gave a result close the one of the C-scan

5.4 Beam Non-uniformity Ratio

This parameter was calculated by using the definition given above, which corresponds to Eq. 9. The results are quite similar and they are in the safe range of 1:6. The calculations for the techniques that use the temperature as the magnitude measured were the same as the C-scan. The acoustic intensity is related to the acoustic pressure and to the increment in temperature, as it can be seen in the next equations:

$$I_x = \frac{p_{rms}^2}{\rho c} \tag{13}$$

where c is the sound velocity. Using Eq. 10 for the temperature increment and substituting in Eq. 13, we have

$$p_{rms}^2 = \frac{C\rho^2 c}{2\alpha} \frac{dT}{dt} \tag{14}$$

Hence, the BNR adjusted for thermographic techniques is

$$BNR = \frac{\Delta T_{max} \cdot ERA}{\Delta T_{average} \cdot a_0} \tag{15}$$

where ΔT_{max} is the maximum temperature increment and the $\Delta T_{average}$ is the average of every temperature increment measured inside the ERA. The results of the calculation of the BNR with the three techniques are registered in Table 4. Again, the similarities of the results of using the thermography with TLC and the C-scan with hydrophone are clear. However, the IR thermography was different.

Technique	BNR
C-scan with hydrophone	1.52
Thermography with TLC	1.69
IR-thermography	1.29

Table 4. Calculations of the BNR. The three techniques had close results. IR thermography was, again, a little different

5.5 Penetration Depth

This parameter was obtained with the IR thermography in order to know the t_{max} to take the pictures. The penetration depth was calculated by using the definition described in section 3.3.3; the radiation pattern of Fig. 11c was used for the calculations. The axial SAR was determined along the beam, and the reduction of 50% of the one calculated at 10 mm was the P_D. Another technique that could be used and which gives accurate results is the invasive thermography by using either thermocouples or thermistors. The thermography in solids with TLC is another option but with the disadvantage of the effect on the acoustic beam caused by the TLC sheets.

The P_D calculated for the transducer radiation on the muscle phantom was 2.086 cm. This indicates that the maximum time to take the picture, in accordance with Eq. 12, is given by

$$13.2(2.086^2) = 57.44 \text{ s.}$$

6. Conclusion

Physiotherapy ultrasonic transducer characterization is required because the patient must be safe. Effects of hot-spots produced by an inhomogeneous beam (large BNR) could injure tissue because of the physiological implications: ablation and cavitation. Moreover, the efficacy of the treatment depends on the device acoustic intensity and this is related to the ultrasonic power and the transducer ERA. Ignorance of these characteristic parameters can generate undesired effects and even tissue damage, as it has been mentioned before.

In this chapter, measurements using each technique were carried out in order to determine the mentioned parameters. By using these techniques, it is possible to determine both the ERA and the BNR of the physiotherapy transducer. The resolutions and the time of acquisition are different for each technique; it was determined that the TLC was the fastest one and the C-scan was the slowest. Even though this comparison does not include other techniques, their use is not excluded. Some improvements are still required so these techniques can be applied confidently in the characterization of ultrasonic transducers, as the reduction of the costs, the uncertainties, and the technological requirements.

The comparison of three of these techniques gave us the possibility to know their characteristics in order to plan the future measurements in accordance with the specific requirements. The C-scan with hydrophone is recommended when a good resolution and high reproducibility of the measurements are required. With this technique, it is also possible to determine the acoustic intensity in every point in the acoustic field, and therefore, to know most of the parameters required in experiments in liquids, i.e., the acoustic pressure, the total power, the attenuation, etc. IR thermography can be used to characterize the US devices when they emit in solid media. It is possible to calculate the desired parameters mentioned before, but taking into consideration that the measurements are the result of the absorption of the same acoustic intensities during a period of time (integrated in time). The technique with TLC is a new proposal to characterize a device quickly. It can be used when fast and high resolution measurements are required. The configuration is similar to that of the C-scan, but this technique uses a sheet to measure the heat produced in an acoustic absorber material. This technique also uses time-integrated magnitudes, but with water between the transducer and the absorber; therefore, it is used to characterize the emission in liquid media. The other variant of the thermography with TLC can be used in solid media, but its application was not mentioned here.

Most of the techniques described along this chapter work adequately under certain conditions, and their use in characterization is chosen in accordance with the necessities. The Schlieren technique has been widely used since their application for quantifying the ultrasound emission. The use of a Michelson interferometer could be another good option, but expensive. However, the challenge is to find an accurate technique that allows characterizing transducers quickly and inexpensively. According to this comparison, the most accurate technique, in regards to IEC standards and FDA definitions, is the C-scan with hydrophone, but as it was mentioned before, it is the slowest one. Techniques as the thermography with TLC and the Schlieren method could be improved to increase its accuracy and to reduce its costs, respectively. It is also required to find a portable system to characterize the transducer *in situ* which does not require a lot of time in the all the process.

7. References

ABNT (1998). "Ultra-som - Sistemas de fisioterapia - Prescriçoes para desempenho e métodos de mediçao na faixa de freqüências de 0,5 MHz a 5 MHz.," 1998, ABNT - Associaçao Brasileira de Normas Técnicas

Águila C. d. (1994). Ultrasonido Terapéutico. In: *Electromedicina*, 291-302, Hispano Americana S.A. Hasa

Andreuccetti D., Bini M., Ignesti A., Olmi R., Priori S. & Vanni R. (1991a). Characterization of hyperthermia applicators by semi-automatic liquid crystal dosimetry. *Physica Medica*, 7, 4, 145-151

Andreuccetti D., Bini M., Ignesti A., Olmi R. & Vanni R. (1991b). Phantom Characterization of Applicators by Liquid-Crystal-Plate Dosimetry. *Int J Hyperther*, 7, 1, 175-183, 0265-6736

Arthur R. M., Straube W. L., Starman J. D. & Moros E. G. (2003). Noninvasive temperature estimation based on the energy of backscattered ultrasound. *Med Phys*, 30, 6, 1021-1029, 0094-2405

Arthur R. M., Straube W. L., Trobaugh J. W. & Moros E. G. (2005). Non-invasive estimation of hyperthermia temperatures with ultrasound. *Int J Hyperther*, 21, 6, 589-600, 0265-6736

Christensen D. A. (1988). *Ultrasonic bioinstrumentation*, John Wiley & Sons, 0471604968

De Poorter J., De Wagter C., De Deene Y., Thomsen C., Stahlberg F. & Achten E. (1995). Noninvasive MRI thermometry with the proton resonance frequency (PRF) method: in vivo results in human muscle. *Magn Reson Med*, 33, 1, 74-81, 0740-3194 (Print)

Fallone B. G., Moran P. R. & Podgorsak E. B. (1982). Noninvasive thermometry with a clinical X-ray CT scanner. *Med Phys*, 9, 5, 715-721, 0094-2405 (Print)

FDA (2008). "Performance Standards for Sonic, Infrasonic, and Ultrasonic Radiation-Emitting Products ", April 1 2008, International Electrotechnical Commission

Feril L. B. & Kondo T. (2004). Biological effects of low intensity ultrasound: the mechanism involved, and its implications on therapy and on biosafety of ultrasound. *Journal of Radiation Research*, 45, 4, 479-489

Field S. B. & Bleehen N. M. (1979). Hyperthermia in the Treatment of Cancer. *Cancer Treat. Rev.*, 6, 2, 63-94, 0305-7372

Gunarathne G. P. P. & Szilard J. (1983). A New Stroboscope for Schlieren and Photo-Elastic Visualization of Ultrasound. *Ultrasonics*, 21, 4, 188-190, 0041-624X

Gutierrez M. I., Leija L. & Vera A. (2008). "Therapy Ultrasound Equipment Characterization: Comparison of Three Techniques," *30th Annual International Conference of the IEEE Engineering in Medicine and Biology Society*, Vancouver, British Columbia, Canada, Aug 20-24 2008, IEEE

Guy A. W. (1971). Analyses of Electromagnetic Fields Induced in Biological Tissues by Thermographic Studies on Equivalent Phantom Models. *IEEE T Microw Theory*, Mt19, 2, 205-&, 0018-9480

Hanafy A. & Zanelli C. I. (1991). "Quantitative real-time pulsed Schlieren imaging of ultrasonic waves," *IEEE 1991 Ultrasonics Symposium Proceedings. (Cat. No.91CH3079-1)*, 1223-1227 vol.1222, Orlando, FL, USA, 8-11 December 1991, IEEE

Hand J. W., Lagendijk J. J. W., Andersen J. B. & Bolomey J. C. (1989). Quality Assurance Guidelines for ESHO Protocols. *Int J Hyperther*, 5, 4, 421-428, 0265-6736

Hekkenberg R. T. (1998). Characterising ultrasonic physiotherapy systems by performance and safety now internationally agreed. *Ultrasonics*, 36, 1-5, 713-720, 0041-624X

Hensley A. B. & Muthuswamy J. (2002). "Ultrasound induced permeabilization of cell membranes as a therapy for cytotoxic neuronal edema," *Conference Proceedings. Second Joint EMBS BMES Conference 2002 24th Annual International Conference of the Engineering in Medicine and Biology Society. Annual Fall Meeting of the Biomedical Engineering Society. Houston, TX, USA. 23 26 Oct. 2002.* 2002, IEEE, Piscataway, NJ, USA

IEC (1991). "Measurement and characterization of ultrasonic fields using hydrophones in the frequency range 0.5 MHz to 15 MHz," 1991, International Electrotechnical Commission

Johns L. D. (2002). Nonthermal effects of therapeutic ultrasound: The frequency resonance hypothesis. *J Athl Training*, 37, 3, 293-299, 1062-6050

Johns L. D., Demchak T. J., Straub S. J. & Howard S. M. (2007). The role of quantitative schlieren assessment of physiotherapy ultrasound fields in describing variations between tissue heating rates of different transducers. *Ultrasound Med Biol*, 33, 12, 1911-1917, 0301-5629

Lu H., Qin L., Cheung W., Lee K., Wong W. & Leung K. (2008). Low-intensity pulsed ultrasound accelerated bone-tendon junction healing through regulation of vascular endothelial growth factor expression and cartilage formation. *Ultrasound Med Biol*, 34, 8, 1248-1260, 0301-5629

Maass-Moreno R. & Damianou C. A. (1996). Noninvasive temperature estimation in tissue via ultrasound echo-shifts. Part I. Analytical model. *Journal of the Acoustical Society of America*, 100, 4, 2514-2521

Mansour T. M. (1979). Evaluation of Ultrasonic Transducers by Cross-Sectional Mapping of the near-Field Using a Point Reflector. *Mater Eval*, 37, 7, 50-54, 0025-5327

Marangopoulos I. P., Martin C. J. & Hutchison J. M. S. (1995). Measurement of Field Distributions in Ultrasonic Cleaning Baths - Implications for Cleaning Efficiency. *Physics in Medicine and Biology*, 40, 11, 1897-1908, 0031-9155

Martin K. & Fernandez R. (1997). A thermal beam-shape phantom for ultrasound physiotherapy transducers. *Ultrasound Med Biol*, 23, 8, 1267-1274, 0301-5629

Mezrich R., Etzold K. F. & Vilkomerson D. (1975). Interferometric Measurement and Display of Ultrasonic-Waves. *IEEE J Quantum Elect*, 11, 9, D9-D10, 0018-9197

Mezrich R., Vilkomerson D. & Etzold K. (1976). Ultrasonic-Waves - Their Interferometric Measurement and Display. *Appl Optics*, 15, 6, 1499-1505, 0003-6935

Nacitarhan V., Elden H., Kisa M., Kaptanogglu E. & Nacitarhan S. (2005). The effects of therapeutic ultrasound on heart rate variability: A placebo controlled trial. *Ultrasound Med Biol*, 31, 5, 643-648, 0301-5629

Obuchi T., Masuyama H., Mizutani K. & Nakanishi S. (2006). Optical computerized tomography for visualization of ultrasonic fields using Michelson interferometer. *Jpn J Appl Phys 1*, 45, 9A, 7152-7157, 0021-4922

Paliwal S. & Mitragotri S. (2008). Therapeutic opportunities in biological responses of ultrasound. *Ultrasonics*, 48, 4, 271-278, 0041-624X

Papadakis E. P. (1999). *Ultrasonic Instruments & Devices: Reference for Modern Instrumentation Techniques, and Technology*, Academic Press

Pernot M., Tanter M., Bercoff J., Waters K. R. & Fink M. (2004). Temperature estimation using ultrasonic spatial compound imaging. *IEEE Transactions on Ultrasonics, Ferroelectrics and Frequency Control*, 51, 5, 606-615, 0885-3010

Pye S. D. & Milford C. (1994). The performance of ultrasound physiotherapy machines in Lothian Region, Scotland, 1992. *Ultrasound Med Biol*, 20, 4, 347-359, 0301-5629 (Print)

Rienitz J. (1975). Schlieren Experiment 300 Years Ago. *Nature*, 254, 5498, 293-295, 0028-0836

Seegenschmiedt M. H. (1995). *Thermo-radiotherapy and Thermo-chemotherapy*, Springer, Atlanta, GA

Selfridge A. R. (1985). Approximate material properties in isotropic materials. *IEEE Transactions on Sonics and Ultrasonics*, SU-32, 3, 381-394

Shiran M. B., Quan K. M., Watmough D. J., Abdellatif K., Mallard J. R., Marshall D. & Gregory D. W. (1990). Some of the Factors Involved in the Sarvazyan Method for Recording Ultrasound Field Distributions with Special Reference to the Application of Ultrasound in Physiotherapy. *Ultrasonics*, 28, 6, 411-414, 0041-624X

Singh V. R., Chauhan S., Yadav S. & Chakarvarti S. K. (1990). Ultrasonic velocity as a non-invasive measure of temperature in biological media. *Applied Acoustics*, 29, 1, 73-80

Speed C. A. (2001). Therapeutic ultrasound in soft tissue lesions. *Rheumatology*, 40, 12, 1331-1336, 1462-0324

ter Haar G. (1999). Therapeutic ultrasound. *European Journal of Ultrasound*, 9, 1, 3-9

ter Haar G. (2007). Therapeutic applications of ultrasound. *Prog Biophys Mol Bio*, 93, 1-3, 111-129, 0079-6107

ter Haar G. & Hand J. W. (1981). Heating techniques in hyperthermia. III. Ultrasound. *The British journal of radiology*, 54, 642, 459-466, 0007-1285 (Print)

Vera A., Moreno E., Leija L. & Vazquez M. (2007). Optimization of hydrophone centering in circular ultrasonic transducer during field characterization using edge waves: A feasibility study. *Jpn J Appl Phys 1*, 46, 7A, 4321-4323, 0021-4922

Watmough D. J., Quan K. M. & Shiran M. (1990). "The Sarvazyan method of mapping ultrasound fields," *IEE Colloquium on `Ultrasound Instrumentation' (Digest No.072)*, 4/1-4/3, London, UK, 10 May 1990, IEE

Watson T. (2008). Ultrasound in contemporary physiotherapy practice. *Ultrasonics*, 48, 4, 321-329, 0041-624X

Zeqiri B. & Bickley C. J. (2000). A new anechoic material for medical ultrasonic applications. *Ultrasound Med Biol*, 26, 3, 481-485, 0301-5629

29

Some Irradiation-Influenced Features of Pericardial Tissues Engineered for Biomaterials

Artur Turek[1] and Beata Cwalina[2]

[1]Department of Biopharmacy, Silesian Medical University, Sosnowiec
Poland
[2]Environmental Biotechnology Department, Silesian University of Technology, Gliwice
Poland

1. Introduction

Engineered xenogeneic tissues are very popular biomaterials used in tissue replacements. For this purpose, various kinds of tissues are exposed to stabilization processes leading to an increase in the biomaterial durability *in vivo* (Ionescu et al., 1982; Khor, 1997; Vesely, 2003). The structure stability is achieved mainly by crosslinking of structural proteins. The main requirements were focused on the reduction of immune response and degradation processes. Such effects have firstly been obtained by the use of formaldehyde (FA) (Paneth & O'Brien, 1966), but resulted crosslinks were reversible. Better results were achieved by the use of glutaraldehyde (GA) being a bifunctional aldehyde. It is widely used from the late 60s of 20th century to reduce the xenografts' antigenicity and proteolytic degradation (Carpentier et al., 1969; Woodroof, 1978). However, the GA cytotoxicity (Gendler et al., 1984; Huang-Lee et al., 1990; Moczar et al., 1994) as well as premature calcification of GA-treated tissues (Golomb et al., 1987; Levy et al., 1991; Thoma & Phillips, 1995) limit the durability of bioprostheses.

These disadvantages of the GA-stabilized biomaterials were a sufficient reason for initializing the tissue stabilization by irradiation being perceived as safer (Mechanic, 1994; Moore el al., 1994). This way of the tissue modification does not cause an incorporation of chemical reagents into the tissue structure, which can be a reason for defects *in vivo* of heart valves stabilized by GA.

Apart from many others, some irradiation methods are proposed as useful for preservation of tissues applied in manufacturing of various biomaterials. The attention has been paid to the tissue stabilization methods based on action of visible (VIS) light or ultraviolet (UV) light, both non-mediated and mediated by a dye (Weadock at al., 1995; Suh et al., 1999; Westaby et al., 1999). The methods using irradiation as modifying or stabilizing factor allow to obtain biomaterials of different durability, both biodegradable and non-biodegradable. The porcine valves or bovine pericardium (BP) irradiation makes it possible to produce non-biodegradable bioprostheses (Westaby et al., 1999; Suh et al., 1999). Irradiation of collagen fibers results in the obtaining biodegradable sponges (Weadock et al., 1996).

2. Photooxidation as a method of tissue stabilization

2.1 Background

It has been well-documented that crosslinking processes in tissues influence their structural modification (Turek et al., 2007), prolongation of durability (Vesely, 2003), increase in biocompatibility (Reardon & O'Brien, 1997) and obtaining sterile products (Stone, 2006).

Photooxidation is one of the methods which make it possible to eliminate the disadvantages of GA (Moore, 1997). Mechanism of photooxidation is still not completely recognized. In the tissues exposed on irradiation, generation of free radicals in the residues of aromatic acids (Fujimori, 1965) and interaction between amino acids residues take place (Mechanic, 1994). One of the hypotheses of crosslinking by photooxidation postulates alteration in the imidazole ring of histidine, leading to the formation of side chains containing aldehyde groups (Weil et al., 1951) or an imidazole peroxide (Au & Madison, 2000).

Dyes may accelerate or facilitate processes of the collagenous materials photomodification (Mechanic, 1994). On the other hand, the presence of dye during photooxidation has a protecting effect on the tissue components against photodegradation (Sionkowska, 2000).

Triplet state catalyst and substrate interact and secondary reactive radicals by electron or hydrogen atom transfer reactions are produced (Spikes & Straight, 1967). In the presence of oxygen electrons and hydrogen atoms the substrates are oxidized. Moreover, dyes, like methylene blue (MB) and riboflavin (RF) generate reactive oxygen species (Halliwell & Gutteridge, 1990; Fernandez et al., 1997). MB, methylene green, rose Bengal, RF and proflavin belong to the group of preferred photocatalysts (Mechanic, 1994).

Photosensitive dyes have been used since 1950s to investigate processes of amino acids oxidation of various proteins (Weil et al., 1952). Following research works indicated that photooxidative process caused modification of methionine (Neumann et al., 1962), tyrosine (Weil et al., 1965), tryptophan (Gurnani et al., 1966) and histidine (Tomita et al., 1969), promoting bonds between the functional groups of the amino acids. One of more attractive and health-safe methods used in biomaterials engineering may be photooxidation of collagenous tissues in the presence of photoactive dyes and VIS light (Mechanic, 1994) or in the presence of UV light (Suh et al., 1999). The photooxidation promotes the forming of covalent bonds between amino acids without cytotoxic linkers.

2.2 Collagen stabilization by photooxidation

Collagens belong to the major proteins group of extracellular matrix which contributes to the structural stability. The name collagen is used for the proteins family forming triple helix of three polypeptide chains (Gelse et al., 2003). In biomaterials engineering, type I collagen plays a key role because of its dominant presence in connective tissues. Collagenous tissues and also isolated collagen as crosslinked or non-crosslinked products are employed in various applications. Native collagen has natural intra- and intermolecular crosslinks which contribute to the stability of collagen fibers. Stabilization processes used in the biomaterials engineering result in introducing additional crosslinks to proteins which influences the decrease in the susceptibility to degradation. The predominant stabilization of xenogeneic collagenous biomaterials may be obtained due to their GA-crosslinking (Jayakrishnan & Jameela, 1996). In the last years attention has been paid to processes using irradiation (Moore, 1997) because of clinical failures of GA-treated tissues (Golomb et al., 1987). It is very important that the collagen photooxidation allows to obtain degradable and non-degradable collagenous materials. Nowadays both bioprostheses and collagenous sponges being obtained as a result of the collagen crosslinking by photomodification are proposed as stabilized biomaterials (Moore, 1997; Chan & So, 2008). Collagen may be photomodified in various ways. Taking into account that photooxidation may be accompanied by degradation processes, the presence of dye as catalyst and protector seems to be correct for obtaining non-degradable bioprostheses, whereas non dye-mediated photooxidation may be used for obtaining the collagen sponges.

In 1969, Gowri and Thomas showed that soluble collagen could be crosslinked in the presence of MB. It was demonstrated by viscosity increase in photooxidized material. Nearly ten years later, Bernstein and Mechanic (1980) noticed that photooxidation transformed soluble collagen into protein insoluble under the most extreme denaturing conditions and resistant to pepsin digestion.

Additional information has been obtained as a result of investigations carried out by Ramshaw et al. (1994). They have shown that MB sensitized photooxidation of tendon led to its stabilization due to crosslinking of collagen fibrils. After this process, an increase in the thermal stability of the collagen as well as a decrease in the amounts of low-weight molecular fragments obtained after cyanogen bromide (CNBr) cleavage of tendon and simultaneous increase in the formation higher molecular components were demonstrated.

Moore et al. (1994) have demonstrated that during the dye-mediated photooxidation of tissue, the crosslinking of collagen fibrils takes place. This effect was shown in electrophoresis studies of soluble collagen isolated from BP (Moore et al., 1994). The dye-mediated photooxidation caused an even multiple increase effect in molecular weight of various collagen types, indicating the formation of intermolecular crosslinks. The resultant tissue was similar to untreated tissue in texture and elasticity (Moore, 1997). Tissues treated with FA and GA (Cwalina et al., 2002) as well as with tannic acid (TA) (Jastrzebska et al., 2005) indicated greater structural complexity, density and bending stiffness as compared with those resulting from dye-mediated stabilization (Cwalina et al., 2000).

UV irradiation of collagen fibers does not introduce cytotoxic reagents into biomaterials and revealed the mechanical properties comparable to the intact human anterior cruciate ligament (ACL). It was also demonstrated that UV-crosslinked collagen fibers exhibited resistance to nonspecific proteases (Weadock et al., 1996). Moreover, significant enhancement of the bending strength and resistance to enzymatic digestion in UV-treated collagen fibers may be obtained due to glucose synergistic effect (Ohan et al., 2002).

Other authors have revealed that photochemical crosslinking improves the physicochemical properties of collagenous scaffolds. In the studies collagen gel was modified with laser in the presence of a photosensitizer. This modification significantly reduced the swelling ratio, improved the stress-strain relationship, peak load, ultimate stress, rupture strain, and also tangent modulus of collagen membranes (Chan & So, 2005).

2.3 Photooxidative crosslinking of collagenous tissues

The growing interest in use of photooxidation to stabilize collagen materials for bioprostheses was observed after patenting this method by Mechanic (1994). His invention relates in particular "to a process for photooxidizing collagenous material in the presence of photocatalyst to crosslink and stabilize that material" as well as "to the resulting crosslinked product". The modified collagenous products resulting from the claimed process may be used as biomaterials for vascular grafts, heart valves, pericardial patches, injectable collagen, or as replacement ligaments. A choice of optimum conditions of photooxidation process, mainly dye concentration, temperature and exposure time, depend both on dye and tissue type as a well as desired application of modified material (Mechanic, 1994).

The BP is a collagenous tissue more often used in studies on dye-mediated photooxidation (Mechanic, 1994; Moore et al., 1994; Bianco et al., 1996; McIlroy et al., 1997). These investigations showed that tissue became stable after treatment with photosensitive dyes. Tissue collagen was resistant to action of chemical and enzymatic agents (Mechanic, 1994; Moore et al., 1994) and to mechanical degradation (Moore et al., 1994). The photooxidized BP maintained the properties of natural tissue, supporting the growth of endothelial cells (Bengtsson et al., 1995), being biocompatible and non-immunogenic (Moore & Phillips, 1997). Moreover, dye-mediated photooxidation of collagen tissues appears to be a feasible way of reducing bioprosthetic heart valves calcification (Mechanic, 1994; Bianco et al., 1996). The stabilization of pericardium by dye-mediated photooxidation was the main objective in investigations carried out by Moore group (Moore et al., 1994; 1996; McIlroy et al., 1997; Moore & Phillips, 1997). To study the efficiency of collagen modification with this method, various collagenous materials were subjected to photooxidation for varying times from 0 to 91 h (Moore et al., 1994) or even to 168 h (McIlroy et al., 1997). Control samples were dye-treated without lighting or were irradiated without the dye. Samples not exposed to either dye or light were studied as untreated material. It was demonstrated that samples photooxidized in the presence of dye were more resistant concerning protein extraction as compared with the control samples. This resistance was shown to be time-increased, which may reflect the kinetic nature of photooxidation. Dye-mediated photooxidation resulted in an alteration of existing crosslinks and a possible addition of new crosslinks in the tissue (McIlroy et al., 1997). Tissue modified was also more resistant to CNBr and pepsin digestion when compared with control tissue (Moore et al., 1994). CNBr-resistance of photooxidized tissue was partially reversible by 2-mercaptoethanol-pretreatment of tissue. This effect may indicate the possibility of methionine photooxidation, which was confirmed in studies carried out by McIlroy et al. (1997). They also indicated that dye-mediated photooxidation of bovine tissues (pericardium, arteries) resulted in a time-dependent reduction of histidine content. Except methionine and histidine, no other amino acid alteration was detected by amino acid analysis (McIlroy et al., 1997).

Other concept was presented by Suh and co-workers (1999; 2000). In the studies the author modified porcine valves by UV irradiation. A decrease in hydroxyproline content as compared with GA-treated tissue and a decrease in the crimp pattern of collagen fibers for UV-modified tissue were observed (Suh et al., 1999). UV-irradiation of porcine valve influenced the reduction of calcification (Suh et al., 2000). The dye-mediated photooxidation processes were also proposed to stabilize acellular BP (de Visscher et al., 2008).

Photooxidation process of tissues results in their smaller immunogenicity and resistance to degradation. It has been demonstrated that allogeneic osteochondral grafts have many disadvantages, like the possibility of diseases transmission, immunogenic response and less complete graft incorporation. Dye-mediated photooxidation may be used to obtain allogeneic and xenogeneic scaffolds to repair damaged or diseased cartilage (Hetherington et al., 2005; 2007; Kawalec-Carroll et al., 2006). In one of the experiments, human and bovine cartilages were photooxidized in the presence of MB and then the grafts were implanted to mice. The photooxidized bovine grafts, native cartilage and photooxidized human grafts did not induce a significant response. Microscopic studies revealed some degree of fibrous encapsulation and inflammatory infiltration in all studied tissue samples. Nowadays, a dye-mediated photooxidation is tested as a method of obtaining xenogeneic osteochondral grafts (Kawalec-Carroll et al., 2006).

2.4 Properties of photooxidized collagenous tissue

Photooxidation processes belong to the alternative tissue stabilization methods. Comparison of the tissues properties resulted from the dye-mediated photooxidation or non dye-mediated photooxidation give grounds to expect correct long term results.

Moore's team (Moore et al., 1994) carried out *in vivo* investigations in which dye-mediated photooxidized collagenous tissues were subcutaneously implanted in rats. It has been shown that modified material indicated higher stability as compared with control samples. After tissues explanation it has been demonstrated that photooxidized material underwent calcification, but this effect was minimal as compared with tissues modified using GA.

Dye-mediated photooxidation has not influence on the sterility of collagenous material. Non-aldehyde method using iodide-based sterilization for dye-mediated photooxidized tissues was proposed by Moore and co-workers (1997). This way of sterilization allows to obtain sterile biomaterial without the changes of collagen structure. Moreover, biocompatibility tests showed that photooxidized and afterwards iodine-sterilized (Moore et al., 1997) BP and porcine pericardium (PP) tissues were non-cytotoxic, non-hemolytic and non-mutagenic (Moore & Phillips, 1997). In contrast, tissues treated with GA were found to be cytotoxic (Nimni et al., 1987; Huang-Lee et al., 1990).

Moreover, no negative symptoms have been observed after dye-mediated photooxidized collagenous material implantation in rabbits. Histopathological studies have not indicated significant macroscopic reaction, but only slight microscopic response (Moore, 1997; Moore & Phillips, 1997). Besides, a lack of the photooxidized collagenous material toxicity has also been demonstrated through tests for intracutaneous toxicity (irritation) and acute systemic toxicity (Moore & Phillips, 1997).

Moore and Phillips (1997) also investigated immunogenicity of BP and PP tissues that were modified using GA or dye-mediated photooxidation and subsequent sterilization in iodine-based solution. Tissues were homogenized and suspensions were injected into rabbits at three-week intervals. Antibody response was determined using a radioimmunoassay. These investigations demonstrated that both controls and modified tissues (photooxidized or treated with GA) showed low antibody levels.

Dye-mediated photooxidation of pericardial tissues was found to be a process which favors the growth of endothelial cells (Bengtsson et al., 1995). Investigations were carried out using BP or PP specimens, on which saphenous vein endothelial cells were seeded and incubated for 1 week. Cultured endothelial cells were grown as a confluent lining similar to native endothelium. This effect was demonstrated by scanning electron microscopy. Results obtained by Bengtsson et al. (1995) may be very important for a long-term durability of implants, manufactured using photooxidized tissues. Dye-mediated photooxidized pericardium did not exhibit any significant increase in thermal stability reflected by shrinkage temperature, but a rise in ultimate tensile strength was indicated (Moore et al., 1996). It was because of the modification and crosslink formation of existing matrix components in pericardial tissue (McIlroy et al., 1997). However, studies in the sheep model of bioprosthetic heart valves manufactured from dye-mediated photooxidized BP have revealed the damages as the result of tissue abrasion on the cloth covering the stent (Butterfield & Fisher, 2000).

Photomodification by UV-irradiation of porcine valves resulted in their resistance to collagenase action and significantly smaller susceptibility to calcification as compared with GA-treated tissue (Suh et al., 1999; 2000).

Dye-mediated photooxidation of allogeneic and xenogeneic ostechondral grafts stabilized the cartilage surface (Kawalec-Carroll et al., 2006). It has been demonstrated that xenogeneic grafts revealed a regeneration effect in the defects but no fusion between the graft and host cartilage took place (Hetherington et al., 2007).

2.5 Possibility of application of photooxidized collagenous products

Photooxidized products based on the collagenous components may found many commercial applications for biomedical uses. Dye-mediated photooxidized pericardial tissue was proposed to manufacture bioprosthetic heart valves. As yet, such valves were implanted into juvenile sheep because of their susceptibility to tissues calcification (Bianco et al., 1996). Since calcification processes represent a major percentage of clinical complications appearing during bioprostheses use, this animal model has been perceived as the most appropriate. Using of them, it was possible to verify early obtained results and to indicate many positive features of dye-mediated photooxidized tissues as compared with GA-stabilized ones. The first and at the same time the most important advantage of dye-mediated photooxidized tissue is that it did not undergo significant calcification. Besides, this tissue indicated high stability when implanted into organism. After explantation, such tissue was flexible and demonstrated collagen structure similar to that of unimplanted tissue (Moore, 1997). Contrary effects have been obtained as a result of investigations carried out on sheep with implanted valves prepared using GA-treated tissues. The valves after explantation showed calcification causing death of animals (Bianco et al., 1996).

Extra advantage of dye-mediated photooxidized pericardial tissues is that such materials (as valve or aorta' section) implanted into organism of juvenile sheep was overspread with layer of flat cells morphologically similar to endothelial cells. Their endothelial character was confirmed by positive staining using von Willebrand's method (Moore & Phillips, 1997). This test showed biocompatibility between cells crept on the implant and endothelial cells. Westaby et al. (1999) have shown in the juvenile sheep model that photomodified valves prepared using dye-mediated photooxidation (PhotoFix™) revealed minimal calcification. The sheep model study started by Carbomedics Inc. was the next important contribution to photooxidized valves investigations. However, clinical failures caused by abrasion of the inflow surface of the leaflets against the cloth-covered inner face of the outer valve frame were revealed (Butterfield & Fisher, 2000). These problems may result from processes of endothelialization which are much more rapid in sheep than in humans (Vesely, 2003). At presence, Carbomedics Inc. offers to sell CardioFix Pericardium obtained by PhotoFix Technology for intra-cardiac repair, great vessels repair, suture lines buttressing and pericardial closure. According to the producer, CardioFix Pericardium exhibits handling and suturability characteristics of autologous tissue.

The most important feature of xenobioprostheses is the initiation of recellularization of the tissues. The concept of a hybrid valve manufactured from a decellularized dye-mediated BP and allogeneic cells may be promising (de Visscher et al., 2008). As such collagenous products are biocompatible they influence a rapid recellularization of hybrid materials both *in vivo* and *in vitro*. Implantation of recellularized dye-mediated BP can result in a reduction of failures noted by Butterfield and Fisher (2000).

Pericardium has more homogenous structure than valve tissues. Photostabilization of pericardium tissues seems to be simpler. However, Suh and co-workers proposed porcine valve modified with UV-irradiation as bioprostheses (Suh et al., 1999; 2000).

Other possible application of photooxidized products includes biodegradable products like sponges or scaffolds. Weadock et al. (1995) have shown that collagen fibers crosslinked by UV irradiation may be used for ACL reconstruction because of mechanical properties, enzymatic resistance and biocompatibility (Weadock et al., 1995; 1996).

Chan and co-workers have demonstrated that collagen crosslinked with rose Bengal under laser light can be used to produce encapsulated structures with proteins for controlled protein release. This method may be useful for the production of collagenous scaffolds (Chan & So, 2005; 2008; Chan et al., 2008a; 2008b).

2.6 Concluding remarks

Summarizing information concerning dye-mediated photooxidation of collagen and collagenous tissues, it may be stated that: (i) photooxidized collagenous tissues do not undergo excessive calcification being the main reason for clinical complications taking place in case of using implants stabilized with GA; (ii) thanks to formation of transversal bonds in the photooxidized collagenous tissues, their strong crosslinking takes place; modified tissue becomes stable, i.e. does not undergo degradation by chemical agents or enzymatic digestion and demonstrate higher mechanical endurance; (iii) photooxidized collagenous tissues are non-toxic, non-immunogenic, biocompatible and maintain the growth of endothelial cells.

Such features of collagen and collagenous tissues photooxidized either in the presence of or without the photoactive dyes confirm the possibility of using these materials in long-term medical implants.

3. Investigated tissues and methods of their photomodification

3.1 Tissues preparation

PP or BP were obtained from the local abattoir directly after animal slaughtering. Before transportation the tissues were rinsed in cooled solution (4°C) of phosphate-buffered saline (PBS; pH 6.5). During transport tissues were placed in the containers with PBS solution in cooler box (4°C). Fibrous part of pericardium was mechanically separated from the pericardial sac. Before photomodification, tissular fat, heavy vasculatures and ligaments were removed.

3.2 Methylene blue-mediated photooxidation of bovine pericardium

The photooxidation process was carried out for 5, 15, 30, 45, 60, 90 and 120 min, using VIS light (12 W light bulb) and 0.05% solution of MB in PBS (pH 6.5), at 23°C. Samples of BP were incubated in 50% solution of saccharose in PBS for 1 h. In the next step, tissues were incubated in the presence of MB and cleaned air. Finally, the tissues were VIS-irradiated in the presence of dye and cleaned air. The distance between the light source and the dye solution level was 15 cm.

3.3 Methylene blue-mediated photooxidation of porcine pericardium

The photooxidation process was carried out for 8 and 24 h. As a control, native tissue and tissue incubated for 24 h with MB without irradiation were used. This photooxidation process took placed in three stages. In the first one PP was incubated (1 h) in 50% solution of saccharose in PBS to improve the efficiency of dye penetration. The second stage was the incubation of tissue with MB (0.05% solution in PBS; pH 6.5) in the presence of cleaned air. In the last stage the tissue was VIS-irradiated (50 W light bulb) for 8 or 24 h in aerated MB-PBS solution, at 15°C.

3.4 Short term riboflavin-mediated photooxidation of porcine pericardium

The samples were exposed to VIS-irradiation (50 W light bulb) for 1, 2, 3 h under aeration in the presence of 0.1% solution of RF in PBS (pH 6.5). Before modification, tissue samples were soaked for 1 h in 50% solution of sacchorose. The photooxidation process was carried out at 15°C. The distance between the light source and the dye solution level was 15 cm.

3.5 Photomodification of porcine pericardium with visible or ultraviolet light

The PP samples were UV or VIS-irradiated (50 W light bulb) for 1, 2 and 3 h, at 15°C. During irradiation the tissue samples were soaked in PBS (pH 6.5; 5 mm solution layer). The distance between the light source and the PBS solution level was 15 cm (Fig. 1).

3.6 Ultraviolet-modification of tannic acid crosslinked porcine pericardium

The samples of PP were stabilized by crosslinking with 2% solution of TA in PBS (pH 6.5; 4°C) for 4, 24 and 48 h. TA-crosslinked tissues were UV-irradiated for 1 h, at 15°C, under 5 mm layer of PBS solution. The distance between the light source and the PBS solution level was 15 cm (Fig. 1).

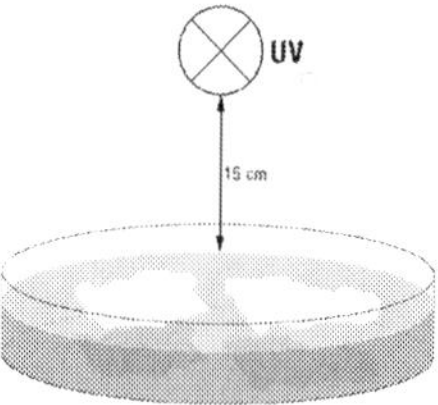

Fig. 1. Photomodification by UV-irradiation of PP.

4. Experiments description

4.1 Density investigation of bovine pericardium modified by methylene blue-mediated photooxidation

Crosslinking reactions in tissues result in an increase in concentrations of additional inter- and intramolecular covalent bonds and also other interactions as compared with native tissue. The modified pericardium tissues indicate the increased strength and simultaneously the decreased chemical degradability, including lower susceptibility to proteolytic enzymes digestion. The aim of the present study was to evaluate (using radioisotopic investigations) the fixation effects in BP tissues modified by the MB-mediated photooxidation or the GA-treatment. One of the stabilization effects, i.e. density increase in the photooxidized tissue due to crosslinking processes was studied by the determination of the $^{60}Co^{2+}$ accumulation in the tissue samples and their permeability to cobalt ions. Photooxidized tissues were compared with both native and GA-treated (0.2% in PBS, 30 min) tissues.

Radioactivity of the tissue samples and the filtrates penetrating through samples were examined using Packard spectrophotometer. The tissue samples were MB-photooxidized or GA-treated, then ^{60}Co (in $^{60}CoCl_2$ solution) accumulation in the tissue samples as well as their permeability to cobalt ions were examined.

Each experiment included three main stages: (i) selection of samples (all of 20 mm diameter) indicating identical permeability to PBS-solution from the tissue pieces of equal masses (0.14+0.01g, 0.21+0.02g or 0.29+0.03g); (ii) crosslinking of tissue samples indicating equal mass and permeability to PBS-solution; (iii) radioisotopic assays for testing binding capacity and permeability to $^{60}Co^{2+}$ of pericardial tissues (native, GA-treated and photooxidized).

4.2 Mechanical properties of porcine pericardium modified by methylene blue-mediated photooxidation

All fibrous proteins determine the mechanical properties of connective tissues. During their modification, important changes occur in interactions between the tissue components. These changes may result in the tissues' better integrity or failures. The aim of present study was the evaluation of the impact of MB-mediated photooxidation on mechanical properties of PP tissues. The results of these measurements were expected to be very useful in the evaluation of conformational changes effects in tissues after irradiation.

The strength tests were performed employing force-meter AFG 25N (Advance Force Gauge; Mecmesin) that was situated on a movable arm of an electromechanical stand.

The tissue was cut up along fibers into stripes. Each tissue stripe was 35 mm long and 10 mm wide. The breaking force (F_b) was performed as a function of time (10 measuring cycles per second). The streeps were subjected to stretching at the speed of 0.3 mm/s. The tissue samples were placed between two handles maintaining the streeps' initial length of 25 mm. During measurements, samples were fully immersed in isotonic NaCl solution to protect the tissue against drying up. These tests were carried out at the room temperature (21±2°C).

Statistical analyses were carried out using the computer program Statgraphic Plus, version 2.1. The normality of analysed variables distribution was examined using the Shapiro-Wilk test. The significance of differences between average values calculated for the modified samples and those not modified was estimated using the t-Student test.

4.3 Stability of porcine pericardium after riboflavin-mediated photooxidation

The purpose of the present work was to investigate the influence of RF and VIS light in the presence of atmospheric oxygen on the structure of PP. Changes in the stability of tissue structure were evaluated on the basis of SDS-PAGE electrophoresis and histological investigations. Impeded extraction of proteins from the tissue was found to be an indicator of its higher stability. It was shown that relations between the proteins extraction and tissues' morphology prove tissue stability (Moore et al., 1996; Cwalina et al., 2002; 2005; Turek et al., 2007). Before electrophoresis, native and irradiated samples (1 g) were homogenised in 50 ml of water (Polytron PT 2100 - Kinematica AG). Next, aliquots of 1.5 ml of tissue homogenates were collected and concentrated by centrifugation (14000 x g) for 10 min. to obtain samples of 0.5 ml volume.

Electrophoretic studies were performed according to SDS/NaCl Laemmli method (1970). Electrophoresis was carried out in 10% separating gel with 4% stacking gel, using voltage 140 V. Separated proteins were visualized in the gel using 0.05% Coomassie Brillant Blue R 250 (CBB) dissolved in solution of methanol : acetic acid : water (25:10:65). For destaining, gels were incubated in the same solution without dye (Cwalina et al., 2005). The qualitative analyses of the electrophoregrams were performed using Biotec Fischer System.

Histological studies were carried out under the Polyvar 2 – Leica light microscope, under magnification 200×. Tissue samples were dehydrated in absolute ethanol, and then embedded in paraffin wax. Six micron samples were stained routinely with Harris hematoxylin and erythrosine. Procedure of preparation-documentation was performed using the Quantament 500 Plus System.

4.4 Stability of porcine pericardium after visible and ultraviolet light irradiation

The aim of the present work was to evaluate the influence of the VIS- and UV-irradiation on the PP structure. Changes in the tissue structure stability were evaluated on the basis of SDS-PAGE electrophoresis and histological investigations (as described in section 4.3).

4.5 Stability of UV-irradiated tannic acid-crosslinked porcine pericardium

The aim of present study was to evaluate the TA-modified PP stability after the tissue UV-irradiation. Changes in the stability of tissue structure were evaluated on the basis of SDS-PAGE electrophoresis and histological investigations (as described in section 4.3). However, two methods were used for staining gels: the first with 0.05% CBB and the second with silver.

Investigated tissue samples were subjected to the SDS/NaCl extraction and to enzymatic digestion in solution containing 1.5 g of pancreatin (P) (5000 U of amylase, 30 U of lipase, 3.7 U of proteases/0.15 g of P) in 100 ml of PBS (pH 6.5), for 3 h (Cwalina et al., 2005).

5. Results

5.1 The influence of tissue modification on its permeability to cobalt ions

Changes in density of native BP and tissues modified by MB-mediated photooxidation or GA-crosslinking were revealed. The efficiency of crosslinking processes was evaluated based on the $^{60}Co^{2+}$ accumulation in the tissue samples and on their permeability to cobalt ions. Decreases in radioactivity (reported as counts per minute; cpm) of the tissue samples of various masses (i.e. thickness) after their photooxidation (Fig. 2A) as well as filtrates penetrating the same samples (Fig. 2B) seem to confirm the tissue crosslinking effect.

The permeability to $^{60}Co^{2+}$ and these ions accumulation in the photooxidized tissues were inversely proportional to the samples' thickness (Figs 2A and 2B). Similar dependence was observed in case of filtrates penetrating GA-treated tissues (Fig. 3), although $^{60}Co^{2+}$ accumulation in tissue samples remained at the same level. The GA-treated tissue samples indicated lower binding capacities as compared with the photooxidized samples of equal mass (thickness), pointing to lower crosslinking efficiency of the photooxidation used.

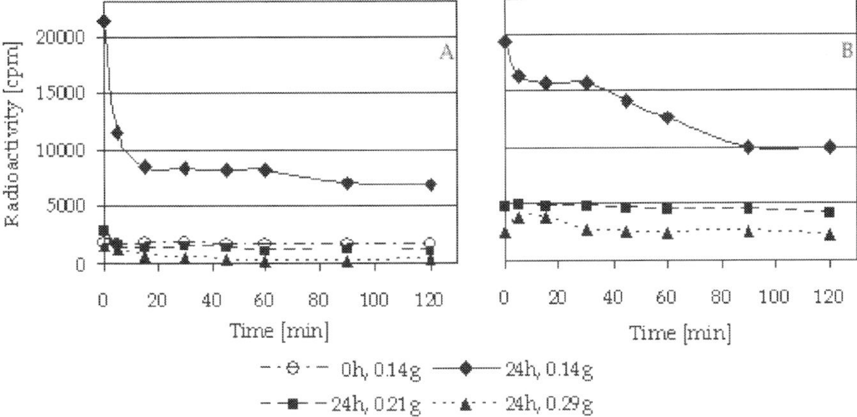

Fig. 2. The influence of photooxidation time on BP density, evaluated by radioactivity of the samples of various weights (0.14, 0.21, 0.29 g) (A); filtrates penetrating these samples (B).

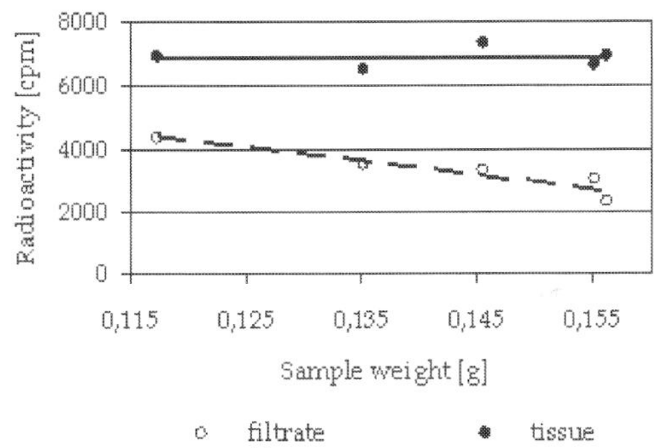

Fig. 3. Radioactivity of the GA-treated BP samples and filtrates penetrating these samples.

Sample weight (mg)	Specific radioactivity [cpm/mg]					
	Tissue samples			Filtrate the tissue samples		
	Native	Photooxidized	GA-treated	Native	Photooxidized	GA-treated
120	-*	-*	57	-*	-*	36
140	139	72	49	152	49	24
160	-*	-*	42	-*	-*	17
210	23	20	-*	14	5	-*
290	9	8	-*	5	1	-*

Table 1. Specific radioactivity of BP samples and filtrates penetrating these samples (* - not measured).

It seemed to be worth recalculating data concerning the tissue samples' permeability to $^{60}Co^{2+}$ and the ions' binding in the tissues in reference to the samples mass. Thus, the values of investigated samples specific radioactivity have been obtained (Table 1).

Almost directly proportional dependence between ^{60}Co-specific activities in crosslinked BP samples (indicative of bound ions) and filtrates penetrating these tissues (indicative of free ions) has been presented in Fig. 4.

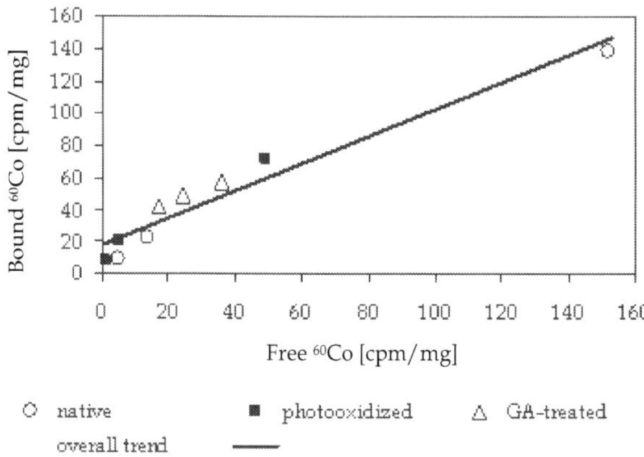

Fig. 4. Dependence between ^{60}Co-specific activities in crosslinked BP samples (bound ions) and filtrates penetrating these tissue samples (free ions).

5.2 The influence of methylene blue-mediated photooxidation on mechanical properties of porcine pericardium

MB-mediated photooxidation leads to significant changes in mechanical properties of modified PP in comparison with native tissue. They are shown in Figure 5 as F_b changes during the PP samples testing, where the most characteristic pictures selected from each series of samples are presented. All F_b–time curves are non-linear and their function graphs are asymmetrical. In case of the modified tissues, wider peaks in the curves were observed. Besides, higher differentiation between graphs representing individual samples in the group of the modified materials was observed than between graphs representing samples of native tissue.

Statistical calculations of F_b have been shown in Table 2. Arithmetic mean and standard deviation of F_b values obtained for six native tissue samples were 1.1±0.13 kG, pointing to their moderate variability (V=11.8%). About three times higher coefficient of variability (V=29.7%) has been calculated for the group of six samples MB-treated without irradiation, where arithmetic mean and standard deviation were 1.18±0.35 kG. The Measured F_b values ranged from 0.6 to 1.7 kG.

The difference between the group of these samples and the group of native tissue samples was not statistically significant. In case of nine samples exposed to MB-action combined with irradiation for 8 h, the mean value of F_b was 0.88±0.16 kG, with coefficient of variability V=18.2%. Prolonged irradiation (24 h) led to the inconsiderable decrease of F_b mean value (0.75±0.19 kG) calculated for eight samples, with coefficient of variability V=25.3%. Results obtained for both groups of irradiated samples treated with MB were statistically different from the group of native tissue samples.

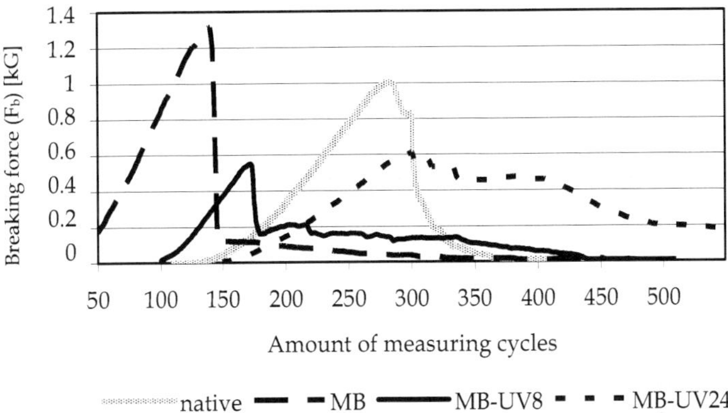

Fig. 5. Breaking force (F_b) measured for tissue samples: native (N); exposed to MB without irradiation (MB); and photooxidized for 8 h (MB-VIS 8) or 24 h (MB-VIS 24).

Sample No.	Breaking force F_b (Kg)			
	N	MB	MB-VIS 8	MB-VIS 24
1	1.0	1.1	0.9	0.8*
2	1.2	1.7	0.7	0.5
3	1.0	0.6	0.9	0.8
4	1.1	1.2*	0.9	0.9
5	1.3	1.2	1.1	0.9
6	1.0*	1.3	1.1	1.0
7			0.8	0.5
8			0.9	0.6
9			0.6*	
X	1.10	1.18	0.88	0.75
SD	0.13	0.35	0.16	0.19
V(%)	11.8	29.7	18.2	25.3
t-Student test (α=0.05)		SNS	SS	SS

Table 2. Breaking force (F_b) measured for pericardial tissues: native (N); exposed to MB without irradiation (MB), and photooxidized for 8 h (MB-VIS 8) or 24 h (MB-VIS 24); X – arithmetic mean; SD – standard deviation; V – coefficient of variability; SS – statistically significant; SNS – statistically not significant; * – values presented in the Figure 5.

5.3 Biochemical and morphological changes in porcine pericardium after riboflavin-mediated photooxidation

The influence of RF-mediated photooxidation on biochemical and morphological features reflecting stability of PP structure has been investigated. Changes in structure stability of the collagenous tissue can be reflected by changes in number of polypeptides of various molecular weight, which are released from photomodified tissues as compared with the native tissue. The electrophoretic profiles of polypeptides extracted from native pericardium and tissues treated with the RF in the presence of VIS light have been shown in Figure 6. Electrophoretic profiles of peptides extracted from all samples indicate similar patterns in range of the molecular weights of 15-160 kDa. Polypeptides of the highest molecular weights (above 200 kDa) were released from native tissue (Fig. 6, line 2) and RF-treated tissues irradiated for 1 h (Fig. 6, line 3). When PP was photooxidized for increasing periods, there was an increase in quantity of polypeptides extracted from the tissues. The peptide bands did not change in quality, although their intensities were increased with longer irradiation time (Fig. 6, lines 2; 4; 5).

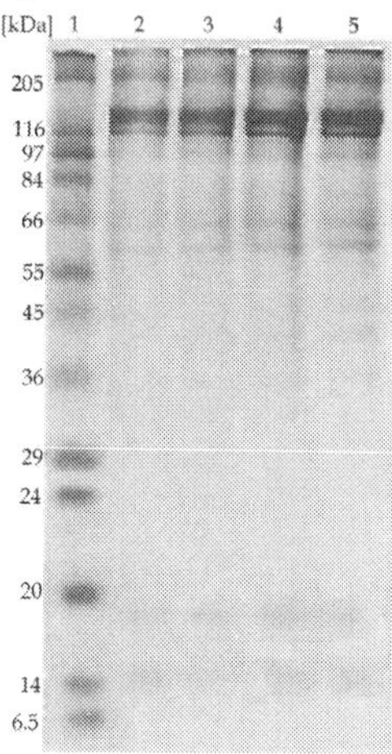

Fig. 6. Electrophoretic profiles of polypeptides extracted from PP samples. Lines: 1 – molecular weight standard; 2 – native tissue; 3; 4; 5 – tissues treated with RF and photooxidized during 1, 2 or 3 h, respectively.

Histological images of the investigated pericardium have been shown in Figures 7-10. Native tissue indicates tight structure with small slits in extracellular matrix. Correct aggregations of fiber bundles of various size and fibroblast nuclei are visible (Fig. 7). The structure of native tissue (Fig. 7) is considerably different from tissue samples treated with RF and VIS-irradiated samples for 1, 2 and 3 h (Fig. 8-10, respectively). Gradual evanishment of some morphological features in the tissues modified by RF-mediated photooxidation was observed as a result of the irradiation period prolongation. After irradiation during 1 h, homogeneous structure of tissue was observed. Moreover, degradation of fibrous structure of pericardium tissue and the disintegration of fibroblast nuclei was noted (Fig. 8). Additionally, after longer RF-mediated photomodification of the tissues a decrease in their cellularity was observed as a result of cell nuclei progressive loss (Fig. 9). After 3 h modification, looser extracellular matrix with evident slits in the tissue structure was visible. Moreover, a lack of fibroblast nuclei as well as the matrix perforation was observed (Fig. 10).

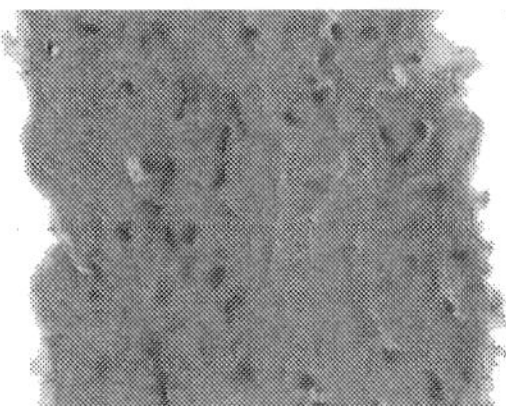

Fig. 7. Native tissue

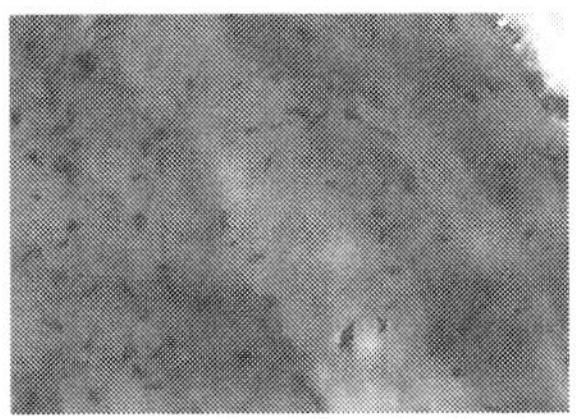

Fig. 8. Tissue treated with riboflavin and light during 1 h.

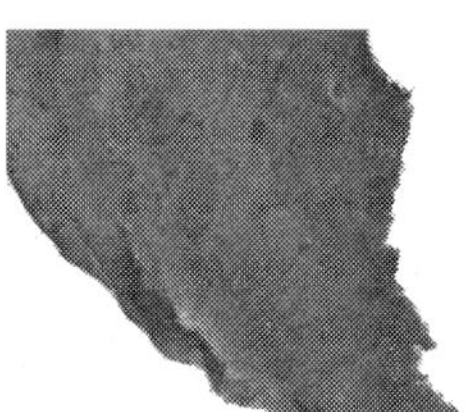

Fig. 9. Tissue treated with riboflavin and light during 2 h.

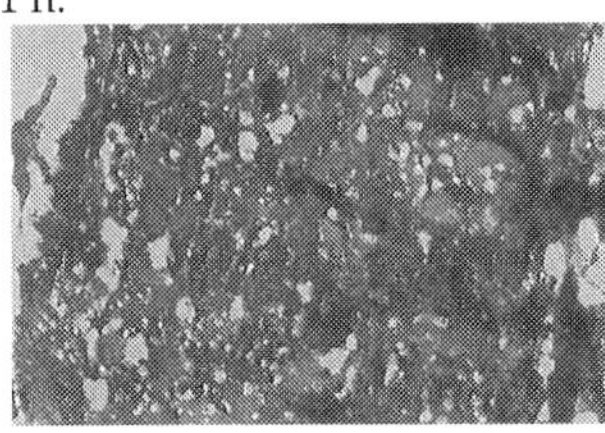

Fig. 10. Tissue treated with riboflavin and light during 3 h.

5.4 Biochemical and morphological changes in porcine pericardium irradiated by visible or ultraviolet light

The influence of the PP irradiation with UV or VIS light on electrophoretic profiles of polypeptides extracted from tissues has been shown in the Figure 11. An electrophoretic pattern representing native tissue (Fig. 11, line 2) comprises of polypeptides with molecular weights of 16-213 kDa. Non significant qualitative and quantitative changes were observed after SDS/NaCl extraction between electrophoretic profiles of tissues: native (Fig. 11, line 2) and irradiated (Fig. 11, lines 3-8).

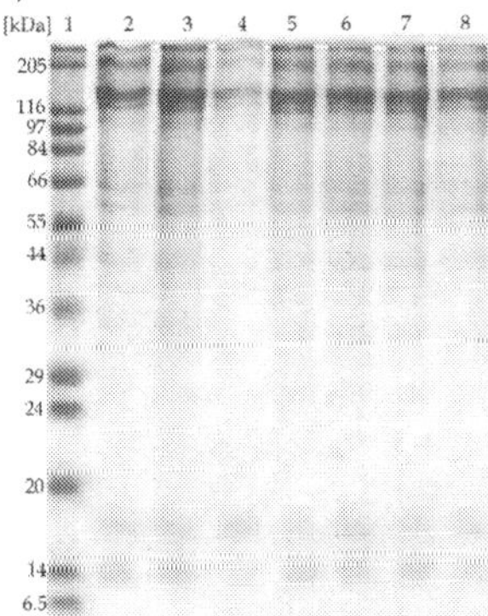

Fig. 11. Electrophoretic profiles of polypeptides extracted from the pericardium samples. Lines: 1 – molecular weight standard; 2 - native tissue; 3; 4; 5 - UV irradiated samples, during 1, 2 or 3 h, respectively; 6; 7; 8 – VIS irradiated samples, during 1, 2 or 3 h, respectively.

Moreover, changes in electrophoretic patterns of samples irradiated with UV and VIS light were also non-significant.

Significant differences were revealed in morphology of tissues irradiated by UV and VIS light. Particularly, it is worth noting the total evanishment of morphological features in the UV-irradiated tissues. Independently of UV-irradiation period, the degradation of PP-morphological components was shown. However, single fragments of connective tissue fibers may be identified. The lack of fibroblast nuclei and the intensive basophilia of extracellular matrix were observed (Fig. 12-14).

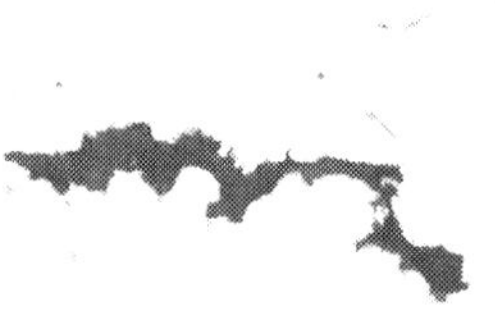

Fig. 12. Tissue irradiated with ultraviolet light during 1 h.

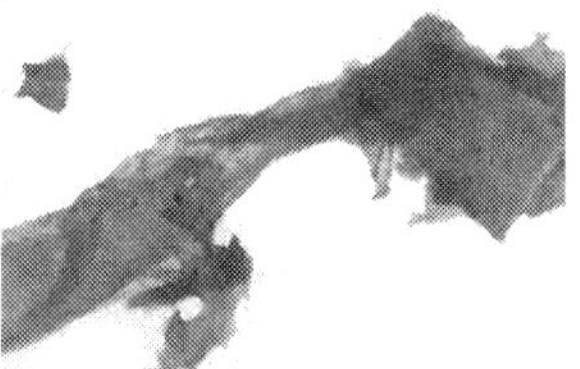

Fig. 13. Tissue irradiated with ultraviolet light during 2 h.

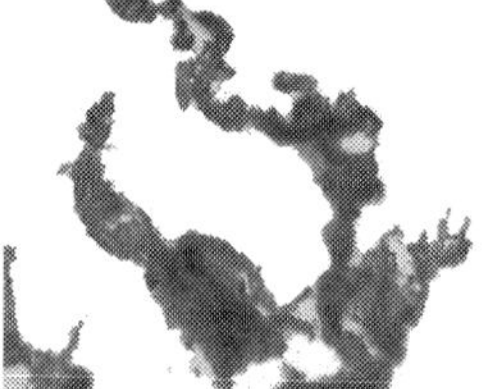

Fig. 14. Tissue irradiated with ultraviolet light during 3 h.

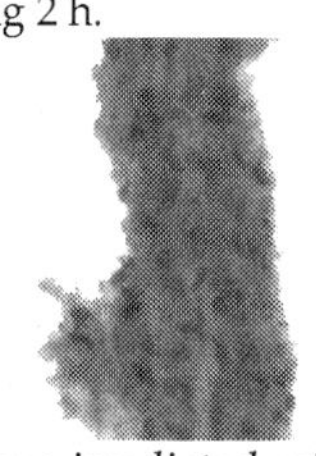

Fig. 15. Tissue irradiated with visible light during 1 h.

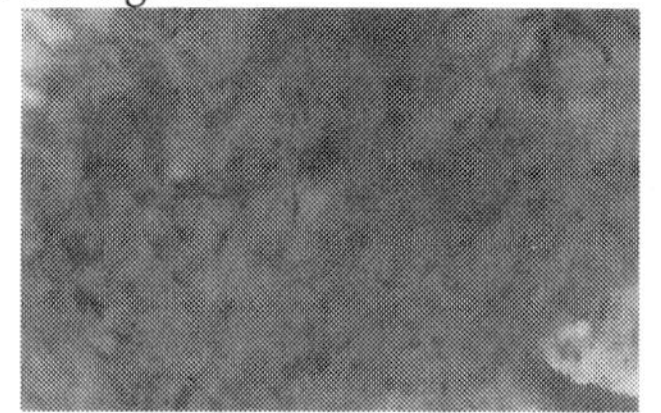

Fig. 16. Tissue irradiated with visible light during 2 h.

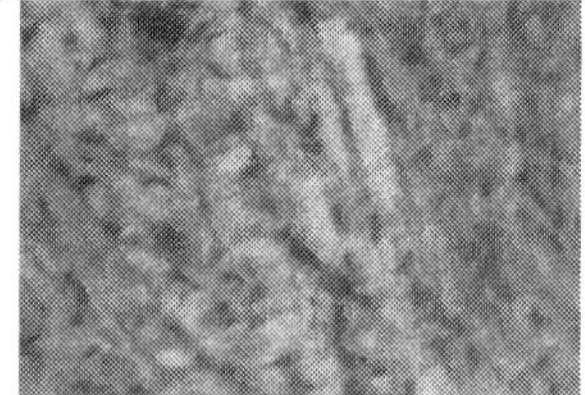

Fig. 17. Tissue irradiated with visible light during 3 h.

More favorable action to the tissue structure by VIS-irradiation was revealed. Irradiation during 1 h makes it possible to maintain fibroblast nuclei and partly fibrous structure (Fig. 15). The prolongation of irradiation period to 2 h and 3 h influences the nuclei disintegration and the appearance of significant swelling of connective tissue fibers (Fig. 16, 17). Diameter of single fibers in this tissue sample is increased as compared with the fibers of native tissue (Fig. 17).

5.5. Effect of tannic acid and UV-irradiation interactions on the biochemical features of porcine pericardium

The electrophoretic profiles of polypeptides stained with CBB or silver, extracted from native and TA-stabilized tissues before and after their irradiation with UV and digestion with P were shown in Figure 18 A and B.

Electrophoretic profiles representing tissues modified with TA and UV-irradiation (Fig. 18. A and B, lines 5, 6, 7) or only UV-irradiated (Fig. 18 A and B, line 3) revealed no significant quantitative changes as compared with native tissues, although some different polypeptides are visualized as the additional bands whereas the other bands are missing in particular lines representing adequate samples in the electrophoregrams obtained using two different staining methods (with CBB or silver). However, significant differences in tissues' structure were revealed in electrophoretic profiles of samples digested with P (Fig. 18 A and B, lines 4 and 8). Higher resistance to enzymatic digestion was shown for the sample modified by TA-crosslinking and UV-irradiation (Fig. 18 A and B, line 8). UV-irradiation and P-digestion of tissue resulted in its destroying and easier removing polypeptides of molecular weights lower than 66 kDa (Fig. 18 A and B, line 4).

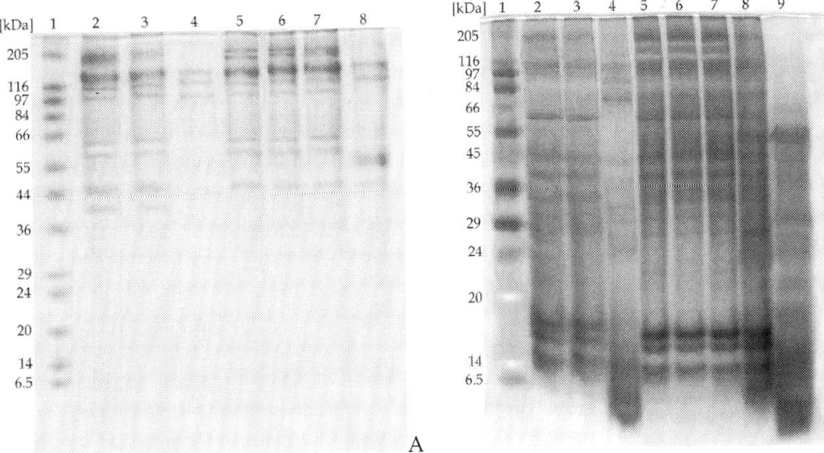

Fig. 18. Electrophoretic profiles of peptides extracted from porcine pericardium samples; A – polypeptides stained with CBB; B – polypeptides stained with silver. Lanes: 1 – molecular weight standard; 2 – native tissue; 3 – UV-irradiated tissue; 4 – UV-irradiated tissue, digested with P; 5 – tissue crosslinked with TA for 4 h and UV-irradiated; 6 – tissue crosslinked with TA for 24 h and UV-irradiated; 7 – tissue crosslinked with TA for 48 h and UV-irradiated; 8 – tissue crosslinked with TA for 4 h and UV-irradiated, digested with P; B – lane 9 – pancreatin.

6. Discussion

6.1. Influence of photomodification on pericardium density

Collagen is responsible for structural integration of collagenous tissues. In the tissue structure, collagen is organized with other proteins and other elements as fine-mesh sieve.

Collagen type I is the main component of pericardium. Density of this tissue is dependent on the crosslinking degree of collagen.

In this study, the BP stability after the MB-mediated photooxidation or GA-treatment was evaluated on the basis of the $^{60}Co^{2+}$ (in $^{60}CoCl_2$ solution) accumulation in the tissue samples as well as on the tissue samples permeability to $^{60}Co^{2+}$. It was shown that both of these characteristics may be useful to confirm the increase of tissue density, which is a result of crosslinking processes and may indicate the tissue fixation effects.

The reduced $^{60}Co^{2+}$-binding capacity in the photooxidized tissues (Fig. 2A) may be the evidence for the decrease in number of free bonding sites due to effective formation of intra- and intermolecular crosslinks between the protein particles in the tissue structure.

On the other hand, the decrease in the photooxidized tissue samples permeability to $^{60}Co^{2+}$ (Fig. 2B) may point to the modified tissue acting as a "molecular sieve" of higher density, in comparison with the native tissue density. The tissues lower binding ability and permeability to $^{60}Co^{2+}$ were attributed both to their higher compactness and thickness.

The ^{60}Co radioactivity in filtrates penetrating the GA-treated tissue samples were also mass-dependent, whereas the cobalt ions accumulation in these tissues was not (Fig. 3).

Changes in the samples' specific activities (Table 1) confirm the mass-dependent increase of the crosslinked tissues compactness as well as their decrease in binding capacities. The specific radioactivity values calculated for tissue-bound and free $^{60}Co^{2+}$ were almost directly proportional regardless of the crosslinking process or the lack of it (Fig. 4).

Concluding, it may be stated that the fixation effects in photomodified pericardium depend on the tissue thickness and time of its exposition to the light and dye. The exposition time is of special importance in case of the thin tissues photooxidation.

6.2. Assessment of mechanical properties of modified pericardium

Mechanical properties of collagenous connective tissues are related to their hierarchical structure, in which type I collagen plays one of the most important role. Pericardium is the tissue consisting mostly of type I collagen. The tensile strength of collagen fibers is the result of the presence of covalent crosslinks. Crosslinking changes the mechanical properties of collagenous materials (Kato & Silver, 1990; Olde Damink et al., 1996; Caruso & Dunn, 2004). It was shown that crosslinking of collagen causes an increase of the elastic modulus and the failure stress of this protein (van der Rijt, 2004).

In our study, the photooxidation of pericardium in the presence of MB resulted in significant changes of mechanical properties after 8 and 24 h modification (Fig. 5; Table 2). Incubation with dye (without irradiation) did not cause significant changes. F_b measured for the photooxidized pericardium was lower. Other authors showed that the breaking stress of individual collagen fibrils increased to 30% after crosslinking by carbodiimide with the N-hydroxysuccinimide and 22% after crosslinking by GA (Yang et al., 2008). However, physical processes and chemical agents influence the mechanical properties in various ways. Moreover different effects after modification of isolated collagen fibers and collagenous tissues may be obtained.

In the studies of Butterfield and Fisher (2000), the failures of heart valves made of photooxidized BP were attributed to this material increased abrasiveness. In our studies, lower F_b measured for MB-mediated tissues as compared with native tissues may correspond to these results. However, Suh et al. (1998) demonstrated that UV-iradiation of the collagen in porcine heart valves led to improvement of their mechanical properties and that this effect was the most advantageous after 24 h UV-exposition.

Generally, the dye-mediated photooxidation is the stabilization method which bases on catalysis of the processes of additional crosslinks formation in all proteins. In case of connective tissues irradiation, border between photostabilization and photodegradation effects may be fluid and it depends on reaction conditions. Undoubtedly, during dye-mediated photooxidation new crosslinks are formed. However, native crosslinks may be influenced by photolysis.

6.3. Assessment of the stability of pericardium photooxidized in the presence of riboflavin

This assessment of the tissue stability was evaluated by the measurement of quantity of polypeptides extracted with SDS/NaCl from PP using the Laemmli method (1970). The quantity of the proteins is inversely proportional to the extent of the tissue stability (McIlroy et al., 1997).

In electrophoretic profiles presented in Figure 6, the time dependent increase in content of peptides indicating almost the same molecular weights in all the tissues tested (both native and modified) has been observed. Surprisingly, the obtained results suggest that modified tissues did not possess the stable structure; the pericardium treatment with RF in the presence of VIS light and atmospheric oxygen resulted in swelling of the tissue structure. This effect was visible as early as after 2 h of the tissue photomodification. It may be due to the aeration of tissues during their treatment. The inhibitory effect of dissolved oxygen on the modification of collagen was also observed by other authors (Kato et al., 1994).

Microscopic observations show disappearances of fibrous structure as well as gradual broadening of extracellular matrix and decrease in cellularity of the tissues modified for 1 and 2 h (Fig. 8 and 9), as compared with the native material (Fig. 7). After 3 h of the tissue treatment, very loose extracellular matrixes as well as evident slits in tissue structure were observed (Fig. 10).

A reason for the cells damage may be the dynamic formation of reactive oxygen species such as superoxide anion, hydrogen peroxide, and the hydroxyl radical in the reaction mixture (Akiba et al., 1994; Sarkar et al., 1997). An electron transfer from the sensitizer triplet state to molecular oxygen is the usual pathway of superoxide anion formation in oxygenated aqueous solutions (Fernadez et al., 1997). On the other hand, it has been shown that UV irradiation of the collagen solution causes the loss of the protein ability to form natural fibrils (Fujimori, 1965). It is possible, that RF-mediated photooxidaton in the presence of VIS light causes the damage of collagen fibrils which build the tissue structure, leading to the effect observed in the Figures 6, 8-10.

Obtained results suggest that tissues modified by RF-mediated photooxidation may be used as biodegradable materials.

6.4. Assessment of the stability of pericardium modified by visible and ultraviolet light

The crosslinking processes catalysed by VIS or UV light do not introduce the exogenous chemical reagents into the structure of proteins (mainly of collagen) and tissular biomaterials, enabling elimination of the disadvantages resulted from the GA-treatment. However, during UV-irradiation both crosslinking and fragmentation of collagen helixes take place. The domination of one of these effects results from process conditions, including the exposure period and distance between light source and collagenous material. The collagen form is also significant in the processing of materials containing this protein (Kaminska & Sionkowska, 1996; Cwalina et al., 2003). Different irradiation effects may be obtained by photomodification of freeze-dried collagen, hydrated collagen and collagenous tissues.

In our studies, the same proteins were extracted from all investigated tissue samples, native and VIS- or UV-treated. Non significant changes in electrophoretic patterns between samples irradiated with UV and VIS light were observed. Thus, electrophoretic studies did not reveal biochemical changes (Fig. 11). However, histological images of the UV-irradiated samples showed the disappearance of tissue structure and the intensive basophilia (Fig. 12-14). Similar effects were observed in case of the VIS-treated samples. Morphological changes point to the processes of the tissue photodegradation during its irradiation without the protective action of dye (Fig. 15-17).

These results indicate that the collagen photomodification in the presence of VIS or UV light may be suitable for obtaining collagenous sponges.

6.5. Influence of ultraviolet irradiation on the stability of tannic acid-crosslinked pericardium

UV-irradiation causes increase in the durability of collagenous materials. However, this method is not as effective as GA treatment at reducing biodegradation. The structure of UV-modified collagenous materials may be strengthened by synergistic interaction of UV-irradiation with TA. This synergistic effect of physical (UV-irradiation) and chemical (TA-treatment) stabilization may be reached by two mechanisms. Firstly, TA belongs to chemical crosslinking reagents. In comparison with GA, TA is less cytotoxic (Insenburg et al, 2004) and does not accelerate tissue calcification (Insenburg et al., 2006). Moreover, TA-modification leads to increase of tissues resistance to enzymatic degradation (Cwalina et al., 2005) and is effective as sterilization method (Latte & Kolodziej, 2000; Akiyama et al., 2001). Secondly, TA is composed of gallic acid residues and glucose molecules. It was demonstrated that the generation of free radicals in the residues of aromatic acids plays a key role in photomodification of collagenous materials (Cooper & Davidson, 1965; Fujimori, 1965). The introduction of additional aromatic residues of TA into the tissue may influence the increased efficiency of its modification. Collagen crosslinking by glucose is also taken into consideration. Moreover, Ohan et al. (2002) have showed that interactions during glucose-treatment and UV-irradiation give positive results in collagen modification.

In this work, the TA-treated PP was influenced by UV-irradiation. Taking into account that some combined treatments of collagenous tissues are effective in their structure stabilization, we expected beneficial effects due to proposed modification procedure including the TA-stabilization followed by UV-irradiation.

Comparison of the electrophoretic patterns (obtained after staining polypeptides with CBB and silver) of the native tissue, the UV-irradiated tissue, the same tissue after digestion with P for 3 h as well as the tissues treated with TA for 4, 24 or 48 h and then UV-irradiated did not confirm our expectations (Fig. 18 A and B). The CBB-stained gel (Fig. 18 A) seemed to indicate the TA-treated tissues crosslinking effect and their structure stability, which was reflected by the increase in number of polypeptides of higher molecular weights (Fig. 18 A). However, the silver-stained polypeptides patterns showed that the TA-crosslinked particles of high molecular weight were more hydrolyzed after UV-irradiation and digestion with P as compared with the native tissue (Fig. 18 B). Simultaneously, a concomitant increase in number of small polypeptides has been observed. Besides, the higher biochemical affinity of P to the TA-treated tissue structural components has been observed (Fig. 18 B). The results also suggest that crosslinked proteins separated from the TA-stabilized PP samples after their UV-irradiation were less tolerant to P-digestion than the native tissue samples.

Obtained results suggest that the TA may be used to attain the prolongation of biodegradation period in the UV-crosslinked collagenous sponges. Besides, release of TA during the sponge biodegradation may in additional way support the biomaterial healing effect on wounds.

6.6. Summary

Irradiation is one from amongst several physical treatments used for collagenous materials stabilization before their utilization in biomaterials. For valve prostheses production, BP and PP may be used. These tissues fixation by chemical substances alone or by their combinations with some physical methods is attributed to the crosslinks formation in proteins, mainly in the collagen. The tissues stabilized due to their crosslinking may act as molecular sieves of higher density in comparison with the native tissue. Increase in the tissues compactness is accompanied by the decrease in number of free bonding sites in structure of crosslinked tissue proteins. In this work it was shown that photooxidation of BP caused decrease in the tissue permeability to $^{60}Co^{2+}$ ions pointing to the tissue higher density. The fixation effects in the pericardium tissues after dye-mediated photooxidation depend on their thickness and time of exposition to the light and dye. The exposition time is of special importance in case of the thin tissues photooxidation. The mechanical properties of photomodified PP were statistically lower as compared with the native tissue. Lower F_b measured for photomodified tissues may result from co-occurrence of crosslinking and photodegradation processes. Both UV- and VIS-irradiation of PP, alone or in the presence of RF resulted in significant changes of the tissue morphological and biochemical features. Especially interesting results have been obtained after the PP treatment with TA and UV light. Such modified tissues were more stable to SDS/NaCl extraction and enzymatic digestion as compared with native (fresh) and UV-treated non-modified tissues.

7. Conclusions

In conclusion, photooxidation permit obtaining bioprostheses being non biodegradable as well as biodegradable biomaterials like collagen sponges. The TA may be used to attain the prolongation of biodegradation period in the UV-crosslinked collagenous sponges. Besides, release of TA during the sponge biodegradation may in additional way support the biomaterial healing effect on wounds.

8. References

Akiba, J., Ueno, N., Chakrabarti, B. (1994). Mechanisms of photo-induced vitreous liquefaction. *Curr Eye Res*, 13, 7, 505-512

Akiyama, H., Fujii, K., Yamasaki, O., Oono, T., Iwatsuki, K. (2001). Antibacterial action of several tannins against *Staphylococcus aureus*. *J Antimicrob Chemother*, 48, 4, 487-91

Au, V., Madison, S.A. (2000). Effects of singlet oxygen on the extracellular matrix protein collagen: oxidation of the collagen crosslink histidinohydroxylysinonorleucine and histidine. *Arch Biochem Biophys*, 384, 1, 133-42

Bengtsson, L.A., Phillips, R., Haegerstrand, A.N. (1995). *In vitro* endothelialization of photooxidatively stabilized xenogeneic pericardium. *Ann Thorac Surg*, 60, (2 Suppl), S365-8

Bernstein, P.H., Mechanic, G.L. (1980). A natural histidine-based imminium cross-link in collagen and its location. *J Biol Chem*, 255, 21, 10414-22

Bianco, R.W., Phillips, R., Mrachec, J., Witson, J. (1996). Feasibility evaluation of a new pericardial bioprosthesis with dye mediated photo-oxidized bovine pericardial tissue. *J Heart Valve Dis*, 5, 3, 317-22

Butterfield, M., Fisher, J. (2000). Fatigue analysis of clinical bioprosthetic heart valves manufactured using photooxidized bovine pericardium. *J Heart Valve Dis*, 9, 1, 161-6

Carpentier, A., Lemaigre, G., Robert, L., Carpentier, S., Dubost, C. (1969). Biological factors affecting long-term results of valvular heterografts. *J Thorac Cardiovasc Surg*, 58, 4, 467-83

Caruso, A.B., Dunn, M.G. (2004). Functional evaluation of collagen fiber scaffolds for ACL reconstruction: cyclic loading in proteolytic enzyme solutions. *J Biomed Mater Res A*, 69, 1, 164-71

Chan, B.P., So, K.F. (2005). Photochemical crosslinking improves the physiochemical properties of collagen scaffolds. *J Biomed Mater Res A*, 75, 3, 689-701

Chan, B.P., So, K.F. (2008). Photochemically crosslinked collagen scaffolds and methods for their preparation. *Patent US 7393437*

Chan, O.C., So, K.F., Chan, B.P. (2008a). Fabrication of nano-fibrous collagen microspheres for protein delivery and effects of photochemical crosslinking on release kinetics. *J Control Release*, 129, 2, 135-43

Chan, B.P., Chan, O.C., So, K.F. (2008b). Effects of photochemical crosslinking on the microstructure of collagen and a feasibility study on controlled protein release. *Acta Biomater*, 4, 6, 1627-36

Cooper, D.R., Davidson, R.J. (1965). The effect of ultraviolet irradiation on soluble collagen. *Biochem J*, 97, 1, 139-47

Cwalina, B., Turek, A., Miskowiec, M., Nawrat, Z., Domal-Kwiatkowska, D. (2002). Biochemical stability of pericardial tissues modified using glutaraldehyde or formaldehyde. *Engineering of Biomaterials*, 23-25, 64-67

Cwalina, B., Turek, A., Nozynski, J., Jastrzebska, M. (2003). Effect of ultraviolet radiation and visible light on structure of porcine pericardium tissue. *Engineering of Biomaterials*, 30-33, 85-88

Cwalina, B., Turek, A., Nozynski, J., Jastrzebska, M., Nawrat, Z. (2005). Structural changes in pericardium tissue modified with tannic acid. *Int J Artif Organs*, 28, 6, 648-53

Cwalina, B., Bogacz, A., Turek, A. (2000). The influence of proteins modification on pericardial tissue permeability to cobalt ions. In: *Wave Methods and Mechanics in Biomedical Engineering*, Panuszka R., Iwaniec M. & Reron E. (Ed.), 115-118, Polish Acoustical Society, Cracow de Visscher, G., Blockx, H., Meuris, B., van Oosterwyck, H., Verbeken, E., Herregods, M.C., Flameng, W. (2008). Functional and biochemical evaluation of a completely recellularized stentless pulmonary bioprosthesis in sheep. *J Thorac Cardiovasc Surg*, 135, 2, 395-404

Fernandez, J.M., Bilgin, M.D., Grossweiner, L.I. (1997). Singlet oxygen generation by photodynamic agents. *J Photochem Photobiol B*, 37, 131-40

Fujimori, E. (1965). Ultraviolet light-induced change in collagen macromolecules *Biopolymers*, 3, 2, 115-9

Gelse, K., Poschl, E., Aigner, T. (2003). Collagens-structure, functions, and biosynthesis. *Adv Drug Deliv Rev*, 55, 12, 1531-46

Gendler, E., Gendler, S., Nimni, M.E. (1984). Toxic reactions evoked by glutaraldehyde-fixed pericardium and cardiac valve tissue bioprosthesis. *J Biomed Mater Res*, 18, 7, 727-36

Golomb, G., Schoen, F.J., Smith, M.S., Linden, J., Dixon, M., Levy, R.J. (1987). The role of glutaraldehyde-induced cross-links in calcification of bovine pericardium used in cardiac valve bioprosthesis. *Am J Pathol*, 127, 1, 122-30

Gowri, C., Thomas, K.T. (1969). Photooxidation of collagen in the presence of methylene blue. *Leather Sci*, 16, 8, 297-300

Gurnani, S., Arifuddin, M., Augusti, K.T. (1966). Effect of visible light on amino acids. I. Tryptophan. *Photochem Photobiol*, 5, 7, 495-505

Halliwell, B., Gutteridge, J.M. (1990). Role of free radicals and catalytic metal ions in human disease: an overview. *Methods Enzymol*, 186, 1-85

Hetherington, V.J., Kawalec J.S., Dockery, D.S., Targoni, O.S., Lehmann P.V., Nadler D. (2005). Immunologic testing of xeno-derived osteochondral grafts using peripheral blood mononuclear cells from healthy human donors. *BMC Musculoskelet Disord*, 6, 36

Hetherington, V.J., Kawalec-Carroll, J.S., Nadler, D. (2007). Qualitative histological evaluation of photooxidized bovine osteochondral grafts in rabbits: a pilot study. *J Foot Ankle Surg*, 46, 4, 223-9

Huang-Lee, L.L., Cheung, D.T., Nimni, M.E. (1990). Biochemical changes and cytotoxicity associated with the degradation of polymeric glutaraldehyde derived crosslinks. *J Biomed Mater Res*, 24, 9, 1185-201

Ionescu, M.I., Smith, D.R., Hasan, S.S., Chidambaram, M., Tandon A.P. (1982). Clinical durability of the pericardial xenograft valve: ten years experiments with mitral replacement. *Ann Thorac Surg*, 34, 3, 265-77

Isenburg, J.C., Karamchandani, N.V., Simionescu, D.T., Vyavahare, N.R. (2006). Structural requirements for stabilization of vascular elastin by polyphenolic tannins. *Biomaterial*, 27, 19, 3645-51

Isenburg, J.C., Simionescu, D.T., Vyavahare, N.R. (2004). Elastin stabilization in cardiovascular implants: improved resistance to enzymatic degradation by treatment with tannic acid. *Biomaterials*, 25, 16, 3293-302

Jastrzebska, M., Barwinski, B., Mroz, I., Turek, A., Zalewska-Rejdak, J., Cwalina, B. (2005). Atomic force microscopy investigation of chemically stabilized pericardium tissue. *Eur Phys J E Soft Matter*, 16, 4, 381 8

Jayakrishnan, A., Jameela, S.R. (1996). Glutaraldehyde as a fixation in bioprostheses and drug delivery matrices. *Biomaterials*, 17, 5, 417-84

Kaminska, A., Sionkowska, A. (1996). The effect of UV radiation on the thermal parameters of collagen degradation. *Polym Deg Stab*, 51, 1, 15-18

Kato, Y., Uchida, K., Kawakishi, S. (1994). Aggregation of collagen exposed to UVA in the presence of riboflavin: a plausible role of tyrosine modification. *Photochem Photobiol*, 59, 3, 343-9

Kato, Y.P., Silver, F.H. (1990). Formation of continuous collagen fibres: evaluation of biocompatibility and mechanical properties. *Biomaterials*, 11, 3, 169-75

Kawalec-Carroll, J.S., Hetherington, V.J., Dockery, D.S., Shive, C., Targoni, O.S., Lehmann, P.V., Nadler, D., Prins, D. (2006). Immunogenicity of unprocessed and photooxidized bovine and human osteochondral grafts in collagen-sensitive mice. *BMC Musculoskelet Disord*, 7, 32

Khor, E. (1997). Methods for the treatment of collagenous tissue for bioprotheses. *Biomaterials*, 18, 2, 95-105

Laemmli, U.K. (1970). Cleavage of structural proteins during the assembly of the head of bacteriophage T4. *Nature*, 227, 5259, 680-5

Latte, K.P., Kolodziej, H. (2000). Antifungal effects of hydrolysable tannins and related compounds on dermatophytes, mould fungi and yeasts. *Z Naturforsch [C]*, 55, 5-6, 467-72

Levy, R.J., Schoen, F.J., Anderson, H.C., Harasaki, H., Koch, T.H., Brown, W., Lian, J.B., Cumming, R., Gavin, J.B. (1991). Cardiovascular implant calcification: a survey and update. *Biomaterials*, 12, 8, 707-714

McIlroy, B.K., Robinson, M.D., Chen, WM., Moore, M.A. (1997). Chemical modification of bovine tissues by dye-mediated photooxidation. *J Heart Valve Dis*, 6, 4, 416-23

Mechanic, G.L. (1994). Cross-linking collagenous product. *Patent US 5332475*

Moczar, M., Mazzucotelli, J.P., Bertrand P., Ginat M., Leandri J., Loisance D. (1994). Deterioration of bioprosthetic heart valves. *ASAIO J*, 40, 3, M697-M701

Moore, M.A. (1997). Pericardial tissue stabilized by dye-mediated photooxidation: a review article. *J Heart Valve Dis*, 6, 5, 521-6

Moore, M.A., Bohachevsky, I.K., Cheung, D.T., Boyan, B.D., Chen, W.M., Bickers, R.R., McIlroy, B.K. (1994). Stabilization of pericardial tissue by dye-mediated photooxidation. *J Biomed Mater Res*, 28, 5, 611-8

Moore, M.A., Chen, W.M., Phillips, R.E., Bohachevsky, I.K., McIlroy, B.K. (1996). Shrinkage temperature versus protein extraction as a measure of stabilization of photooxidized tissue. *J Biomed Mater Res*, 32, 2, 209-14

Moore, M.A., McIlroy B.K., Phillips R.E. (1997). Nonaldehyde sterilization of biologic tissue for use in implantable medical devices. *ASAIO J*, 43, 1, 23-30

Moore, M.A., Phillips, R.E. (1997). Biocompatibility and immunologic properties of pericardial tissue stabilized by dye-mediated photooxidation. *J Heart Valve Dis*, 6, 3, 307-15

Neumann, N.P., Moore, S., Stein, W.H. (1962). Modification of the methionine residues in ribonuclease. *Biochemistry*, 1, 68-75

Nimni, M.E., Cheung, D., Strates, B., Kodama, M., Sheikh, K. (1987). Chemically modified collagen: a natural biomaterial for tissue replacement. *J Biomed Mater Res*, 21, 6, 741-71

Ohan, M.P., Weadock, K.S., Dunn, M.G. (2002). Synergistic effects of glucose and ultraviolet irradiation on the physical properties of collagen. *J Biomed Mater Res*, 60, 3, 384-91

Olde Daminink, L.H., Dijkstra, P.J., van Luyn, M.J., van Wachem, P.B., Nieuwenhuis, P., Feijen, J. (1996). Cross-linking of dermal sheep collagen using a water-soluble carbodiimide. *Biomaterials*, 17, 8, 765-73

Paneth, M., O'Brien M.F. (1966). Transplantation of human homograft aortic valve. *Thorax*, 21, 2, 115-7

Ramshaw, J.A., Stephens, L.J., Tulloch, P.A. (1994). Methylene blue sensitized photo-oxidation of collagen fibrils. *Biochem Biophis Acta*, 1206, 2, 225-30

Reardon, M.J., O'Brien, M.F. (1997). Allograft valves for aortic and mitral valve replacement. *Curr Opin Cardiol*, 12, 2, 114-22

Sarkar, B., Das, U., Bhattacharyya, S., Bose, S.K. (1997). Studies on the aerobic photooxidation of cysteine using riboflavin as a sensitizer: evidence for the photogeneration of a superoxide anion and hydrogen peroxide. *Biol Pharm Bull*, 20, 8, 910-12

Sionkowska, A. (2000). The influence of methylene blue on the photochemical stability of collagen. *Polym Deg Stab*, 67, 1, 79-83

Spikes, J.D., Straight, R. (1967). Sensitized photochemical processes in biological systems. *Annu Rev Phys Chem*, 18, 409-36

Stone, K.R. (2006). Immunochemically modified and sterilized xenografts and allografts. *Patent US 20070010897*

Suh, H., Hwang, Y.S., Park, J.C., Cho, B.K. (2000). Calcification of leaflets from porcine aortic valves crosslinked by ultraviolet irradiation. *Artif Organs*, 24, 7, 555-63

Suh, H., Lee, W.K., Park, J.C., Cho, B.K. (1999). Evaluation of the cross-linking in UV irradiated porcine valves. *Yonsei Med J*, 40, 2, 159-65

Suh, H., Park, J.C., Kim, K.T., Lee, W.K., Cho, B.K. (1998). Mechanical properties of the UV irradiated porcine valves. *J Biomat Res*, 2, 3, 95-9

Thoma, R.J., Phillips, R.E. (1995). The role of material surface chemistry in implant device calcification: a hypothesis. *J Heart Valve Dis*, 4, 3, 214-21

Tomita, M., Irie, M., Ukita, T. (1969). Sensitized photooxidation of histidine and its derivatives. Products and mechanism of the reaction. *Biochemistry*, 8, 12, 5149-60

Turek, A., Cwalina, B., Pawlus-Lachecka, L., Dzierzewicz, Z. (2007). Influence of tannic acid and penicillin on pericardium proteins stability. *Engineering of Biomaterials*, 69-72, 82-84

van der Rijt, J.A.J. (2004). Micromechanical testing of single collagen type I fibrils. Ph. D thesis, University of Twente, Enschede, The Netherlands, ISBN 90-365-2082-7

Vesely, I. (2003). The evolution of bioprosthetic heart valve design and its impact on durability. *Cardiovasc Pathol*, 12, 5, 277-86

Weadock, K.S., Miller, E.J., Bellincampi, L.D., Zawadsky, J.P., Dunn M.G. (1995). Physical crosslinking of collagen fibers: comparison of ultraviolet irradiation and dehydrothermal treatment. *J Biomed Mater Res*, 29, 11, 1373-9

Weadock, K.S., Miller, E.J., Keuffel, E.J., Dunn, M.G. (1996). Effect of physical crosslinking methods on collagen-fiber durability in proteolytic solution. *J Biomed Mater Res*, 32, 2, 221-6

Weil, L., Burchert, A.R., Maher, J. (1952). Photooxidation of crystalline lysozyme in the presence of methylene blue and its reaction to enzymatic activity. *Arch Biochem Biophys*, 40, 2, 245-52

Weil, L., Gordon, W.G., Burchert, A.R. (1951). Photooxidation of amino acids in the presence of methylene blue. *Arch Biochem,* 33, 1, 90-109

Weil, L., Seibles, T.S., Herskovits, T.T. (1965). Photooxidation of bovine insulin sensitized be methylene blue. *Arch Biochem Biophys,* 111, 2, 308-20

Westaby, S., Bianco, R.W., Katsumata, T., Termin, P. (1999). The Carbomedics "Oxford" Photofix stentless valve (PSV). *Semin Thorac Cardiovasc Surg,* 11, 4 Suppl 1, 206-9

Woodroof, E.A. (1978). Use of glutaraldehyde and formaldehyde to process tissue heart valves. *J Bioeng,* 2, 1-2, 1-9

Yang, L., van der Werf, K.O., Fitie, C.F., Bennink, M.L., Dijkstra, P.J., Feijen, J. (2008). Micromechanical bending of single collagen fibrils using atomic force microscopy. *Biophys J,* 94, 6, 2204-11

30

Non-invasive Localized Heating and Temperature Monitoring based on a Cavity Applicator for Hyperthermia

Yasutoshi Ishihara[1], Naoki Wadamori[1] and Hiroshi Ohwada[2]
[1]Nagaoka University of Technology, [2]Niigata Sangyo University
Japan

1. Introduction

Hyperthermia, which heats cancer tissue to around 43 °C, is an effective therapeutic technique that is used with radiotherapy or carcinostatic procedures. However, the regression mechanism and therapeutic effect on cancer tissue are not always clear when heating is carried out independently. Moreover, some have expressed skepticism about the clinical value of hyperthermia (Perez et al., 1989; 1991). One reason for this is that it is difficult to heat a local region of a living body to the required temperature in clinical experiments. Furthermore, it has been pointed out that it is difficult to perform non-invasive and precise measurements of the temperature change inside a target object. Currently, therefore, the effect of hyperthermia on cancer tissue in a living body cannot be accurately evaluated and analyzed. Thus, unfortunately, it is sometimes concluded that hyperthermia essentially has few therapeutic effects on cancer.

Hence, it is indispensable to develop an integrated system capable of both heating and quantitative temperature monitoring (temperature measurement) under *in-vivo* conditions in order to identify the factor that specifies the heat sensitivity of cancer tissue, to determine the mechanism of thermal necrosis, and to achieve a completely non-invasive cancer treatment.

Previously, various heat therapies have been proposed that apply wave energy from outside the body to selectively and non-invasively treat localized cancers. Some of these non-invasive methods involve the application of heat to object using dipole antennas (Turner, 1999; Wust et al., 2000) or patch antennas (Paulides et al., 2007a; 2007b) with different amplitudes and phases, or high-temperature thermal ablation using focused ultrasound (FUS) (Lynn et al., 1942; Hynynen et al., 2004; McDannold et al., 2006). Clinical experiments utilizing both methods have been conducted and some good results have been obtained. However, in the method that uses an array antenna, the localized heating of a deeper region is difficult as a relatively larger region can be heated due to the limitations of the electromagnetic wavelength, which, in principle, is determined according to the size of the antenna. Another drawback of this method is that a water bolus is required to prevent excess heating at the surface of the human body (Nadobny et al., 2005). On the other hand, it is difficult to apply the method that uses FUS to internal organs and tissues surrounded by bones due to the limitations of the characteristics of ultrasound.

In order to non-invasively heat a deep region in a human body, we have proposed a heating applicator that uses an electric field distribution generated by a reentrant cylindrical cavity (Fig. 1), which is widely used in microwave devices, such as cavity-based transducers (Tsubono et al., 1977), linear accelerators (Fujisawa 1958), and electron spin resonance (ESR) spectrometers (Giordano et al., 1983). A reentrant cylindrical cavity is a resonator in which inner cylinders (known as reentrant electrodes) are attached to the upper and lower sides of a cylindrical cavity. Since an intensive electric field is produced in the gap between these reentrant electrodes, a standing wave of the electric field distribution is formed in a heating object when it is placed in this gap, allowing a deep region in a living body to be heated effectively.

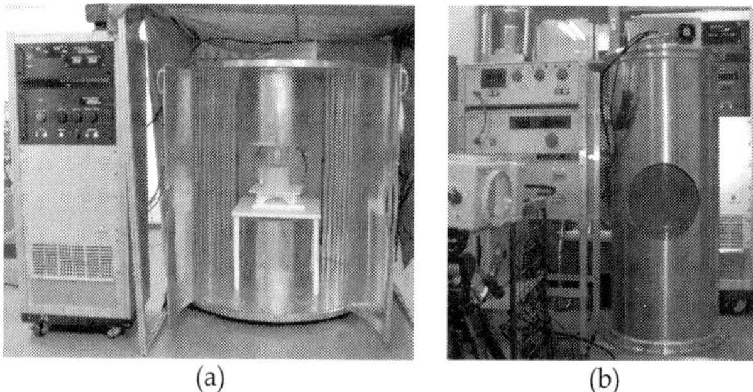

(a)   (b)

Fig. 1. Localized heating applicator based on a reentrant cylindrical cavity for abdominal organs (a), and head and neck (b).

Through numerical and experimental analyses, we have already reported that localized heating is possible with this method (Matsuda et al., 1988; Kato et al., 1989; 2003; Wadamori et al., 2004). Moreover, in order to improve the therapeutic effects for a localized cancer, we attempted to miniaturize the applicator (Ishihara et al., 2007a; 2008a), as well as optimize the size of the applicator by using experimental design methods (Ishihara et al., 2008b). As a result, we found that the electric field distribution generated between the reentrant electrodes can be localized within a spatial region with a diameter of 70–90 mm. However, when the subject of the treatment is a small cancer localized in the head or neck region, a localized region with a diameter of 30–50 mm must be selectively heated; and thus the heating characteristics achieved in the previous studies were still insufficient. To deal with this issue, we proposed rotating the beam-shaped electric field distribution generated by the reentrant cylindrical cavity, and showed that it is possible to produce focused localized heating by concentrating the electric field distribution in the region around the rotating axis (Ishihara et al., 2008c; 2009; Kameyama et al., 2008).

Thus, although investigations for heating systems are ongoing, the development of non-invasive thermometry is progressing slowly. In most cases during hyperthermia, therefore, only a thermocouple or an optical fiber type thermometer has been used to confirm the heating and treatment effect.

Recently, we proposed non-invasive thermometry using magnetic resonance imaging (MRI) (Ishihara et al., 1992; 1995; Kuroda et al., 1996). The internal temperature change in the object was imaged with a measurement error of less than 1 °C by measuring the water proton chemical shift change observed with MRI. This procedure is performed with a therapeutic device using the techniques mentioned above: focused ultrasound (McDannold et al., 2006) and radiofrequency (RF) waves (Gellermann et al., 2006), as an almost standard non-invasive temperature monitoring method during hyperthermia and cancer ablation treatments. However, a large setup and expensive MRI equipment are necessary for monitoring the temperature change.

Therefore, we focused on the changes in the electromagnetic field distribution inside the heating applicator based on a cavity with temperature changes, and proposed a new non-invasive thermometry method using the temperature dependence of the dielectric constant (Ishihara et al., 2007b; 2007c; Ohwada et al., 2009). Using this concept, after measuring the phase information of the electrical field inside a cavity spatially, an image of the temperature change distribution inside a body is reconstructed by applying the computed tomography (CT) algorithm (Gordon et al., 1970; Goitein 1972; Gordon 1974). Accordingly, since it is easy to fuse this temperature monitoring method with a heating applicator based on a cavity resonator, a novel integrated treatment system is achieved that treats cancer effectively while non-invasively monitoring the heating effect.

By a numerical analysis using a three-dimensional finite element method (FEM) and an experiment using the prototype heating applicator, this study demonstrated the possibility of focusing the electric field distribution by rotating the reentrant cylindrical cavity. The results indicated that when the beam-shaped electric field distribution formed in the reentrant gap was rotated, the heated region became more focused as compared to that without rotating the applicator. In addition, the reconstruction algorithm for the temperature change distribution is discussed in this paper and the efficacy of this method is shown by numerical analyses.

2. Localized heating method

2.1 Principle of the heating system with a reentrant cylindrical cavity

The principle of the heating applicator based on a reentrant cylindrical cavity is explained by the schematic diagram shown in Fig. 2. In this applicator, the reentrant electrodes are attached to the upper and lower sides of a cylindrical cavity. The RF power required for heating is supplied by the loop antenna attached to the upper surface of the cavity, and the characteristic electromagnetic field distribution is formed in a cavity resonator. This field distribution can be explained and compared with that of the conventional radio frequency (RF) capacitive heating system that is commonly used in clinics by using Fig. 3.

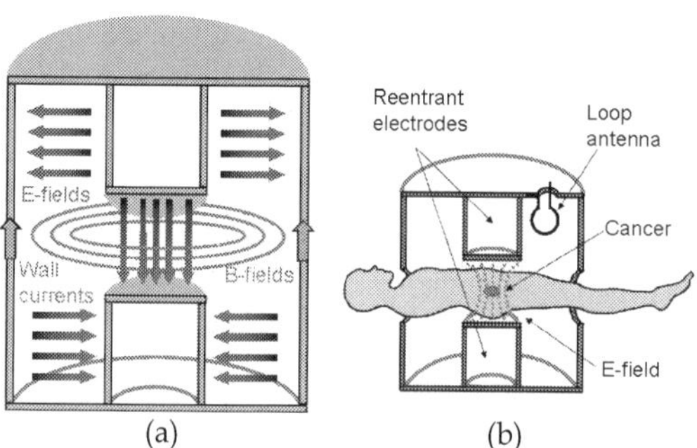

Fig. 2. Electromagnetic field distribution in a reentrant cylindrical cavity (a), and the setup for a heating target (b).

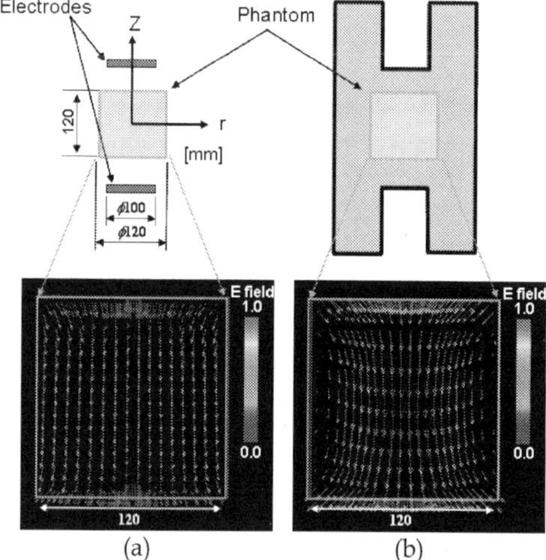

Fig. 3. Comparison of electric field distributions in a heating object between traditional capacitive heating system (a) and reentrant cylindrical cavity (b).

In an RF capacitive heating system, the electric field distribution is uniform between the electrodes along both the radius (r) and longitudinal (Z) axes; this distribution is expressed by Laplace's equation. Hence, not only the cancer tissue but also the healthy tissues located between the electrodes might become heated. In addition, the electric field tends to concentrate at the ends of the electrodes, and hence the tissues in these areas may be heated excessively; therefore, a water bolus is required to cool the surface of the human body in many cases during treatments. On the other hand, the electromagnetic distribution inside a cavity resonator is expressed by the Helmholtz equation (Eq. (1)). Further, when an electromagnetic distribution is formed inside a reentrant cylindrical cavity resonator with the lowest resonant mode, the electric field distribution is concentrated in the gap between the reentrant electrodes.

$$\Delta E + k^2 E = 0$$
$$\Delta H + k^2 H = 0 \tag{1}$$
$$k^2 = \omega^2 \varepsilon \mu$$

Here, Δ represents the Laplacian; E, the electric field vector; H, the magnetic field vector; ω, the angular frequency (rad/s); ε, the complex dielectric constant (F/m); and μ, the permeability (H/m). With this heating system, a standing wave will be generated and concentrated between the reentrant electrodes; further, the electric field strength is the highest at the center of the electrode, and decreases rapidly along the r-direction. In addition, since a standing wave of the electric field distribution is also formed in a heating object when it is placed between the reentrant electrodes, the electric field at the midpoint between the electrodes along the Z-direction will also be higher than that closer to the electrodes, unlike RF capacitive heating systems. Thus, by placing a treatment region between the reentrant electrodes for treatment, a deep lesion in a human body can be heated locally, noninvasively, and without contact. By using such a heating system, we confirmed that not only agar phantoms (cubical, oblate spherical, and human-like in shape) but also a dog brain could be heated locally (Kato et al., 2003; Wadamori et al., 2004; Ishihara et al., 2008b).

2.2 Focusing the electric field by rotating the applicator

If the electric field distribution between the reentrant electrodes can be further localized, it will be possible to achieve more localized heating compared to the use of the current applicators. To achieve this, we proposed a method that involves the loading of dielectrics between the reentrant electrodes and a target object, like an electric field absorber (Kroeze et al. 2003), and showed that this method is useful to narrow the electric field distribution and improve the localized heating characteristics, particularly along the r-direction of the applicator (Ishihara et al., 2008d). However, by loading dielectrics, the electric field distribution generated inside a target object became beam-shaped; thus we found that the convergence of the electric field in the Z-direction was more difficult than that in the r-direction due to the formation of this beam-shaped electric field distribution in the Z-direction.

Here, therefore, we propose that the rotation of such a beam-shaped electric field distribution would make it possible to focus the electric field distribution in the region around the rotating axis that is common to the rotating beam-shaped electric field distribution (Ishihara et al., 2008c; 2009; Kameyama et al., 2008). Fig. 4 shows a conceptual schematic image of a rotatable heating applicator.

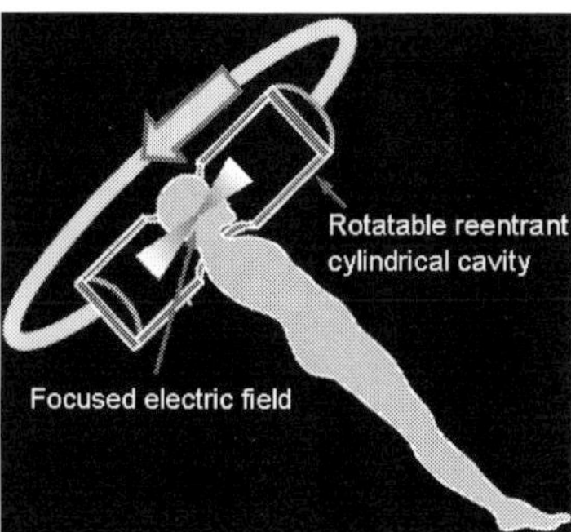

Fig. 4. Concept of a rotatable heating applicator to localize the electric field distribution at the center of a heating target.

3. Non-invasive temperature measurement method

3.1 Measurement of the phase information of the electromagnetic field

Even if non-invasive heating can be achieved, a temperature probe would need to be inserted into the heating target region to measure the temperature change. We therefore considered the temperature dependence of a dielectric constant. For example, the temperature dependence of pure water is given by Eq. (2) (Buckley et al., 1958), allowing the resonant frequency change due to the change in this dielectric constant with temperature to be detected.

$$\varepsilon_r = 87.74 - 0.40\ T + 9.40 \times 10^{-4}\ T^2 - 1.41 \times 10^{-6}\ T^3 \tag{2}$$

Here, T represents a temperature (°C). The dielectric constant of a target material is measured based on the resonant frequency change due to its temperature dependence by using the cavity resonator in the field of material analysis (Pointon et al., 1971; Karikh 1977). However, since it is necessary to measure a frequency change of only tens of kHz, in contrast to a resonant frequency of hundreds of MHz, such a measurement is dramatically difficult when a living body is the target. In such cases, the frequency change with temperature is not measured directly and spatially, but the phase change due to a frequency change may be detected. Thus, the minute frequency change with temperature is detectable as an expanded phase change, that is, $\Delta\theta$, by adjusting the observation time (time delay from when an external electromagnetic wave is applied) for the electromagnetic waves, as expressed in Eq. (3). Accordingly, it is expected that the dynamic range of the detectable temperature change can be improved.

$$\Delta\theta(T(r)) \cong 2\pi[f(T(r)) - f(T_0(r))]t_{delay} \tag{3}$$

Here, T_0 represents the reference temperature (°C); r, the spatial vector; and t_{delay}, the time delays from the reference time (s).

3.2 Introduction of the CT algorithm

Here, electromagnetic waves can be observed only outside the target body. Therefore, it is necessary to estimate the phase change distribution inside a target body and convert this phase change to a temperature change. An example of such an application is the concept that is illustrated in Fig. 5. The phase change distribution of the electromagnetic waves formed between the reentrant gaps is mainly distributed in the direction parallel to an electrical field, which will be shown later. In this case, the projection data reflecting the line integral value of the phase change distribution along the electrical field is similar to the projection data showing X-ray absorption in the case of X-ray CT. Therefore, it is believed that the phase distribution within an object can be estimated by rotating a cavity resonator, in contrast to that obtained in an object with the X-ray CT shown in Fig. 6. We then indicate that the CT algorithm based on the back-projection could be applied by considering the characteristics of the electrical field formed between the reentrant electrodes and the temperature dependence of the dielectrics. In order to evaluate this possibility, a numerical analysis using the finite difference time domain (FDTD) method was carried out and a basic examination of thermometry, which can be easily fused with a heating applicator based on a cavity resonator, was performed.

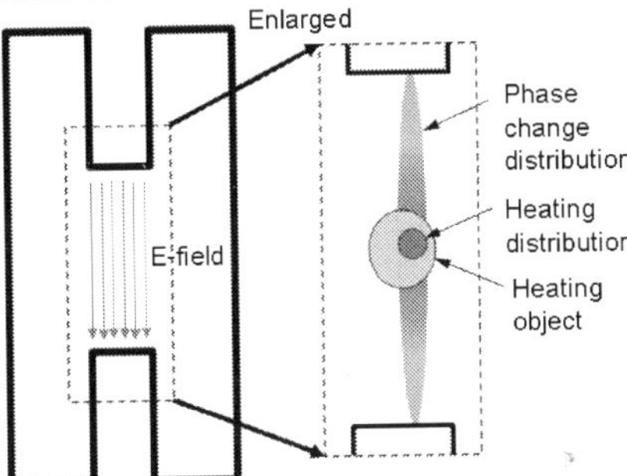

Fig. 5. Phase change distribution before and after the temperature change in a cavity resonator.

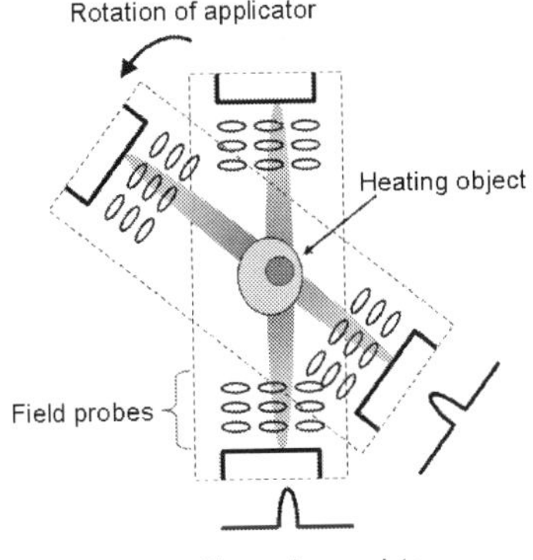

Fig. 6. Reconstruction of a phase change distribution from the projection data by introducing the CT algorithm.

4. Materials and Methods

4.1 Localized heating
4.1.1 Numerical analysis of focused electric field and temperature distributions

To confirm the electric field focusing effect achieved by rotating an applicator, we analyzed the electromagnetic distribution in a reentrant cylindrical cavity model (applicator height: 950 mm, outer diameter: 400 mm, reentrant diameter: 50 mm, and reentrant gap: 350 mm), which is shown in Fig. 7, using a three-dimensional FEM with 15,000 nodes and 1,000 elements. We assumed that the applicator container was an ideal conductor, and an element region corresponding to this assumption was considered to be the perfect electric conductor (PEC) by applying boundary conditions. The size of this model was determined according to our prototype applicator (Ishihara et al., 2009). The target object was a cylindrical phantom with a radius of 160 mm and a height of 160 mm, and we selected a relative permittivity of 63 and an electric conductivity of 0.47 S/m assuming cerebral hyperthermia treatment (Hartsgrove et al., 1987). After the resonant condition inside the cavity was analyzed when the phantom was loaded between the reentrant electrodes, the electromagnetic distribution was calculated.

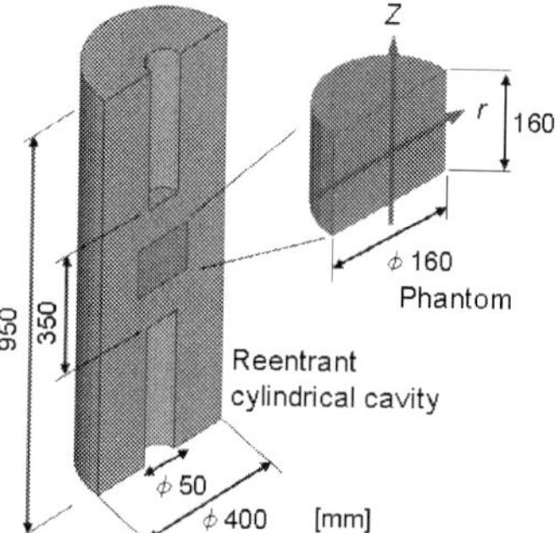

Fig. 7. Numerical heating applicator model with FEM.

The focusing effect of the electric field distribution was evaluated by the full width–half maximum (FWHM) of the normalized SAR distribution along the r- and Z-directions of the phantom inside the applicator.

After obtaining the electromagnetic fields inside the cavity resonator, we calculated the temperature distribution in the phantom based on the coupled analysis of the heating distribution due to the electromagnetic distribution using the three-dimensional FEM with the same model. In this study, it was assumed that the electric field distribution applied to the inside of a phantom did not change at each direction with an applicator's rotation. Then, the SAR distributions formed for each angle of the applicator were overlapped as a heating source, and the temperature distribution was analyzed. The RF power was set up so that the SAR at the center of the phantom became 20 W/kg, and this power was supplied to the phantom from five directions spaced 45 degrees apart with a heating period of 4 minutes for each direction. A comparison with the temperature distribution in the case where the applicator does not rotate (the total heating period was 20 min) was performed. Table 1 showed the values for the thermal parameters of the phantom (Hamada et al., 1998) used in the temperature distribution analysis.

Heat conductivity	[W/m(m K)]	0.55
Specific heat	[J/(kg K)]	4200
Coefficient of heat transfer	[W/(m³ K)]	20
Volume density	[kg/m³]	980

Table 1. Heat characteristics of the phantom.

4.1.2 Experimental evaluation of the localized heating effect

To experimentally confirm the focused electric field distribution by rotating a cavity resonator, we developed the prototype system shown in Fig. 8 and performed a phantom experiment. This heating system consists of a reentrant cylindrical cavity, impedance-matching circuit (NCS-04A and NMO1A200M-01; Noda RF Technologies, Suita, Japan), power amplifier (BSA 0125-250; BONN Elektronik, Ottobrunn, Germany), and signal generator (E4430B; Agilent Technologies, Santa Clara, CA, USA). To efficiently transmit the RF power to the cavity resonator, we measured the resonant frequency using a network analyzer (E5061A; Agilent Technologies, Santa Clara, CA, USA), and then the matching circuit was adjusted before the RF power was fed. However, since the matching conditions changed with the rotation of the applicator, the frequency of the applied RF power and the matching conditions at a given angle needed to be re-adjusted with rotation. A cylindrical phantom with a radius of 160 mm and a height of 160 mm (agar: 4%, NaCl: 0.24%, and NaN$_3$: 0.1%) was fixed on a Teflon table set at the center of the applicator. The electric field strength around the sides of the phantom was measured using an electric field intensity meter (EMR-20; Narda Safety Test Solutions, Pfullingen, Germany); further, the RF power supplied to the applicator was adjusted (20–50 W) so that the SAR value at the center of the phantom was approximately 20 W/kg. To evaluate the heating characteristics, the temperature distribution on a cross-section of the phantom was measured immediately after heating using thermography (TH7102MX; NEC Avio Infrared Technologies, Tokyo, Japan), with a temperature resolution of 0.1 °C and an accuracy of ±0.25 °C.

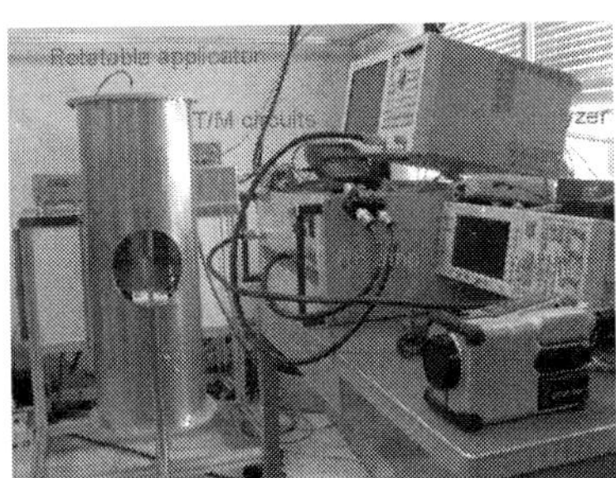

Fig. 8. Experimental system setup to confirm a focusing effect by rotating an applicator.

4.2 Non-invasive temperature measurement
4.2.1 Numerical model on FDTD

In order to analyze the changes in the transitional electromagnetic field distribution, a three-dimensional FDTD method was used. In this basic examination, the numerical calculation was carried out using a rectangular cavity resonator (1.0 x 1.0 x 1.0 m), since such an analysis was simple, and the electrical field distribution between the reentrant electrodes in the reentrant cylindrical cavity could be simulated with this rectangular cavity resonator. A cubic solid phantom (0.2 x 0.2 x 0.2 m) was placed in the center of a rectangular cavity resonator, as shown in Fig. 9.

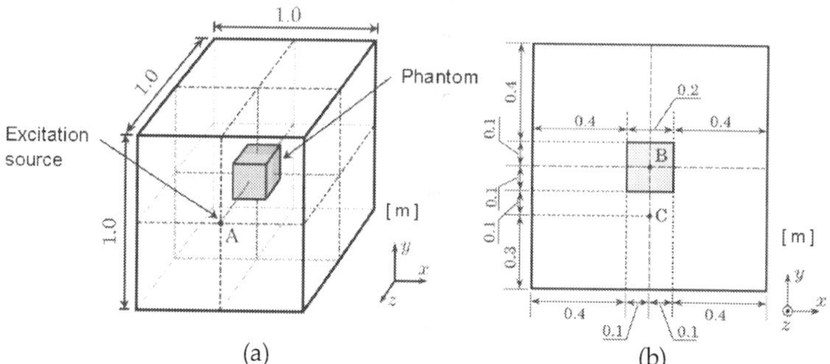

Fig. 9. Numerical rectangular cavity model for FDTD shown in a perspective diagram (a) and front elevation (b).

In order to increase the analysis accuracy using the FDTD method, the smaller cell size used in this analytic model was preferable, but since the computational resources and computation time required for a simulation become huge when there are a large number of cells, it was necessary to choose an adequate number of cells. Therefore, the resonant frequency estimation error for the number of cells used for the resonator was evaluated in advance, and 95 x 95 x 95 cells were chosen for the abovementioned model, which could achieve a resonant frequency estimate with an error of 0.5% or less. Moreover, the number of cells used for a phantom was set to 19 x 19 x 19. The values shown in Tables 2 and 3 were used as the dielectric constant, conductivity, and permeability for each part. The temperature dependence of the phantom was set to the value of pure water, as shown in Eq. (2).

Parameters	Air	Phantom	Cavity
Permittivity [F/m]	$1.00059\varepsilon_0$	Ref. Table 3	$1.00059\varepsilon_0$
Permeability [H/m]	$1.00000\mu_0$	$0.99999\mu_0$	$0.99998\mu_0$
Electric conductivity [S/m]	0.0000	0.0005	6.1000×10^7

Table 2. Electromagnetic characteristics for FDTD.

Temperature [°C]	Permittivity [F/m]
38.0	$73.81600\varepsilon_0$
43.0	$72.16600\varepsilon_0$

Table 3. Permittivity with temperature of phantom.

Since the electrical field component E_z parallel to a reentrant electrode (called the TM010 mode) was formed in the abovementioned heating applicator shown in Fig. 2, in order to achieve an equivalent electric field distribution in a rectangular cavity resonator, the excitation source expressed with Eq. (4) was used. By applying this exciting pulse, the electric field distribution *Ey* was formed in the perpendicular direction of a rectangular cavity resonator (called the TE101 mode). Then, the phase change distribution on the x-y plane parallel to an electric field vector was observed.

$$H_x(t) = A \exp\{-[(t - T_B)/0.29T_B]^2\} \sin(2\pi f_0 t) \tag{4}$$

Here, $T_B = 0.646/f_B$, f_B represents the excitation frequency band (Hz), A is the amplitude of the excitation pulse, and f_0 is the resonant frequency (Hz).

4.2.2 Numerical analysis of the phase change distribution

The phase change distribution with temperature (38–43 °C) was computed. In this study, the time delay from the reference time was set at around 200 ns, which provided a high sensitivity for detecting a phase change with temperature.

In order to estimate the temperature distribution inside a phantom using just the phase distribution of the external region, projection data for 32 directions were prepared from the phase distributions calculated for the rectangular cavity resonator, which rotated in 11.25 degree steps. The projection data for each column were determined as integrated values of the phase change along a projection direction (y-direction) within the line integral range shown in Fig. 10; however, the phase changes within the phantom region were not integrated into the projection data. The phase change distributions inside a phantom with temperature changes were reconstructed by a simple back projection and a filtered back projection with a Shepp-Logan filter (Shepp et al., 1974).

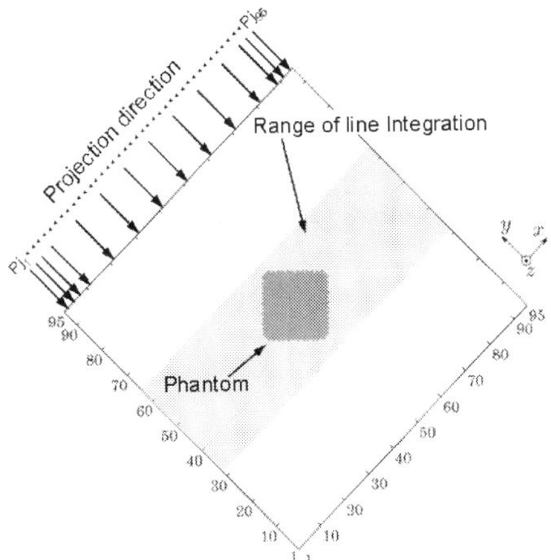

Fig. 10. Integration region to determine projection data (in a case where the applicator angle was 45°).

5. Results and discussion

5.1 Localized heating effect by rotating the applicator

The results of electromagnetic field and modal analyses showed that the electromagnetic field distribution in the reentrant cylindrical resonator shown in Fig. 11 had a resonant frequency of 226.5 MHz. Fig. 12 shows the normalized SAR distributions at the central plane (r–Z plane) of the phantom. The FWHM in the r and Z directions were 60.0 mm and 101.2 mm, respectively. When considering the normalized SAR distribution in the Z-direction, the convergence of the electric field in the Z-direction is more difficult than that in the r-direction without rotating the applicator.

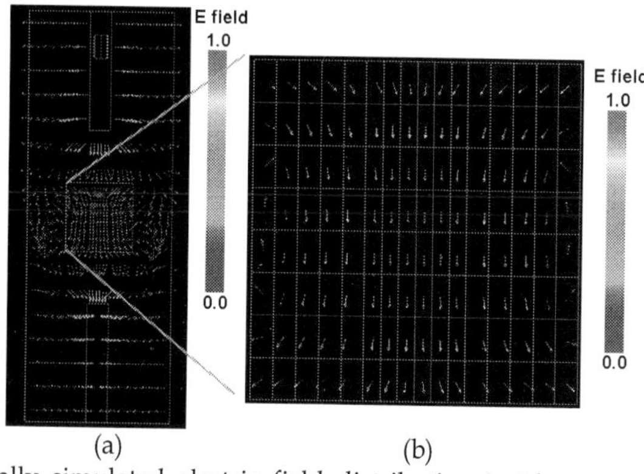

Fig. 11. Numerically simulated electric field distribution inside an applicator (a), and a phantom (b).

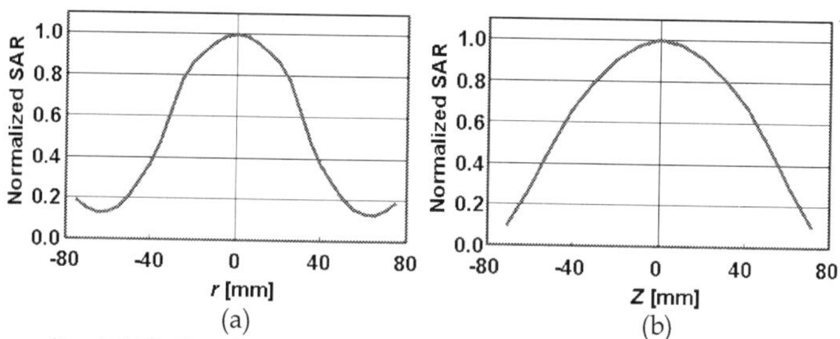

Fig. 12. Normalized SAR distribution in the r (a) and Z (b) directions.

Therefore, we evaluated the focusing effect by rotating the beam-shaped electric field distribution, and showed the temperature distribution of a cross-section (r–Z plane) at the center of the agar phantom with and without rotation of the applicator, as shown in Fig. 13. We evaluated the heating region by the FWHM of the temperature distribution and confirmed that the localized heating region could be improved by approximately 16% by rotating in the Z-direction; the FWHM was 107.1 mm without rotating the applicator, while it was 92.5 mm when the applicator was rotated (Fig. 14).

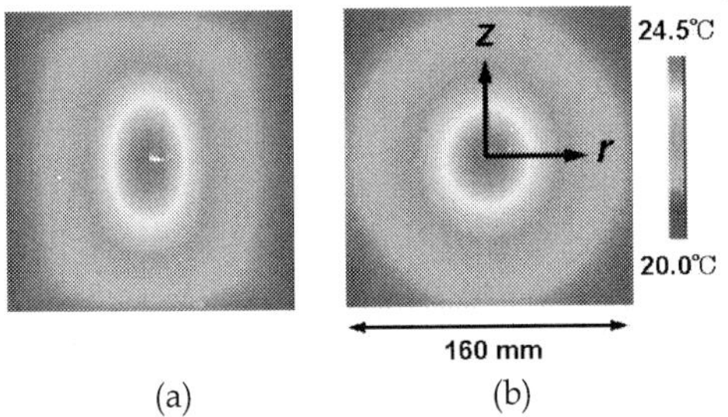

(a)   (b)

Fig. 13. Temperature distributions of a cross-section at the center of the phantom without rotation (a) and with rotation (b).

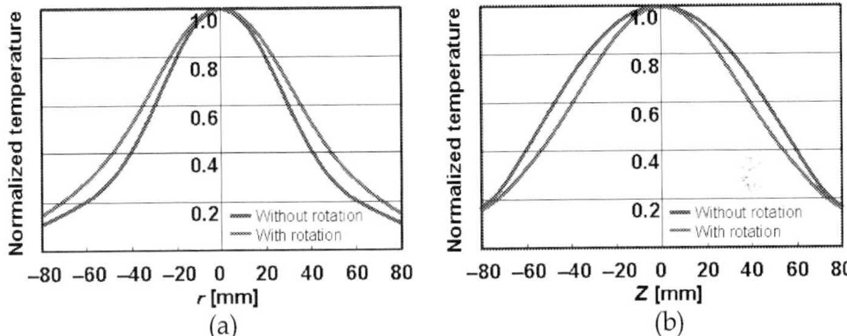

(a)   (b)

Fig. 14. Temperature profile along the r (a) and Z (b) directions normalized with the maximum temperature corresponding to that shown in Fig. 13.

In addition, Fig. 15 shows an example of a fundamental experiment to confirm the possibility of focusing the electric field distribution by rotating the applicator. These temperature distributions show a cross-section (r–Z surface) at the center of the agar phantom with and without rotation of the applicator with an incident RF power of approximately 25 W, which corresponds to an SAR of 20 W/kg at the object center and a total heating period of 20 min. Fig. 16 shows the temperature distribution along the r and Z directions. These figures indicate that the results of the numerical analysis and those obtained in the experiment were almost identical. From these experimental results, we evaluated the heating region by the FWHM of the temperature distribution and confirmed that the localized heating region could be improved by approximately 21% by rotating an applicator in the Z-direction; the FWHM was 101.2 mm without rotation, while it was 83.7 mm when the applicator was rotated.

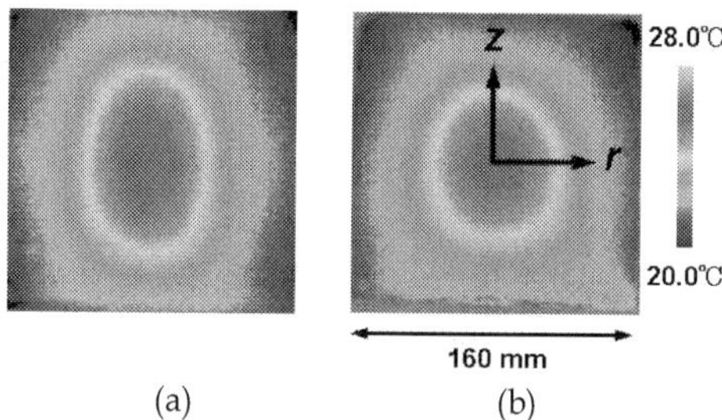

(a)   (b)

Fig. 15. Temperature distributions of a cross-section at the center of the phantom without rotation (a) and with rotation (b).

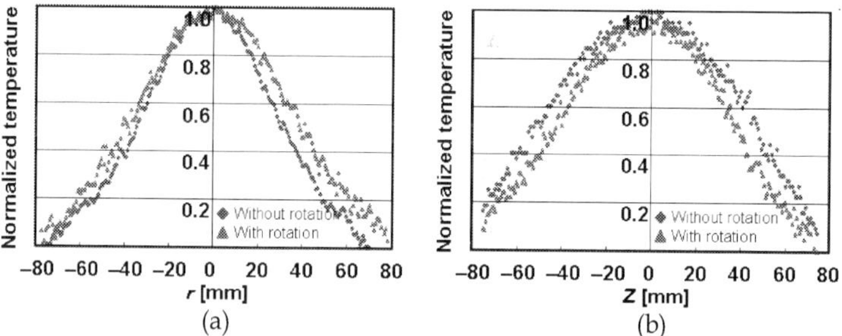

(a)   (b)

Fig. 16. Temperature profile along the r (a) and Z (b) directions normalized with the maximum temperature corresponding to that shown in Fig. 15.

These results indicated that the heating region was focused in the Z-direction, although the narrowing effect degrades in the r-direction due to the averaging of the electric fields by the rotation of the heating region. One idea is to focus such a narrowed electric field distribution in the Z-direction after narrowing the electric field distribution in the r-direction by loading dielectrics (Ishihara et al., 2008d). In addition to this complementary procedure, miniaturizing the diameter of the reentrant electrodes is another potential way to greatly improve the localized heating characteristics. However, since the narrowing effect of the electric field in the r-direction and the concentration effect of the electric field in the Z-direction have a trade-off relationship, it is necessary to optimize these parameters, taking into consideration the rotation of the applicator.

By using the abovementioned methods and optimizing both the size and rotation conditions of the heating applicator, we could predict that the localized heating region would be an area with a diameter of 50–60 mm.

5.2 Noninvasive temperature measurement

When a temperature change of 5 °C (from 38 to 43 °C) was generated in the phantom, there was a phase change in the electric field formed in the rectangular cavity resonator (t_{dealy} = 200 ns), as indicated in Fig. 17. According to this figure, the phase change with temperature was produced mainly as a distribution along the electrical field direction (y-direction in Fig. 18(b)), corresponding to the region at which the temperature change was produced compared with the direction (x-direction in Fig. 18(a)) perpendicular to the electric field. It was confirmed that such behavior for an approximate distribution did not change when the applied field direction was changed by rotating the cavity resonator, as shown in Fig. 19. Then the phase projection data in the direction of the electrical field were computed according to the line integral, as in the X-ray CT mentioned above, and the phase change distribution within the target object was estimated.

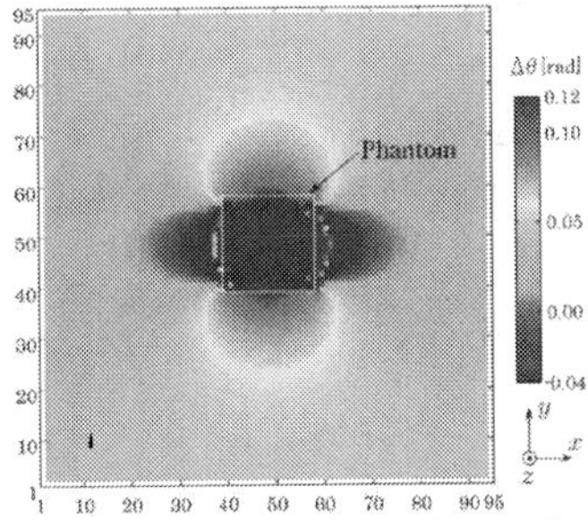

Fig. 17. Phase change distribution with temperature change from 38 to 43 °C at the center of the x-y plane.

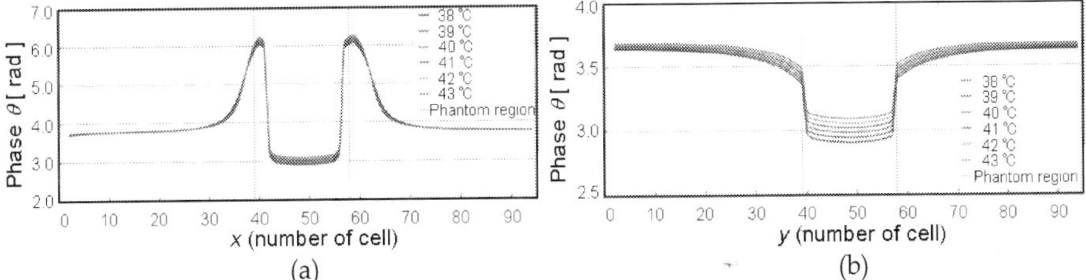

(a)

(b)

Fig. 18. Phase change distribution with temperature change from 38 to 43 °C along the x (a) and y (b) directions on the center x-y plane.

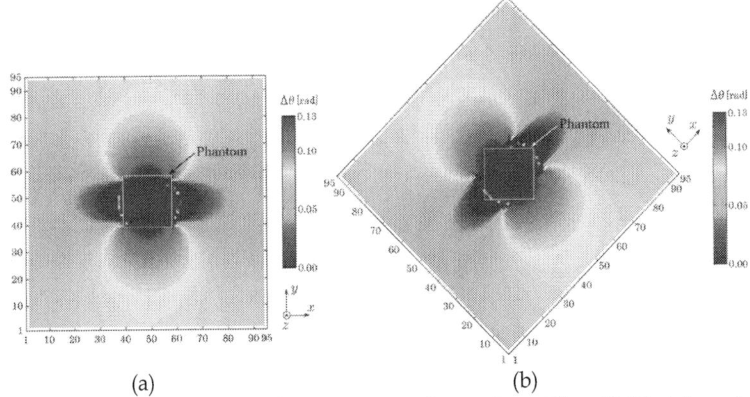

(a)

(b)

Fig. 19. Phase change distribution with temperature change from 38 to 43 °C at the rotation angles of 0 degree (a) and 45 degrees (b) at the center of the x-y plane.

Fig. 20 shows the reconstructed phase change distributions with a simple back-projection CT algorithm when the number of projections was 32. As anticipated, the surroundings of the reconstructed phase change distribution were blurred due to the point spread function of the simple back-projection. Therefore, in order to compensate for such broadening of the phase distribution, a filtered back projection with a Shepp-Logan filter was applied to the projection data (Fig. 21). As a result of this filtering, the reconstruction error due to image blurring was reduced by approximately 60%. Although degradation of the spatial resolution resulting from the broadening of the phase distribution was mentioned as a problem under the current circumstances, and an evaluation of the thermometry accuracy was difficult due to the still large image blurring, it was shown that the detection of a 1 °C temperature change, which is required of hyperthermia (Delannoy et al., 1991), can be sufficiently measured by the phase change with temperature. However, since it is expected that the temperature dependence of a dielectric constant changes with tissues (Jaspard et al., 2002), for clinical application it will be necessary to devise a method to convert from a phase value to temperature and to evaluate the measurement error generated in the required temperature range.

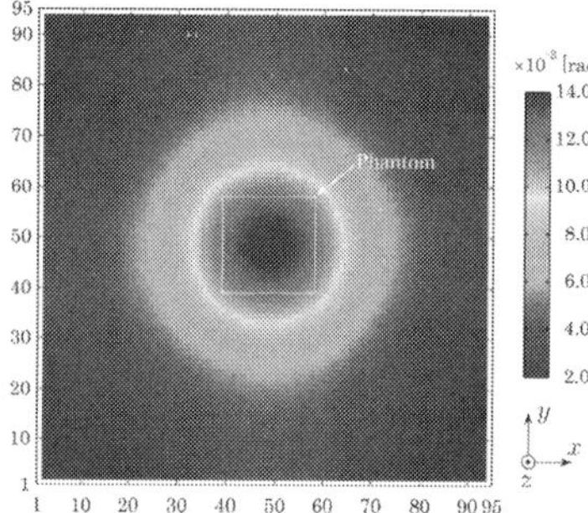

Fig. 20. Reconstructed phase change distribution with a simple back projection.

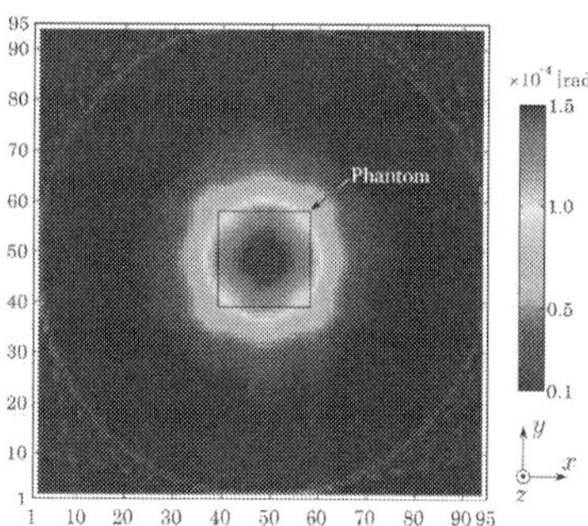

Fig. 21. Reconstructed phase change distribution with a Shepp-Logan filter.

In addition, the reconstruction error regarding the detected position was evaluated when the measurement subject was shifted from the center position of the cavity resonator. Fig. 22 shows the reconstructed results with the simple back projection and filtered back projection methods, respectively. When the shifted distance of a phantom was set at 4.21 cm (which corresponded to 4 cells of the FDTD numerical model), the detected distance from the reconstructed phase distribution with a simple back-projection was 5.15 cm, which corresponded to a relative error of 23.3% compared to the true value. In contrast, the detected distance from the reconstructed phase distribution with a filtered-back-projection was 4.69 cm, which corresponded to a relative error of 11.3%. Consequently, it became clear that the position of a heating region was detectable with this method, with an accuracy corresponding to a spatial resolution of one or less cell. Conversely, since this detection accuracy may be restrained by the size of the cell used with this FDTD, it is necessary to investigate spatial resolution while including other factors in the future.

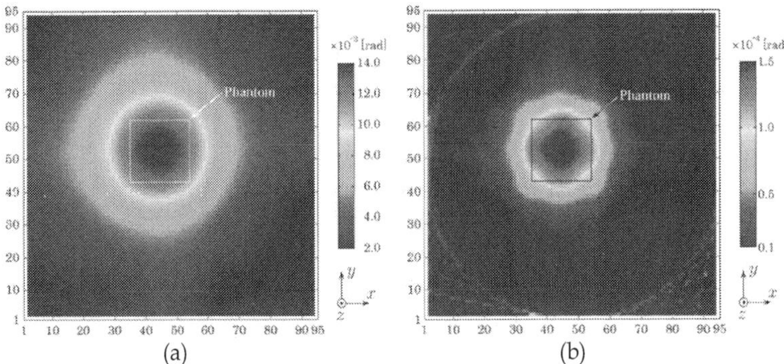

Fig. 22. Reconstructed phase change distributions by a simple back projection (a) and filtered back projection (b) when the phantom position was shifted from the center of the cavity resonator.

6. Conclusions and Future Research

A heating region with a diameter of approximately 85–90 mm was obtained by rotating a beam-shaped electric field distribution. This corresponded to an improvement in the heating region of 15–20%, compared to a case in which heating was carried out without rotating the applicator. Although this is insufficient to heat a cancer localized in the head or neck region, such a heating method has the potential of achieving a heating region with a diameter of less than 50 mm by optimizing the beam-shaped electric field distribution and rotation conditions. However, further improvement in the localized characteristics may be difficult due to the restrictions of the trade-off between the convergence of electric fields in the r and Z-directions.

On the other hand, it is possible to achieve more localized heating by noninvasive real-time temperature measurement and active temperature control since the heat source generated by the heating applicator based on a reentrant cylindrical cavity indicates an approximately concentrated spherical distribution whose intensity is maximum at the center of the heating target body. Since the proposed method to measure temperature distribution from the information on the electromagnetic waves inside a cavity resonator can be easily embedded in our heating applicator, a novel cancer treatment system that combines the localized heating of cancer with non-invasive temperature monitoring can be established.

Consequently, a cancer treatment for a lesion with a diameter of approximately 30–50 mm, which is required to heat a cancer localized in the head or neck region, can be achieved.

7. Acknowledgement

This study was supported by the Industrial Technology Research Grant Program 2006 from the New Energy and Industrial Technology Development Organization (NEDO) of Japan, and a Grant-in-Aid for Scientific Research (B), 20300155, 2008 from the Japan Society for the Promotion of Science (JSPS).

8. References

Buckley, F. & Maryott, A. A. (1958). Tables of Dielectric Dispersion Data for Pure Liquids and Dilute Solutions. *Natl. Bur. Stand. Circ.* 589, US Government Printing Office, 10–18353, Washington, DC

Delannoy, J.; Chen, C., Turner, T., Levin, R. L. & Le Bihan, D. (1991). Noninvasive temperature imaging using diffusion MRI. *Magn. Reson. Med.*, Vol. 19, No.2, Jun. 1991, 333–339, 0740–3194

Fujisawa, K. (1958). General treatment of klystron resonant cavities. *IRE Trans. Microwave Theory and Tech.*, Vol. 6, No. 4, Oct. 1958, 344–358, 0097–2002

Gellermann, J.; Wlodarczyk, W., Hildebrandt, B., Ganter, H., Nicolau, A., Rau, B., Tilly, W., Fähling, H., Nadobny, J., Felix, R. & Wust, P. (2006). Noninvasive magnetic resonance thermography of recurrent rectal carcinoma in a 1.5 tesla hybrid system. *Cancer Res.*, Vol. 63, No. 13, Jul. 2005, 5872–5880, 0008–5472

Giordano, M.; Momo, F. & Sotgiu, A. (1983). On the design of a re-entrant square cavity as resonator for low-frequency ESR spectroscopy. *J. Phys. E: Sci. Instrum.*, Vol. 16, No. 8, Aug. 1983, 774–779, 0022–3735

Goitein, M. (1972). Three-dimensional density reconstruction from a series of two-dimensional projections. *Nuclear Instruments and Methods*, Vol. 101, No. 3, Jun, 1972, 509–518, 0168–9002

Gordon, R.; Bender, R. & Herman, G. T. (1970). Algebraic reconstruction techniques (ART) for three-dimensional electron microscopy and X-ray photography. *J. Theor. Biol.*, Vol. 29, No. 3, Dec. 1970, 471–481, 0022–5193

Gordon, R. (1974). A tutorial on ART. *IEEE Trans. Nucl. Sci.*, Vol. NS-21, No. 3, Jun. 1974, 78–93, 0018–9499

Hamada, L.; Furuya, K. & Ito, K. (1998). Biological tissue-equivalent phantom for microwave hyperthermia. *Jpn. J. Hyperthermic Oncol.*, Vol. 14, No. 1, Mar. 1998, 31–40, 0197–8462, 0911–2529 (Japanese)

Hartsgrove, G.; Kraszewski, A. & Surowiec, A. (1987). Simulated biological materials for electromagnetic radiation absorption studies. *Bioelectromag*, Vol. 8, No. 1, Jan. 1987, 29–36, 0197–8462

Hynynen, K.; Clement, G. T., McDannold, N., Vykhodtseva, N., King, R., White, P. J., Vitek, S. & Jolesz, J. (2004). 500-element ultrasound phased array system for noninvasive focal surgery of the brain: a preliminary rabbit study with ex vivo human skulls. *Magn. Reson. Med.*, Vol. 52, No. 1, Jul. 2004, 100–107, 0740–3194

Ishihara, Y.; Calderon, A., Watanabe, H., Mori, K., Okamoto, K., Suzuki, Y., Sato, K., Kuroda, K., Nakagawa, N. & Tsutsumi, S. (1992). A precise and fast temperature mapping using water proton chemical shift, *Proceedings of Society of Magnetic Resonance in Medicine, 11th Annual Meeting*, pp. 4804, Berlin, Germany, Aug. 1992

Ishihara, Y.; Calderon, A., Watanabe, H., Okamoto, K., Suzuki, Y., Kuroda, K. & Suzuki, Y. (1995). A precise and fast temperature mapping using water proton chemical shift. *Magn. Reson. Med.*, Vol. 34, No. 6, Dec. 1995, 814–823, 0740–3194

Ishihara, Y.; Gotanda, Y., Wadamori, N. & Matsuda, J. (2007a). Hyperthermia applicator based on reentrant cavity for localized head and neck tumors. *Rev. Sci. Inst.*, Vol. 72, No. 2, Feb. 2007, 024301.1–024301.8, 0034–6748

Ishihara, Y.; Endo, Y. Wadamori, N. & Ohwada, H. (2007b). A noninvasive temperature measurement regarding the heating applicator based on a reentrant cavity, *Proceedings of 2007 Joint Annual Meeting of the. World Conference on Interventional. Oncology (WCIO) and the Society for. Thermal Medicine (STM)*, pp. 232–233, Washington, DC, USA, May 2007

Ishihara, Y.; Endo, Y., Ohwada, H. & Wadamori, N. (2007c). Noninvasive thermometry in a reentrant resonant cavity applicator, *Proceedings of the IEEE of the 29th Annual International Conference of the Engineering in Medicine and Biology Society, 2007*, pp. 1487–1490, Lyon, France, Aug. 2007

Ishihara, Y. & Wadamori, N. (2008a). Localized heating characteristics of hyperthermia using a reentrant cavity. *J Med Eng*, Vol. 32, No. 5, Sep. 2008, 348–357, 0309–1902

Ishihara, Y. & Wadamori, N. (2008b). Heating applicator based on reentrant cavity with optimized local heating characteristics. *Int. J. Hyperthermia*, Vol. 24, No. 8, Dec. 2008, 694–704, 0265–6736

Ishihara, Y. & Wadamori, N. (2008c). Improvement in the localized heating characteristics by the rotation of a heating applicator based on a reentrant cavity, *Proceedings of 10th International Congress on Hyperthermic Oncology*, pp. 1487, Munich, Germany, Apr. 2008

Ishihara, Y.; Kameyama, Y., Ino, Y. & Wadamori, N. (2008d). Improvement in localized heating characteristics by loading dielectrics in a heating applicator based on a cylindrical reentrant cavity. *Thermal Med.*, Vol. 24, No. 2, Aug. 2008, 61–72, 1882–2576

Ishihara, Y.; Kameyama, Y. & Wadamori, N. (2009). Localized heating method by a rotatable applicator based on a reentrant cylindrical cavity, *Proceedings of Society for Thermal Medicine 2009 Annual Meeting*, pp. 172, Tucson, AZ, USA, Apr. 2009

Jaspard, F. & Nadi, M. (2002). Dielectric properties of blood: an investigation of temperature dependence. *Physiol. Meas.*, Vol. 23, No. 3, Aug. 2002, 547–554, 0967–3334

Kameyama, Y. & Ishihara, Y. (2008). Regional heating by insertion of dielectrics and rotation of the focused electric field in the hyperthermia, *Proceedings of the IEEE of the 30th Annual International Conference of the Engineering in Medicine and Biology Society, 2008*, pp. 4380–4383, Vancouver, Canada, Aug. 2008

Karikh, N. M. (1977). Method of calculating dielectric permittivity in a partly filled resonator cavity. Measurement Techniques, Vol. 20, No. 5, May 1977, 68–71, 0543–1972

Kato, K.; Matsuda, J. & Saitoh, Y. (1989). A re-entrant type resonant cavity applicator for deep-seated hyperthermia treatment, *Proceedings of the Annual International Conference of the IEEE Engineering in Medicine and Biology Society, 1989*, pp. 1712–1713, Seattle, WA, USA, Nov. 1989

Kato, K.; Wadamori, N., Matsuda, J., Uzuka, T., Takahashi, H. & Tanaka, R. (2003). Improvement of the resonant cavity applicator for brain tumor hyperthermia, *Proceedings of the IEEE of the 25th Annual International Conference of the Engineering in Medicine and Biology Society, 2003*, pp. 3271–3274, Cancun, Mexico, Sep. 2003

Kroeze, H.; Van Vulpen M., De Leeuw, A. A. C., De Kamer, J. B. & Lagendijk, J. J. W. (2003). Improvement of absorbing structures used in regional hyperthermia. Int. J. Hyperthermia, Vol. 19, No. 6, Nov. 2003, 598–616, 0265–6736

Kuroda, K.; Suzuki, Y., Ishihara, Y. Okamoto, K. & Suzuki, Y. (1996). Temperature mapping by water proton chemical shift obtained with 3D-MRSI -Feasibility in vivo-. *Magn. Reson. Med.*, Vol. 35, No. 1, Jan. 1996, 20–29, 0740–3194

Lynn, J. G.; Zwemer, R. L., Chick, A. J. & Miller, A. E. (1942). A new method for the generation and use of focused ultrasound in experimental biology. *J. Gen. Physiol.*, Vol. 26, No. 2, Nov. 1942, 179–193, 0022–1295

Matsuda, J.; Kato, K. & Saitoh, Y. (1988). The application of a re-entrant type resonant cavity applicator to deep and concentrated hyperthermia. *Jpn. J. Hyperthermia Oncol.*, Vol. 4, No. 2, Jun. 1988, 111–118, 0911–2529 (in Japanese)

McDannold, N.; Tempany, C. M., Fennessy, F. M., So, M. M., Rybicki, F. J., Stewart, E. A., Jolesz, F. A. & Hynynen, K. (2006). Uterine leiomyomas: MR imaging-based thermometry and thermal dosimetry during focused ultrasound thermal ablation. *Radiology*, Vol. 240, No. 1, Jul. 2006, 263–272, 0033–8419

Nadobny, J.; Wlodarczyk, W., Westhoff, L., Gellermann, J., Felix, R. & Wust, P. (2005). A clinical water-coated antenna applicator for MR-controlled deep-body hyperthermia: a comparison of calculated and measured 3-D temperature data sets. *IEEE Trans. Biomed. Eng.*, Vol. 52, No. 3, Mar. 2005, 505–519, 0018–9294

Ohwada, H. & Ishihara, Y. (2009). Noninvasive thermometry on the heating applicator based on the reentrant cavity. *The IEICE transactions on information and systems (Japanese edition)*, Vol. 92-D, No. 4, Apr. 2009, 562–570, 1880–4535 (in Japanese)

Paulides, M. M.; Bakker, J. F., Zwamborn, A. P. M. & Van Rhoon, G. C. (2007a). A head and neck hyperthermia applicator: Theoretical antenna array design. *Int. J. Hyperthermia*, Vol. 23, No. 1, Feb. 2007, 59–67, 1464–5157

Paulides, M. M.; Bakker, J. F., Neufeld, E., Van Der Zee, J., Jansen, P. P., Levendag, P. C. & Van Rhoon, G. C. (2007b). The HYPERcollar: A novel applicator for hyperthermia in the head and neck. *Int. J. Hyperthermia*, Vol. 23, No. 7, Nov. 2007, 567–576, 1464–5157

Perez, C. A.; Gillespie, B., Pajak, T., Emami, N. B. & Rubin, P. (1989). Quality assurance problems in clinical hyperthermia and their impact on therapeutic outcome: a report by the Radiation Therapy Oncology Group. *Int. J. Radiat. Oncol. Biol. Phys.*, Vol. 16, No. 3, Mar. 1989, 551–558, 0360–3016

Perez, C. A.; Pajak, T., Emami, B., Hornback, N. B., Tupchong, L. & Rubin, P. (1991). Randomized phase III study comparing irradiation and hyperthermia with irradiation alone in superficial measurable tumors. Final report by the Radiation Therapy Oncology Group. *Am. J. Clin. Oncol.*, Vol. 14, No. 2, Apr. 1991, 133–141, 0277-3732

Pointon, A. J. & Woodman, K. F. (1971). A coaxial cavity for measuring the dielectric properties of high permittivity materials. *J. Phys. E: Sci. Instrum.*, Vol. 4, No. 3, Mar. 1971, 208–210, 0022-3735

Shepp, L. A. & Logan, B. F. (1974). The Fourier reconstruction of a head section. *IEEE Trans. Nucl. Sci.*, Vol. NS-21, No. 3, Jun. 1974, 21–43, 0018-9499

Tsubono, K.; Hiramatsu, S. & Hirakawa, H. (1977). Cavity transducer for subatomic mechanical vibration. *Jpn. J. Appl. Phys.*, Vol. 16, No. 9, Sep. 1977, 1641–1645, 0021-4922

Turner, P. F. (1999). MRI integration with 3D phased array BSD-2000 3D hyperthermia system, *Proceedings of the 1st Joint BMES/EMBS Conference*, pp. 1278, Atlanta, GA, USA, Oct. 1999

Wadamori, N.; Matsuda, J., Takahashi, H., Grinev, I., Uzuka, T. & Tanaka, R. (2004). Heating properties of a re-entrant cavity-type applicator for deep regional hyperthermia treatments, *Proceedings of 9th International Congress on Hyperthermic Oncology*, pp. 169, St. Louis, MO, USA, Apr. 2004

Wust, P.; Beck, R., Berger, J., Seebass, M., Wlodarczyk, W., Hoffmann, W. & Nadobny, J. (2000). Electric field distributions in a phased–array applicator with 12 channels: Measurements and numerical simulations. *Med. Phys.*, Vol. 17, No. 11, Nov. 2000, 2565–2579, 0094-2405

31

Wireless Body Area Network (WBAN) for Medical Applications

Jamil. Y. Khan and Mehmet R. Yuce
School of Electrical Engineering & Computer Science
The University of Newcastle
Australia

1. Introduction to WBAN

With the rapid advancements of wireless communication and semiconductor technologies the area of sensor network has grown significantly supporting a range of applications including medical and healthcare systems. A Wireless Body Area Network (WBAN) is a special purpose sensor network designed to operate autonomously to connect various medical sensors and appliances, located inside and outside of a human body. Introduction of a WBAN for medical monitoring and other applications will offer flexibilities and cost saving options to both health care professionals and patients. A WBAN system can offer two significant advantages compared to current electronic patient monitoring systems. The first advantage is the mobility of patients due to use of portable monitoring devices. Second advantage is the location independent monitoring facility. A WBAN node being an autonomous device can search and find a suitable communication network to transmit data to a remote database server for storage. It is also possible that a WBAN will connect it self to the internet to transmit data in a non-invasive manner.

The health care sector is increasingly looking for advanced ICT (Information & Communication Technology) systems to efficiently administer the healthcare delivery for a range of services. Advanced ICT systems will be able to deliver healthcare not only to patients in hospitals and medical centres; but also in their homes and workplaces thus offering cost savings, and improving the quality of life of patients. A WBAN will consist of a number of tiny sensor nodes and a Gateway node used to connect to the external database server. The Gateway node could connect the sensor node to a range of telecommunication networks. These communication networks could be either a standard telephone network, mobile phone network, a dedicated medical centre/hospital network or using public WLAN (Wireless Local Area Network) hotspots also known as WiFi. A WBAN can also take advantage of widely deployed mobile data networks such as the 3G/4G data networks to transmit patient data. A WBAN could allow a user to store its collected data on his/her PDA (Personal Digital Assistant) or iPod or any other portable devices and then transfer those information to a suitable computer. Future applications of WBAN introduce numerous possibilities to improve the health care and sports training facilities. The WBAN concept in recent years has attracted attention of medical and ICT researchers. ICT systems are already in use in medical areas but their applications are limited. The main drawback of current systems is the location specific nature of the system due to the use of fixed/wired systems. There are many existing medical monitoring systems using specialised equipments which could send data using either standard telephone lines or specially designed network for medical applications. However, these systems are not location independent and in most cases they are clumsy in nature due to use of wired sensors. Use of a WBAN can introduce location independent monitoring systems. WBAN applications can also be extended to sports training areas where athletes or players can be monitored to find their deficiencies or to improve their skills.

This chapter presents the WBAN hardware and network design techniques. Section 2.0 presents medical applications scenarios by introducing the roles of different wireless networking standards. Section 3.0 presents hardware design techniques of WBAN nodes and networks. This section also discusses basic architecture of a WBAN node. Design of other nodes such as GATEWAY and CCU (Central Control Unit) is also presented in this section. Some basic performance result is also discussed in this section. Section 4 discusses WBAN network design technique. This section discusses several fundamental design techniques and introduces different MAC (Medium Access Control) protocols suitable for WBAN applications. Section 4 also discusses the link budget design issues. Section 5 presents a multi-patient monitoring system based on the WBAN architecture. This section also discusses various design features of a multi-patient monitoring system. Section 6 presents simulation results of the multi-patient WBAN system. Results presented in this section explain various operational features of the WBAN. Section 7 presents some future WBAN development issues. Summary of the chapter is presented in section 8.

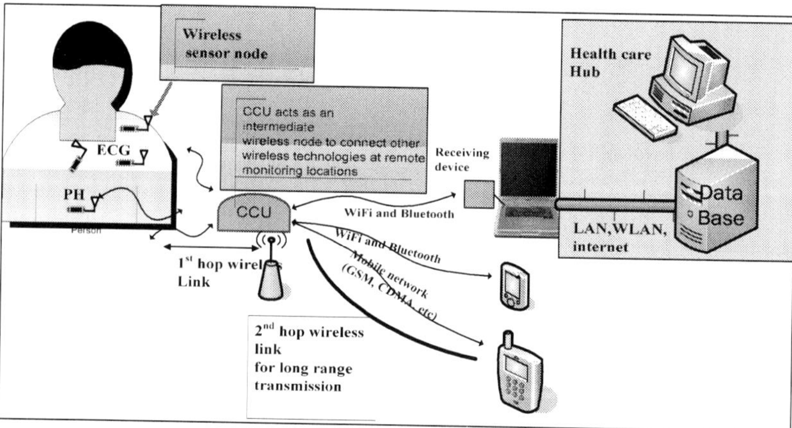

Fig. 1. A wireless body area network system. Collecting and monitoring data from individual wireless sensor nodes from a single human body via the gateway CCU.

2. Medical Application Scenarios

The application of Wireless Body Area Networks (WBAN) in medical environments may consist of sensor nodes attached to or implanted into a human body. These sensor nodes have wireless transmission capability and sense biological information from human body to transmit over a short distance to a control device worn on the body or placed at an accessible location. A sensor node electronics should be miniaturized, low-power and detect medical signals such as electrocardiogram (ECG), photoplethysmogram (PPG), electroencephalo-graphy (EEG), pulse rate, blood flow, pressure, and temperature. The collected data from the control devices are then transferred to remote destinations in a wireless body area network for diagnostic and therapeutic purposes incorporating another wireless network for a long range transmission (See Figure 1). There are a vast majority of monitoring systems developed and already being used in medical systems. Currently available systems are based on wired connection and their electronics are bulky, particularly when many sensors are wired to a wireless device. Any wire connection in a monitoring system becomes cumbersome and is not suitable to be worn by patients which could restrict their mobility. Thus WBAN requires individual wireless sensor node without any wire connections. Each individual sensor nodes will directly transfer the sensed physiological data to a control unit (CCU) and then to remote stations for diagnostic and health care purposes.

So far there is no available standard for a wireless body area network specifically targeting healthcare applications. Most popular wireless technologies used for medical monitoring are ZigBee/IEEE892.15.4, WLAN, GSM (Global System for Mobile), Bluetooth (802.15.1) (Otto et.al., 2006, Soomro et.al., 2007, Anliker et.al., 2004, Proulx et.al., 2006). All these technologies are commercially available and optimized for short range communications except the GSM standard. These wireless standards are targeting general purpose sensor network applications and thus are not optimum solutions for medical environments. If these devices are used for wireless body area network applications, they should deal with the interference and coexistence issues (Howitt et.al., 2003, Sikora et.al., 2005). In addition to unlicensed ISM (Instrumentation Scientific and Medical) bands, there are other medical bands such as MICS (Medical Implant Communication Service) and WMTS (Wireless Medical Telemetry Service) that are specifically regulated for medical monitoring by communication commissions around the world (Yuce et.al., 2008). Recently developed short-range low data rate ultra-wideband (UWB) technology is another attractive technology that could be used for body area network applications due to its low transmitter power (Ho et.al., 2008).

In order to monitor medical implant devices and status of inner organs, a frequency around 400 MHz have been used as a popular transmission band in recent systems (Bradley 2007). The MICS is an ultra-low power, unlicensed, mobile radio service for transmitting data to support diagnostic or therapeutic functions associated with implanted medical devices. This frequency range can be used to enable the wireless communication of medical implant devices to deliver high level of comfort, mobility and better patient care (FCC, 2003). To treat a large number of patients wearing implanted systems in the same environment (e.g. hospital) require a reliable wireless networking in order to monitor and differentiate each individual implanted device and a patient. Thus implanted wireless nodes in a patient's body should form a wireless body area network so that one or more implanted devices inserted in the bodies of a number of patients in a hospital environment can be controlled with minimum complexity. The system presented in (Bradley 2007) uses a RF (Radio Frequency) transceiver that is specifically designed to be used for in-body communication systems. The device uses the new medical band MICS together with the 433 MHz ISM band to form a medical sensor network of implant devices. More of such miniaturized low power RF transceivers should be designed in future in order to use in a medical sensor network as the MICS band is gaining more popularity. The successful implementation of a complete WBAN system will provide: wearable, wireless (no wire connections), easy to remove and attach sensor nodes, leading to increased mobility of patients and flexibility. A WBAN should operate and co-exists with other network devices operating in similar frequency bands. It is thus very important to ensure an interference-free, reliable wireless link from sensors that incorporates and interacts with the existing wireless technologies to form a heterogeneous networking environment.

One of the main applications of a WBAN is in medical care environment where conditions of a large number of patients could be continuously monitored. Figure 2 shows a WBAN based monitoring scenario applicable to a hospital environment. The figure represents several rooms at a single hospital floor. As can be seen, for a large scale deployment of WBANs, several controlled units (CCUs) are required to organize the collection of medical data from patients' body. Presence of several CCU is also useful for free movement of patients in hospitals. In fact monitoring many physiological signals from a large number of patients presents some challenges in both software and hardware designs. Some of those challenges are as follows: reliable communication by eliminating collisions of multi-patients' signals, and interference from other external wireless devices, low-cost, low power consumption, and providing flexibility to the patients so that patients can be relocated anytime (Yuce & Ho, 2008). Most of the existing schemes in the literature deal with a single patient monitoring or designed for monitoring one or few physiological signals.

The system in figure 2 includes individual wireless sensor nodes that can transfer a person's physiological data such as heart rate, blood pressure, ECG, EEG EMG via a wireless link, without the need of any wired connection. Each sensor will have wireless capability and its design will be optimized in terms of the physical characteristics of the physiological signal. The sensor nodes use a dedicated wireless link to eliminate the strong interference from other communication devices in a healthcare area; as reliable communication and accurate monitoring are very crucial for patients' safety. Hardware and software designs are being developed for a high performance and fault tolerant wireless communication and monitoring system.

Currently we are developing a complete wireless body area network that is based on different frequencies in order to eliminate interference issues as well as to apply different environments (Yuce & Ho, 2008). We use MICS, WMTS and 433 ISM bands to transmit signals from the sensors on the body. For the applications that require monitoring of many continuous signals such as ECG/EEG/EMG, we incorporate UWB (Ultra Wide Band) technology since a high data rate wireless link will be required (Ho et.al., 2008). The selection of wireless scheme for sensor nodes will depend on very much on the environment of the sensors nodes to be used and its signal characteristic. In addition, we also interfaced our devices with IEEE 802.15.4 (Zigbee) and WiFi links to cover a large area of a body area network, as depicted in Figure 2. As these short ranges wireless standards are already available and in use for different applications in medical centers, incorporating a WBAN implementation with these standards will be an added advantage. As an example when installed in CCUs, these existing wireless standards can be used in a WBAN gateway to provide a networking between the CCUs and the remote stations.

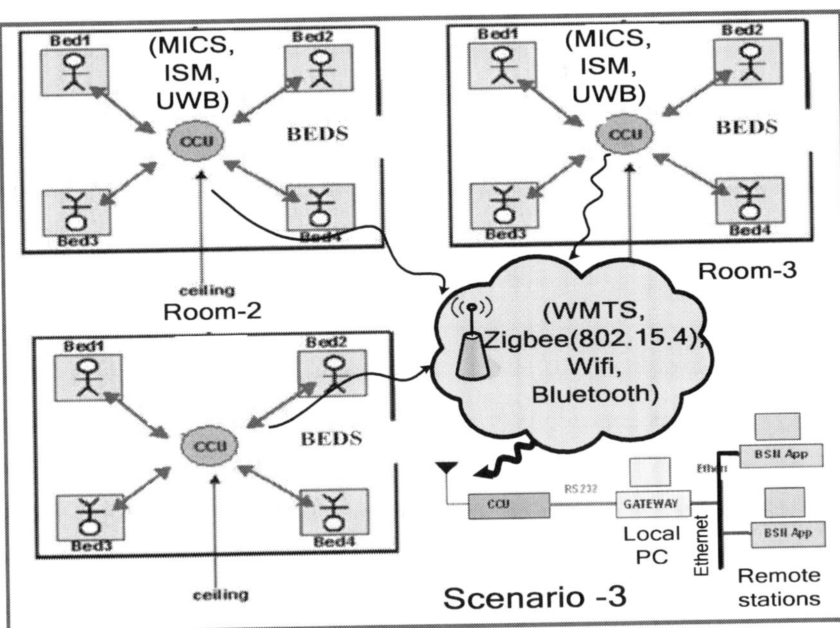

Fig. 2. A multi-patient monitoring scenario in a medical center, representing one room and one floor respectively.

In next section, we will describe a WBAN based medical monitoring prototyping system as a part of our wireless body area network project. The body area network prototyping system uses a multi-hopping structure to implement the scenario given in Figure 2.

3. Implementation of WBAN and Hardware Issues

A WBAN system that has been designed for healthcare applications is presented in this section. Hardware electronics and software programs are developed for the scenario presented in Fig. 2. In the implementation, one of the medical or ISM bands-MICS (Medical Implant Communication Service) or WMTS (Wireless Medical Telemetry Systems) or 433 ISM bands will be used between one CCU and its sensor nodes (the first wireless link). CCUs will interface with one of existing wireless standards such as Bluetooth, ZigBee, and WiFi for a remote monitoring system using a mobile network or the internet. Two pieces of software have been created in this project. The software residing at the local PC is named as the GATEWAY. The job of GATEWAY is to gather data from the CCU through RS232/USB cable and forwards it to the remote PC using TCP/IP connections over an Ethernet network. The software residing at the Remote PC is named as BSN Application. The BSN Application will collate data from the local PC, convert and stores them onto the remote PC to be analyzed later by health professionals. The receiver station (i.e. the remote PC) is capable of displaying all the received data on a User Display Graphic (GUI) and is also capable of storing all the data in the database system of a medical center.

A hardware setup to realize the medical scenario presented in section 2 is depicted in Figure 3. Patients' physiological parameters are sent to intermediate CCUs and then to the base station. We are using a multi-hopping network technique that consists of three networking levels in the system. A network between sensors CCU, another network level is between CCUs-base station, and the last communication link is between base stations in the medical centers. The first wireless link is usually less than 10 meters. The second link targets a distance of more than 100 m. Distribution of data to remote destinations is sent via the internet. A CCU can be used for one individual in the medical center or can be used privately in a patient home. If more than one patient shares a CCU box, the CCU can either be connected to a local PC in the room or it can transmit data to another remote CCU box that is attached to a local PC via another wireless link using the WMTS (600 MHz) link as depicted in Figure 2.

The WBAN in Figure 3 is a multi-hopping wireless medical network that uses MICS band to obtain data from sensors placed on or in the body. The WMTS band is used in the intermediate node for a remote wireless communication link. The data is transferred to remote stations through the local area network or the internet already available in medical centers. Unlike the other medical sensor networks (usually operate at 2.4 GHz ISM band), we mainly use medical standards occupying the frequency bands that are usually assigned to medical applications. Both frequency bands are internationally available and are permitted for a remote monitoring of multiple patients simultaneously. The MICS band has a low emission power of 25 µW, comparable to the UWB. The lower power consumption feature is suitable for medical sensor nodes. Hardware and software designs are realized in the system to provide a multi-patient monitoring system with data transfer ability over a network or the internet to a remote computer. A media access layer (MAC) has been implemented on the developed hardware to support multi-patient monitoring facility.

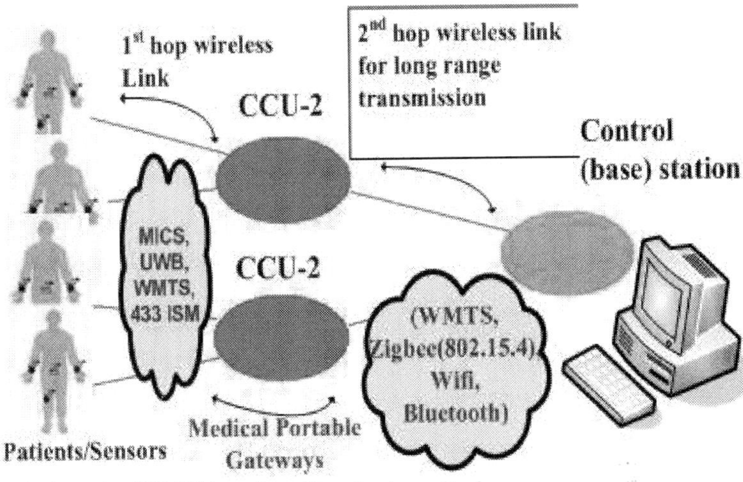

Fig. 3. Multi-hopping WBAN based multi-patient monitoring.

3.1 Sensor nodes Design

Sensor nodes are designed to collect raw signals from a human body. A sensor node undertakes three tasks: detecting signal via a front-end, digitizing/coding/controlling for a multi access communication and finally wireless transmission via a radio transceiver technology, as shown in Figure 4. In addition data acquisition and processing, the microcontroller maintains a power management scheme to control the distribution of the energy from battery in an optimized manner. It should be programmed to turn battery connections OFF for the blocks that are not functioning (i.e. during sleep mode). The signal from a human body is usually weak and coupled with noise. First, the signal should go through an amplification process to increase the signal strength. It then passes through a filtering stage to remove unwanted signals and noise. After which, it will go through an Analog to Digital conversion (ADC) stage to be converted into digital for digital processing. The digitized signal is then processed and stored in the microprocessor (i.e. microcontroller). The microcontroller will then pack those data and transmit over the air via a transceiver. Sensor nodes are designed to be small and power efficient so that their battery last for a long time. Figure 5 shows the hardware implementation of a sensor node containing all the blocks shown in Fig.4.

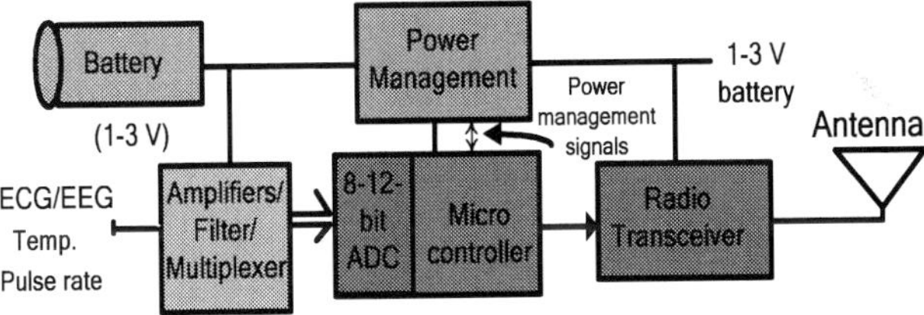

Fig 4. Block diagram of a wireless sensor node in a WBAN.

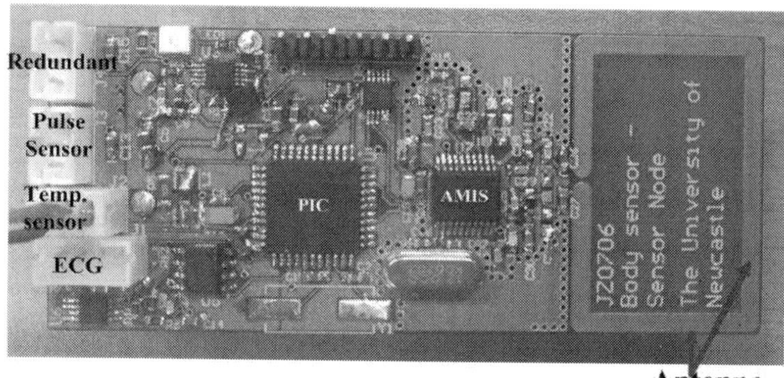

Fig. 5. A 4-channel sensor node.

A sensor node electronics is designed to detect and transmit the physiological signals listed in Table 1. Characteristics of these physiological signals are obtained from the public domain available on the internet. Most physiological signals are low frequency in nature and occupy a small information bandwidth. At such low frequencies and low amplitudes, some problems inherent to circuits need additional attention. For reliable information transfer it is necessary that the interface electronics in the sensor nodes detect physiological signals in the presence of noise and increase the signal-to-noise ratio (SNR) of the detected signal for processing by the subsequent blocks of the sensor nodes. Considering the signal bandwidths given in Table 2, a sampling rate of around 200-400 Hz will be necessary for the analog-to-digital converter (ADC) in the microcontroller (the sampling rate should be at least twice the highest frequency of the signal that is digitized). The tradeoff between the reduction in sampling rate and the total power consumption of the ADC is determined by the choice of the specific physiological parameter used in the sensor node.

Parameter	Range of Parameter	Signal Frequency
ECG signal	0.5-4mV	0.01 – 250 Hz
Respiratory rate	2-50breaths/min	0.1 –10 Hz
Blood Pressure (BP)	10-400mm Hg	0-50 Hz
EEG	3µV-300µV	0.5-60 Hz
Body Temperature	32-40 ^{0}C	0 - 0.1Hz
EMG(Electromyogram)	10µV-15mV	10-5000 Hz
GSR(Galvanic Skin Reflex)	30µV-3mV	0.03-20 Hz

Table 1. Physiological parameter range and signal frequencies.

3.2 CCU and Gateway Design

The primary function of the CCU is to collect data from sensor nodes via the wireless MICS band link and forward these data to a local as well as to a remote PC for further analysis. As explained in the scenario given in Fig. 1, two CCU devices are needed in order to provide a complete WBAN transmission coverage in medical centers. One CCU is designed to be connected to a computer (Fig. 6) via the USB port while the other CCU is used to function as an intermediate device (Fig. 7) that presents a second wireless link for a longer range wireless sensor network. The latter case is more suitable for large medical centers and functions as an intermediate device. Although both CCUs can be used for multiple patients monitoring, the first CCU type (CCU-1) can also be useful for private usage at home or in a room of a hospital for a single patient monitoring.

The sensor nodes/CCU hardware requires a microcontroller and a wireless transceiver to coordinate all activities. The CCU-1/sensor nodes consist of the wireless link (AMI52100 IC) from AMI semiconductor used for the MICS band generation (we also used CC1000 in some sensor nodes to generate 433 MHz ISM and WMTS bands for sensors-CCU wireless connection) and the microcontroller PIC16F87. In addition to these chips, we use another transceiver the CC1010 chip from Chipcon (this chip contains CC1000 and a microcontroller built in) on the intermediate CCU (CCU-2) board to develop a wireless transmission and networking with the WMTS band. The CC1010 and CC1000 transceiver chips have the capability to transmit anywhere within 300 and 1000MHz (It was tuned to WMTS band in our prototype system). The wireless chips AMI52100 IC (Integrated Circuit) and CC1000 family are selected in the project for following reasons: overall cost saving, low-power consumption, size, and the suitability of operating at the MICS, WMTS, and 433 MHZ ISM bands. The AMIS IC has a data rate capability of 19 kbps while CC1010 provides 76 kbps. The CCU-2 device in a WBAN can be comprised of the standards such Zigbee and the 802.11 Wi-Fi standards to accommodate and interface with different wireless platforms and to connect to internet for remote monitoring.

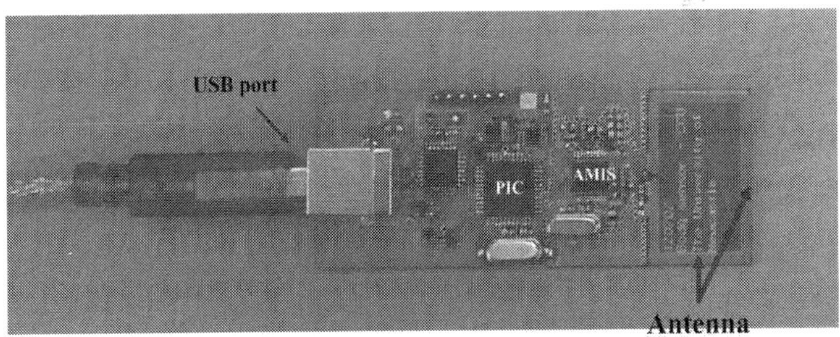

Fig. 6. CCU-1: a central control unit (CCU) used individually.

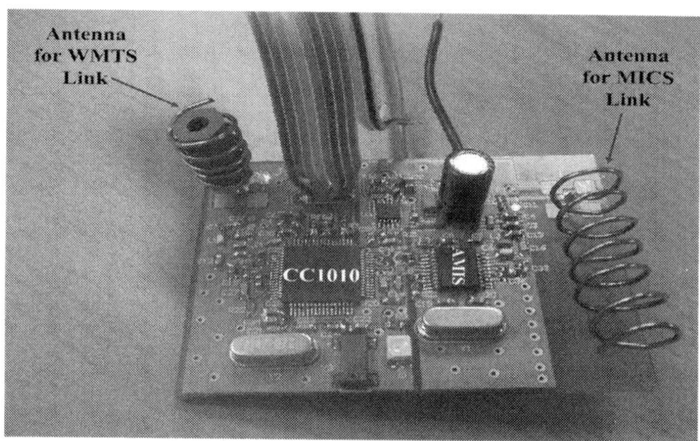

Fig. 7. CCU-2: Intermediate Central Control Unit (CCU). This device is shared by more than one patient and portable. It contains a dual wireless transceiver to support two directional wireless links.

3.3 Medium Access Control Protocol (MAC) and Monitoring

A number of MAC protocols have been proposed for medical sensor networks. Main requirements of a MAC protocol of a medical wireless sensor network are reliability, flexible transmission mechanism and high channel efficiency. Mainly three classes of MAC protocols have been considered for medical applications. They are TDMA (Time Division Multiple Access), polling protocol, and the contention based protocol also known as the random access protocol (Yuce et.al., 2008).

The contention based protocols such as ALOHA and CSMA have been proposed and used for many low power sensor network applications. A combination of a polling protocol and CSMA/CA (Carrier Sense Multiple Access with Collision Avoidance) MAC protocol to transmit the sensor data from multiple sensors to the CCU could be a good mechanism for both power saving as well as for reliable communication of critical medical data. The CSMA/CA MAC protocol is used by the IEEE802.11 WLAN (Wireless Local Area Network) based WiFi and the IEEE802.15.4 based WPAN (Wireless Personal Area Network) standards. The CSMA/CA protocol is a contention based protocol which could offer lower delay and reliable transmission of packets in small size networks like a wireless medical network.

The signals in Table 1 are grouped by the CCU into critical data and non-critical data during the transmission. The wireless protocol will be designed such that the priority will be given to critical data. A critical data packet (such as ECG, it could change according to status of a patient) in a CSMA/CA based sensor network can be immediately transmitted without waiting for its turn. Thus such a mechanism will allow the sensor nodes collecting crucial physiological data (i.e. ECG) to CCU without any collision, loss and delay. For non critical data like temperature, the polling network will be used for the node so that the information will be sent whenever it is needed. A polling structure can be very power efficient and is utilized for the sensor nodes in the WBAN where the data collection is not necessary all the time. By using a polling structure, we can keep the power consumption of the sensor nodes significantly low so that a battery can last several years.

The CCU will collect information and control its flow using the developed communication protocols. The mode of information transmission of a sensor node will depend on the application and the signal type. The sensor nodes in polling scheme will sleep most of the time and wake up for a duration required for a reliable data transfer. Sleep and wake up patterns can be controlled by the acquired signal and by the application. Wake up pattern could be periodic or it can be demand driven. Only the ASIC processor in the microcontroller, which operates with a very low clock rate, always stays awake in the system and will trigger the awakening process. As a result of this process, significant power saving is achieved hence, the battery life is extended. Sensor nodes that are configured in a polling scheme will enter CSMA/CA communication scheme during data transmission so that it will not affect the transmission of the critical data. One of the main objectives is to conserve power within each node and to keep active power to a minimum level so that smaller batteries can be utilized in sensor nodes. Since the time spent in sleep mode is very long compared to the active period, keeping the power consumption as low as possible will greatly increase the battery life of each node.

In order to monitor data, several computer programs have been developed in this project. The necessary software programs have been identified in Figure 2. The software called GATEWAY is developed at the monitoring PC to control the communication with the CCU to get readings from sensors and then forward them through the network/internet to an application on a remote PC. While performing this task, the GATEWAY also verifies the data integrity and schedules retransmission if required. Another software was developed at the remote PC (called BSN) that collects readings from GATEWAY via the network/internet. These readings are stored in the remote PC for analysis. The BSN application can collect and store readings automatically so that no manual intervention is required. It can undertake the administration of patients' particulars such as assigning new sensor ID to patients, segregating sensor readings from different patients and storing them into the data base. The GUI also allows the medical personnel to enter the patient's information.

A graphical user interface (GUI) at the local PC as well as at remote PCs is also designed to display medical data. Both the data received from the CCU and the data sent to the BSN can also be displayed by the GUI in a text or graphical formats. The physiological signals of patients can be accessed by medical staff anywhere in the medical center as long as their computers are connected to the local area network in the building. An example of live monitoring from two patients scenario is shown in Figure 8. It displays temperature and pulse rate information of two patients at the same time. The graph allows up to 20 readings to be displayed. Every sensor device has a unique Sensor ID and must be registered under a patient name before they are used (Yuce et.al., 2008). In the event that an unregistered sensor node is used, all its readings received will be discarded by the BSN application.

The monitoring of the continuous signal like ECG, EMG and EEG is more complicated compared to parameters such as pulse rate and temperature signals. Unlike temperature and pulse rate, the information sent to the CCU requires a continual and undisturbed sampling period as high as 400 samples per second, each sample of size 10 bits will require a connection speed of 4000 bps. To allow for MAC overhead and packet retransmission, the baud rate (i.e. data rate) for the RF link should be at least twice this rate. The use of Manchester encoding is advisable to help maintain data integrity and a stable connection, which halves the data rate of the link. As shown in Table 1 amplitude and frequency information of the continuous physiological signals are similar and thus the same analog front end is used to detect these signals with similar signal amplification and filtering. Typically ECG and EEG signal has amplitude of less than 500μV with frequency less than 100 Hz. The front-end of the sensor node (.e. interface electronics) uses an instrumental amplifier (INA321) and an active low pass filter (LTC6081) (TI 2009). When operating in shut down mode it consumes less than 3μA. Figure 9 is an ECG signal obtained from our set up. Each sensor node representing only one patient can only have one ECG. In order to eliminate the DC noise (50 Hz/60 Hz interference) a recursive filter has been implemented at the PC to obtain an accurate ECG signal. Shown in Figure 9, by clicking on 50 Hz filter, the recursive notch filter operates on the received ECG signal.

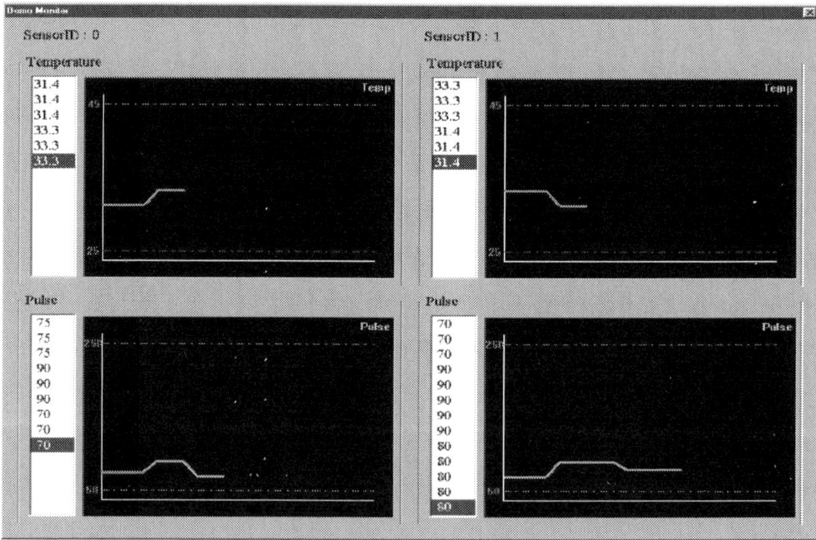

Fig. 8. Live monitoring of multi-patients (physiological data presented in a graphical form at the remote PC). SensorID is used to define each patient.

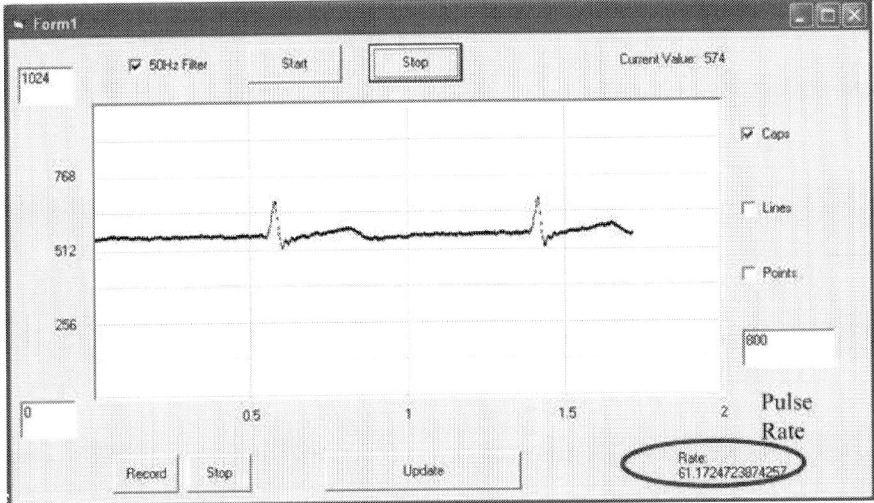

Fig. 9. A clean wireless ECG monitoring showing pulse rate is displayed.

3.4 Ultra Wideband Based WBAN

We design sensor node electronics using the low data rate ultra wideband (UWB) wireless transmission for wireless body area network (UWB-WBAN) (Ho & Yuce, 2008). The UWB is a narrow pulse based transmission system whose spectrum is spread across a wide range of frequencies. Low data rate UWB is suitable for vital signs monitoring system as it transmission power is lower than WLAN, Bluetooth and Zigbee systems, which is less likely to affect human tissue and causes interference to other medical equipments. Furthermore, it is able to transmit at higher data rate which is suitable for real time continuous monitoring of many physiological signals. In this part of the project, we developed the sensor node electronics using the low data rate UWB transmission technique and investigate its characteristics when operating in or around the human body. The ultimate goal is to integrate UWB sensor nodes together with our narrow band medical based sensor nodes to form a wireless body area network application for healthcare systems.

4. WBAN Network Design Techniques

A WBAN which could collect critical and non-critical data from different parts of a patient body needs to be designed considering a number of important issues. In a patient monitoring system data transmission reliability and latency is extremely important. Reliability and latency of a WBAN will depend on the design of physical and MAC (Medium Access Control) layers. Design of these layers determines the power consumption profile of a WBAN which is an important design issue. The MAC layer also plays an important role to determine network efficiency and resource utilization issues which ultimately determine a system and operating costs of a WBAN. At the same time the PHY (Physical) layer also determines reliability of a WBAN. A PHY layer could select appropriate modulation and coding techniques to combat against transmission channel variability. Performance of a WBAN can be defined in terms of reliability, power efficiency and scalability. Section 6 presented a particular implementation of a MAC protocol for a WBAN. This section presents a more general MAC design approach and design rules.

Reliability:

Reliability of a WBAN is directly related to the packet loss probability and the packet transmission delay. Packet loss probability is influenced by the BER (Bit Error Rate) of a channel and the MAC layer transmission procedures. The PHY layer of a WBAN can reduce the effective bit error rate of a transmission link by using adaptive modulation and coding techniques to suit the transmission channel conditions. Details on the BER values for various modulation techniques can be found in references (Mark et.al., 2003). Use of forward correction error (FEC) technique can reduce the effective bit error rate however, the use of a FEC technique requires transmission of additional redundant bits which could increase the power budget of a WBAN node due to transmission of additional bits. Careful design of modulation and coding techniques is essential for the optimum operation of a WBAN. The MAC layer has also important role for the reliability of a WBAN related to the channel access technique, packet size selection and packet retransmission strategy used in a WBAN. The reliability and power budget of a WBAN also depends on the interference situation of a network. If the interference and noise floor of a network is high, in order to successfully transmit packets, a node needs to transmit at a higher transmitter power level. MAC layer design techniques are further discussed in section 9.

Power Efficiency:

Power management in a WBAN is a very important operational issue. Power usage can be minimized by optimizing the PHY and MAC layer processes. A PHY layer can increase the probability of successful transmissions by selecting appropriate modulation and coding techniques. Higher packet transmission success probability reduces the end-to-end packet delay as well as the power budget of a WBAN node. Power budget of a node could be optimized by increasing successful packet transmission probability. Power optimization scope at the PHY layer is generally limited and fixed. On the other hand a MAC layer can introduce much higher level of power savings by using a range of techniques including packet transmission scheduling and channel access techniques, use of optimal packet structure, and intelligent signaling techniques. Since a WBAN will be operating in a shared communication environment it is necessary to minimize the contentions and interference.

Scalability:

A WBAN needs to be scalable which is essential for a patient monitoring system. For patient monitoring it is quite often necessary to change the number of WBAN nodes to collect various physiological data from a patient. A scalable WBAN will allow health care professionals to easily reconfigure a WBAN by either adding or removing nodes without affecting the operation of the WBAN. Scalability will largely depend on the MAC protocol design.

In an installed WBAN generally PHY layers are fixed hence, the MAC layer can take a major role to maintain QoS (Quality of Service) and reliability under variable transmission and traffic conditions. In this chapter we examine the MAC protocol design issues for a WBAN based patient monitoring system. Before moving into the discussion of network and MAC design issues first we examine the network and MAC protocol design requirements. Some of the main requirements of a WBAN design are listed below.

- A WBAN should be able to support a range of medical applications including acquiring periodic and non-periodic data sources, and transmitting to a service node (figure 1) in a multihop network within a maximum fixed delay without any loss of critical information (Golmie et.al., 2006). At the same time a WBAN should be able to support exchange of non-medical and control information to remotely supervise various appliances when operating in a remote patient monitoring environment.

- A WBAN should be able to operate in a power constrained environment where power sources such as battery could last for a reasonably longer period of time. Power optimization for the implantable nodes is more critical than other nodes. Power savings can be achieved by combining appropriate PHY and MAC layer procedures.

- A WBAN should be self healing, secure and reliable which may include implantable and external nodes.

- A WBAN should support data rates between few tens of kbs to several Mbs to host a range of applications such as images and video clips.

- A WBAN should support QoS management features to offer priority services. Particularly when a critical patient is monitored, the system must guarantee delivery of critical physiological data to a service node. For medical data the main QoS features will be the transmission delay and the packet loss.

- A WBAN should operate and co-exists with other network devices operating in similar frequency bands. Also, a WBAN should be able to operate in a heterogeneous networking environment where different wireless networks can co-exist and may offer similar or different services.

There are a number of classes of MAC protocols exist which are used for different networking applications (Golmie et.al., 2006). MAC protocols are mainly classified into two categories; scheduled and random access protocols. The scheduled access protocols offer deterministic packet delay and packet loss thus offering higher quality of service (QoS). On the other hand the random access protocols are dynamic in nature where transmission resources are allocated to the communication nodes only when a node has any information to transmit. A random access protocol introduces variable delay and sometime packet losses. However, the delay and packet loss figures depend on the traffic volume and application scenarios. For a low traffic volume such as the WBAN scenario a random access protocol may offer pseudo deterministic performance which will be similar to scheduled access protocols. Another main advantage of a random access protocol is the ability to use of adaptive sleep cycle control and resource management techniques which reduce power consumption of sensor nodes (Omeni et.al., 2008).

4.1 MAC Protocols for Wireless Body Area Networks

Wireless Body Area Network is a special purpose wireless sensor network with several specific requirements as mentioned in previous sections. A short range wireless system such as the body area network can be developed using either a scheduled or a random medium access control protocol. In a WBAN, the MAC protocol determines the packet or information delivery schedule as well as the packet loss probability. These two QoS factors are also influenced by the transmission channel and traffic/data characteristics in a network. Figure 1 showed a typical WBAN with multiple sensor nodes and a single Central Coordinator Unit (CCU) which collects data from all sensor nodes as well as controls the operation of these sensor nodes. In order to transmit information among these nodes and to coordinate these transmissions, it is necessary to develop a suitable MAC protocol. This particular WBAN shown in figure 1 is operating in a star configuration where all the sensor nodes are connected to the CCU by using a single hop connection. A star configuration allows all sensor nodes to directly transmit data to the CCU.

Sensors on the body will collect different physiological data where the data sampling rate and data sample size will vary. Table-2 lists the characteristics of physiological data. The table shows that the data rate and data generation times of different physiological signals are quite variable. Generally these signals are periodic in nature but their rate could vary based on the physiological condition of a patient. Some of the signals ideally appears to be periodic but may turn into a non-periodic or a random signal based on a patient condition. For example, if a patient develops an abnormal heart condition then the heartbeat sensor could generate an aperiodic or a random signal. A MAC protocol of a WBAN should be able to efficiently handle these variations. Also, a body sensor node generally have very limited storage capacity, hence it will be necessary to transmit data within a specified time delay to avoid any data loss due to the buffer overflow. Time delay constraint will also be determined by the priority status of a data stream. For example, if a critical patient is monitored then some of the physiological data could be more important than other data and hence, the high priority data stream requires a quick channel access. To support information transmission within a WBAN it is necessary to develop a dynamic MAC protocol which not only transmit information reliably but also the protocol needs to be energy efficient and scalable. Next section we review three classes of protocols such are scheduled TDMA (Time Division Multiple Access), polling and random access protocols. Beside these three protocols another class of protocols known as the reservation protocol is also used in the sensor networking applications however, this class of protocol is not well suited for WBAN applications due to higher signaling requirements. Additional signaling traffic not only consumes extra bandwidth but also consumes significant amount of energy. Below we briefly discuss the scheduled and random access protocol features for WBAN applications.

Physiological Signal	Parameter range	Maximum Frequency (Hz)	Sample Interarrival time (sec)	Payload /sample(bits)	Required data rate (kbs)
Blood flow	1-300ml/s	20	0.025	12	0.48
ECG signal	0.5-4mV	250	0.002	12	6.0
Respiratory rate	2-50breaths/min	10	0.05	12	0.24
Blood Pressure (Direct Arterial)	10-400mm Hg	50	0.01	12	1.2
Blood pH	6.8-7.8pH units	2	0.25	12	.048
Nerve Potentials	0.01-3mV	10,000	5E-06	12	2400
Body Temperature	32-40 ^{0}C	0.1	5	12	.0024

Table 2. Physiological data characteristics.

4.1.1 Scheduled TDMA MAC Protocol

A scheduled MAC protocol can offer deterministic delay and no packet loss due to absence of any transmission channel contention. The Time Division Multiple Access (TDMA) is a scheduled multiple access technique where transmission of packets are managed in the form of time frame and slots. A time slot can be seen as a dedicated transmission resource used to carry patient data with minimum or no overhead. A central controller which is the CCU in case of a WBAN will allocate time slots to each sensor nodes to transmit data. Figure 10 shows a typical TDMA frame and slot structure. Slots could be allocated on a permanent basis to each sensor node to transmit information from a sensor node to the CCU. When time slots are allocated by the CCU then packet overhead of the information transfer can be eliminated resulting fewer bits to transmit. A TDMA based MAC protocol could be suitable for a small WBAN with a limited number of sensors generating data at a fixed rate and transmitting fixed block of data.

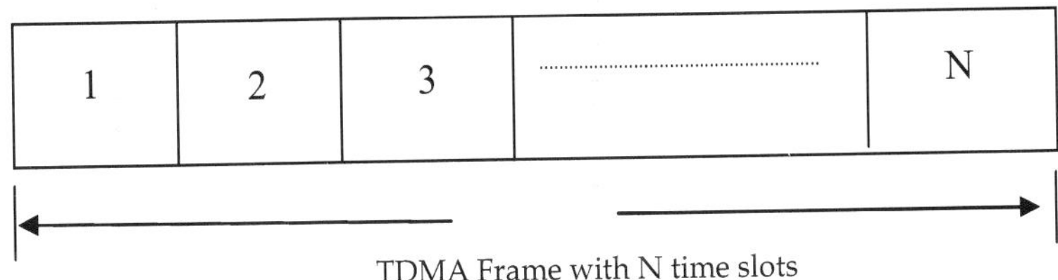

Fig. 10. TDMA frame and slot structure.

A TDMA based WBAN can be made energy efficient where transmitter circuit of a sensor node is only activated in the specified slot. Also, a sensor node does not need to listen to the transmission channels all the time hence, energy consumptions for the communication circuits will be minimized. A fixed timer based sleep cycle control scheme can be used for a TDMA based system. However, a TDMA based WBAN has two major resource allocation problems. One of the main problems is supporting different sensors with different data inter-arrival time i.e. handling non-periodic data. In a TDMA based system generally a time slot will be allocated on a fixed basis to a particular sensor node and allow that node to transmit in the specified time slot without any possibility of collisions. As shown in the table 2 that a typical WBAN needs to cater for different sampling rates to gather various physiological data. Whereas in a TDMA system time slots are allocated on a fixed basis designed to handle synchronous information. For example, one can see from table 2 that for each blood flow sample a sensor node transmits 12 ECG samples. If these samples are generated from different nodes and they are allocated with separate time slots then the blood flow sensor node will not utilize transmission resources (time slots) efficiently. Resource utilization may not be a major problem for a WBAN because when sensor nodes are not transmitting any data, they will not utilize the transmission slot but will remain in the idle state to save energy. However, in this situation some system resources will be under utilized and the cost of a system may increase. The main problem of a TDMA based system is the scalability. The TDMA is a centralized protocol which requires changes in the central controller setup to accommodate any extra sensor node in a WBAN which could be the main drawback for a patient monitoring system; because the number of sensor nodes could vary depending on the condition of a patient. For example, should medical staff wants to add more monitoring devices on a patient body who is under observation then it will be necessary to modify the design of the TDMA time frame from the main controller. From a WBAN design point of view, a TDMA based system can be used to implement a patient monitoring system using a fixed number of nodes.

4.1.2 Polling MAC Protocol

Polling based MAC protocols are based on scheduled transmission technique utilizing the master slave architecture to transmit data. In a polling network, a central controller schedules all transmissions in the network thus avoiding any contention probability. Figure 11(a) shows a typical polling network architecture where all transmissions are controlled by the CCU. A polling network is more flexible than a fixed assignment based TDMA network where traffic sources with different interarrival rates can easily be accommodated. As shown in figure 11(a) the CCU will send polling messages to all nodes which in response to the poll can either transmit a message or can send a short NACK (Negative ACKnowledgement) when a node has no data to transmit. An ACK (Acknowledgement) for the previous transmission could be included in the polling message to improve data reliability. The polling frequency can be varied and optimized to support traffic sources of different information inter-arrival rate. Figure 11(b) shows the polling cycle and the polling sequence. It shows a round robin polling scheme where nodes are polled in a sequential manner. Figure also shows an additional polling slot is kept in at the end of the poll cycle which is used to support the scalability feature of the protocol. New nodes can either join or depart a network by simply sending a message to the central controller. Number of nodes in a network will vary the polling cycle time as well as the packet transmission delay. The propagation delay is insignificant and can be ignored for a WBAN application. A polling network offers two main advantages. They are the deterministic and bounded transmission delay, and the scalable network architecture. When a new sensor node needs to be added in a WBAN, the new unregistered sensor node will send a JOIN message when the new poll slot appears in the polling cycle. When the controller receives the JOIN message then it creates a new polling slot and data slot for the new terminal. Similarly, when a node departs the network by sending a DEPART message the controller will remove the allocated poll and data slots. This simple process will allow a WBAN to accommodate variable number of sensor nodes. In a polling network the queuing and the packet transmission delay is largely determined by the traffic volume and the number of active nodes. When a new node joins a WBAN then the polling cycle length will increase thus increasing the packet delay by a fixed value (assuming fixed size slots are used). Power consumption of a polling network can be controlled by organizing the polling and data transmission sequences. For example, when a WBAN transmits data with different interarrival times then the polling sequence can be synchronized with the sampling rate. Similar to the TDMA MAC protocol, a node can wake up before its poll message then transmits or receives data in the specified time. The CCU could broadcast the polling and transmission schedules to maximize the node sleep time.

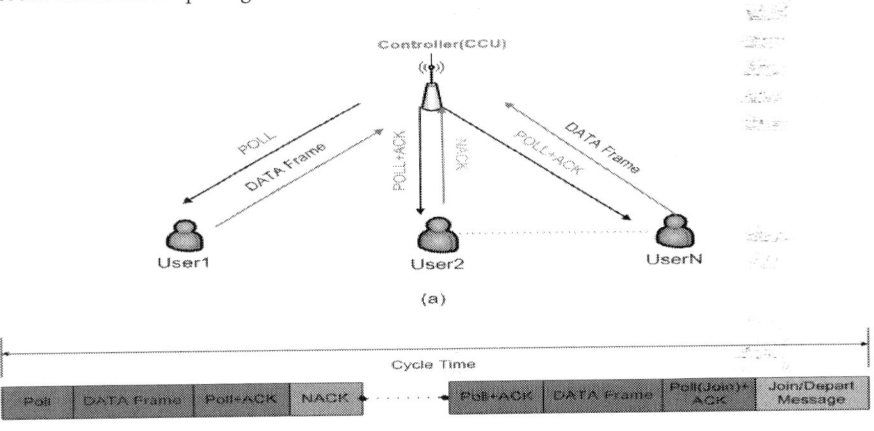

Fig. 11. A polling MAC based transmission sequence.

4.1.3 Random Access MAC Protocol

Random access protocols are commonly known as the ON DEMAND access protocol widely used in wireless local area and sensor networks designed for short range communications. These protocols are suitable for distributed systems with no or minimal control signaling. There are many random access protocols are in use among them the CSMA/CA (Collision Sense Multiple Access with Collision Avoidance) protocol is suitable for the short range wireless communication (Karl et.al., 2008). A CSMA/CA protocol based sensor accesses a transmission channel only when it needs to transmit any information. A node using the MAC protocol will check a transmission channel status only when it has data in its transmission buffer. If it finds a transmission channel to be free then the node initiates a packet transmission using a contention based procedure. Because of the contention nature of the protocol a transmitted packet may collide and may require retransmission(s) to successfully transmit the packet. There are a number of advantages a random access protocol can offer for WBAN applications. Main advantages include lower signaling overhead, scalability, distributed control which allows the network to accommodate traffic sources with different interarrival rate and data rates. The CSMA/CA protocol also allows network to optimize power and transmission resources locally at each sensor node. For example, if a node generates any urgent data in a non-scheduled manner then a TDMA or a polling based system will have difficulties to transmit those data immediately. Whereas, as soon as the non-scheduled data is generated at a node the random access protocol based system can transmit the data provided the node have the necessary priority. However, the main disadvantage of a random access protocol could introduce a variable and longer delay if the traffic load is high. For a WBAN design it is not expected that the traffic load will be higher because of the system's transmission capacity. If the traffic load remains fairly stable and lower than about 70~80% of a network capacity then a random access based protocol offers reasonably lower delay. The average packet delay of a random access protocol based network is given by (1). Propagation delay is ignored in the equation. The first term of the right hand side of the equation represents the access delay (T_{access}) which is the time required by a CSMA/CA node to access the channel. Detail description of the CSMA/CA based channel access procedure can be found in the reference (Golmie et.al., 2006). The access delay depends on the traffic load of a network. The second terms represents the retransmission delay (T_{retry}). During the access phase if a packet experiences a collision then the transmitting node will backoff for a certain duration and then try to transmit the packet. The backoff period will be randomly distributed to minimize the collision probability. In case of a collision multiple retransmission attempts may be needed to resolve the collision. A packet could be dropped if the packet cannot be transmitted successfully after multiple collisions. The queuing delay (T_{queue}) represents the buffering delay at a node. The last term of the equation represents the packet transmission delay (T_{packet}) whose value depends on the packet size and the transmission data rate. From the discussion it is clear that the first three components could introduce delay jitter if the incoming traffic volume varies significantly over the time or the received signal to noise ratio (SNR) varies significantly over the time.

$$T_{d(random)} = T_{access} + T_{retry} + T_{queue} + T_{packet} \qquad (1)$$

To summarise the review of MAC protocols we compare the key features of three classes or protocols in Table 3. In the next section we examine the IEEE802.15.4 standard which defines the physical and MAC layers of the Zigbee standard. The Zigbee standard can be potentially applied for WBAN patient monitoring applications. The IEEE802.15.4 standard supports both random and schedules access protocols. Also, the IEEE802.1.5.6 working group is working on develops PHY and MAC layers with strong similarity with the IEEE802.15.4 standard (TG6). As mentioned earlier that a WBAN can be seen as a special purpose sensor network whose operational characteristics will be very similar to a wireless personal network (WPAN). The IEEE802.15.4 MAC protocol also supports the WPAN features using the star network topology.

MAC Features	Scheduled MAC: TDMA	Scheduled Mac: Poll	Random Access MAC: CSMA/CA
Packet Delay	Deterministic and fixed.	Deterministic, varies with the network traffic load (volume of data).	Variable, varies with network traffic load, priority and application type.
Packet Loss[*]	Deterministic and fixed.	Deterministic, varies with the network traffic load.	Variable, varies with the network traffic load and application type.
Traffic handling capability	Efficiently handle periodic traffic. For non-periodic traffic efficiency is lower due to variable delay.	Efficiently handle periodic traffic. Also, can handle non-periodic data by adjusting the polling cycle.	Can handle non-periodic traffic more efficiently than scheduled MAC protocols.
Energy Efficiency	Fixed transmission sequence can introduce fixed sleep cycle. However, energy efficiency could be low when handling non-periodic traffic.	Fixed transmission sequence can introduce fixed sleep cycle. Energy efficiency is better than the TDMA protocol where a node may wake up from sleep and send NACK to reduce the transmission cycle time.	Can offer much better energy efficiency compared to scheduled MAC protocols. Transmitting nodes remain in sleep mode until it is necessary to actually transmit data.
Transmission[#] efficiency	Very low or no overhead involve in this transmission.	High overhead due to the polling mechanism used. However, for WBAN applications the overhead is lower due to shorter propagation delay.	For WBAN applications the ratio of overhead to payload is normally high unless the aggregation technique is used.
Network Scalability	Poor scalability feature, particularly with non-periodic traffic.	Scalability property is good. Scalability margin is limited by the delay.	Scalability feature is good.

Table 3. Summary of yey features of WBAN MAC protocols.

*: Assuming a low BER channel and the effect of transmission errors are not considered.
#: Transmission efficiency is defined as the ratio of number of information bits transmitted to the total number of transmitted bits (data and overhead bits).

4.2 IEEE802.15.4 MAC Protocol

In this section we introduce the IEEE802.15.4 MAC standard which could be used to design first generation WBAN for medical and other health monitoring applications. The main objective of the IEEE802.15.4 standard is to provide a low-cost, reliable and low power wireless protocol to support a range of sensor networks and home networking solutions. The standard defines the lower two layers functionalities i.e. the PHY and MAC layer functionalities (Gutierrez et.al. 2001, Khan et.al., 2006). Both these layers have been designed to prolong the battery life requirement. Tables 4-(a) and 4-(b) lists the key PHY and MAC layers features of the IEEE802.15.4 standard respectively.

Frequency	*868 – 868.6 MHz (Europe)*	*901 – 928 MHz (North America)*	*2.4 – 2.4835 GHz (World Wide)*
Channel Bandwidth	0.3 MHz	0.6 MHz	2 MHz
No. of RF Channels	1	10 (separation 2 MHz)	16 (separation 5 MHz)
Maximum Data Rate	20 kbs	40 kbs	250 kbs
Modulation Technique	BPSK	BPSK	O-QPSK
Transmission Power	1 mw (min)	1 mw (min)	1 mw (min)
BER requirements	< 1%	< 1%	< 1%

Table 4-(a). Key PHY layer features of the IEEE802.15.4 standard.

Feature	*Description*
MAC Protocol	CSMA/CA (Carrier Sensing Multiple Access/Collision Avoidance)
Address	16 bit (short) or 64 bit (extended)
Transmission mode	Fully acknowledged mode
Energy Detection	Yes with the cooperation of the physical layer
Link Quality Indication	Yes with the cooperation of the physical layer

Table 4-(b). Key MAC layer features of the IEEE802.15.4 standard.

The standard supports two network topologies; these are star and peer-to-peer topologies as shown in the Figure 12. The star topology is a typical centralized architecture where a coordinator controls activities of various nodes. The star configuration will typically operate in a WPAN configuration. The peer-to-peer configuration can support a multi-hop network and the range can be extended by incorporating the mesh network architecture using the configuration. The IEEE802.15.4 standard divides transmission nodes in two categories, which determines the topology and the media access used by the network. One class of nodes are classified as a Full Functional Device (FFD) which can directly communicate with any other node and can act as a PAN coordinator as shown in Figure 13. The other class of node is known as a Reduced Function Devices (RFD) which can only communicate with FFDs.

A Personal Area Network (PAN) structure as shown in Figure 13 is controlled by the PAN coordinator. In a WBAN design the CCU can take the role of a PAN coordinator. The coordinator periodically sends beacon signals that identify the PAN. The PAN is identified by a 16 bit PAN identifier. The beacon frame also contains information such as a list of outstanding frames, and other system related parameters. The time interval between these beacon signals is constant and users can select a value which is a multiple of 15.38 ms. The maximum beacon interval time could go up to 252 ms. Two consecutive beacon signals forms a *superframe* separated by 16 equally sized time slots as shown in the Figure 13. The superframe is subdivided into active and inactive periods. All nodes including the coordinator can turn off its transceivers and go into a sleep state during the inactive period of a superframe. The active period which consists of 16 timeslots, where each timeslot is divided into two groups. One set of slots forms the *contention access period* **(CAP)** and the rest of the slots become part of the *Guaranteed Time Slots* **(GTS)**. The length of the active and inactive periods is configurable hence, allowing system design flexibility to accommodate different types of applications. The CAP slots can be accessed using the standard CSMA/CA procedure whereas the GTS slots are allocated by the coordinator when a request is made by a node. The flag in the request packet indicates whether the slot will be used to transmit or to receive. Upon receiving a slot request the coordinator will allocate a GTS slot when appropriate resources are available. When GTS slots are used for transmission a node can schedule its sleep cycle and wakes up just before the time slot starts and sends the packet. On the other hand when a CAP slot is used then the node must wake up in advance and perform carrier sensing or other collision avoidance procedures before it can initiate a transmission. The CAP slots can be used to support both periodic and non-periodic data sources such as irregular heart beat or pulses. Whereas the GTS slots can be used to transmit high priority information from critical patients to guarantee data transfer. Both access modes can be configured to support acknowledgement based connections to improve the reliability. From the MAC architecture point of view it can be seen that the 802.15.4 standard is well suited for a WBAN applications.

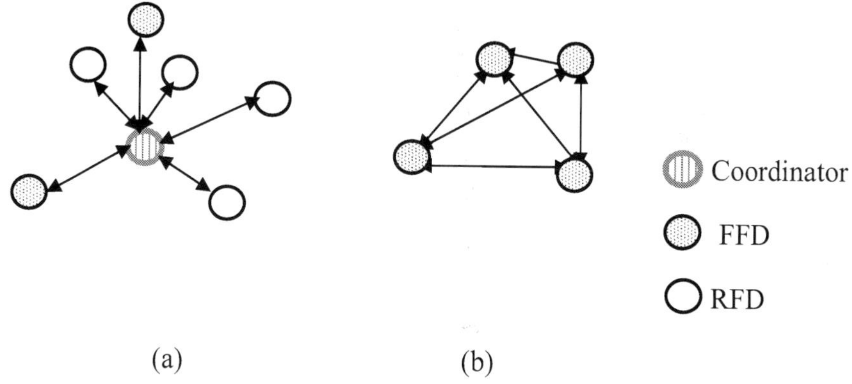

Fig. 12. Network topologies. (a) star topology, (b) peer to peer topology.

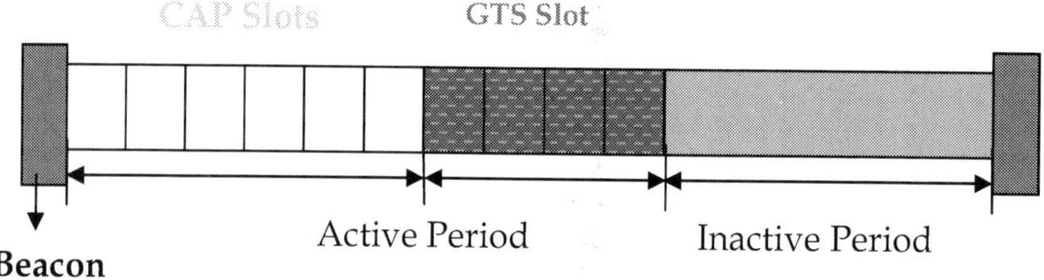

Fig. 13. Super frame structure of the IEEE802.15.4.

4.3 Basics of Link Budget Calculation

For every wireless network it is important to properly design the wireless link in order to maximize the packet transmission success rate and to minimize the energy consumption of nodes. The link budget of a WBAN will depend on the radio propagation conditions and packet transmission techniques used in a WBAN. The packet transmission issue has already been discussed in the previous sections. The radio propagation condition is dictated by the path loss and fading processes. Fading can be classified as a large scale and small scale fading. Small scale fading occurs due to the relative position of a transmitter and a receiver, whereas the large scale fading is attributed to the mobility of a node which is not very relevant for a WBAN node. The path loss in a WBAN environment will depend on the location of a node. An implanted node will experience a different path loss value compared to an external node for the same transmitter receiver separation distance due to the presence of various body tissues and fluids. A transmitter's energy requirements will be directly influenced by the path loss environment of a node. The task force TG6 of the IEEE802.15.6 work group has extensively studied the channel modeling issues for the WBAN (Yazdandoost et.al., 2009). The work divided WBAN nodes in three different categories:

Implant node, body surface node and the external node. An implant node could reside immediately under the skin or deep inside a body surrounded by various tissues. A body surface node is placed on the surface of human skin with a maximum permissible distance of 2 cm from the body. An external node will be generally away from the body upto a distance of 5 meters. The standards committee also considered that an implant device will operate in the MICS band only. The body surface and external nodes are allowed to use a range of frequencies available for WBAN applications.

The maximum power limitation of a medical devices decided by various regulatory bodies. The ETSI (European Telecommunication Standards Institute) set the maximum to 25 µwatt ERP (Equivalent Radiated Power), whereas FCC (Federal Communication Commission) and the ITU-R (International Telecommunications Union – Radio) set the maximum power to 25 µwatt EIRP (Equivalent Radiated Isotropic Power) which is 2.2 dB lower than the ETSI value. With this limitation it is very important to design nodes and place them strategically to obtain physiological information from various part of the body. The power budget of a WBAN node is also affected by the selection of antenna used on these nodes. In a WBAN two types of antenna's could be used; one is the dipole antenna and the other type is the loop antenna. The radiation patterns of these antennas will also influence a link delay budget. The total path loss between a WBAN implant transmitter and a receiver can be calculated by the equation 2. The path loss for a body surface node can be approximated by using the free space path loss model for a short link distance.

$$PL(d) = PL(d_0) + 10n \log_{10}\left(\frac{d}{d_0} \right) + S$$

$$S \alpha N(0, \sigma_s)$$

(2)

Where $PL(d_0)$ is the measured path loss at a reference distance d_0 from the transmitter, d is the distance in meter, n is the path loss exponent, and S is the loss due to the shadow fading which is normally distributed with a zero mean value with a standard deviation of σ_s. One of TG6 groups established test beds using a multi-thread loop antenna to measure various loss components of (1) for implant to implant and implant to body surface transmissions. Measured values of various loss components are listed in Table 5. A number of other research groups have measured different path loss components for different operating environments. More detail information can be obtained from following references (Yazdandoost et.al., 2009).

Communication Environment	PL(d₀) dB		n		σs dB	
	Implant to Implant	Implant to Body Node	Implant to Implant	Implant to Body Node	Implant to Body Node	Implant to Body Node
Deep tissue	35.04	47.14	6.26	4.26	8.18	7.85
Near Surface	40.94	49.81	4.99	4.22	9.05	6.81

Table 5. Measured values of path loss components (Yazdandoost et.al., 2009).

For a WBAN design it is very important to calculate the path loss and fading values to determine the minimum transmission power of a node. Minimum transmission power of a node can be approximately determined by(3)

$$P_{Tx}(\min) = P_L(total) + P_{Rx}(\min) \qquad (3)$$

Where P_L(total) represents total power loss between a transmitter and a receiver, P_{Rx} represents the minimum power required by a receiver in to order to receive a packet successfully. The minimum received power value will depend on the receiver's sensitivity which is largely determined by the SNR/BER (Signal to Noise Ratio/Bit Error Rate) profile of the modulator/demodulator used. In some cases instead of measuring SNR values, the SNIR (Signal to Noise Interference Ratio) is used which takes care of the interference generated by other transmitters in the vicinity. Interference could be generated by other wireless devices operating in the same or adjacent frequency bands. For example, for the 2.4 GHz operation there could be potentially many interfering sources in hospital environment. Figure 14 shows the BER profile of different modulation techniques which could be used in a WBAN node. Simpler modulation technique which supports moderate data rate offers reasonable BER value when the SNR value is above 7 dB. The effective BER measured at the MAC layer could be reduced by using appropriate FEC technique. For a high quality medical monitoring system it is necessary to maintain the packet error rate (PER) close to zero. Packet error rate of a link can be derived using (4).

$$PER = 1 - (1 - p)^L \qquad (4)$$

Where p is the bit error probability and L is the packet length expressed in bits. As shown in (4) that PER value depends on the transmission link condition and the packet length selection. For example, a packet size of 100 bits will introduce a PER value of 9.5% when the BER is 10^{-3} which is a typical transmission channel condition, whereas the PER value drops to zero if the channel BER is 10^{-5}. For a BPSK modulator for a change of 3 dB SNR could result in such a significant improvement of PER values. Hence it is important to notice that the selection of physical layer parameters and link budget value will significantly influences the quality of a WBAN monitoring system.

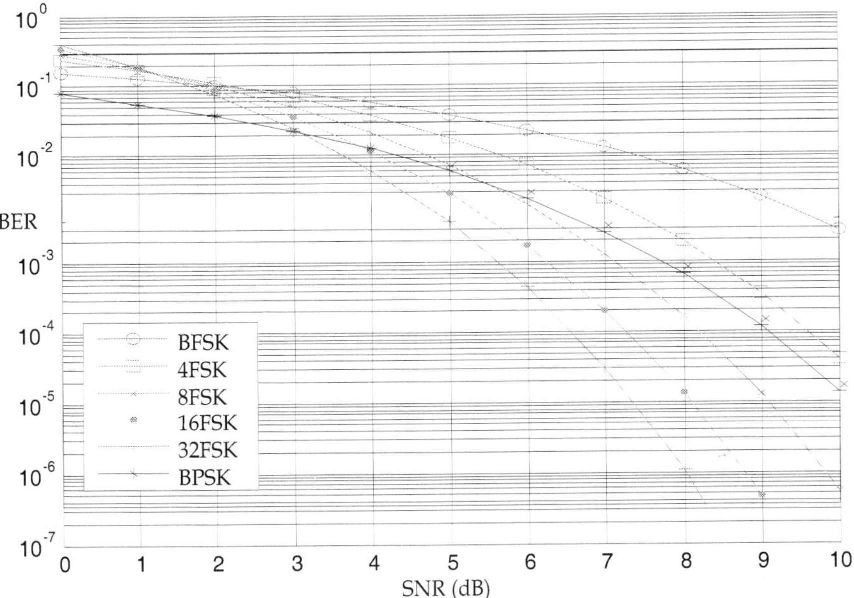

Fig. 14. BER profile of different modulation scheme using coherent receivers (Doong-Sun et.al., 2009).

In the next section we examine a ZigBee based patient monitoring system which can be configured to support single or multi-patient monitoring applications. The ZigBee standard is based on the IEEE802.15.4 PHY and MAC layers (Zigbee).

5. A WBAN Based Patient Monitoring System

In this section we present a ZigBee based muti-hop patient monitoring system which illustrates a WBAN network architecture is proposed in Figure 15 where multiple sensors are placed on each patient. The data from sensors are transmitted to the PCU (Patient Coordinator Unit-A wearable device that can be carried or wearable by the patient). The PCU aggregates sensor data and transmit them to the CCU (Central Coordination Unit). The CCU acts as an intermediate network device that forward the collected medical data to a patient database (DB) where remote monitoring devices can retrieve patients' data for healthcare professions. Each patient body forms a PAN (Personal Area Network) where PCU acts as the PAN coordinator. Similarly the CCU acts as the PAN coordinator for all PCUs which can be considered as a second tier network. All nodes in each PAN will synchronize with their PAN coordinators. In case of signaling failure, a coordinator may not be able to form a PAN in time resulting in transmission failures. The network operates in a multi-hop fashion where each link transmits data using the CSMA/CA protocol. Relay nodes such as the PCU and the CCU can be configured in two ways. One of the configurations is that these nodes simply act as forwarding node i.e. it receives a packet and simply forwards the packet to the next link. Other configuration is that these nodes receive multiple packets from sensor nodes, and then encapsulates multiple packets and forward a larger packet. The former approach can be implemented with nodes with low processing capability whereas later approach reduces the number of transmission access on the forward link thus reducing probability of collisions for a ZigBee based system.

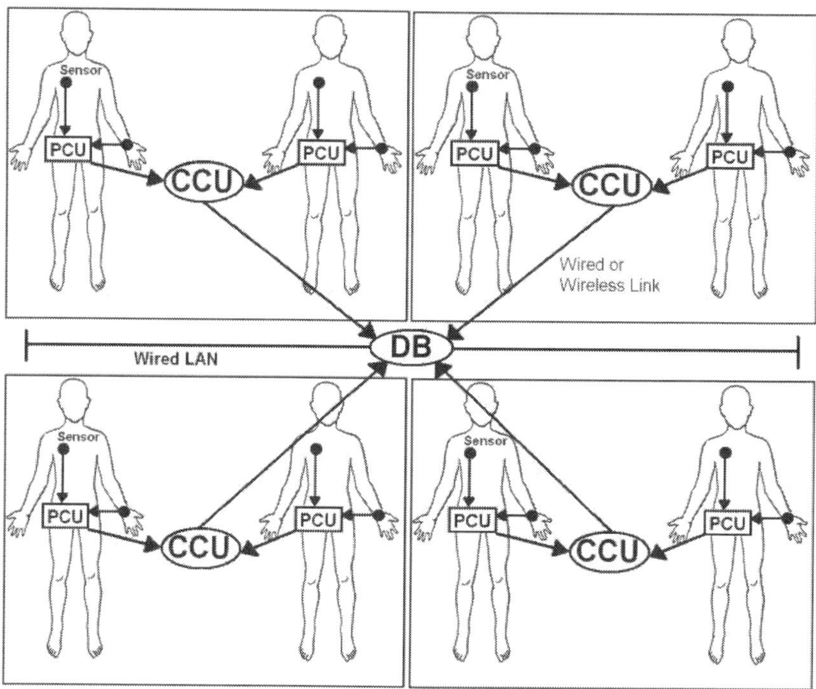

Fig. 15. A WBAN based multi-hop patient monitoring system. Each patient's body forms a PAN and consists of sensor nodes and the PCU.

In a Zigbee based system it will be necessary to reduce the number of packets transmitted from sensor nodes to reduce the contention level in a network. To achieve that, the sensor nodes may aggregate multiple physiological data and transmit in a single packet. As seen from Table-2 that data sample sizes are quite small only 12 bits/sample which is much smaller than the minimum 802.15.4 packet header length. Sending each sample separately will increase the contention level significantly, which will result in an increase in the packet loss and delay. In order to reduce the contention level it will be prudent to opportunistically combine multiple samples and transmit these samples in a single packet. Later in the performance analysis section, the effectiveness of data aggregation technique will be further discussed. The multi-hop network shown in the Figure 15 may have interference problem when the CSMA/CA protocol is used. A transmission on a path can interfere another transmission on a different path. For example, a sensor node to PCU transmission can interfere with the transmission between the CCU to DB. To avoid this problem, it is necessary to control power levels of each transmission and in addition, some form of loose scheduling is necessary to avoid or to reduce collision levels. Also, the relay configuration could reduce the problem. Figure 16 shows the IEEE802.15.4 sensor node transmit profile. The power profile of the sensor node was generated using the path loss model only, fading effects were not considered in this calculation. Based on the power-distance relationship, sensor nodes on the body will transmit at an appropriate power level depending on the proximity of receivers and transmitters.

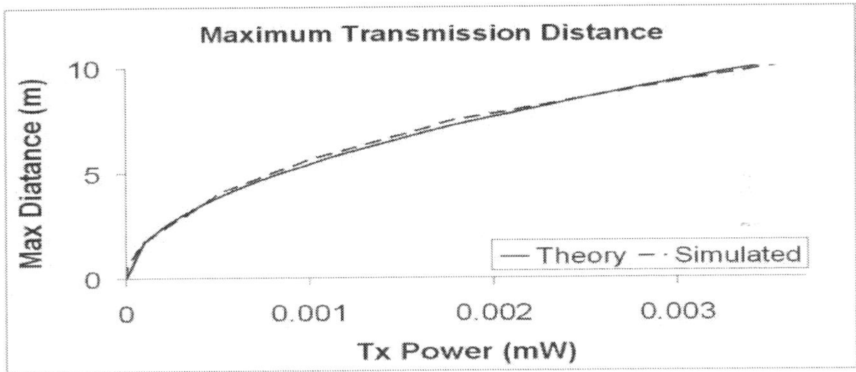

Fig. 16. IEEE802.15.4 Sensor node power transmission profile.

6. Performance Analysis of WBAN

In this section we analyze the performance of the proposed WBAN for patient monitoring applications using a simulation model (Bulger, 2008). We use this model to analyze the performance of a multi-hop network where patient data is transmitted from sensors to the data base (DB) using the PCU and the CCU as relay nodes. In the body area network model, we simulated all sensors but the nerve potential traffic generators listed in Table 2. In the initial simulation model all sensors are connected using individual ZigBee transmitters. When the aggregate data model was used then a number of sensors are connected to a single transmitter. In the later section we discuss the effect of data aggregation on the WBAN performance. Figure 17 shows the packet structure used in the simulation.

The physical layer generates the packet by encapsulating the MPDU (MAC Protocol Data Unit) with the physical layer overheads. The minimum header length is 18 bytes long. Considering the transmission efficiency, such a large overhead introduces a design constraint for the WBAN. As discussed before that each physiological signal sample is only 12 bits long hence, it will be inefficient to transmit a single sample in a packet. Sending a short payload not only reduces the transmission efficiencies but also increases the probability of collisions consequently increasing packet delay and losses. Increasing contention level in a random access network has further consequences on the power consumption of sensor nodes. Higher contention level in a CSMA network introduces more collisions and retransmissions. When packets are retransmitted more frequently, then a node consumes higher power level thus decreasing the battery life. During retransmission, the energy consumption increases because same information is transmitted multiple times before a packet is successfully received. Most of the ZigBee Integrated Circuits (IC)'s will consume highest power when the device is transmitting data (Khan et.al., 2006). So, it is necessary to optimize the number of transmission and retransmission of packets to reduce the packet delay and loss as well as to reduce the power consumption requirements of sensor nodes. As discussed, minimizing energy consumption of a WBAN is one primary objective of the MAC design process hence, it is necessary to design packet transmission process taking into account of energy consumption issues. Although the CSMA/CA protocol introduces the contention/collisions in a network which may results in packet losses or delay but this protocol handles both periodic and non-periodic data with equal efficiencies. Later we will show that by appropriately selecting parameters and traffic levels the QoS parameters of patient monitoring system can be improved.

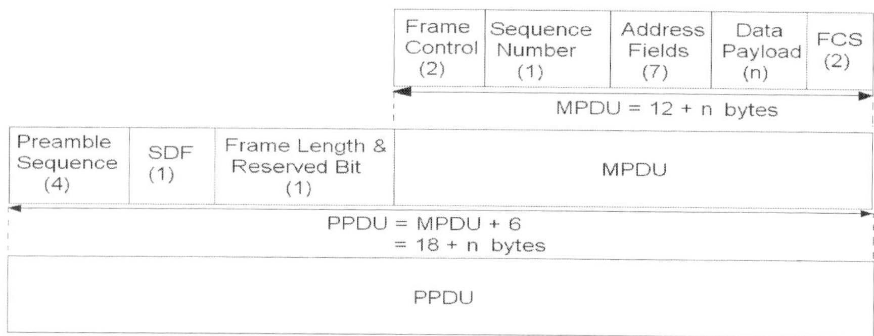

Fig. 17. Zigbee packet structure used in the simulation model. The MPDU represents MAC protocol data unit and PPDU represents the physical layer protocol data unit.

Multiple useful simulation results are obtained using the developed simulation model. In this simulation a single CCU is used which connects a number of sensor nodes. Both the CCU and sensor nodes are implemented using the Zigbee Standard. Figure 18 shows the packet loss and packet generation rate of the simulated WBAN for different payload sizes. Result shows that with the increasing payload size the throughput of WBAN increases due to fewer transmission attempts. The figure shows that with single sample/payload the network only manages to successfully transmit 120 packets offering a success rate of 40%. When the average payload size is increased to 120 bits/packet then the number of transmission attempts is dropped to 50 packets/sec offering 100% throughput in the network. The improvement in the efficiency can be achieved due to lower contention level in the network which resulted fewer packet losses due to the packet dropping threshold. In this simulation, we used five retransmission attempts as the packet dropping threshold, which means if a packet is unable to successfully transmit a packet in five successive attempts then the packet is dropped from the transmission queue.

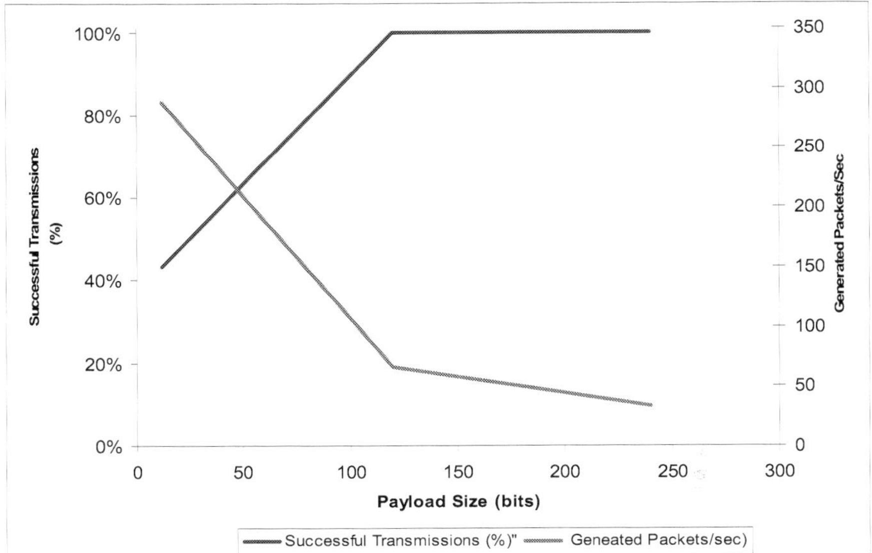

Fig. 18. WBAN packet loss and packet generation rate for different data aggregation rate/payload size.

The delay profile of the WBAN for different payload sizes is investigated and presented in Figure 19. The plot shows that the average packet delay decreases with the increasing payload size. Both results (Figure 18 & 19) show the same trend. The delay profile shows that delay decreases more sharply when the payload size is between 12 to 120 bits. This characteristic can be explained using the equation (1). As shown in the equation the end-to-end delay has four major components. The first three delay components T_{access}, T_{retry} and T_{queue} are contention level dependent. For a smaller payload the contention level increases due to the frequent network access causes significant rise in all these delay components. As the payload size exceeds the total header size the packet transmission delay T_{packet} becomes the dominant component of the overall delay. During the simulation it was observed that when single sample is used as the payload per packet some of the ECG sensor nodes are not able to get any access to the network. From Table 1 it can be seen that the ECG node is a demanding node in terms of transmission access. It requires the transmission channel access after every 2 ms with a data rate requirement of 6 kbs. However, when the overhead bits of a packet is considered the actual data rate for the ECG links become 72 kbs. One can see from these results that the selection of packet size and frequency of packets transmissions in a WBAN is very important from the reliability and QoS point of view.

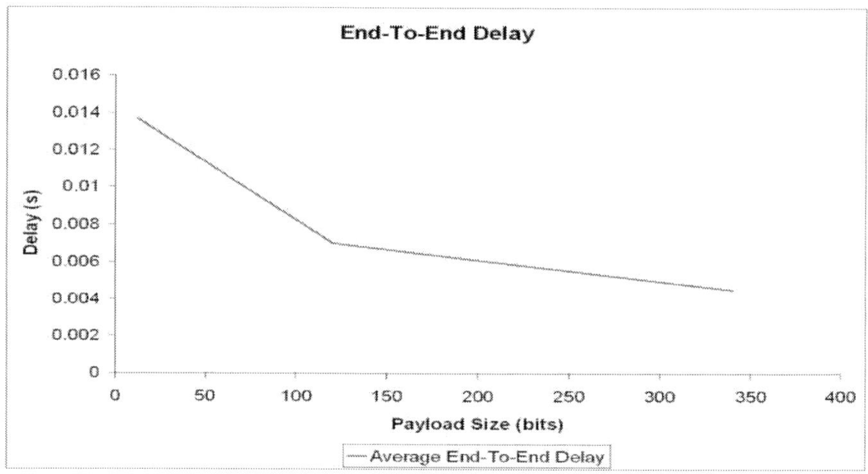

Fig. 19. WBAN delay profile for different payload sizes.

It is important to investigate the performance of an in interconnected WBAN to analyze the performance of a multi-patient monitoring system. In the proposed scenario, it is assumed that all patients' sensor nodes transmit their data via the PCU and CCU to the DB. As discussed earlier that in this model PCUs and CCUs are simply acting as a relay node and forwarding those data to the DB. In order to minimize the number of packets we use the data aggregation technique at the source node. In this simulation we connect all sensors to two sensor nodes which transmits data using the data aggregation technique. One of the sensor nodes (sensor 1) aggregates ECG, body temperature and blood pH data and transmits these data after every 145 ms generating 7 packets/sec. The other sensor node (sensor 2) aggregates data from the blood flow, blood pressure and respiratory rate sensor and transmit these data after every 485 ms generating 3 packets/sec. This aggregated packet structure allows 73 data samples with a payload size of 880 bits/packet. Using the aggregating technique each PAN now generates only 10 packets/sec. The effective data rate requirement of sensor 1 and sensor 2 becomes 6.05 kbs and 1.92 kbs respectively.

The delay profile for a multipatient networking scenario is depicted in Figure 20. The plot shows the average end-to-end delay which is the total delay over 3 hops (sensor→PCU, PCU→CCU and CCU→DB). It is observed that the delay increases with increasing number of patients. In this case the main reason for the increase in delay is caused by the contention or interference from different PANs. For an operating ZigBee network, sensor nodes on each patient's body forms a working PAN with the PCU as the coordinator. In a multi-hop networking, collisions can happen either within a PAN or between PANs when simultaneous transmission goes on in different PANs. Also, transmission from the PCU to CCU or from the CCU to DB transmissions can be interfered by the transmissions from other PANs if the IEEE802.15.4 MAC is used on all the links. In our simulation all the wireless links used the CSMA/CA protocol. Figure 20 shows the end-to-end delay which the sum of the all hop delays is as represented in (5). The delay plot shows that the delay profile for up to 6 patients is quite acceptable where the average packet delay is about 170 ms. Within this 170 ms the monitoring system will be able to transmit large number of samples due to the aggregation technique used.

$$T_{ee} = \sum_{i=1}^{N} T_{d(random)i}$$ (5)

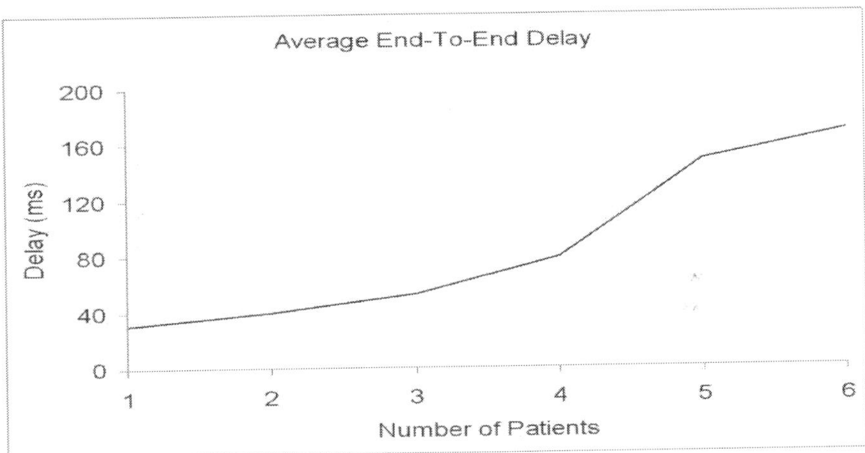

Fig. 20. Delay profile of the multi-patient monitoring system.

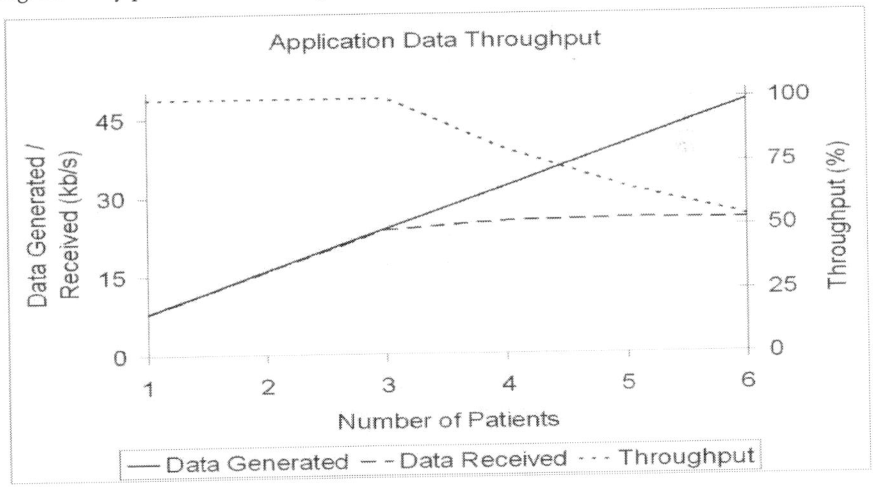

Fig. 21. Data generation and application throughput profile in a multi-patient monitoring system.

The application throughput profile of the monitoring system which is presented in Figure 21 was obtained using the simulation model presented in figure 15. Figure 21 shows that the application throughput remains 100% for upto three patients. The application throughput starts to drop due higher end to end delay and the contention level. In this network each packet crosses three links and these packets may experience collisions on all links depending on the transmission status of other networks. Application throughput can be increased if higher end-to-end delay is tolerated. Both the application throughput and delay can be tuned by controlling the backoff parameters and the number of allowable retransmission attempts used to resolve collisions. For a WBAN based system design one needs to tune the traffic and MAC protocol parameters to compromise between the delay and the throughput. When contention level increases, packets are lost due to two main reasons; one is expiry of packet lifetime due to fixed number of retransmission attempts, and secondly due to the PAN formation error as depicted in Figure 22. If sensor nodes are unable to communicate with its PAN coordinator then a PAN formation error occurs. When the PAN formation error occurs then sensor nodes in that PAN can not transmit any packets. A PAN error can occurs due to the failure of signaling packet transmission which can be caused by the collisions or interference from other PANs or links in a multi-hop network.

Figure 22 shows that the PAN formation error starts to appear when the number of patients exceeds three. To minimize the effect of collision and interference on other links in this simulation we incorporated variable transmission power technique as shown in Table 6. The table shows that the PCU and CCU are transmitting at higher levels than the sensor nodes because CCU and PCU will need to cover longer distances. Higher transmission power of CCU and PCU is mainly responsible for interfering with other PAN transmissions. A suggested method for a ZigBee based design approach would be to use the GTS slots for PCU and CCU transmissions and use the CAP slots for the sensor nodes. This means that higher power nodes will not interfere with the sensor nodes and hence the contention levels will significantly drop.

Node Type	Maximum Transmission Distance (m)	Power Constraint	Transmit Power (dBm)
Sensor	0.5	High	-50
PCU	8	Medium	-26.6
CCU	8	Low	0
DB	10	Low	0

Table 6. Node transmission power.

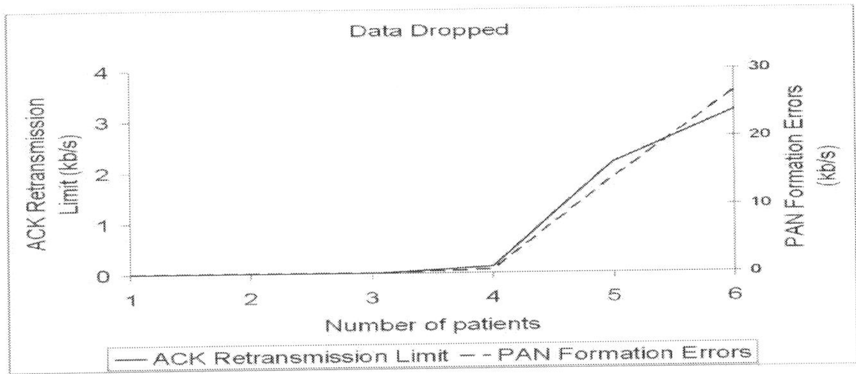

Fig. 22. Packet dropping profile in a multi-patient monitoring system. Figure shows packet dropping rate due to expiry of retransmission threshold and the PAN formation error.

7. Future Application Prospects and Development for WBAN

Future WBAN designs should concentrate a number of areas including the hardware and protocols design. The hardware development area should focus on design of very small and miniaturized wireless sensor nodes so that they can be used as a wearable device or could be implanted in the body. The hardware design should also concentrate on the development low power sensor nodes possibly by harvesting energy from body movements or using some other intelligent technique to generate its own power. The sensor nodes should be able to transmit the medical data in a reliable and secure method. A sensor node should also be able to incorporate with other wireless systems such as Bluetooth, WiFi and short-range wireless sensor networks such as Zigbee. Seamless interconnection feature of WBAN means the protocol stack should be developed intelligently so that a WBAN node can adapt itself in any operating environment. Developing an interference free wireless medical network for monitoring physiological parameters is one of the most important issues for a WBAN application. A future WBAN system should incorporate the following enhanced features:

- Low cost and tiny sensor node electronics design with wireless capability.
- A dedicated wireless transmission standard to eliminate possible interference issues.
- **Wireless Security**-Key software components should be developed to accommodate secure and effective wireless transmission. Medical data should only be accessible by authorized medical professionals without any possibility of eves dropping on the radio link.
- A WBAN should include alarm mechanism to define critical level of physiological signals monitored and can interact with other medical instrument.
- A dedicated adaptive wireless protocol should be designed for WBANs to accommodate critical and non critical data in the same platform with a low latency and information loss probability.

The selected wireless technologies and the frequency for transmission are very critical for future implementation of WBAN systems. Some of the recommendations made in this section are also being investigated by the IEEE802.15.6 working group (TG6). The group started their work in December 2007 and expected to produce a draft ready standard for sponsor ballot in December 2009. It is expected that the development of an unified IEEE standard could lead to many commercial development and deployment of WBANs in many healthcare and aged care applications.

8. Summary

This chapter has introduced the WBAN technology as well as main concepts and relevant design techniques. To develop an efficient WBAN system it is necessary to use advanced design concepts to develop its hardware and protocols. Hardware and protocol design techniques presented in this chapter can be used to develop an efficient WBAN system. The performance analysis section presented some results which will give an idea to researchers and system developers how a WBAN will perform in a multi-patient monitoring environment. Further work will be necessary in future to develop fully autonomous, long life, multimedia WBAN systems which could be used to support advance medical diagnostic systems.

Acknowledgements

We like to thank the following students Anthony Bott and Farbod Karami for their help in WBAN projects especially for the developing the database and OPNET simulation setup.

9. References

Anliker, U. *et al.* (2004) AMON: a wearable multiparameter medical monitoring and alert system. *IEEE Trans. Information Tech. In Biomedicine*, December 2004, vol. 8, no: 4, pp.415-427, ISSN: 1089-7771

Bradley PD. (2007) Implantable ultralow-power radio chip facilitates in-body communications. (Zarlink semiconductor) RF Dessign 2007; 20-24, Zarlink

Bugler G. and Yuce M. R. "Communication protocols for a multi-hoping wireless body sensor network," Technical Document, University of Newcastle, November, 2008

Dong-Sun, K., et.al, (2009) Block Based PHY and Packet transmission for low data rate in-body WBAN, IEEE802.15.6 group working document: IEEE802.15-09-0317-0006, May 2009.

FCC, (2003) FCC Rules and Regulations, "MICS Band Plan," Table of Frequency Allocations, Part 95, Jan. 2003

Golmie, N., Cypher, D. & Rebala, O. (2006), Performance analysis for low rate wireless technologies for medical applications, *Computer Communications*, vol:28, no: , pp. 1266-1275, ISSN: 0140-3664

Gutierrez, G. A., et.al, (2001) IEEE802.15.4: a developing standard for low-power low-cost wireless personal area networks, *IEEE Network*, Sept/Oct-2001, vol: 15, issue: 5, pp: 12-19, ISSN: 0890-8044

Ho C. K. and M. R. Yuce, (2008) Low Data Rate Ultra Wideband ECG Monitoring System, *Proceedings of the IEEE Engineering in Medicine and Biology Society Conference (IEEE EMBC08)*, pp. 3413-3416, August 2008, IEEE, Vancouver, British Columbia, Canada

Howitt, I.; Gutierrez, J. A. (2003) IEEE 802.15.4 low rate - wireless personal area network coexistence issues. *IEEE Wireless Commun. and Networking Conf. (WCNC)*, 2003, pp. 1481-1486, IEEE, New Orleans, Louisiana, USA

Karl, H. and Willig, B.T., (2008) Dynamic Duty Cycle Adaptation to Real-Time Data in IEEE802.1.5.4 based WSN, *Proceedings of the 5th IEEE Conference on Consumer Communications & Networking Conference*, pp. 353-357, IEEE, Las Vegas, Nevada, USA

Khan, J.Y., Hall, D.F. and Turner, P. D. (2006) Development of a Wireless Sensor Network System for Power Constrained Applications", *IEEE Asia Pacific Conferences on Circuits and Systems*, 2006, pp. 147-150, IEEE, Singapore

Mark, J.W. & Zhuang W. (2003). Wireless Communications and Networking, pp. 63-116, Prentice Hall, 0-13-040905-7, USA.

Omeni, O., Wong, A. C. W, Burdott A. J. & Toumazou, C. (2008) Energy Efficient Medium Access Protocol for Wireless Medical Body Area Sensor Networks, *IEEE Transactions on Biomedical Circuits and Systems*, vol:2, no:4, December 2008, pp. 251-258, ISSN: 1932-4545

Otto, C. A., Jovanov, E., and Milenkovic, E., (2006) A WBAN-based system for health monitoring at home. *Proceedings of the 3rd IEEE/EMBS Int. Summer School, Medical Devices and Biosensors*. Sept, 20-23, 2006, IEEE, Cambridge, MA, USA.

Proulx, J.; Clifford, R.; Sorensen, S.; Lee, D. J.; Archibald, J. (2006) Development and evaluation of a bluetooth EKG monitoring system. *Proceedings of the 19th IEEE Symposium on Computer-Based Medical Systems*, 2006, pp. 507 – 511, IEEE, Salt Lake city, Utah, USA.

Sikora A.; Groza V. F. (2005) Coexistence of IEEE802. 15.4 with other Systems in the 2.4 GHz-ISM-Band. *Proceedings of IEEE Instrumentation and Measurement*, May 2005, pages 1776-1791, IEEE, Ottawa, Ontario, Canada

Soomro, A; Cavalcanti, D. (2007) Opportunities and Challenges in Using WPAN and WLAN Technologies in Medical Environments. *IEEE Communications Magazine*, February 2007, vol:45, no:2, pp. 114-122, ISSN:0163-6804

TG6, http://www.ieee802.org/15/pub/TG6.html, IEEE

TI, http://focus.ti.com/lit/ds/sbos168d/sbos168d.pdf pg 14. 2009.

Yazdandoost, K. Y. & Sayrafian-Pour, K. (2009) Channel Model for Body Area Network, IEEE802.15.6 group working document: IEEEP802.15-08-0780-09-006, April 2009

Yuce M.R.; Ho C. K. (2008) Implementation of Body Area Networks Based on MICS/WMTS Medical Bands for Healthcare Systems. *IEEE Engineering in Medicine and Biology Society Conference (IEEE EMBC08)*, August 2008, page(s): 3417-3421, IEEE, Vancouver, British Columbia, Canada

Yuce, M. R.; Ng, P. C.; Khan, J. Y. (2008) Monitoring of physiological parameters from multiple patients using wireless sensor network. *Journal of Medical Systems*, 2008, vol. 32 , pp. 433-441, ISSN: 0148-5598

Zigbee, http://www.zigbee.org, Zigbee

32

Dynamic Wireless Sensor Networks for Animal Behavior Research

Johannes Thiele[1], Jó Ágila Bitsch Link[2], Okuary Osechas[1],
Hanspeter Mallot[1] and Klaus Wehrle[2]
[1]Tübingen University
Germany
[2]RWTH Aachen University
Germany

Introduction

Wireless sensor networks have developed into a variety of applications where data is obtained from restrictive environments. Data acquisition in biological systems is often constrained by the necessity to avoid wired connections, encouraging the use of radio communication between a mobile sensor unit and a data sink.

If several different data sources have to be surveyed simultaneously, a multitude of sensor units can be involved, this often results in wireless networks with a predictable and static structure. Changes in connectivity of these networks occur rarely and are undesirable because they slow down the data flow. However, in social networks, the dynamics in network connectivity are the actual focus of interest.

Because of their flexibility, we decided to use wireless sensor networks (i.e. radio equipped microcontrollers) to explore various aspects in the behavior of rodents nesting in subterranean habitats, such as the social structure or the structure of their burrows. Thus we model the social structure of a group of animals tagged with our sensor nodes using the changes in network topology, while, on the other hand, we use a customized sensor suite to obtain additional information about the activity of the animals in their burrows. In this contribution we will present some concepts that proved to be useful for such a network, in terms of the acquisition and pre-processing of sensor data in order to decrease the network load and the data transmission protocol that provides a good trade-off between overall data loss and redundancy, between data loss and redundancy and the post-processing of data that achieves meaningful models for animal behavior analysis.

We chose Norway rats (*Rattus norvegicus*) as a model system because they are abundant and easy to handle in laboratory and outdoor environments. Our sensor network application however, will not be limited to rats alone and our goal is to provide a system that is applicable for a broad spectrum of animal species, whenever their lifestyle requires the observation of many individuals and/or their localization is hampered due to subterranean, underwater or otherwise difficult structured habitats.

1. Norway Rat Behavior

Norway rats live closely socialized to humans, presumably since the latter began to settle down and store resources. Similar to humans they live in groups with flexible social structures, and just like them they are curious and explorative and were able to adapt to almost all terrestrial habitats worldwide. When humans discovered the utility of their rodent commensals as a model system for clinical and behavioral studies during the early 20th century, rats became one of the most abundant species in laboratories, too (see Whishaw & Kolb, 2004 for an overview over rat behavior in the laboratory). Although rats' behavior and cognitive capabilities have been studied extensively since that time in laboratory studies, only little is known about the behavior of rats in their natural habitat.

A fundamental reason for that is the fact, that rats – like many other rodents – spend a significant part of their life in burrows that are located underground, which so far could not be investigated without destroying them. The most extensive work that tried to scrutinize the community and life history of rats in their subterranean burrows is already more than 40 years old (Calhoun, 1963). In this work rats were kept in an enclosure, almost without any interferences by the observer, where they started to build burrows. In lack of better methods, observations of behavior in this study were restricted to that part of behavior that takes place over ground. Information about the behavior of the animals inside their burrows was only accessible during the final phase of the research, when the burrows were mapped and destroyed. The artifacts that were found during the excavation – like food stores, straw and droppings allowed a rough reconstruction of behavioral habits in the burrow but they only represent a snapshot of the burrow structure at the time of destruction and not much information about the social interactions between individuals that lived in the burrow.

More recent investigations of rodent ecology in the field normally use radiotelemetry but they are also limited to the observation of the animals' above ground activities. In addition, classic radiotelemetry systems require a high amount of manpower and their spatial accuracy is often appalling: Usually the results are limited to home-range analysis, overlap and population-based questions (Turchin, 1998). Sporadically researchers have started to use combinations of radiotelemetry and the aforementioned destructive methods by implanting radios into individual animals that record and transmit for example the activity cycles of the animals, whilst the burrows are only destroyed by successive digging by the researcher, keeping parts of the burrow intact during the study (Skliba et al, 2008). The radios in these kinds of studies are very simple VHF-transmitters without memory or data processing functions. Nevertheless the findings of these studies and the background of knowledge about subterranean rodents already show that there is a high frequency of social interactions in these populations with complex dynamics in group structure that hasn't been accessible to detailed research up to now (Dowding & Murphy, 1994).

The use of wireless sensor network technology for rodent observation will establish a new methodology for the investigation and mapping of subterranean burrows as well as for the observation and recording of animal behavior in species that are hard to observe, due to their lifestyle or an impenetrable habitat structure. We expect to obtain significant new insights into the natural behavior of the Norway rat, particularly about the function of its cognitive abilities and their implications for behavioral ecology.

Rodents are the largest order among mammals and the subterranean lifestyle of the Norway rat is not at all unique among rodents. In fact there are about 250 different species that live partly or even exclusively underground. They live in a variety of climates and ecosystems

(See Begall et al, 2007 for an overview). This variety is a promising basis for a series of comparative studies about social systems in rodents.

We decided to use the laboratory rat in our study, because the available breeding lines for lab use make them much easier to handle in contrast to most wild animals. Nevertheless the development of our sensor network is oriented towards a broader spectrum of applications.

2. A short presentation of the Hardware we used so far

The most stringent constraints on our hardware are the size and weight of the sensor nodes (often referred to as "motes"), which translates into a trade-off between battery size and its capacity.

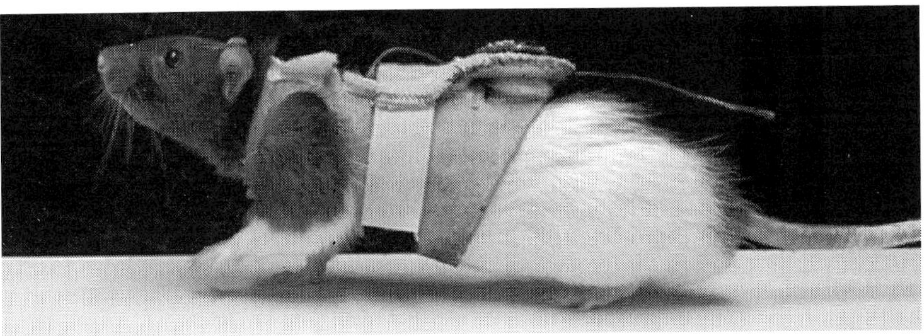

Fig. 1. An example of a laboratory rat wearing a mica2dot sensor node on a removable harness

So far we have used two different kinds of commercially available motes: The Crossbow mica2dot MPR500 which uses a radio frequency of 915 MHz for data propagation and the radiocrafts RC2301 transceiver module which communicates in the 2.45 GHz ISM band. Both devices run on 3.3 V power supply which we provided either with a CR2354 Lithium battery or customized Lithium-polymer rechargeable batteries. So far the motes and the customized sensor hardware were attached to the animals using a custom leather harness, which contains the sensing equipment in a pocket (Fig. 1). Our goal is to sketch out specifications for a system-on-chip implementation and move towards an implantable solution when the development of the prototype is completed

3. Mapping network structure on social structure

Social network analysis is an upcoming domain in animal behavior research since automatic observation techniques become more and more detailed and individual-specific. In contrast to the hitherto quantitative studies of animal movements based on population statistics, social network analysis is the study of social groups as networks of nodes connected by social ties, thereby disclosing association patterns, dominance hierarchies and the fluctuations of in groups (Wey et al, 2008). The basic ideas and terminology of social network analysis are in many respects identical to the terminology used in descriptions of the topology of technical communication networks. In the following section we will therefore show that the subterranean burrows of Norway rats are suited to study social networks of animals with wireless sensor network technology.

In an underground environment the effective communication range is limited, so forwarding of measurement data can be achieved using a technique known as Delay-Tolerant Networking, or Pocket-Switched Networking. We exploit the physical meetings of different rats as opportunities to transfer data between their attached sensor nodes. These meetings are also the focus of interest in the effort to understand the social structure of the animals. Data forwarding therefore utilizes the social structure and, vice versa, the social structure of an animal community can be reconstructed by the routing data of the network.

3.1. Radio Propagation in Artificial Rat Burrows

A typical rat burrow system consists of a number of segments with a mean diameter of 8.3 cm (see Calhoun, 1963) and a mean length of 30 cm. The propagation of electromagnetic waves is very important for the adequate design of an efficient network protocol. Predicting the communication range between two nodes theoretically is difficult, as we have to assume the burrow tunnel will act as a lossy wave guide in which the conductivity of the soil depends heavily on the exact composition, humidity, and surface.

As our nodes are based on the CC2420 radio chip, we work in the 2.4 GHz ISM radio band. This chip employs direct sequence spread spectrum (DSSS) technology, which is particularly well-suited for environments suffering from a high degree of multi-path propagation.

To be able to better characterize radio propagation in rat burrows we built an artificial burrow system out of drainage pipes, depicted in Fig. 2. As a test field, we selected a 10 by 10 m field of loose ground, consisting of mold, small stones and some sand, as would be expected for a rat burrow. We selected flexible drainage pipes with a diameter of 8 cm and 10 cm and a stiff drainage pipe with a diameter of 7 cm. The drainage pipes were buried at a depth of about 1 m. We then tied a number of sensor nodes to a small rope, which allowed us to pull them through the pipe. The sensor nodes were programmed to record all received messages to flash memory, along with the received signal strength and link quality indicators. The flash memory was later read out via USB.

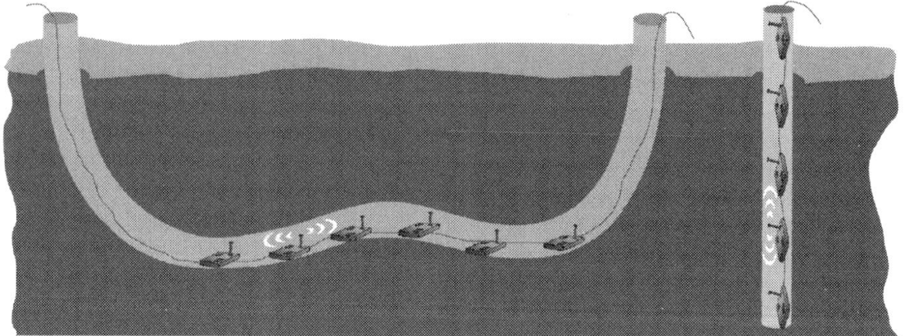

Fig. 2. Experimental setup for radio propagation measurements

The experimental results for an output power setting of 0 dBm can be found in Table 1. The packet reception rate(PRR) signifies the percentage of received packets. The received signal strength indicator(RSSI) indicates how much the packets have been damped by the tunnel. The lowest signal strength the used hardware can still properly decode is about -90dBm. Finally, the link quality indicator (LQI) is calculated using the number of errors in the preamble of a packet. It ranges from 55 (worst) to 110 (best). The results clearly demonstrate that the main factor limiting the range is the dampening effect of the burrow bit walls. The effective range is between 60 and 90 cm. This is significantly larger than radio propagation through solid earth, which we measured to be about 20 to 30 cm.

Tube diameter [cm]	Distance [m]	PRR [%]	RSSI [dBm]	LQI
10	0.8	0.91	-78.50 ± 0.50	105.17 ± 1.28
	0.6	0.91	-60.23 ± 0.42	106.26 ± 0.82
	0.4	0.91	-47.29 ± 0.93	106.22 ± 0.94
	0.2	0.87	-27.26 ± 0.44	106.27 ± 0.91
8	0.6	0.90	-90.09 ± 0.30	85.59 ± 4.80
	0.4	0.91	-66.05 ± 0.21	106.79 ± 0.90
	0.2	0.87	-42.39 ± 0.49	107.00 ± 0.81
7	0.6	0.92	-68.92 ± 0.27	107.00 ± 0.99
	0.4	0.92	-54.95 ± 0.79	107.36 ± 0.74
	0.2	0.92	-33.40 ± 0.85	107.26 ± 0.92

Table 1. Packet Reception Rates, Received Signal Strengths and Link Quality for different tube diameters and different distances between sender and receiver

We can thereby conclude that radio connectivity in an underground rat burrow can be used as an indicator of physical proximity. This allows us to make use of the radio as both, a method to transmit data and a proximity sensor. In the following subsections, we discuss, how this sporadic connectivity can be exploited for data forwarding, while at the same time investigating the social structure of the animals under observation.

3.2. Using Pocket Switched Networking for Data Forwarding

The term Pocket Switched Networking (PSN) was coined by Jon Crowcroft in 2005 (see Hui, 2005). PSN makes use of a nodes' local and global communication links, but also of the mobility of the nodes themselves. It is a special case of Delay/Disruption Tolerant Networking. However, it focuses on the opportunistic contacts between nodes. The key issue in the design of forwarding algorithms is to deal with and possibly foresee human - or in this case - rat mobility. In general, the complexity of this problem is strongly related to the complexity of the network, i.e. uncertainties in connectivity and movement of nodes. If the complexity of a network becomes too high, traditional routing strategies based on link-state schemes will fail due to the frequency of changes. To cope with these uncertainties in high dynamic networks we need to discover some structures that help to decide which neighbor is an appropriate next hop. An illustration of the concept of DTN can be found in Fig. 3.

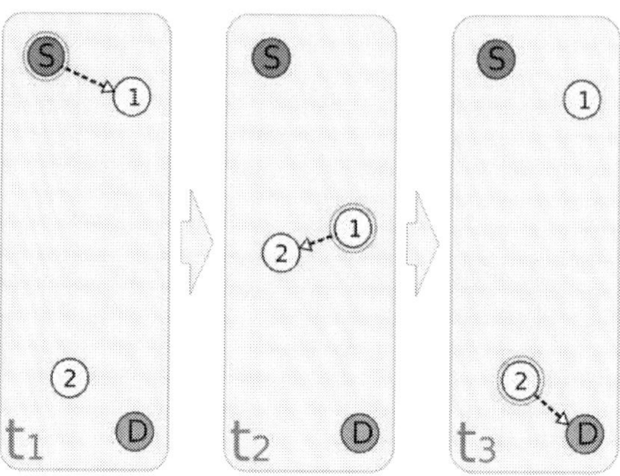

Fig. 3. A packet from S to D is forwarded via node 1 and node 2. There is no direct connection between S and D and so the packet is stored at node 1 (t1) until a connection with node 2 is available (t2). When node 2 finds a connection to D (t3), the packet is delivered.

3.3. Making Use of the Social Structure

In the field of social network analysis, a variety of measures have been defined to characterize social networks. These measures describe specific aspects of nodes in such a network. Daly et al., 2007 presented a routing strategy based similarity and betweenness centrality. We extended this routing scheme to better follow the temporal changes in social structure.

To illustrate the intuition of social network based forwarding algorithms, let us consider the following example: Alice, a student at a university wants to forward a token to Bob. If Alice meets Bob directly, she can just give the token directly; we call this simplistic approach Direct Delivery. In cases where the token is immaterial, e.g. a message, Alice could decide to give a copy of the message to anyone she meets and instruct them to do the same. This approach is called Epidemic Forwarding. Bob will eventually receive the message, but in resource constrained systems, this approach is prohibitively expensive in the number of transmissions and used buffer space.

Let us suppose, the token can only be forwarded, not copied. Alice could give the token to a person who shares many friends with Bob. This person is very likely to meet Bob, or a good friend of Bob. This metric is called similarity and we will later define it in more detail.

If Alice only knows of the existence of Bob, but doesn't know Bob directly, she may either give the token to anyone who knows of Bob or to someone who knows a lot of people in general. We call the former directed betweenness and the latter betweenness centrality.

Combining similarity, directed betweenness, and betweenness centrality, we came up with a useful forwarding strategy for this kind of opportunistic contact based networks, see (Viol, 2009).

Similarity in social networks can be defined as the number of common acquaintances of two nodes. This metric is inherently based on local knowledge. In the following, N_1 denotes the 1-hop neighborhood of a node.

$$S(u,v) = \left| N_1(u) \cap N_1(v) \right| \qquad (1)$$

Betweenness centrality of a node u is generally defined as the proportion of all shortest paths in a graph from any node v to any other node w, which pass through u. Also this metric is global in principal, (Daly, 2005) showed that an ego-centric adaption considering only nodes v and w from the 1-hop neighborhood of u, does retain the necessary properties to properly route on them.

$$BC_u = \sum_{\substack{v \neq w \neq u \\ v,w \in N_1(u)}} \frac{g_{v,w}(u)}{g_{v,w}} \qquad (2)$$

Classic social network analysis considers social networks binary: Either a person knows another person, or not. While this is a useful abstraction if relatively short periods of time are considered, intuition demands for dynamics and degrees in that relation: People might have been best friends in kindergarten but haven't seen each other in years now. Data from longer running traces, e.g. (Scott, 2006) show that these variations indeed reflects in the network structure, as illustrated in the next figure (Fig. 4), depicting the changing network structure of about 50 people over the course of a conference.

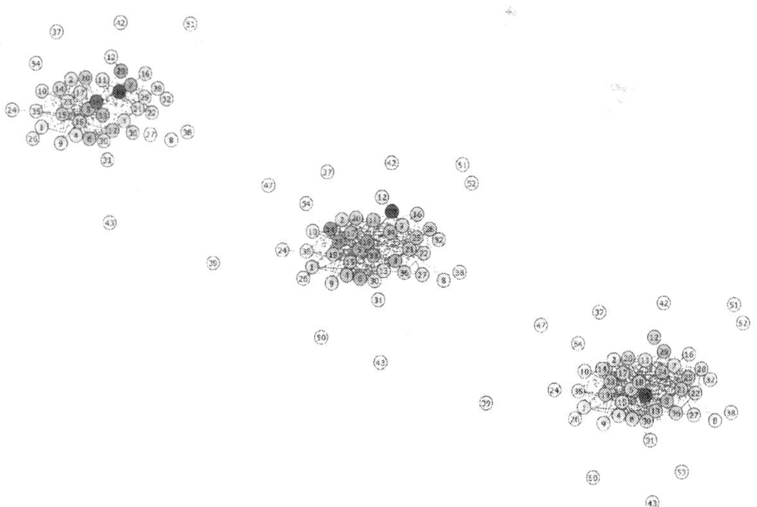

Fig. 4. Social structures changes over time (source data from Scott, 2006)

To better reflect these changes over time, we don't use a binary graph but assign weights to the edges. A weight of 0 signifies no acquaintance, while 1 signifies constant connection. If two nodes meet, their weight is updated using logistic growth:

$$\omega_{new} = \omega_{old} + \left(1 - \omega_{old}\right) \cdot \alpha \tag{3}$$

If nodes don't meet for a time, the weight of the edge decays exponentially:

$$\omega_{new} = \omega_{old} \cdot \gamma^{\Delta t} \tag{4}$$

Similarity, as defined above, must be adapted to reflect the weight of the edges. To do so, we define the weighted similarity as the sum of the product of the weight edges to a common neighbor.

Also, the above definition of Betweenness Centrality cannot be applied to weighted graphs without modifications. (Freeman, 1991) introduced the concept of Flow Betweenness Centrality. The intuition behind this change is realization that communication in social networks does not necessarily follow the shortest path between two nodes, but rather all links that there are with varying preference. This allows us to step back from shortest paths and consider flows on weighted edges instead. Details of this can be found in (Viol, 2009).

Furthermore, when we combine Similarity, Directed Betweenness and Betweenness Centrality, in this order of prevalence, the resulting delivery rates are significantly improved with respect to the original SimBet algorithm by (Daly, 2007), while being able to maintain a egocentric world view per node. In Fig. 5, the first 4 algorithms are trivial or taken from related work, while the last 3 are variants of the above described. SimBetAge considers Similarity and Betweenness Centrality in a weighted graph as described above, while DestSimBetAge also considers the directed betweenness. Dest2SimBetAge uses only local knowledge to calculate the directed betweenness and is thereby completely egocentric.

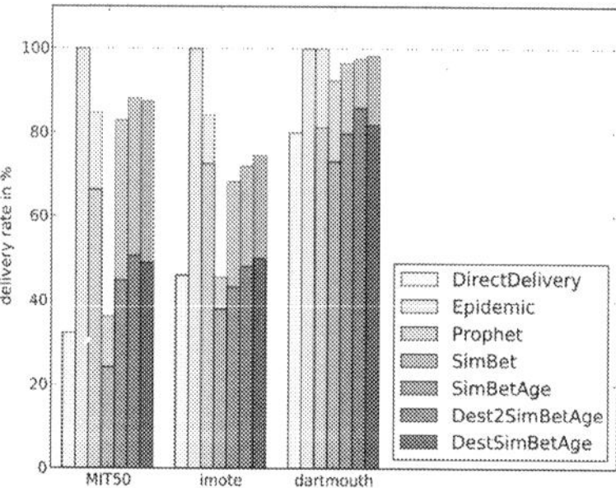

Fig. 5. Delivery rates for 3 different traces by algorithm used. Direct Delivery, Epidemic, Prophet and SimBet are taken from related work, while the remaining three are variants of our algorithm.

4. Vocalization classification

Rats share their subterranean burrows in loose assemblies of varying group size and communicate via olfactory, tactile and acoustic signals. Inter-individual rat calls are variable but can easily be classified and most of these call types are associated to a well-defined internal state of an animal and the kind of interaction between the animals emitting them. As this phenomenon is very useful to classify interactions of individuals in laboratory setups, a number of studies already bear a rich 'vocabulary' of calls and the behavioral context in which they occur - e.g. resident-intruder, mother-child interactions or post-ejaculatory and other mating sounds (e.g. Kaltwasser, 1990; Voipio 1997). An analysis of the vocalizations that occur when two rats meet in the burrow will therefore allow us to classify the kind of relationship in which the participating individuals are. This additional information should allow us to detect details of the social network inside a burrow, like dominance structures, kinship relations and hierarchies and will broaden the knowledge of social networks in addition to the network-reconstructions based on the analysis of message routing data mentioned in section 3.3.

4.1. Characterization of acoustic signals by Zero Crossing Analysis

In our aim to analyze and classify the rats' vocalizations, we have to consider the limited computing capacities and the limitations that result from the sparse connectivity in our network. Our goal is to analyze the call structure in real-time and on the mote, in order to keep the network load for the data transmission as low as possible.

To realize that, a drastic data reduction is required.

As our hardware needs to be small and energy-efficient, we developed a classification method based on zero-crossing analysis (ZCA) as a much simpler method for the prior evaluation of call structure, compared to other common methods, like Fourier analysis. In ZCA, the ultrasonic signals of the rats, which occur predominantly in the range between 20 and 90 kHz are extensively filtered and then digitized by a comparator. The cycle period of the resulting square-wave signal is measured with a 1 MHz clock. The measured period is registered in a histogram which is updated every 15ms. The combined histogram vectors of one sound event result into a matrix that contains enough information for a final classification of the call into behaviorally relevant categories. In order to cope with ambient noise, an additional buffer holds the average for each of the histogram bins from previous measurements and compares them with the actual results in order to detect sounds of interest. Fig. 6 gives an overview over the hardware required for such pre-processing.

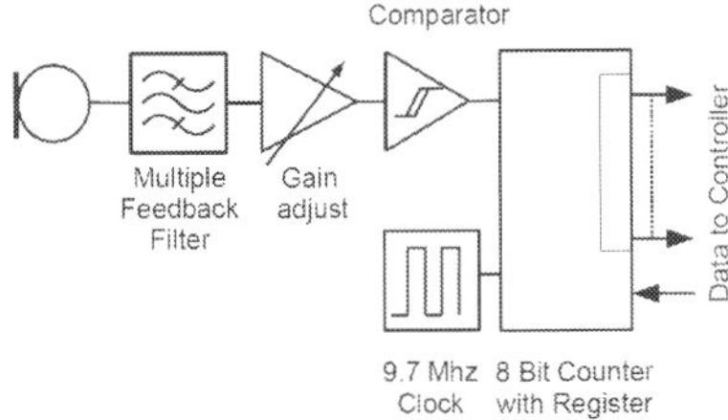

Fig. 6. Block Diagram of the ZCA sensor hardware

Fig. 7 shows examples of how different calls are represented by the ZCA algorithm in comparison with an FFT exposition. Although the ZCA is less detailed, each call type has distinctive parameters that allow a distinction between call classes. A classifier software, based on the ZCA cluster counts and temporal call parameters is under way.

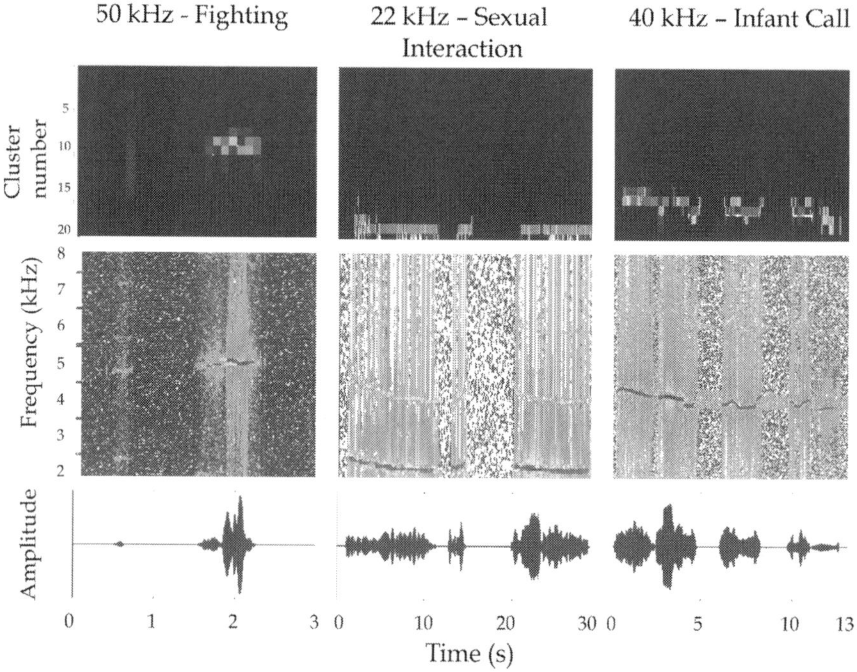

Fig. 7. Comparison between 3 rat calls that are analyzed by ZCA (upper row), by spectrograms (mid row) or by their amplitude (lower row). The behavioral classification of the calls is following (Voipio, 1997). The results shown here were realized on a test setup running on a mica2dot mote with 10 times delayed playback.

5. Position Estimation

Knowing how rats move about in the environment may enable us to describe their foraging habits, as well as the layout of their burrows. This may also allow us to draw conclusions about the actual use of different sections of the burrow in a non-destructive fashion.

Many technical systems feature pose estimation in 6 degrees of freedom, using a combination of inertial measurements, satellite navigation systems and magnetic sensors. A number of factors make 6-DOF tracking unfeasible for studying rat movement. For one, the processing power required by that method exceeds our current capabilities, as they ultimately translate on heavier and bulkier batteries, for another, and more important is, that radio signals for satellite based navigation, are not available in underground burrows. Finally, our sensor nodes are attached to rats at the torso (rather than implanted), and as a consequence the orientation of the inertial sensors may change in time, as they sag off the rats' backs, causing drift in the readings. It is currently not feasible for us to implant sensor nodes into rats.

As an alternative, we have used an approach following some ideas on pedestrian navigation(Fang 2005), to be used with rats, and allow for an estimation of their position in 2 dimensions. The original approach measures human stepping for distance measurements and combines them with azimuth measurements from a fusion of compass and gyrometer readings.

Thus we distinguish two main issues in estimating the position of a rat: Estimating the velocity at which it moves and its orientation in time. Knowledge of these two quantities would allow us to calculate the position of the rat in time, which would in turn yield important behavioral information such as activity profiles or the layout of the burrow.

5.1. Pseudo-steps

Although there are similarities between our system and existing pedestrian navigation systems, they are optimized for different scenarios, the main differences between our approach and step counting with human subjects, are:

i. Accelerometers cannot be attached to the rats' feet as they are in some pedestrian navigation systems, thus the use of the term *step* is not accurate. The periodicity of the signal does not correlate with individual steps of one paw, but with a cycle of four steps. In fact, the number of actual steps in a cycle is neither relevant, nor can it be inferred from the signals. Thus we often refer to one cycle as a pseudo-step.

ii. Our setup has a lower ratio of *"step"* time to available sample period, making period detection more difficult. In human step counting, it is possible to detect the phases of a step, with a signal that offers strong features and thus reliable time measurements and even context information. In comparison, our signal offers fewer features for time-domain measurements.

These constraints have led to a method that estimates the velocity of rats by measuring the time between peaks in the signal of the accelerometer in the transverse plane of the rat. Laboratory experiments have shown that the time between two peaks correlates with the velocity (Fig. 8), under the knowledge that the rat is actually walking (as opposed to exploratory movements that do not involve displacement).

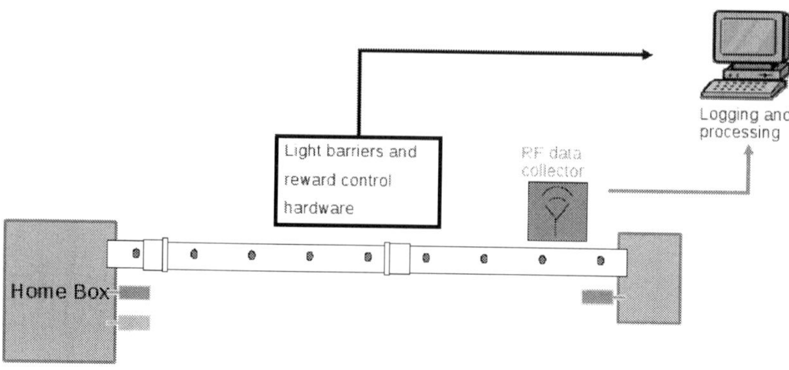

Fig. 8. Drain-pipe setup with light barriers to monitor rat movement

5.2. Implementation

The pseudo-step detection is done in hardware, using one channel of an ADXL330 accelerometer, the signal goes to an analog low-pass filter and is passed to a comparator, sampled at 10 Hz. The rats were free to move about in an artificial burrow, constructed from drain pipes and fitted with light barriers (Fig. 8), allowing to reconstruct the velocity at which the rats move.

Measuring the time between pseudo-steps, and calculating the estimated speed is done in firmware. When no stepping is measured, the system is able to record the estimated elevation (or pitch) angle relative to gravity, a feature that is useful in characterizing rats' exploratory habits.

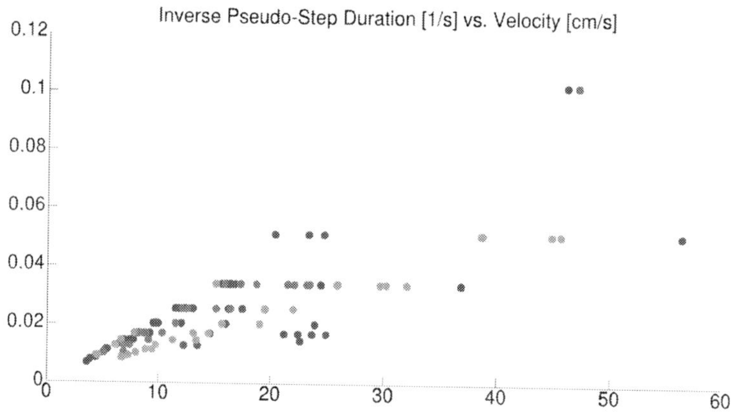

Fig. 9. The inverse of the duration of a pseudo-step correlates with the velocity of the rat

The time between two pseudo-steps has been observed to correspond with the velocity measurement obtained from the light-barrier data. Fig. 9 shows a scatter plot of the inverse of the step duration versus measured speed, with a least squares fit showing regression of R^2 = 0.6. This represents an improvement with respect to (Osechas et al., 2008), achieved through the exclusion of artifacts caused by insufficiencies in the light barrier setup.

5.3. Integration with Heading Estimation

It is common practice to combine gyrometer and compass readings to yield improved heading estimation (Fang 2005). In our case, the processing was simplified as much as possible, in order to save computational power, replacing the commonly used Kalman-filter-based integration by a simpler approach.

In order to prove the viability of the approach, the previously described test setup with drain pipes was expanded to include turns (Fig. 10), see also: Zeiß, 2009). Again, the pipes were fitted with light barriers to verify the rat's actual position at key points.

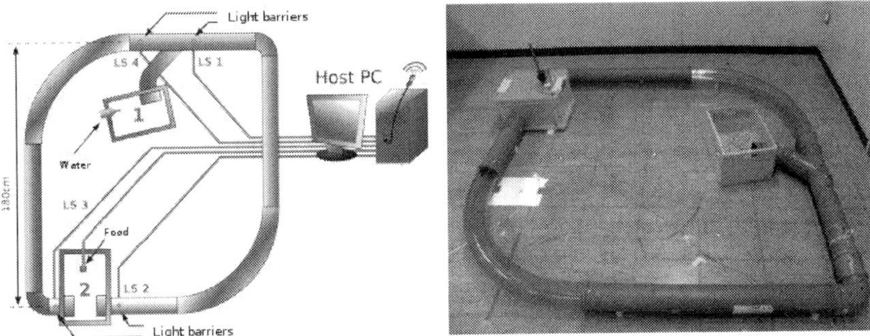

Fig. 10. Setup for testing position estimation

So far our experiments have been carried out indoors, inside a concrete building. In consequence, the earth's magnetic field is disturbed at the experiment site, in some places the disturbance is up to 55°. As the final deployment scenario is outdoors, we introduced a correction for the local disturbances of the magnetic field. The field was characterized for the whole of the experiment site and for each compass reading, the sample was corrected according to the current location. This correction would not be required in an eventual outdoor deployment.

Fig. 11 shows the average over 129 runs of two rats over 20 days in the setup. It is evident that, while there is room for improvement, the system could be used to study the layout of rat burrows, if enough data are gathered. The striking differences in accuracy on the left (x<0) of the setup, as compared to the right side, can be attributed to intricacies in the magnetic field disturbances that could not be corrected by our approach.

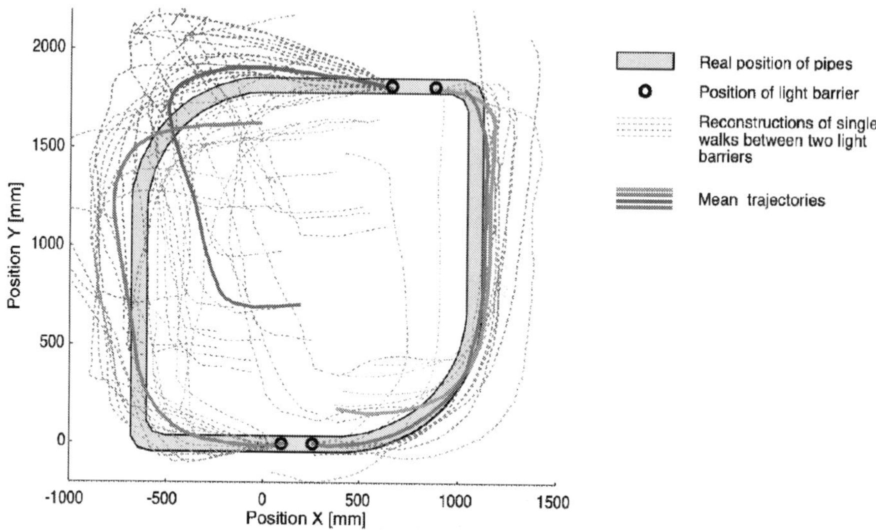

Fig. 11. Result of the 2-D position estimation

Current work is focused on context recognition, to differentiate acceleration events due to displacement, from events due to exploration. This knowledge is important to increase the reliability of the velocity estimation. Furthermore, the knowledge of when a rat is not walking enables us to analyze their exploratory behavior, as they stand on their hind legs while sniffing out unknown environments, or sleeping habits. This is the main reason for using 3-D acceleration measurements, even though lateral measurements are sufficient to characterize stepping. Measuring the pitch angle, between the gravity vector and the longitudinal axis of the rat, may yield information on the height of a chamber in a burrow.

6. Conclusion

This contribution sums up two years' development work on the RatPack project. The aim is to develop a system that will enable researchers to study the ecology of otherwise inaccessible animals, or populations, that are difficult to monitor, with a focus on animals that live in underground burrows and show social interactions. As the approach is based on dynamic wireless sensor networks, the work focused on designing sensing capabilities on the individual nodes and on data forwarding schemes on a network level.

The project has produced a set of proof-of-concept modules that provide capabilities in areas such extracting information on social structure, both from vocalizations and from the dynamic network topology, and estimating position without relying on satellite navigation, based on the animals' stepping.

On the sensing side, the working paradigm has been to trade measurement precision for simplicity, relying as much as possible on hardware pre-processing. On the networking side, the main challenge is dealing with dynamic connectivity, as the network topology is not predictable over time.

The single biggest challenge remains the envisioned outdoor deployment. It presents a major hardware challenge, as there is a trade-off between the reliability of the system and its obtrusion of the animals. Thus, efforts are focused on further miniaturization of the system, as well as on studying its behavioral disruption of the subjects.

In the long run, the RatPack should provide a tool for studying wild subterranean animal behavior, exploiting the synergy between the underlying ecology and the capabilities of disruption-tolerant networks, resulting from information fusion on various levels of abstraction, in turn yielding networking protocols that adapt to the given social scenarios to transport data efficiently and reliably from the animals to the collection stations.

7. References

Begall S, Burda H, Schleich CE (2007) *Subterranean Rodents: News from the Underground*, ISBN 978-3540692751, Springer, Berlin.

Calhoun JB (1963) *Sociology and Ecology of the Norway Rat* – US Health Serv. Publications No. 1008. Bethesda, Maryland.

Daly EM, Haahr M (2007) Social network analysis for routing in disconnected delay-tolerant manets. In *MobiHoc'07: Proceedings of the 8th ACM international symposium on Mobile ad hoc networking and computing*, ISBN 978-1-59593-684-4, pp. 32-40, Montreal, Quebec, Canada, September 2007, ACM Press, New York City, NY, USA.

Dowding JE, Murphy EC (1994) Ecology of ship rats (*Rattus rattus*) in a kauri (*Agathis australis*) forest in northland, New Zealand. *New Zealand Journal of Ecology*, 18 (1): 19-28.

Fang L, Antsaklis PJ, Montestruque LA, Mickell MB, Lemmon M, Sun Y,

Koutroulis HI, Haenggi M, Xie M, Xie X (2005) *Design of a Wireless Assisted Pedestrian Dead Reckoning System – The NavMote Experience* IEEE Transactions on Instrumentation and Measurement, Vol. 54, No. 6

Hui P, Chaintreau A, Scott J, Gass R, Crowcroft J, Diot C (2005) Pocket switched networks and human mobility in conference environments. In *Proceedings of the 2005 ACM SIGCOMM workshop on Delay-tolerant networking*, ISBN 1-59593-026-4, pp. 224-251, Philadelphia, Pennsylvania, USA, August 2005, ACM Press, New York City, NY, USA.

Kaltwasser, M-T, (1990) Acoustic signaling in the black rat (*Rattus rattus*), Journal of Comparative Psychology. 104(3):227-232.

Kausrud KL, Mysterud A, Steen H, Vik JO, Østbye E, Cazelles B, Framstad E, Eikeset AM, Mysterud I, Solhøy T & Stenseth NC (2008). Linking climate change to lemming cycles. *Nature* 456:93-97.

Osechas O, Thiele J, Bitsch J, Wehrle K (2008) *Ratpack: Wearable Sensor Networks for Animal Observation. Proceedings of EMBC 2008, Vancouver, Canada. IEEE.*

Scott J, Gass R, Crowcroft J, Hui P, Diot C, Chaintreau A (2006) *CRAWDAD data set cambridge/haggle (v. 2006-09-15).* Downloaded from http://crawdad.cs.dartmouth.edu/cambridge/haggle

Skliba J, Sumbera R, Chitaukali WN, Burda H (2008) Home-Range Dynamics in a Solitary Subterranean Rodent, *Ethology* 115:217–226.

Turchin, P (1998) *Quantitative Analysis of Movement: Measuring and Modeling Population Redistribution in Animals and Plants*, Sinauer Associated Publishers, ISBN: 0-87893-847-8, Sunderland, Massachusetts.

Viol, N (2009) SimBetAge, *Design and Evaluation of Efficient Delay Tolerant Routing in Mobile WSNs* , RWTH Aachen University, Diploma Thesis. Aachen, Germany.

Voipio, HM (1997) How do rats react to sound? *Scandinavian Journal of Laboratory Animal Science. Supplement* 24(1):1-80.

Wey T, Blumstein DT, Shen W, Jordán F (2008) Social network analysis of animal behavior: a promising tool for the study of sociality. *Animal behavior* 75: 333-344.

Whishaw IQ, Kolb B (2004) *The behavior of the laboratory rat: a handbook with tests*, Oxford University Press, ISBN 0-19516-285-4, Oxford.

Zeiß, M (2009) *Rekonstruktion von natürlichen Laufbewegungen der Ratte mit Hilfe von Magnet- und Inertialsensoren*, Tübingen University, Diploma Thesis. Tübingen, Germany.

33

Complete Sound and Speech Recognition System for Health Smart Homes: Application to the Recognition of Activities of Daily Living

Michel Vacher[1], Anthony Fleury[2], François Portet[1],
Jean-François Serignat[1] and Norbert Noury[2]

[1]*Laboratoire d'Informatique de Grenoble, GETALP team, Université de Grenoble*
France
[2]*Laboratory TIMC-IMAG, AFIRM team, Université de Grenoble*
France

1. Introduction

Recent advances in technology have made possible the emergence of Health Smart Homes (Chan et al., 2008) designed to improve daily living conditions and independence for the population with loss of autonomy. Health smart homes are aiming at assisting disabled and the growing number of elderly people which, according to the World Health Organization (WHO), is forecasted to reach 2 billion by 2050. Of course, one of the first wishes of this population is to be able to live independently as long as possible for a better comfort and to age well. Independent living also reduces the cost to society of supporting people who have lost some autonomy. Nowadays, when somebody is loosing autonomy, according to the health system of her country, she is transferred to a care institution which will provide all the necessary supports. Autonomy assessment is usually performed by geriatricians, using the index of independence in Activities of Daily Living (ADL) (Katz & Akpom, 1976), which evaluates the person's ability to realize different activities of daily living (e.g., doing a meal, washing, going to the toilets ...) either alone, or with a little or total assistance. For example, the AG-GIR grid (*Autonomie Gérontologie Groupes Iso-Ressources*) is used by the French health system. Seventeen activities including ten discriminative (e.g., talking coherently, orientating himself, dressing, going to the toilets...) and seven illustrative (e.g., transports, money management, ...) are graded with an A (the task can be achieved alone, completely and correctly), a B (the task has not been totally performed without assistance or not completely or not correctly) or a C (the task has not been achieved). Using these grades, a score is computed and, according to the scale, a geriatrician can deduce the person's level of autonomy to evaluate the need for medical or financial support.

Health Smart Home has been designed to provide daily living support to compensate some disabilities (e.g., memory help), to provide training (e.g., guided muscular exercise) or to detect harmful situations (e.g., fall, gas not turned off). Basically, an health smart home contains sensors used to monitor the activity of the inhabitant. The sensors data is analyzed to detect the current situation and to execute the appropriate feedback or assistance. One of the first steps to achieve these goals is to detect the daily activities and to assess the evolution of the monitored person's autonomy. Therefore, activity recognition is an active research area (Albinali et al., 2007; Dalal et al., 2005; Duchêne et al., 2007; Duong et al., 2009; Fleury, 2008; Moore & Essa, 2002) but, despite this, it has still not reached a satisfactory performance nor led to a standard methodology. One reason is the high number of flat configurations and available sensors (e.g., infra-red sensors, contact doors, video cameras, RFID tags, etc.) which may not provide the necessary information for a robust identification of ADL. Furthermore, to reduce the cost of such an equipment and to enable interaction (i.e., assistance) the chosen sensors should serve not only to monitor but also to provide feedback and to permit direct orders. One of the modalities of choice is the audio channel. Indeed, audio processing can give information about the different sounds in the home (e.g., object falling, washing machine spinning, door opening, foot step ...) but also about the sentences that have been uttered (e.g., distress situations, voice commands). Moreover, speaking is the most natural way for communication. A person, who cannot move after a fall but being concious has still the possibility to call for assistance while a remote controller may be unreachable.

In this chapter, we present AUDITHIS— a system that performs real-time sound and speech analysis from eight microphone channels — and its evaluation in different settings and experimental conditions. Before presenting the system, some background about health smart home projects and the *Habitat Intelligent pour la Santé* of Grenoble is given in section 2. The related work in the domain of sound and speech processing in Smart Home is introduced in section 3. The architecture of the AUDITHIS system is then detailed in section 4. Two experimentations performed in the field to validate the detection of distress keywords and the noise suppression are then summarised in section 5. AUDITHIS has been used in conjunction with other sensors to identify seven Activities of Daily Living. To determine the usefulness of the audio information for ADL recognition, a method based on feature selection techniques is presented in section 6. The evaluation has been performed on data recorded in the Health Smart Home of Grenoble. Both data and evaluation are detailed in section 7. Finally, the limits and the challenges of the approach in light of the evaluation results are discussed in section 8.

2. Background

Health smart homes have been designed to provide ambient assisted living. This topic is supported by many research programs around the world because ambient assisted living is supposed to be one of the many ways to aid the growing number of people with loss of autonomy (e.g., weak elderly people, disabled people ...). Apart from supporting daily living, health smart homes constitute a new market to provide services (e.g., video-conferencing, tele-medicine, etc.). This explains the involvement of the major telecommunication companies. Despite these efforts, health smart home is still in its early age and the domain is far from being standardised (Chan et al., 2008). In the following section, the main projects in this field — focusing on the activity recognition — are introduced. The reader is referred to (Chan et al., 2008) for an extensive overview of smart home projects. The second section is devoted to the Health Smart Home of the TIMC-IMAG laboratory which served for the experiments described further in this chapter.

2.1 Related Health Smart Home Projects

To be able to provide assistance, health smart homes need to perceive the environment — through sensors — and to infer the current situation. Recognition of activities and distress situations are generally done by analyzing the evolution of indicators extracted from the sensors raw signals. A popular trend is to use as many as possible sensors to acquire the most information. An opposite direction is to use the least number of sensors as possible to reduce the cost of the smart home. For instance, the Edelia company[1] evaluates the quantity of water used per day. A model is built from these measurements and in case of high discrepancy between the current water use and the model, an alert to the relatives of the inhabitant is generated. Similar work has been launched by Zojirushi Corporation[2] which keeps track of the use of the electric water boiler to help people stay healthy by drinking tea (which is of particular importance in Japan). In an hospital environment, the Elite Care project (Adami et al., 2003) proposed to detect the bedtime and wake-up hours to adapt the care of patients with Alzheimer's disease.

These projects focus on only one sensor indicator but most of the research projects includes several sensors to estimate the *'model'* of the lifestyle of the person. The model is generally estimated by data mining techniques and permits decision being made from multisource data. Such smart homes are numerous. For instance, the project *House_n* from the Massachusetts Institute of Technology, includes a flat equipped with hundreds of sensors (Intille, 2002). These sensors are used to help performing the activities of daily living, to test Human-Machine Interfaces, to test environment controller or to help people staying physically and mentally active. This environment has been designed to easily assess the interest of new sensors (e.g., RFID, video camera, etc.). A notable project, *The Aware Home Research Initiative* (Abowd et al., 2002) by the Georgia Institute of Technology, consists in a two-floor home. The ground floor is devoted to an elderly person who lives in an independent manner whereas the upper floor is dedicated to her family. This family is composed of a children mentally disabled and his parents who raise him while they work full-time. This house is equipped with motion and environmental sensors, video cameras (for fall detection and activity recognition (Moore & Essa, 2002) and short-term memory help (Tran & Mynatt, 2003)) and finally RFID tags to find lost items easily. Both floors are connected with flat screens to permit the communication of the two generations. The AILISA (LeBellego et al., 2006) and PROSAFE (Bonhomme et al., 2008) projects have monitored the activities of the person with presence infra-red sensors to raise alarms in case of abnormal situations (e.g., changes in the level of activities). Within the PROSAFE project, the ERGDOM system controls the comfort of the person inside the flat (i.e., temperature, light...).

Regarding the activity detection, although most of the many researches related to health smart homes is focused on sensors, network and data sharing (Chan et al., 2008), a fair number of laboratories started to work on reliable Activities of Daily Living (ADL) detection and classification using Bayesian (Dalal et al., 2005), rule-based (Duong et al., 2009; Moore & Essa, 2002), evidential fusion (Hong et al., 2008), Markovian (Albinali et al., 2007; Kröse et al., 2008), Support Vector Machine (Fleury, 2008), or ensemble of classifiers (Albinali et al., 2007) approaches. For instance, (Kröse et al., 2008) learned models to recognize two activities: *'going to the toilets'* and *'exit from the flat'*. (Hong et al., 2008) tagged the entire fridge content and other equipments in the flat to differentiate the activities of preparing cold or hot drinks from hygiene. Most of these approaches have used Infra-red sensors, contact doors, videos, RFID tags etc. But, to the best of our knowledge, only few studies include audio sensors (Intille, 2002) and even less have assessed what the important features (i.e. sensors) for robust classification of activities are (Albinali et al., 2007; Dalal et al., 2005). Moreover, these projects considered only few activities while many daily living activities detection is required for autonomy assessment. Our approach was to identify seven activities of daily living that will be useful for

---

[1] www.edelia.fr/
[2] www.zojirushi-world.com/

the automatic evaluation of autonomy, and then to equip our Health Smart Home with the most relevant sensors to learn models of the different activities (Portet et al., 2009). The next section details the configuration of health smart home.

2.2 The TIMC-IMAG's Health Smart Home

Since 1999, the TIMC-IMAG laboratory in Grenoble set-up, inside the faculty of medicine of Grenoble, a flat of $47m^2$ equipped with sensing technology. This flat is called *HIS* from the French denomination: *Habitat Intelligent pour la Santé* (i.e., Health Smart Home). The sensors and the flat organization are presented in Figure 1. It includes a bedroom, a living-room, a corridor, a kitchen (with cupboards, fridge...), a bathroom with a shower and a cabinet. It has been firstly equipped with presence infra-red sensors, in the context of the AILISA project (LeBellego et al., 2006) and served as prototype for implementation into two flats of elderly persons and into hospital suites of elderly people in France. Important features brought by the infra-red sensors have been identified such as mobility and agitation (Noury et al., 2006) (respectively the number of transitions between sensors and the number of consecutive detections on one sensor) which are related to the health status of the person (Noury et al., 2008). The HIS equipment has been further complemented with several sensors to include:

- *presence infra-red sensors* (PIR), placed in each room to sense the location of the person in the flat;
- *door contacts*, for the recording of the use of some furniture (fridge, cupboard and dresser);
- *microphones*, set in each room to process sounds and speech; and
- *large angle webcams*, that are placed only for annotation purpose.

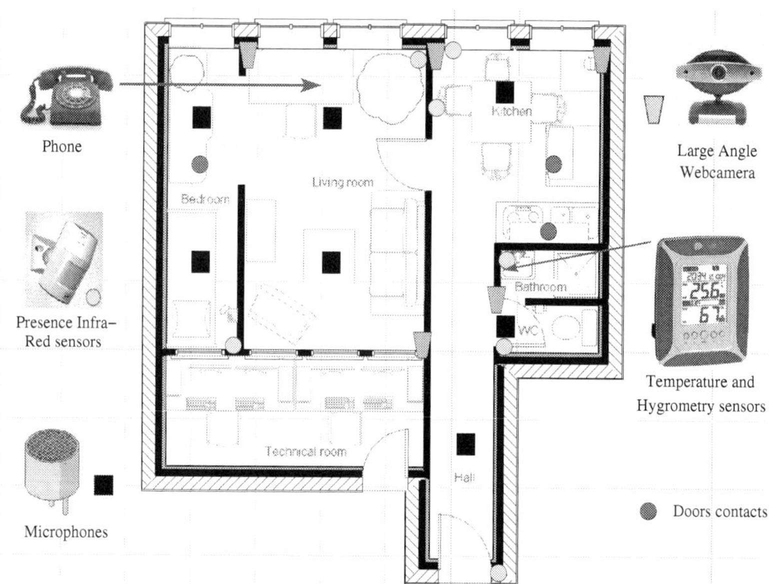

Fig. 1. The Health Smart Home of the TIMC-IMAG Laboratory in Grenoble

The cost of deployment of such installation is reduced by using only the sensors that are the most informative. This explains the small number of sensors compared to other smart homes (Intille, 2002). The technical room contains 4 standard computers which receive and store, in real time, the information from the sensors. The sensors are connected with serial port (contact-doors), USB port (webcams), wireless receiver (PIRs) or through an analog acquisition board (microphones). Except for the microphones these connections are available on every (even low-cost) computer. These sensors were chosen to enable the recognition of activities of daily living, such as sleeping, preparing and having a breakfast dressing and undressing, resting, etc. The information that can be extracted from these sensors and the activities they are related to are summarised in Table 5 presented in section 7.

It is important to note that this flat represents an hostile environment for information acquisition similar to the one that can be encountered in real home. This is particularly true for the audio information. For example, we have no control on the sounds that are measured from the exterior (e.g., the flat is near the helicopter landing strip of the local hospital). Moreover, there is a lot of reverberation because of the 2 important glazed areas opposite to each other in the living room. The sound and speech recognition system presented in section 4 has been tested in laboratory and gave an average Signal to Noise Ratio of 27dB in-lab. In the HIS, this fell to 12dB. Thus, the signal processing and learning methods that are presented in the next sections have to address the challenges of activity recognition in such a noisy environment.

3. State of the Art in the Context of Sound and Speech Analysis

Automatic sound and speech analysis are involved in numerous fields of investigation due to an increasing interest for automatic monitoring systems. Sounds can be speech, music, songs or more generally sounds of the everyday life (e.g., dishes, step,...). This state of the art presents firstly the sound and speech recognition domains and then details the main applications of sound and speech recognition in smart home context.

3.1 Sound Recognition

Sound recognition is a challenge that has been explored for many years using machine learning methods with different techniques (e.g., neural networks, learning vector quantizations,...) and with different features extracted depending on the technique (Cowling & Sitte, 2003). It can be used for many applications inside the home, such as the quantification of water use (Ibarz et al., 2008) but it is mostly used for the detection of distress situations. For instance, (Litvak et al., 2008) used microphones to detect a special distress situation: the fall. An accelerometer and a microphone are both placed on the floor. Mixing sound and vibration of the floor allowed to detect fall of the occupant of the room. (Popescu et al., 2008) used two microphones for the same purpose, using Kohonen Neural Networks. Out of a context of distress situation detection, (Chen et al., 2005) used HMM with the Mel-Frequency Cepstral Coefficients (MFCC) to determine the different uses of the bathroom (in order to recognize sequences of daily living). (Cowling, 2004) applied the recognition of non-speech sounds associated with their direction, with the purpose of using these techniques in an autonomous mobile surveillance robot.

3.2 Speech Recognition

Human communication by voice appears to be so simple that we tend to forget how variable a signal speech is. In fact, spoken utterances even of the same text are characterized by large differences that depend on context, speaking style, the speaker's dialect, the acoustic environment... Even identical texts spoken by the same speaker can show sizable acoustic differences. Automatic methods of speech recognition must be able to handle this large variability in a fault-free fashion and thus the progress in speech processing are not as fast as hoped at the time of the early work in this field.

The phoneme duration, the fundamental frequency (melody) and the Fourier analysis have been used for studying phonograph recordings of speech in 1906. The concept of short-term representation of speech, where individual feature vectors are computed from short (10-20 ms) semi-stationary segments of the signal, were introduced during the Second World War. This concept led to a spectrographic representation of the speech signal and to underline the importance of the formants as carriers of linguistic information. The first recognizer used a resonator tuned to the vicinity of the first formant vowel region to trigger an action when a loud sound were pronounced. This knowledge-based approach were abandoned by the first spoken digit recognizer in 1952 (Davis et al., 1952). (Rabiner & Luang, 1996) published the scaling algorithm for the Forward-Backward method of training of Hidden Markov Model recognizers and at this time modern general-purpose speech recognition systems are generally based on HMMs as far as the phonemes are concerned. Models of the targeted language are often used. A Language model is a collection of constraints on the sequence of words acceptable on a given language and may be adapted to a particular application. The specificities of a recognizer are related to its adaptation to a unique speaker or to a large variety of speakers, and to its capacities of accepting continuous speech, and small or large vocabularies. Many computer softwares are nowadays able to transcript documents on a computer from speech that is uttered at normal pace (for the person) and at normal loud in front of a microphone connected to the computer. This technique necessitates a learning phase to adapt the acoustic models to the person. That is done from a given set of sentences uttered by the speaker the first time he used the system. Dictation systems are capable of accepting very large vocabularies, more than ten thousand words. Another kind of application aims to recognize a small set of commands, i.e. for home automation purpose or on a vocal server (of an answering machine for instance). This can be done without a speaker adapted learning step (that would be too complicated to set-up). Document transcription and command recognition use speech recognition but have to face different problems in their implementation. The first application needs to be able to recognize, with the smallest number of mistakes, a large number of words. For the second application, the number of words is lower, but the conditions are worst. Indeed, the use of speech recognition to enter a text on a computer will be done with a good microphone, well placed (because often associated to the headphone) and with relatively stable conditions of noise on the measured signal. In the second application, the microphone could be, for instance, the one of a cell phone, that will be associated to a low-pass filter to reduce the transmissions on the network, and the use could be done in every possible conditions (e.g., in a train with a baby crying next to the person).

More general applications are for example related to the context of civil safety. (Clavel et al., 2007) studied the detection and analysis of abnormal situations through fear-type acoustic manifestations. Two kinds of application will be presented in the continuation of this section: the first one is related to people aids and the second one to home automation.

3.3 Speech and Sound Recognition Applied to People Aids

Speech and sound recognition have been applied to the assistance to the person. For example, based on a low number of words, France Telecom Research and Development worked on a pervasive scarf that can be useful to elderly or dependant people (with physical disabilities for instance) in case of problem. It allows to call, easily (with vocal or tactile commands) a given person (previously registered) or the emergencies.

Concerning disabled or elderly people, (Fezari & Bousbia-Salah, 2007) have demonstrated the feasibility to control a wheel chair using a given set of vocal commands. This kind of commands uses existing speech recognition engines adapted to the application. In the same way, Renouard et al. (2003) worked on a system with few commands able to adapt continuously to the voice of the person. This system is equipped with a memory that allows the training of a reject class.

Finally, speech recognition can be used to facilitate elderly people access to new technologies. For example, Kumiko et al. (2004) aims at assisting elderly people that are not familiar with keyboards through the use of vocal commands. Anderson et al. (1999) proposed the speech recognition of elderly people in the context of information retrieval in document databases.

3.4 Application of Speech and Sound Recognition in Smart Homes

Such recognition of speech and sound can be integrated into the home for two applications:

- Home automation,
- Recognition of distress situations.

For home automation, (Wang et al., 2008) proposed a system based on sound classification, this allows them to help or to automatize tasks in the flat. This system is based on a set of microphones integrated into the ceiling. Classification is done with Support Vector Machines from the MFCC coefficients of the sounds.

Recognition of distress situations may be achieved through sound or speech analysis; a distress situation being recognized when some distress sentences or key words are uttered, or when some sounds are emitted in the flat like glass breaking, screams or object falling. This was explored by (Maunder et al., 2008) which constructed a database of sounds of daily life acquired by two microphones in a kitchen. They tried to differentiate sounds like phone, dropping a cup, dropping a spoon, etc. using Gaussian Mixture Models. (Harma et al., 2005) collected sounds in an office environment and tried unsupervised algorithms to classify the sounds of daily life at work. Another group, (Istrate et al., 2008), aimed at recognizing the distress situations at home in embedded situations using affordable material (with classical audio sound cards and microphones).

On another direction, researches have been engaged to model the dialogue of an automated system with elderly people (Takahashi et al., 2003). The system performs voice synthesis, speech recognition, and construction of a coherent dialogue with the person. This kind of research have application in robotics, where the aim is then to accompany the person and reduce his loneliness.

Speech and sound analyses are quite challenging because of the recording conditions. Indeed, the microphone is almost never placed near the speaker or embedded, but often set in the ceiling. Surrounding noise and sound reverberation can make the recognition very difficult. Therefore, speech and sound recognition have to face different kind of problems. Thus a signal processing adapted to the recording conditions is requested. Moreover, automatic speech recognition necessitates acoustic models (to identify the different phonemes) and languages models (recognition of words) adapted to the situation. Elderly people tends to have voice characteristics different from the active population (Wilpon & Jacobsen, 1996). (Baba et al., 2004) constructed specifically acoustic models for this target population to asses the usefulness of such adaptation.

Our work consists in a complete sound recognition system to identify the different sounds in the flat in order to recognize the currently performed activity of daily living, associated to a speech recognition system in French to search for distress keywords inside the signal measured. The implementation and test of this complete system is described in the next sections.

4. The AUDITHIS and RAPHAEL Systems

The term AUDITHIS is built from the names audit and audition, and the acronym HIS (*Habitat Intelligent pour la Santé* - Health Smart Home) and the merger of audio and audit, because the system aims at sound and speech analysis in a health smart home. Therefore, AUDITHIS is able to analyze, in real-time, information from eight microphones placed at different location of a smart home. Figure 2 depicts the general organization of the AUDITHIS audio analysis system and its interaction with the Autonomous Speech Recognizer RAPHAEL.

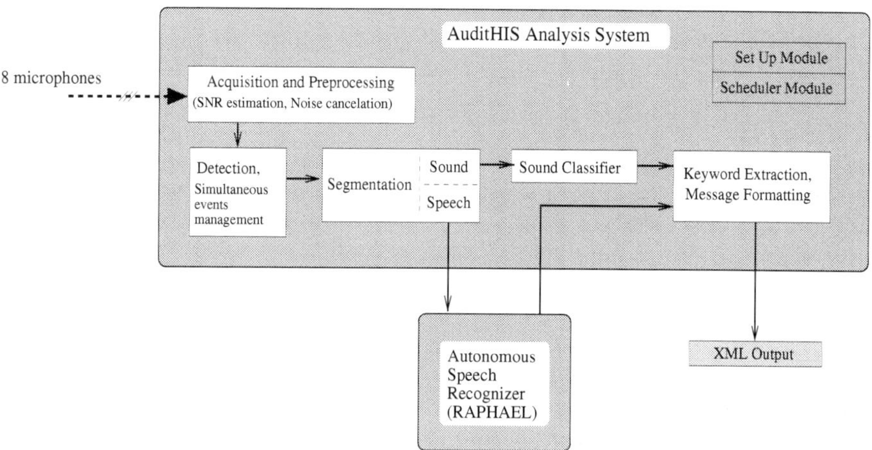

Fig. 2. Architecture of the AUDITHIS and RAPHAEL systems

Both systems are running in real-time as independent applications on the same GNU/Linux operating system and they are synchronized through a file exchange protocol. Each of the 8 microphones is connected to an analog input channel of the acquisition board. Each sound is processed independently and sucessively by the different modules thanks to a queuing management protocol:

1. **Data Acquisition and preprocessing**, which is in charge of signal acquisition, SNR estimation, noise cancellation;
2. **Detection**, which estimates the beginning and end of a sound to analyse and manage the simultaneous audio events;
3. **Segmentation**, which classifies each audio event as being speech or sound of daily living;
4. **Sound classification or Speech Recognition** (RAPHAEL), which determines which class of sound or which phrase has been uttered; and
5. **Message Formatting**.

These modules run as independent threads synchronized by a scheduler. The following sections detail each of the modules.

4.1 Data Acquisition and preprocessing

Data acquisition is operated on the 8 input channels simultaneously at a 16 kHz sampling rate by the first module. Data of each channel is stored in a buffer and processed sequentially and separately. Noise level is also evaluated by this module to assess the Signal to Noise Ratio (SNR) of each acquired sound. The SNR of each audio signal is very important for the decision system to estimate the reliability of the corresponding analysis output. Moreover, noise suppression techniques are incorporated in this module in order to suppress on the fly the noise emitted by known sources like TV or radio; this part of the module is described in section 4.2.

4.2 Known Source Noise Suppression

Listening to the radio and watching TV are very frequent everyday activities; this can seriously disturb a sound and speech recognizer. Because of that, sound and speech analysis must solve two problems: firstly, sounds or speech emitted by the person in the flat can be altered by the loudspeaker and badly recognized, and secondly, radio and TV sounds will be analyzed as well although their information is not relevant. It will be then mandatory to take into account the fact that the radio or the TV is up to suppress this noise or to exploit the resulting information in an other way. Sound $x(n)$ emitted by a loudspeaker in the health smart home is a noise source that will be altered by the room acoustics depending on the position of the microphone in the room. The resulting noise $y(n)$ of this alteration may be expressed by a convolution product in the time domain (Equation 1), h being the impulse response and n the discrete time.

$$y(n) = h(n) * x(n) \tag{1}$$

This noise is then superposed to the interesting signal $e(n)$ emitted in the room: speech uttered by the person or everyday life sound. The signal recorded by the microphone is then $y(n) = e(n) + h(n) * x(n)$. Various methods were developed in order to cancel the noise (Michaut & Bellanger, 2005), some methods attempt to obtain $\widehat{h}(n)$ an estimation of the impulse response of the room in order to remove the noise as shown on Figure 3. The resulting output is given in Equation 2.

$$v(n) = e(n) + y(n) - \widehat{y}(n) = e(n) + h(n) * x(n) - \widehat{h}(n) * x(n) \tag{2}$$

These methods may be divided into 2 classes: Least Mean Square (LMS) and Recursive Least Square (RLS) methods. Stability and convergence properties are studied in (Michaut & Bellanger, 2005). The Multi-delay Block Frequency Domain (MDF) algorithm is an implementation of the LMS algorithm in the frequency domain (Soo & Pang, 1990). In echo cancellation systems, the presence of audio signal $e(n)$ (double-talk) tends to make the adaptive filter diverge. To prevent this problem, robust echo cancellers require adjustment of the learning rate to take the presence of double talk in the signal into account. Most echo cancellation algorithms attempt to explicitly detect double-talk but this approach is not very successful, especially in presence of a stationary background noise. A new method (Valin & Collings, 2007) was proposed by the authors of the library, where the misalignment is estimated in closed-loop based on a gradient adaptive approach; this closed-loop technique is applied to the block frequency domain (MDF) adaptive filter.

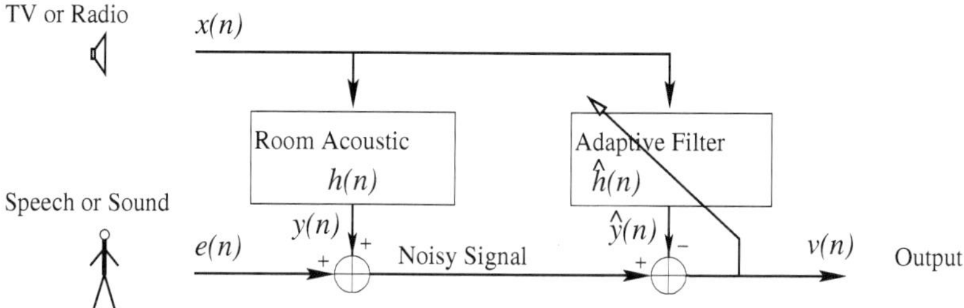

Fig. 3. Echo Cancellation System used for Noise Suppression

The echo cancellation technique used introduces a specific noise into the $v(n)$ signal and a post-filtering is requested. This algorithm is implemented in the SPEEX library under GPL License (Valin, 2007) for echo cancellation system. The method implemented in this library is the Minimum Mean Square Estimator Short-Time Amplitude Spectrum Estimator (MMSE-STSA) presented in (Ephraim & Malah, 1984). The STSA estimator is associated to an estimation of the *a priori* SNR. The formulated hypothesis are following:

- added noise is Gaussian, stationary and the spectral density is known;
- an estimation of the speech spectrum is available;
- spectral coefficients are Gaussian and statistically independents;
- the phase of the Discrete Fourier Transform follows a uniform distribution law and is amplitude independent.

Some improvements are added to the SNR estimation (Cohen & Berdugo, 2001) and a psycho-acoustical approach for post-filtering (Gustafsson et al., 2004) is implemented. The purpose of this post-filter is to attenuate both the residual echo remaining after an imperfect echo cancellation and the noise without introducing *'musical noise'* (i.e. randomly distributed, time-variant spectral peaks in the residual noise spectrum as spectral subtraction or Wiener rule does (Vaseghi, 1996)). The post-filter is implemented in the frequency domain, which basically means that the spectrum of the input signal is multiplied by weighting coefficients. Their weighted values are chosen by taking into account auditory masking. Noise is inaudible if it is too close to the useful signal in frequency or time; therefore noise components which lie below the masked threshold of the ear are inaudible and can thus be left unchanged. This method leads to more natural hearing and to less annoying residual noise.

4.3 Detection

The detection module is in charge of signal extraction, i.e. to detect the beginning and the end of the audio event. The first step detects the portion of signal that corresponds to a sound segment. It evaluates the background noise of the room and determines a threshold of detection from this. If this adaptive threshold is exceeded by the energy of wavelet trees of highest order level (3 level depth), the signal of the channel is recorded until its energy becomes lower than a second adaptive threshold. Each event is stored in a file for further analysis by the segmentation and recognition modules. The complete method for the detection of the bounds of a given event and also the associated evaluations is described in (Istrate et al., 2006).

4.4 Segmentation

The segmentation module is a Gaussian Mixture Model (GMM) classifier which classifies each audio event as everyday life sound or speech. The segmentation module was trained with an everyday life sound corpus (Vacher et al., 2007) and with the Normal/Distress speech corpus recorded in our laboratory (Vacher et al., 2008). Acoustical features are Linear-Frequency Cepstral Coefficients (LFCC) with 16 filter banks; the classifier uses 24 Gaussian models. These features are used because life sounds are better discriminated from speech with constant bandwidth filters, than with Mel-Frequency Cepstral Coefficients (MFCC), on a logarithmic Mel scale (Vacher et al., 2007). MFCC are the most widely used features for speech recognition. Acoustical features are evaluated using frames whose width is of 16 ms, with an overlap of 50%.

4.5 Sound Classification

Everyday life sounds are classified with either a GMM or Hidden Markov Model (HMM) classifier; the classifier is chosen at the beginning of the experiment. The models were trained with our corpus containing the eight classes of everyday life sounds, using LFCC features (24 filter banks) and 12 Gaussian models. The sound classes are: dishes sounds, door lock, door slap, glass breaking, object falls, ringing phone, screams and step sounds. This corpus is made of 1985 sounds and its total duration is 35 min 38 s. The HMM classifier gives best results in noiseless conditions but we chose the GMM classifier that gives best results when the SNR is under +10 dB. The models could be extended to include more daily living sounds requested to operate in the real life.

4.6 Speech Recognition: the RAPHAEL ASR

The autonomous speech recognizer RAPHAEL (Vacher et al., 2008) is running as an independent application. It analyzes the speech events resulting from the segmentation module, through a file exchange protocol. As soon as an input file is analyzed, it is deleted, and the 5 best hypothesizes are stored in a file. This event allows the AuditHIS scheduler to send the next queued file to the recognizer. Moreover, each sentence file is stored in order to allow future analysis with different recognition parameters of the recognizer. The architecture of the ASR is described by Figure 4. The first stage is the audio interface in charge of acoustical feature extraction in each 16 ms frame with a 50% overlay. The next 3 stages working together are:

- the phoneme recognizer stage;
- the word recognition stage constructing the graph of phonemes; and
- the sentence recognition stage constructing the graph of words.

The data associated with these stages are respectively the *acoustic models* (HMMs), the *phonetic dictionary* and the *language models* (tri-grams). The output of the recognizer is made of the 5 best hypothesis lattices.

The training of the *acoustic models* was made with large corpora in order to ensure good speaker independence. These corpora were recorded by 300 French speakers by our team (BRAF100) (Vaufreydaz et al., 2000) and at the LIMSI laboratory (BREF80 and BREF120) (Gauvain et al., 1990). The phonetic dictionary consists in the association of each word in French with its phoneme sequence using the SAMPA coding. Some phonetic variants were added to take into account the possible liaison between word or a possible incorrect pronunciation (e.g., the confusion between the closed vowel [e] and the open vowel [E]).

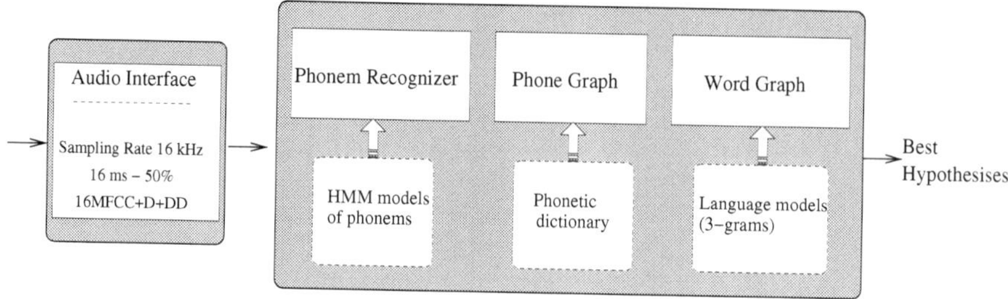

Fig. 4. Architecture of the AUDITHIS and RAPHAEL systems

Sample	Domotic Order	Distress Sentence	Usual Sentence
1	Allume la lumière	A l'aide	Allo c'est moi
2	Eteins la lumière	Je suis tombé	Allo c'est qui
3	Ferme la porte	Une infirmière vite	Bonjour Monsieur
4	Ouvre la porte	Appelez une ambulance	Dehors il pleut
5	Fermez les volets	Aïe aïe aïe	Euh non
6	Ouvrez les volets	Je ne peux plus bouger	J'ai bu du café
7	Il fait très chaud	Je ne me sens pas bien du tout	J'ai fermé la fenêtre
8	Il fait très froid	Je me sens très mal	J'ai sommeil
9	J'ai très chaud	J'ai mal	Tout va bien
10	J'ai très froid	J'ai de la fièvre	A demain

Table 1. Excerpt of the colloquial corpus

The *language model* of this system is a small vocabulary statistical system (299 words in French). The language model is made of 299 uni-grams, 729 bi-grams and 862 trigrams, it is obtained using textual information of a colloquial corpus in French. Our main requirement is the correct detection of a possible distress situation through keyword detection, without understanding the patient's speech. This colloquial corpus contains the sentences in the Normal/Distress speech corpus (Vacher et al., 2006), along with sentences currently uttered during a phone conversation: 'Allo oui', 'A demain', 'J'ai bu ma tisane', 'Au revoir' etc. and sentences that may be a command for a home automation system. The Normal/Distress language corpus is composed of 126 sentences in French in which 66 are every day sentences: 'Bonjour' ('Hello'), 'Où est le sel?' ('Where is the salt?') …and 60 are distress phrases: 'Aouh !', 'Aïe !', 'Au secours !' ('Help !'), 'Un médecin vite !' ('A doctor! hurry!') along with incorrect grammatically phrases such as 'Ça va pas bien' ('I'm not well')…The entire colloquial corpus is made of 415 sentences: 39 home automation orders, 93 distress sentences, the others are usual sentences. Examples of phrases are given in Table 1.

5. Distress Situation Detection Evaluation

The next sections present the evaluation of the AUDITHIS and RAPHAEL systems. Our evaluation is oriented to distress situation detection. First the results of the evaluation of the sound recognition system and the performances of our ASR in the recording conditions of a flat are assessed. During this experiment, a person is alone in his home and is uttering sentences which are or not distress sentences; this experiment aims to evaluate AUDITHIS and especially the distress keyword detection by RAPHAEL as explained in section 4.6.

Speaker Identifier	1	2	3	4	5	6	7	8	9	10
Sentences with distress keyword (197)	21	19	20	18	20	19	17	21	21	21
Sentences without distress keyword (232)	24	25	23	24	22	24	23	20	24	23

Table 2. Experimental Recorded Corpus: best SNR sentences

Secondly the known source noise suppression system presented in section 4.2 is evaluated in presence of music or radio broadcasting.

5.1 Sound Recognition and Normal/Distress Sentence Recognition
5.1.1 Experiment set up

To validate the system in uncontrolled conditions, we designed a scenario in which every subject had to utter 45 sentences (20 distress sentences, 10 normal sentences and 3 phone conversations made up of 5 sentences each) and to perform different sounds inside the flat. For this experiment, 10 subjects volunteered, 3 women and 7 men (age: 37.2 ± 14 years, weight: 69 ± 12 kg, height: 1.72 ± 0.08 m). To realize these successions of sentences, we chose 30 typical sentences from the colloquial corpus that we randomly scrambled 5 times; then we realized 5 real phone conversations containing 5 successions of sentences, and we picked randomly 3 of the 5 phone conversations.

The experiment took place during daytime – hence we did not control the environmental conditions of the experimental session (such as noises occurring in the hall outside the flat). The sentences were uttered in the flat, with the subject sat down or stood up. The subjects were situated between 1 and 10 meters away from the microphones and have no instruction concerning their orientation with respect to the microphones (they could choose to turn their back to the microphone direction). Microphones were set on the ceiling and directed vertically to the floor. The phone was placed on a table in the living room. The uttered sentences were chosen from the colloquial corpus presented in section 4.6.

Each subject was asked to first enter the flat and close the door, and then to play a scenario (close the toilet door, make a noise with a cup and a spoon, let a box fall on the floor and scream '*Aïe !*'). This whole scenario was repeated 3 times for each subject. Then, he had to go to the living room, and close the communication door between the kitchen and the living room, go to the bed room and read the first half of one of the lists of sentences containing 10 normal and 20 distress sentences. Afterwards, he had to go to the living room and utter the second half of the set of sentences. Each subject was finally called 3 times and must answer the phone and read the phone conversation given (5 sentences each).

Every audio signal was recorded by the application, analyzed on the fly and finally stored on the computer. Each detected signal was first segmented (as sound or speech), and then classified (as one of the eight classes) for a sound, or, in case of a speech event, the 5 more probable hypothesis were stored. For each sound, an XML file was generated, containing the important information.

During this experiment, 2,019 audio signals with an SNR of less than 5 dB were not kept; this 5 dB threshold was chosen because of the poor results given by classification and recognition under this value (Vacher et al., 2006). The number of audio signals collected in this experiment was 3,164 with an SNR of 12.65 ± 5.6 dB.

After classification, 1008 sounds and 2156 sentences were kept with a mean SNR of 14.4 ± 6.5 dB. When a sentence was uttered by the speaker, more than one audio signal was recorded

		Results								
		Clap	Step	Phone	Dishes	Lock	Break	Falls	Scream	Speech
Action	Clap	**81.25 %**	0 %	0 %	0 %	0 %	0 %	18.75 %	0 %	0 %
	Phone	0 %	0 %	**100 %**	0 %	0 %	0 %	0 %	0 %	0 %
	Dishes	0 %	0 %	0 %	**42.86 %**	0 %	0 %	0 %	4.76 %	52.38 %
	Falls	19.05 %	0 %	0 %	4.76 %	0 %	0 %	**76.19 %**	0 %	0 %
	Scream	8.7 %	0 %	0 %	8.7 %	0 %	0 %	30.43 %	**30.43 %**	21.74 %

Table 3. Confusion matrix for sound classification (bold values corresponds to the well classified sounds, some sounds are classified as speech).

by the 7 microphones, depending on his position in the room, but only the signal with the best SNR was kept. At the end, the recorded speech corpus was composed of 429 sentences (7.8 minutes of signal), 7 sentences were not kept because of signal saturation (see Table 2). The repartition of the sentences among the speakers is quite well balanced. This corpus was then indexed manually because the speakers did not follow strictly the instructions given at the beginning of the experiment. Moreover, when two sentences were uttered without a sufficient silence between them, some of these couples were considered as one sentence by the audio analysis system. For these reasons, the number of sentences with and without distress keyword was not the same for each speaker.

This first experiment will be used in the two following sections for the evaluation of first the sound recognition and then the identification of distress keywords in the transcribed speech of the AuditHIS system.

5.1.2 Normal/Distress Situation Recognition from Sounds

The results of this experiment are summed-up in the confusion matrix of the global system (Table 3). Rows are the actions performed, and columns give the result. The bold values are the correct decisions that were taken by the system.

This table shows the classes that are (e.g. object fall and doors clapping or dishes and normal sentences) difficult to separate. Some of the classes are very well recognized (phone ringing for instance) but dishes sounds for instance is very difficult to identify, especially because it is not correctly segmented (it is recognized as speech instead of sound). To complete this table, we could add that the global performances of the system are 89.76% of good differentiation sound/speech and 72.14% of well-classified sounds.

5.1.3 Normal/Distress Situation Recognition from Speech

The 429 sentences were analysed by RAPHAEL using both acoustical and language models presented in section 4.6. The uttered sentences were recorded at various input levels depending on the position of the speaker in the room; therefore the dynamic of the signal was increased; the maximal input level for each file was set to 50% of the maximal level if requested. These sentences are distress sentences (DS) or normal sentences (NS).

Distress keywords are extracted by a subsequent process from the complete recognized sentences: it is a Missed Alarm (MA) if the uttered sentence is a distress sentence and if there is no distress keyword in the recognized sentence. In the opposite way, it is a False Alarm (FA) if the uttered sentence is a usual conversation sentence or a home automation order sentence and if the recognized sentence contains a distress keyword. We define the Missed Alarm Rate (MAR), the False Alarm Rate (FAR) and the Global Error Rate (GER) in Equation 3 as:

Error Type	MAR	FAR	GER
Error Rate	29.5%	4%	15.6%

Table 4. Distress Keyword Performance for the Experimental Corpus

$$MAR = \frac{nMA}{nDS} \quad , \quad FAR = \frac{nFA}{nNS} \quad , \quad GER = \frac{nMA + nFA}{nDS + nNS} \tag{3}$$

n referring to the 'number of'.

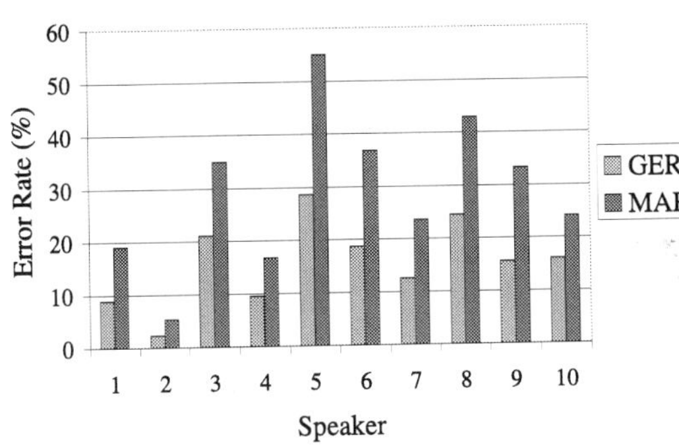

Fig. 5. GER and MAR as a function of the speaker

The results are shown as a function of the speaker on Figure 5 and given overall in Table 4. The FAR is too low to be displayed as a function of the speaker. MAR and GER highly depend on the speaker. For one speaker the MAR is about 5% but for another one, it is above 50%; this speaker uttered distress sentences like a film actor, so some sentences are very different from the sentences of the corpus and this led to errors. For example the French article 'je' was not uttered at the beginning of one sentence. For another speaker, a woman, the MAR is upper 40%. This speaker walked when she uttered the sentences and made noise with her high-heeled shoes, this noise was added to the speech signal. More generally, one distress sentence is 'help!', this sentence is well recognized if it was uttered with a French pronunciation but not with an English pronunciation because the phoneme [h] does not exist in French. When a sentence was uttered in the presence of an environmental noise or after a tongue clicking, the first phoneme of the recognized sentence will be preferentially a fricative or an occlusive and the recognition process may be altered.

5.2 Noise Suppression Evaluation

TV and radio signals are perturbing the hearing in the room but a speaker can distinguish easily this noise from speech even if the SNR is about 0 dB. It is not the case for automatic systems, thus it is of great interest to evaluate their performances in conjunction with suppression techniques.

5.2.1 Noise Suppression Experiments

Two microphones were set in a room, the Reference Microphone in front of the Speaker System in order to record music or radio news (radio broadcasting news all the day) and the Signal Microphone in order to record a speaker uttering sentences in the room as shown on Figure 6. The two microphones are connected to AUDITHIS in charge of echo-cancellation; the resulting signal after echo-cancellation with or without post-filtering is then sent to RAPHAEL and stored for further analysis. For this experiment the French speaker is standing in the centre of the recording room, he is not facing the signal microphone. He has to speak with a normal voice level, the level of the radio is set to be rather strong and then the SNR may be approximately 0 dB but there is no real control of the SNR.

Another way is to record separately the reference and the noise after propagation in the room. The speech signal may then be added to the resulting noise at different SNR levels; the Normal/Distress corpus recorded during precedent studies (Vacher et al., 2006) may be used for this purpose. Echo-cancellation is operated in batch accorded to the reference and the addition of speech and noise. So it is possible to proceed with the same signal using different settings of the echo-canceller. This mixing experiment allows a full control of the SNR.

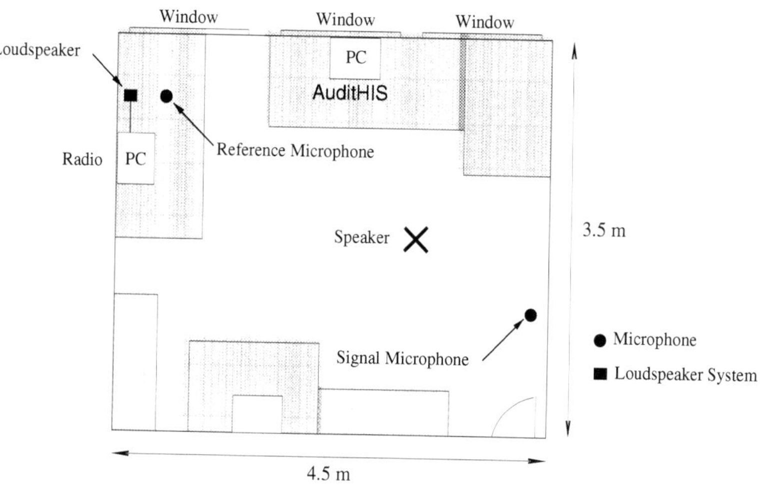

Fig. 6. Setting of the microphones and speaker system in the recording room

5.2.2 Noise Cancellation Results for the Mixing Experiment

The reference signal and the resulting noise in the room were recorded on the 2 microphones during 30 minutes at 16 kHz sampling rate. 126 sentences uttered by one speaker were extracted from the Normal/Distress corpus and mixed with the resulting noise at 9 SNR levels: -12, -9, -6, -3, 0, 3, 6, 9 and 12 dB. Each SNR level was obtained by adjusting the level of both the recorded noise and the audio file of the corpus. The resulting signal was then processed by the echo-cancellation system and the 126 sentences were extracted and sent to the ASR. This process was iterated a second time by the echo-cancellation system with post-filtering. The language model of the ASR was a medium vocabulary statistical system (9958 words in

French). This model is obtained by extraction of textual information from the Internet and from the French newspaper *"Le Monde"*. Then it was optimized using our conversation corpus (refer to Table 1). The recognition results for these two processing methods are presented on Figure 7. The buffer size of the algorithm was 256 samples in order to improve the processing time; the filter size was 8192 samples enough to take into account the size of the room and the delay after reverberation on walls and windows.

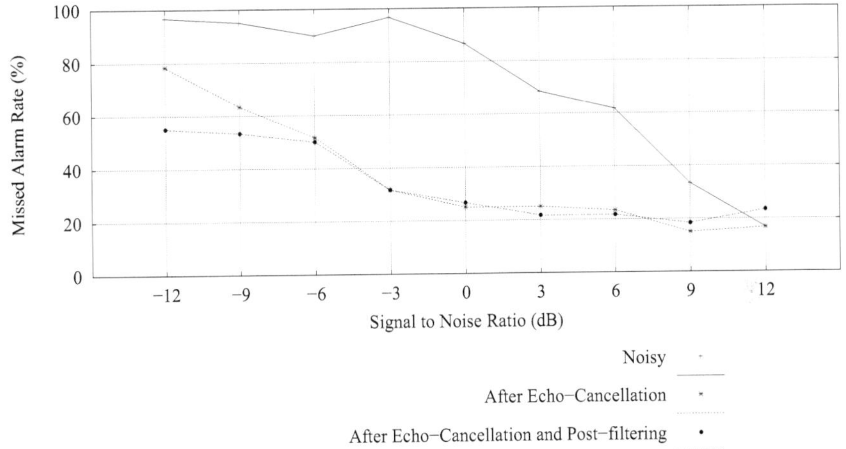

Fig. 7. MAR with France-Info broadcast news

In the absence of echo-cancellation, distress keywords are badly recognized, the MAR is fast increasing under +10 dB SNR. The MAR curve is nearly flat between -3 dB and + 12 dB when echo-cancellation is processed, the post-filtering does not improve significantly speech recognition in this interval, the MAR is even greater at +12 dB. On the contrary, the post-filtering is important below -6 dB and allows the MAR to be 55% (78% for echo-cancellation alone).

The echo-cancellation system was tested with the same corpus with 2 different noise sources: classical music (The 3rd symphony opus 55 by Beethoven) and pop music (Artificial Animals Riding on Neverland by AaRON). Results are displayed on Figure 8, they are very different from the results obtained with the news and the error rate increases linearly with noise level. Thus this kind of noises, and especially pop music, are more difficult to suppress because of the presence of large band sources like percussion instruments.

5.2.3 Noise Cancellation Results for the Real-Time Experiment

In complement, 4 speakers (3 men, 1 woman, between 22 and 55 years old) uttered 20 distress sentences of the Normal/Distress corpus in the recording room, this process was operated by each speaker 2 or 3 times. The echo-cancellation was operated in real-time by the Audio System analysis. Results are shown on Figure 9. The level of the radio France-Info was set in order to achieve a near 0 dB SNR level, each speaker was standing in the centre of the recording room. The MAR, global for all the speakers, is 27%. The results depend on the voice level of the speaker during this experiment and on the speaker himself. Resulting noise at

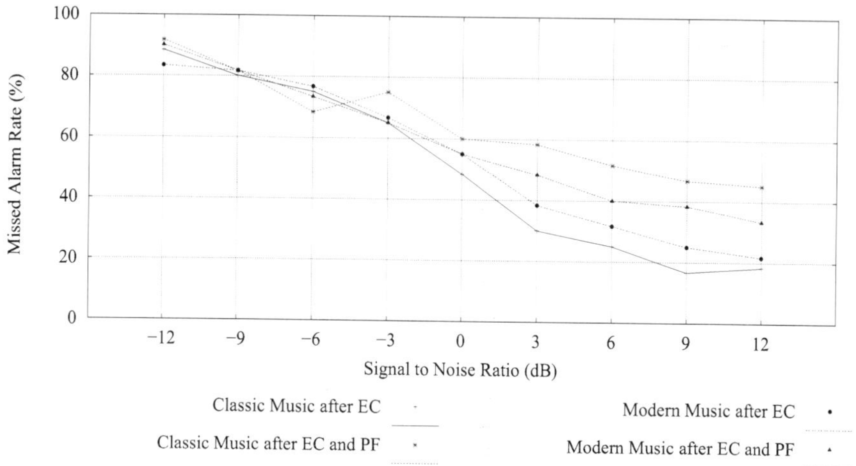

Fig. 8. MAR with Music as Noise Source

the beginning and at the end of the sentence alters the recognition; it may then be useful for detecting these 2 moments with a good precision to use shorter silence intervals.

6. Method for Assessment of the Usefulness of Sound and Speech Recognition for Classification of Activities of Daily Living in Health Smart Homes

To assess the impact of the sound and speech processing on the ADL classification, we have applied several feature selection methods with numerous machine learning schemes. Attribute selection (also called feature selection) is the process of finding a subset of attributes that leads to a good representation of the original data generally for classification (Saeys et al., 2007). Apart from reducing the data set which eases the learning (i.e., less time and memory used) this often leads to better classification performance as useless information (i.e., noise) can degrade the learning phase. This also leads to a more compact classifier representation which is more humanly interpretable (according to the model learned). The usefulness of the audio processing for ADL classification is assessed by the number of audio attributes selected by the attribute selection methods and the impact of this selection on the learning performance. This section presents the machine learning methods retained and the attribute selection techniques applied.

6.1 Supervised Learning

Supervised learning consists in building a classifier *Model* from a learning set L composed of N instances (also called examples or individuals) described by M attributes $A_1 \times A_2 \times \cdots \times A_M$, where A_m represents the domain of the mth attribute, plus a specific attribute C, which represents the class (i.e., concept to learn) in a finite discrete domain (i.e., no regression). The *Model* is then used to predict the class of new unclassified instances (i.e., for which C is unknown). The prediction results, on a specific testing set, is used to assess the *score* of *Model*.

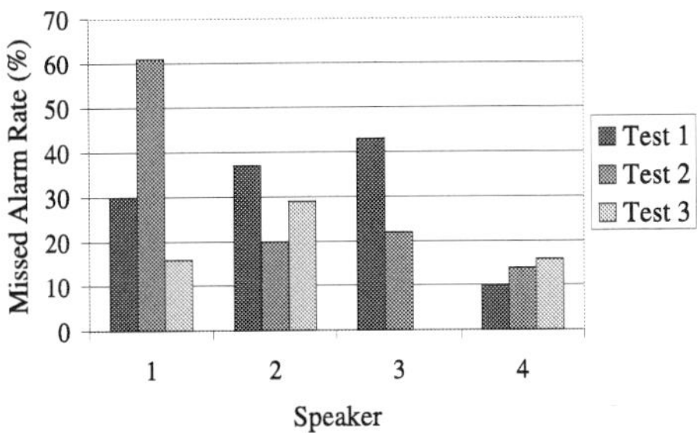

Fig. 9. MAR with Echo-Cancellation in Real-Time

In this work, the learning induction algorithms used are: *Decision Tree (C4.5)*, *Decision Table Majority (DTM)*, *Naïve Bayesian Network (NBayes)* and *Support Vector Machine (SVM)*. They have been chosen for their popularity in data mining applications and because they represent quite different approaches to learning.

Although most of the chosen algorithms can handle numerical attributes (C4.5, NBayes, SVM), L has been discretized using supervised discretization. The method consists in dividing the continuous domain of the attribute with respect to the class into discrete intervals containing the smallest information as possible (i.e., the sub-interval values are similar). As our numerical attributes are derived from categorical ones and as they do not respect normal distribution, this transformation is clearly justified.

6.2 Attribute Selection

Attribute selection techniques are generally divided into two families *filter* and *wrapper* (*embedded* attribute selection is sometimes considered as another family) (Saeys et al., 2007). Broadly speaking, supervised attribute selection by *filter* consist in either ranking each attribute according to its value with respect to C or finding a subset $SA \subseteq A_1 \times A_2 \times \cdots \times A_M$ which describes the most the class C. *Wrapper* method consists in finding a subset $SA \subseteq A_1 \times A_2 \times \cdots \times A_M$ for which the *Model* learned with the target learning algorithm leads to a score better than or close to *Model* learned with L. Single attribute evaluation (for ranking) makes only use of a specific metrics. To test the impact of attribute selection on the learning performance a small subset of each method type has been chosen.

- *Correlation-based Attribute Selection (CorrFA)* searches for subsets of attributes that are highly correlated with the class but with minimal inter-correlation with each other. This method is thus well suited to discover non redundant attributes sets such as one could expect in health smart home.
- *Consistency-based Attribute Selection (ConsFA)* searches for subsets of attributes that are consistent with C. An attribute subset is inconsistent if there are more than one instance with same attribute values but associated with different classes.
- *Wrapping* method is an attribute subset selection method that uses the targeted learning algorithm score at each node as evaluator. This method is more time consuming but leads generally to higher performance than the previous described as it fits the learning algorithm.

Sensors	Attributes	Number	Domain value	Information
Seven	Nb_sound_w	7	$\mathbb{N}$	Number of times a sound is detected in a room during the time window.
Microphones	Nb_sound_x	9	$\mathbb{N}$	Number of times a detected sound has been classified in one of the 9 classes.
Seven Presence	in_y	7	[0,1]	Ratio of time spent in each room (room occupation) during the time window.
Infra-Red sensors	Nb_in_y	7	$\mathbb{N}$	Number of detections in each room (agitation) during the time window
Three Doors	z_state	3	{open, close}	Most used position in the window (Cooking: use of the cupboard and fridge; dressing: use of the dresser).
contacts	Nb_z_open	3	$\mathbb{N}$	Number of times the doors have been opened during the time window.
One in-home weather station	temperature, hygrometry	2	$\mathbb{R}^+$	Differential measure for the last 15 minutes for temperature and hygrometry (use of the shower).

$w \in \{$ kitchen, WC, corridor, bedroom_window, bedroom_wall, living_room_window, living_room_wall $\}$, $x \in \{$ foot_step, dishes_sound, door_closing, door_locker, glass_breaking, speech, scream, phone_ring, object_fall $\}$, $y \in \{$ doorway, bathroom, corridor, WC, living_room, bedroom, kitchen $\}$, $z \in \{$ fridge, dresser, cupboard $\}$.

Table 5. Sensors and their associated attributes and information

7. Evaluation of the Impact of Audio Processing for Activity of Daily Living Classification

The assessment method has been applied to data acquired in the Health Smart Home of Grenoble (see Section 2). The data acquisition and the results of the application of the method on this data are described in the following sections.

7.1 Data Collection in 'Daily Living Conditions'

An experiment has been run to acquire data in the Health smart home of the TIMC-IMAG lab located in the Faculty of Medicine of Grenoble (Fleury, 2008). Thirteen healthy participants (6 women, 7 men) were asked to perform 7 activities, at least once, without condition on the time spent. The average age was 30.4 ± 5.9 years (24-43, min-max), height 1.76 ± 0.08 meters (1.62-1.92, min-max) and weight 69 ± 7.42 kg (57-80, min-max). The mean execution time of the experiment was 51min 40s (23min 11s – 1h 35min 44s, min–max). A visit, previous to the experiment, was organized to ensure that the participants will find all the items necessary to perform the seven ADLs. Participants were free to choose the order with which they wanted to perform the ADLs to avoid repetitive pattern. The 7 activities were defined based on the ADL scale: (1) Sleeping; (2) Resting: watching TV, listening to the radio, reading a magazine...; (3) Dressing and undressing; (4) Feeding: realising and having a meal; (5) Eliminating: going to the toilets; (6) Hygiene activity: washing hands, teeth ...; and (7) Communicating: using the phone.

The flat (cf. Fig. 1) contains 18 sensors from which 38 attributes have been derived and are presented in Table 5. Data has been annotated by cutting down each ADL interval into 3-minute windows (the adequate time to perform the shortest activity) labelled with the name of the activity. This process resulted in 232 windows for which: 1) 49 were sleeping; 2) 73

Rank	CorrFA	ConsFA	Global Filter
1	in_bathroom (100%)	in_bathroom (100%)	in_bathroom (100%)
2	in_living_room (100%)	in_WC (100%)	in_living_room (100%)
3	in_bedroom (100%)	in_living_room (100%)	in_bedroom (100%)
4	in_kitchen (100%)	in_bedroom (100%)	in_kitchen (100%)
5	Nb_in_kitchen (100%)	in_kitchen (100%)	Nb_in_kitchen (95%)
6	Nb_sounds_bedroom_-window (90%)	Nb_in_living_room (100%)	in_WC (90%)
7	in_WC (80%)	Nb_in_bedroom (100%)	Nb_sounds_bedroom_-window (85%)
8	Nb_sounds_living_-room_window (80%)	dresser_state (100%)	NB_sound_speech (75%)
9	(≤ 50%)	Nb_in_kitchen (100%)	dresser_state (70%)
10		NB_sound_speech (100%)	Nb_sounds_living_-room_window (65%)
11		till the 16th selected	Nb_in_living_room (60%)

Table 6. Attribute ranking for filter attributes selection methods

were resting; 3) 16 were dressing; 4) 45 were eating; 5) 16 were eliminating; 6) 14 were hygiene activity; and 7) 19 were communicating (phone). The final dataset was thus composed of 232 examples of 3-minute activity described by 38 attributes (i.e., attributes) plus the class attribute (i.e., the activity label).

7.2 Attribute Selection Results

Table 6 gives the results of the filter selection method applied on the whole set with a 10-fold stratified cross-validation. For each method the rank of the attribute is given and the number in brackets indicates the percentage of time it has been selected during the cross-validation. The number of retained attributes varies with the method employed but a global trend appears. Four PIR attributes are always in the top of the list (in_bathroom, in_living_room, in_bedroom and in_kitchen) followed by two others (Nb_in_kitchen and in_WC) and by two microphone attributes (sound bedroom, and speech). A rapid analysis of the projection of these attributes against the classes shows that in_bathroom is correlated with hygiene; in_kitchen with eating, in_WC with elimination, in_bedroom with sleeping, dressing and resting, and in_living_room with resting and communicating. This is not surprising as each room is related to several ADLs and thus the presence of someone in a room has a high predictive value about what s/he is doing in it. Regarding the sound attributes, Nb_sounds_bedroom_window and NB_sound_speech are correlated with dressing and communicating. Thus, the audio attributes were found to be informative according to these two activities.

Attribute selection results using the wrapper methods are given in Table 7. The most noticeable changes with the filter method is the dresser_state rank and the disappearance of all bedroom attributes. The former is a Boolean attribute which has a low entropy which is true (i.e., open) only in case of dressing, making it quite interesting for classification. in_bedroom attribute is not discriminative enough to distinguish sleeping from dressing and the configuration of the flat (see Fig. 1) makes this sensor fire sometimes when the participant is resting. Regarding the sound attributes, only Nb_sound_object_fall has been selected as globally useful for ADL classification due to its high correlation with communicating.

Rank	C4.5	DTM	NBayes	SVM (γ=0.8, greedy hill-climbing)	Global Wrapper
1	in_WC (100%)	in_WC (100%)	in_bathroom (100%)	in_bathroom (100%)	in_WC (100%)
2	in_living_room (100%)	in_living_room (100%)	in_WC (100%)	in_WC (100%)	in_living_room (100%)
3	in_kitchen (100%)	in_kitchen (100%)	in_living_room (100%)	in_living_room (100%)	in_kitchen (100%)
4	dresser_state (80%)	dresser_state (80%)	in_kitchen (100%)	in_kitchen (100%)	dresser_state (90%)
5	in_bathroom (70%)	Nb_in_bathroom (70%)	dresser_state (100%)	dresser_state (100%)	in_bathroom (77.5%)
6	($\leq$ 40%)	Nb_sounds_living_room_window (60%)	Nb_sound_object_fall (80%)	Nb_sound_object_fall (100%)	Nb_sound_object_fall (60%)
7		($\leq$ 40%)	Nb_sounds_living_room_window (80%)	Nb_sound_door_closing (80%)	
8			Nb_in_bathroom (60%)	($\leq$ 50%)	
9			($\leq$ 50%)		

Table 7. Attribute ranking for wrapper attribute selection methods with best-first search

method	Whole set	No sound	PIR only	Sound only	GF	GW
C4.5	83.28	76.77**	71.65**	51.50**	82.46	83.41
DTM	79.95	75.73**	71.34**	51.20**	82.59	83.02*
NBayes	85.27	77.37**	72.90**	50.78**	85.06	84.49
SVM ($\gamma = 0.8$)	82.91	78.88*	75.00**	51.94**	81.29	84.57
average	82.85	77.19	72.72	51.35	82.85	83.87

$^{*}p < .05;^{**}p < .01$

Table 8. Correctly classified Instances (%) for different learning algorithms and data sets

7.3 Impact on the Supervised Learning

The impact of the attribute selection has been assessed by learning from the data sets composed from subsets of attributes using a 10-fold stratified cross-validation repeated 10 times in the same learning conditions as for the wrapping selection. Table 8 summarises the results. Performance with the whole set is the reference for corrected paired student T-test.

Results with the whole set give the lowest performances for DTM (79.95%). NBayes and C4.5 have significantly higher performance than DTM ($p < .05$) but no significant difference is observed between them nor with SVM. When the sound attributes are removed (i.e., 'No sound' data set), the performances are significantly lower. This shows that the sound processing does present essential information to perform activity recognition. Data set composed of PIR attributes (i.e., 'PIR only' data set) only gives significantly reduced performances but still reasonable which emphasizes the location information impact for the classification. Whereas sound sensor should provide information redundant with the PIR sensors at a higher level (foot step, speech), the data set composed only of sound attributes (i.e. 'sound only' data set) leads to very poor performances. However, the Signal-To-Noise ratio of the sound signal must be improved to reach satisfying performance in this flat which has poor noise insulation (Fleury, 2008). This shows that each modality seems to play a different role for activity classification.

The data set composed of the attributes selected by Global Filtering (GF) attribute selection method leads to performances that are not significantly different from the ones with the whole set. This data set contains less than 29% of the original data (using only 7 sensors). No learning scheme is significantly better than the others. The data set composed of the attributes selected by Global Wrapping (GW) attribute selection method leads to performances that are significantly better for the DTM learning scheme ($p < .05$) but not for the other schemes when compared with the whole set. No significant difference is observed when compared to the GF performances. This data set contains less than 16% of the original data (using only 6 sensors). No learning scheme is significantly better than the others. Overall the GW method leads to higher average performance (83.87%) than with the Whole set (82.85%) and than the GF method (82.85%) but this is not significant and is mainly led by the DTM learning scheme. The main result of the study is that it is possible to keep high performance for automatic classification of ADL when selecting a relevant subset of attributes. About 33% of the sensors (and less than 16% of the attributes) are enough to classify ADL with same (and sometime superior) performance as with the whole data set. But the retained sensors are of different nature (location, sound, contact door) and thus complement each other. The selected attributes were mainly related to PIR sensors and microphones. While these sensors seem to be the most informative, contact door attached to the dresser was essential for classifying dressing activity. Indeed, the chosen ADLs were all related to a location (e.g.: sleeping in the bedroom, eating in the kitchen ...) and when two activities are usually done in the same room (e.g., sleeping and dressing) a strict location sensor is not enough to distinguish them. Thus, realistic ADLs should include activities in unusual location (e.g., eating while watching TV, sleeping on the sofa ...) to challenge the learning process and acquire more accurate models. This is illustrated by the eliminating and hygiene activities which, due to their natural interrelation (e.g., WC and then washing hand) and the flat configuration, challenged the learning.

Globally, sound sensors attributes have a good predictive power and the study shows that this information is essential for ADL classification. But the study also showed the limit of the current audio processing. Indeed, the sound attribute should deliver the same information as the PIR sensors while adding higher semantic level attributes (speech, footstep ...) but the very hostile sound conditions of the experiment shows that the robustness of the current audio processing needs to be improved. However, the presented results confirmed the information power of this modality at least for support to classical smart home sensors.

8. Discussion

The main outcome of this work is the demonstration that acceptable multisource audio processing performances are reachable, in real time, in a noisy environment. Moreover, although the audio processing performances are still not perfect, the study showed that the audio system (AUDITHIS) provides information essential for automatic identification of activity of daily living. This preliminary work, the first, to the best of our knowledge, that includes real-time sound and speech processing tested in a health smart home, is very encouraging. Of course the approach can be improved in many ways and the experimentations helped us to identify a number of limitations and challenges that need to be overcome.

Regarding the sound processing, the experiments generated very mixed results. Only two classes have been correctly recognized (`Clap` and `Phone`). The `Dishes` is very often confused with `Speech` because the training set doesn't include examples of spoon hitting a cup. This has a fundamental frequency in the spectral band of speech, hence the error of the segmentation module of AUDITHIS. `Scream` is often confused with `Falls of objects` and `Speech`. The former has been learned from a very small training set which explains the misclassification. The latter is more related to a design choice. Indeed, `Scream` is both a sound and a speech and difference between these two is quite vague. For example '*Aïe!*' is an intelligible scream that has been learned by the ASR (RAPHAEL) but a scream could also consist in '*Aaaa!*' which, in this case, should be handled by the sound recognizer. We still not have today a method to handle these situations and investigations about this problem is part of our research agenda. However, most of the poor performances can be explained by the too small training set. Our next goal is to extend this set to include more examples with more variation as well as more classes (such as water sounds and a reject class for unknown or non-frequent sounds). This is mandatory because GMM is a probabilistic approach which relies on a high number of instances to learn correctly each class. With a 'design-for-all' aim — which is reasonable considering that many homes in several countries generate the same kinds of sound — a probabilistic approach seems to be the most suited. However, other approaches, such as (Niessen et al., 2008) which relies on non-statistical techniques are worth being considered and we plan to compare our approach to some of the literature such as the ones base on soundscape (Aucouturier et al., 2007; Guastavino, 2006).

The speech recognition for the detection of distress situation led to interesting results in-lab but still needs to be improved. Indeed, the experiments during which persons were asked to utter normal and distress speech sentences in two different rooms showed how degraded the speech recognition is in hostile condition. The error rate for the recognition of distress sentences in this situation reached 30%. This can be partly explained by the very bad acoustic of the flat (with a mean SNR of about 12 dB instead of 27 dB for the learning corpora). Another limitation of the RAPHAEL system is that its language model is constructed with our colloquial speech corpus. We plan to refine this model by adding expressions and words frequently used in daily conditions. This should give better results and make the distress situation detection tool more adapted to real conditions. The experiments have been performed with young healthy people but it is well known that the voice characteristics vary with the age. Thus, a second challenge is to adapt the acoustic model of RAPHAEL to the target population: the elderly people. We plan to collect speech uttered by a large corpus of elderly people to obtain a system usable for elderly. Other way of improving the speech recognition would be to use acoustic models learned directly from the person which would be more adapted to her voice. However, we believe that a speaker independent approach makes more sense for this kind of application which necessitates to be easily integrable to the flat with a minimal setting period. But, an approach that would automatically adapt the speaker independent models to the person's voice would offer an interesting compromise. The speech processing also offers an interesting approach to deal with the presence of several persons in the flat. This problem is often neglegted, because many works consider that the person lives alone. But an aged person is visited many times and one of the aims of the new technology is to fight loneliness by augmenting the number of daily communications. Thus we need to distinguish what the data that belongs to the monitored person is. Speaker diarization (Fredouille et al., 2006) could be adapted to deal with this problem.

Both sound and speech processings are highly perturbed by audio source of daily living (e.g., TV, radio). The tests of the noise cancellation technique gave a better understanding of the kinds of noise source that may be the most difficult to deal with. The test has been performed only in laboratory and future work includes the test of this method in the health smart home conditions. This will give more conclusive insight about the method performances in this condition.

Sound and speech recognition system is used, *in fine*, for the automatic learning and recognition of activities of daily living together with other modalities. We have shown that the audio modality in health smart home for the recognition of ADL has a significant impact on recognition performance. The evaluation showed that the most informative sensors were the PIR ones. However, the audio channel should provide information not only redundant with the PIR one (e.g., presence in one room) but also higher level (e.g., washing machine spinning). Thus we expect that the improvement of the audio processing will lead to higher performance in activity of daily living recognition. The presented results come from a short number of young and healthy participants in only one flat. Future work should include data from elderly people in more that one flat to test the influence of the disposition of a flat on the results. Such supplementary experimentations would be useful to confirm the relative importance of each sensor. One of the limits of the study is to not have taken the time into account. Indeed, activities such as eating may be repeated at regular time. However, this information is useful only when the resident is following his usual routine and may not challenge the learning to acquire more accurate models. Moreover, as in many data acquired from volunteers outside their home, the time information does not respect the participants' routine. Finally, many applications assess the inhabitant's autonomy by computing the deviance from a routine pattern of activities. But, a deviance may not be a sign of autonomy loss. Microphones can thus play a central role to remove the ambiguity by adding some context detection from the sentences uttered during the day (e.g., multiple voices, plumber intervention . . .).

Audio is not a modality much employed in the domain due to its intrusive nature, but sociological studies (Rialle et al., 2008) have shown that the degree of acceptance of sensors in one's home is idiosyncratic and depend on the level of distress of the person and his relatives. Moreover, the current approach does not record what the speakers are saying but only uses speech processing to detect distress situations. Microphone for sound and speech processing is thus a very interesting sensor to acquire information about human activities which has also the capacity of being used as voice command for domotic purposes.

Finally, it should be emphasized that data acquisition in such environment is a very hard task. Although the number of projects related to ambient assisted living is high, only few datasets are from real data (i.e., aged people with loss of autonomy) and dataset acquisition in this non-standardised domain is a challenge by itself.

9. Conclusion

This chapter presents the AUDITHIS system which performs real-time sound analysis from eight microphone channels in Health Smart Home associated to the autonomous speech analyzer RAPHAEL. The evaluation of AUDITHIS and RAPHAEL in different settings showed that audio modality is very promising to acquire information that are not available through other classical sensors. Audio processing is also the most natural way for a human to interact with his environment. Thus, this approach particularly fits Health Smart Homes that include home automation (e.g., voice command) or other high level interactions (e.g., dialogue). The originality of the work is also to include sounds of daily living as indicators to distinguish distress from normal situations. First development gave acceptable results for the sound recognition (72% correct classification) and we are working on the reduction of missed-alarm rate to improve performance in the near future.

Although the current system suffers a number of limitations and that we raised numerous challenges that need to be addressed, the pair AUDITHIS and RAPHAEL is, to the best of our knowledge, one of the first serious attempts to build a real-time system that consider sound and speech analysis for ambient assisted living. This work also includes several evaluations on data acquired from volunteers in a real health smart home condition. Further work will include refinement of the acoustic models to adapt the speech recognition to the aged population as well as connexion to home automation systems.

Acknowledgment

The authors would like to thank Hubert Glasson that accomplished an amazing work on AU-DITHIS and Noé Guirand who worked on the noise suppression. They also are very grateful to the participants who took part to the different experiments. Thanks are also extended to Christophe Villemazet and the RBI company for their support during the AILISA project.

10. References

Abowd, G., Mynatt, E. & Rodden, T. (2002). The human experience [of ubiquitous computing], *IEEE Pervasive Computing* 1(1): 48–57.

Adami, A., Hayes, T. & Pavel, M. (2003). Unobtrusive monitoring of sleep patterns, *Proc. 25th Annual Int. Conference of the IEEE-EMBS 2003*, Vol. 2, pp. 1360–1363.

Albinali, F., Davies, N. & Friday, A. (2007). Structural learning of activities from sparse datasets, *5th IEEE Int. Conference on Pervasive Computing and Communications*.

Anderson, S., Liberman, N., Bernstein, E., Foster, S., Cate, E., Levin, B. & Hudson, R. (1999). Recognition of elderly speech and voice-driven document retrieval, *Proc. IEEE Int. Conference on Acoustics, Speech, and Signal Processing*, Vol. 1, pp. 145–148.

Aucouturier, J., Defreville, B. & Pachet, F. (2007). The bag-of-frames approach to audio pattern recognition: a sufficient model for urban soundscapes but not for polyphonic music, *Journal of Acoustical Society of America* 122(2): 881–891.

Baba, A., Yoshizawa, S., Yamada, M., Lee, A. & Shikano, K. (2004). Acoustic models of the elderly for large-vocabulary continuous speech recognition, *Electronics and Communications in Japan, Part 2, Vol. 87, No. 7, 2004* 87(2): 49–57.

Bonhomme, S., Campo, E., Estève, D. & Guennec, J. (2008). Prosafe-extended, a telemedicine platform to contribute to medical diagnosis., *J. Telemedicine and Telecare* 14(3): 116–119.

Chan, M., Estève, D., Escriba, C. & Campo, E. (2008). A review of smart homes- present state and future challenges., *Computer Methods and Programs in Biomedicine* 91(1): 55–81.

Chen, J., Kam, A. H., Zhang, J., Liu, N. & Shue, L. (2005). Bathroom activity monitoring based on sound, *in* S. B. . Heidelberg (ed.), *Pervasive Computing*, Vol. 3468/2005 of *Lecture Notes in Computer Science*, pp. 47–61.

Clavel, C., Devillers, L., Richard, G., Vasilescu, I. & Ehrette, T. (2007). Detection and analysis of abnormal situations through fear-type acoustic manifestations, *IEEE Trans. on Speech and Audio Processing* 4: 21–24.

Cohen, I. & Berdugo, B. (2001). Speech enhancement for non-stationary noise environments, *Signal Processing* 81: 2403–2418.

Cowling, M. (2004). *Non-Speech Environmental Sound Classification System for Autonomous Surveillance*, PhD thesis, Griffith University.

Cowling, M. & Sitte, R. (2003). Comparison of techniques for environmental sound recognition, *Pattern Recognition Letter* **24**(15): 2895–2907.

Dalal, S., Alwan, M., Seifrafi, R., Kell, S. & Brown, D. (2005). A rule-based approach to the analysis of elders' activity data: detection of health and possible emergency conditions, *AAAI 2005 fall symposium, workshop on caring machines: AI in eldercare*.

Davis, K. H., Biddulph, R. & Balashek, S. (1952). Automatic recognition of spoken digits, *The Journal of the Acoustical Society of America* **24**(6): 637–642.
    URL: *http://link.aip.org/link/?JAS/24/637/1*

Duchêne, F., Garbay, C. & Rialle, V. (2007). Learning recurrent behaviors from heterogeneous multivariate time-series, *Artificial Intelligence in Medicine* **39**: 25–47.

Duong, T., Phung, D., Bui, H. & Venkatesh, S. (2009). Efficient duration and hierarchical modeling for human activity recognition, *Artificial Intelligence* **173**(7–8): 830–856.

Ephraim, Y. & Malah, D. (1984). Speech enhancement using a minimum-mean square error short-time spectral emplitude estimator, *IEEE Trans. on Acoustic, speech and Signal Processing* **32**(3): 1109–1121.

Fezari, M. & Bousbia-Salah, M. (2007). Speech and sensor in guiding an electric wheelchair, *Automatic Control and Computer Sciences* **41**(1): 39–43.

Fleury, A. (2008). *Détection de motifs temporels dans les environements multi-perceptifs – Application à la classification des Activités de la Vie Quotidienne d'une Personne Suivie à Domicile par Télémédecine.*, PhD thesis, University Joseph Fourier, Grenoble.

Fredouille, C., Moraru, D., Meignier, S., Bonastre, J.-F. & Besacier, L. (2006). Step-by-step and integrated approaches in broadcast news speaker diarization, *Computer Speech and Language Journal* **20**(2–3): 303–330.

Gauvain, J.-L., Lamel, L.-F. & Eskenazi, M. (1990). Design considerations and text selection for BREF, a large french read-speech corpus, *ICSLP'90*, Kobe, Japan, pp. 1097–1100.

Guastavino, C. (2006). The ideal urban soundscape: investigating the sound quality of french cities, *Acta Acustica* **92**: 945–951.

Gustafsson, S., Martin, R., Jax, P. & Vary, P. (2004). A psychoacoustic approach to combined acoustic echo cancellation and noise reduction, *IEEE Trans. on Speech and Audio Processing* **10**(5): 245–256.

Harma, A., McKinney, M. & Skowronek, J. (2005). Automatic surveillance of the acoustic activity in our living environment, *Proc. IEEE Int. Conference on Multimedia and Expo ICME 2005*, pp. 634–637.

Hong, X., Nugent, C., Mulvenna, M., McClean, S. & Scotney, B. (2008). Evidential fusion of sensor data for activity recognition in smart homes, *Pervasive and Mobile Computing* pp. 1–17.

Ibarz, A., Bauer, G., Casas, R., Marco, A. & Lukowicz, P. (2008). Design and evaluation of a sound based water flow measurement system, *Smart Sensing and Context*, Vol. 5279/2008 of *Lecture Notes in Computer Science*, Springer Verlag, pp. 41–54.

Intille, S. (2002). Designing a home of the future, *IEEE Pervasive Computing* **1**(2): 76–82.

Istrate, D., Castelli, E., Vacher, M., Besacier, L. & Serignat, J.-F. (2006). Information extraction from sound for medical telemonitoring, *IEEE Trans. on Information Technologies in Biomedicine* **10**(2): 264–274.

Istrate, D., Vacher, M. & Serignat, J.-F. (2008). Embedded implementation of distress situation identification through sound analysis, *The Journal on Information Technology in Healthcare* 6(3): 204–211.

Katz, S. & Akpom, C. (1976). A measure of primary sociobiological functions, *International Journal of Health Services* 6(3): 493–508.

Kröse, B., van Kasteren, T., Gibson, C. & van den Dool, T. (2008). Care: Context awareness in residences for elderly, *Int. Conference of the Int. Soc. for Gerontechnology*, Pisa, Tuscany, Italy.

Kumiko, O., Mitsuhiro, M., Atsushi, E., Shohei, S. & Reiko, T. (2004). Input support for elderly people using speech recognition, *IEIC Technical Report* 104(139): 1–6.

LeBellego, G., Noury, N., Virone, G., Mousseau, M. & Demongeot, J. (2006). A model for the measurement of patient activity in a hospital suite, *IEEE Trans. on Information Technology in Biomedicine* 10(1): 92–99.

Litvak, D., Zigel, Y. & Gannot, I. (2008). Fall detection of elderly through floor vibrations and sound, *Proc. 30th Annual Int. Conference of the IEEE-EMBS 2008*, pp. 4632–4635.

Maunder, D., Ambikairajah, E., Epps, J. & Celler, B. (2008). Dual-microphone sounds of daily life classification for telemonitoring in a noisy environment, *Proc. 30th Annual International Conference of the IEEE-EMBS 2008*, pp. 4636–4639.

Michaut, F. & Bellanger, M. (2005). *Filtrage adaptatif : théorie et algorithmes*, Lavoisier.

Moore, D. & Essa, I. (2002). Recognizing multitasked activities from video using stochastic context-free grammar, *Proc. of American Association of Artificial Intelligence (AAAI) Conference 2002*, Alberta, Canada.

Niessen, M., Van Maanen, L. & Andringa, T. (2008). Disambiguating sounds through context, *Proc. Second IEEE International Conference on Semantic Computing*, pp. 88–95.

Noury, N., Hadidi, T., Laila, M., Fleury, A., Villemazet, C., Rialle, V. & Franco, A. (2008). Level of activity, night and day alternation, and well being measured in a smart hospital suite, *Proc. 30th Annual Int. Conference of the IEEE-EMBS 2008*, pp. 3328–3331.

Noury, N., Villemazet, C., Barralon, P. & Rumeau, P. (2006). Ambient multi-perceptive system for residential health monitoring based on electronic mailings experimentation within the AILISA project, *Proc. 8th Int. Conference on e-Health Networking, Applications and Services HEALTHCOM 2006*, pp. 95–100.

Popescu, M., Li, Y., Skubic, M. & Rantz, M. (2008). An acoustic fall detector system that uses sound height information to reduce the false alarm rate, *Proc. 30th Annual Int. Conference of the IEEE-EMBS 2008*, pp. 4628–4631.

Portet, F., Fleury, A., Vacher, M. & Noury, N. (2009). Determining useful sensors for automatic recognition of activities of daily living in health smart home, *in Intelligent Data Analysis in Medicine and Pharmacology (IDAMAP2009)*, Verona, Italy .

Rabiner, L. & Luang, B. (1996). *Digital processing of speech signals*, Prentice-Hall.

Renouard, S., Charbit, M. & Chollet, G. (2003). Vocal interface with a speech memory for dependent people, *Independent Living for Persons with Disabilities* pp. 15–21.

Rialle, V., Ollivet, C., Guigui, C. & Hervé, C. (2008). What do family caregivers of alzheimer's disease patients desire in health smart home technologies? contrasted results of a wide survey, *Methods of Information in Medicine* 47: 63–69.

Saeys, Y., Inza, I. & Larrañaga, P. (2007). A review of feature selection techniques in bioinformatics, *Bioinformatics* 23: 2507–2517.

Soo, J.-S. & Pang, K. (1990). Multidelay block frequency domain adaptive filter, *IEEE Trans. on Acoustics, Speech and Signal Processing* 38(2): 373–376.

Takahashi, S.-y., Morimoto, T., Maeda, S. & Tsuruta, N. (2003). Dialogue experiment for elderly people in home health care system, *Text Speech and Dialogue (TSD) 2003*.

Tran, Q. T. & Mynatt, E. D. (2003). What was i cooking? towards déjà vu displays of everyday memory, *Technical report*.

Vacher, M., Fleury, A., Serignat, J.-F., Noury, N. & Glasson, H. (2008). Preliminary evaluation of speech/sound recognition for telemedicine application in a real environment, *The 9thAnnual Conference of the International Speech Communication Association, INTER-SPEECH'08 Proceedings*, Brisbane, Australia, pp. 496–499.

Vacher, M., Serignat, J.-F. & Chaillol, S. (2007). Sound classification in a smart room environment: an approach using GMM and HMM methods, *Advances in Spoken Language Technology, SPED 2007 Proceedings*, Iasi, Romania, pp. 135–146.

Vacher, M., Serignat, J.-F., Chaillol, S., Istrate, D. & Popescu, V. (2006). Speech and sound use in a remote monitoring system for health care, *Lecture Notes in Computer Science, Artificial Intelligence, Text Speech and Dialogue, vol. 4188/2006*, Brno, Czech Republic, pp. 711–718.

Valin, J.-M. (2007). On adjusting the learning rate in frequency domain echo cancellation with double talk, *IEEE Trans. on Acoustics, Speech and Signal Processing* 15(3): 1030–1034.

Valin, J.-M. & Collings, I. B. (2007). A new robust frequency domain echo canceller with closed-loop learning rate adaptation, *IEEE Int. Conference on Acoustics, Speech and Signal Processing, ICASSP'07 Proceedings Vol. 1*, Honolulu, Hawaii, USA, pp. 93–96.

Vaseghi, S. V. (1996). *Advanced Signal Processing and Digital Noise Reduction, 1996*.

Vaufreydaz, D., Bergamini, C., Serignat, J.-F., Besacier, L. & Akbar, M. (2000). A new methodology for speech corpora definition from internet documents, *LREC'2000, 2nd Int. Conference on Language Ressources and Evaluation*, Athens, Greece, pp. 423–426.

Wang, J.-C., Lee, H.-P., Wang, J.-F. & Lin, C.-B. (2008). Robust environmental sound recognition for home automation, *IEEE Trans. on Automation Science and Engineering* 5(1): 25–31.

Wilpon, J. & Jacobsen, C. (1996). A study of speech recognition for children and the elderly, *IEEE Int. Conference on Acoustics, Speech and Signal Processing*, pp. 349–352.

34

New emerging biomedical technologies for home-care and telemedicine applications: the *Sensorwear* project

Luca Piccini, Oriana Ciani and Giuseppe Andreoni
Politecnico di Milano, INDACO Department
Italy

1. Introduction

The *Grey Booming* phenomenon is one of the major issues indicated by the European Union as a problem to be analysed and faced by the Seventh Framework Programme (FP7). Statistics highlighted that elderly people (over 65 years old) should double in the next 40 years. The medical and health care to such an 'older' society means growing expenditures for the UE national health systems, which already amount to significant percentages of the Gross Domestic Product (GDP) in the different countries. The UE Healthcare Systems risk to collapse if strong countermeasures will not be undertaken. Agreeing with this assumption, the European Commission included among its priorities the stimuli to deeply remodel the national healthcare systems. France, United Kingdom, Holland, Austria, Italy and other countries drafted national programs in order to face this emerging problem. More in detail, cardiac and respiratory diseases have been identified as some of the most frequent causes of hospitalization; telemedicine and home-care have been therefore selected to face the negative evolution of these pathologies, both in clinical and economical terms, assuring domestic assistance for older people as well as disabled or chronic patients. The rationale of this choice is the opportunity of reducing the overall costs while maintaining high quality of care and providing an easy access to care from any place, at any time. Moreover the focus of healthcare consequently shifts from treatment to prevention and early diagnosis, thanks to the contribution of parallel wellness programs, too.

Increasing the impact of home-care solutions is a difficult challenge, since technological issues, such as biosignals monitoring, data communications and basic automated signal analysis coexist with the efforts to improve new technologies' acceptability by the patients, who need to interact with them for long time. Generally these users are not technologically skilled therefore textile sensors platforms represent an ideal way to develop the telemedicine approach.

Under these perspectives, the research and development of Wearable Health Systems (WHS) become even relevant. They are expected to play a significant role on the spreading of 'extra-hospital' cares, thus improving the national health policies effectiveness and the citizens' quality of life, too.

WHS are integrated systems on body-worn platforms, such as wrist-worn devices or biomedical clothes, offering pervasive solutions for continuous health status monitoring trough non-invasive biomedical, biochemical and physical measurements (Lymberis & Gatzoulis, 2006). In other words, they provide not only a remote monitoring platform for prevention and early diagnosis, but also a valid contribution to disease management and support of elderly or people in need; in particular, they enable multi-parametric monitoring including body-kinematics, vital signs, biochemical as well as emotional and sensorial parameters in a defined social and environmental context.

The integration of electronics and clothing is an emerging field which aims to the development of multi-functional, wearable electro-textiles for applications together with body functions monitoring, actuation, communication, data transfer and individual environment control. Furthermore, the integration of advanced microsystems at the fibre core, in conjunction with user interfaces, power sources and embedded software, make R&D in this field extremely challenging. Moreover, current research is dealing with the development of stretchable conductive patterns and soft-touch substrates for component textile mounting and interconnection.

As a matter of fact, WHS cope with a variety of challenging topics, whose complexity increases with their integration: wireless communication, power supply and management, data processing, new algorithms for biosignal analysis, connection, sensors' cleaning and stability over time and external conditions, sensors positioning on the human body, user's interface, garment's elasticity and adherence to the skin and other minor themes.

Surely the first issue to be managed is the technological one - current state of the art has achieved a good level of maturity to be industrialized and brought to the market - but another key factor, that is still not mature enough, is the ergonomic or human factor in terms of device's usability, comfort and acceptance by the end user. According to the authors, *design for wearability* is necessary for the real and definitive acknowledgment of WHS in clinical applications, telemedicine and more (Andreoni, 2008). That's the reason why, besides the main objectives of developing healthcare wearable devices, meeting the aforementioned requirements for enhanced user-friendliness, affordability and unobtrusive monitoring in several clinical applications is becoming a growing topic of worldwide research about WHS.

In order to let WHS regularly break into the healthcare practice this and other issues should be solved, for example, from the commercial and industrial point of view, the consolidation of R&D results in different domains and their integration (David, 2007). The *Sensorwear* project tries to organically coordinate the emerging technologies in the field of wearable biomedical devices, conductive yarns or garments, embedded monitoring devices, automated alarm systems and ICT channels optimizations, in order to design a complete, automated service for home and clinical cardiac monitoring applications.

2. The international scenario of wearable telemonitoring systems

Wearable solutions for biophysical conditions monitoring can address many of the emerging issues previously described for a broad cross-section of user groups. Elderly care and disease management are just the immediate application, in addition to wellness and sport which represent significant segments that can benefit from continuous, remote and personal monitoring solutions.

During the last years, different research projects all over the European Union were dedicated to the creation of telemonitoring systems based on wearable or standard sensors. MyHeart is one of the most important and complete among them. Notwithstanding the relevant efforts that have been made since 2000 by the granted projects of the Seventh Framework Program (FP7), researchers and industries are still trying to improve patients' condition monitoring at home using unobtrusive sensors built into everyday objects able to automatically report to clinicians[1] (Lymberys & De Rossi, 2004). These examples and other projects demonstrated both the importance of such applications and the technological problems related to the creation of such a systems.

On the other side, pilot studies were lead in order to evaluate the potential impact of home-care monitoring in terms of costs through a comparison with standard instrumentation. The EU Commission, in fact, has underlined the economical potentialities of such solutions, but also has pointed out doubts with the achievement of the potential results and the effective introduction of these technologies in the healthcare systems (COM 689, 2008).

All the predictive models, analysis and studies confirmed the importance of the wearable telemonitoring scenario, but many problems occur if one aims to the implementation of an industrial project and not only to a research prototype (Lymberis & Paradiso, 2008).

The Sensorwear project tries to avoid the segmentation of technologies and competences, concentrating a small, skilled group of people for the creation of a wearable, unobtrusive, low cost and fully automated solution whose usability, reliability and release of brief information are the most peculiar qualities.

The market analysis has shown there are no commercial solutions able to assure those requirements with a complete wearable system for daily clinical monitoring. It is not uncommon reading about prototypes or finding patents about wearable systems for health care and catching poor information coming from military applications context, not accessible by definition (Pantepopulous & Bourbakis, 2008). To date, the main companies involved in the development of wearable monitoring systems such as Body Media Inc., Sensatex Inc., Textronics Inc. and Vivometrics Inc., experience every day the need for more consistent and remote monitoring of individuals for a variety of purpose: from elderly care to chronic disease management and others. Their solutions are just beginning the transition from the development phase into commercialization, facing the barrier of the regulatory approval, which remains critical for many of the producers.

Just to give an example, a common electrocardiograph, the instrument allowing the execution of an electrocardiogram exam, costs about 600€ in the UE market and cannot be used with wearable sensors to provide unobtrusive measures. The paradigm of measures transparency requires solutions' refinement or improvement or the design of new integrated systems when noise, artefacts or ergonomic deficiencies enlarge.

The Sensorwear system points at achieving these crucial objectives.

---

[1] For more details, go to: http://heartcycle.med.auth.gr and http://www.ehealthnews.eu .

3. The Sensorwear project

The Sensorwear project focuses on design and development of a low-cost, industrial solution for smart home-monitoring and hospital applications. The objective is not to create a life-support system, but a reliable, cost effective solution able to monitor biosignals detecting specific conditions requested by clinicians and to transmit them consequently through a long-range communication channel.

The project is granted by the Regione Lombardia and it involves the Politecnico di Milano - INDACO Department -, three technological partners (STMicroelectronics, Microsystems and SXT-Sistemi per Telemedicina), one clothes manufacturer (MCS – Manifatture Cotoniere Settentrionali), a service provider company for the textile and clothing sector (Centro Tessile Cotoniero) and the Mater Domini Hospital in Castellanza (IT), the project's clinical partner. We will illustrate the main aspects related to the project's objectives, technical solutions, applications and expected results in the following paragraphs.

3.1 Objectives and overall architecture

The Sensorwear project aims at developing a complete home monitoring service able to collect a set of different biosignals in a transparent way during the spontaneous activity of the subjects: this paradigm is known as unobtrusive measure. An important part of the project is the creation of a Body Sensor Network (BSN) dedicated to the health state monitoring trough record, process and transmission of the biosignals and some useful parameters obtained from them. BSN is mainly based on wearable sensors for the collection of biopotentials (like the electrocardiographic signals, the ECG) and integrated and miniaturized electronic solution based on Bluetooth® technology.

The detailed objectives of the project are (Fig. 1):

- Research, development and production of a System in Package (SIP) solution for monitoring, processing and transmission.
- Research, development and production of embedded sensors.
- Creation of fully featured t-shirts with integrated SIP devices to be tested and used both at home and in hospital.
- Development of software and algorithms for the processing and management of signals, data and alarm for the different applications.
- Development of software for remote data receiving and database integration.

In order to fulfil those items, the fundamental point of the product industrialisation, which is a peculiarity of the Sensorwear project, is continuously kept into consideration. In this way, the final solution is expected to be compliant with the specifications for medical devices of class IIa. Garments' testing, which is an ongoing concern, is an unavoidable step in order to ensure biocompatibility.

The architecture of the system is essentially composed by four main systems:

1. t-shirt with embedded electrodes for the collection of bio-potentials
2. preconditioning and acquisition system
3. processing and transmission device
4. remote data management software.

The second and third systems compose a body gateway able to directly control a mobile phone without requiring the user interaction. Actually, the possibility to act in a fully automated way is another significant feature of the Sensorwear device.

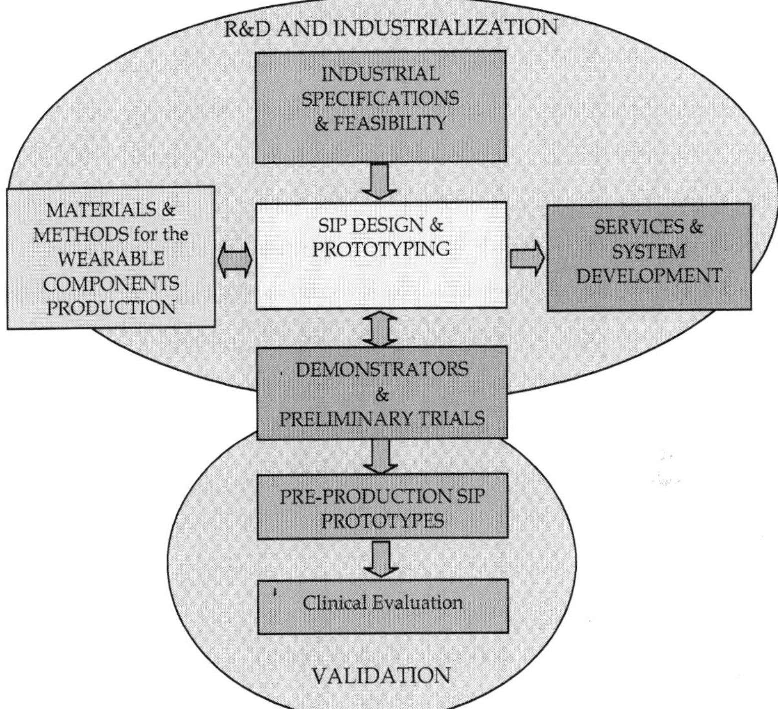

Fig. 1. Sensorwear main activities: different tasks and their relationships.

The signals identified for the specific purpose of the telecardiology application are:
- Three ECG leads
- Body movement
- Respiratory frequency
- Cardiac output monitoring.

The ECG signal is the most important one allowing the device to detect useful parameters like Heart Rate (HR), arrhythmias and their classification, ST line anomalies. ECG is a primary source of indications about health condition, so it receives, at least at early stages, greater attention.

The body movement is recorded through a three-axial accelerometer, whose properly processed signals allow determining the number of steps and the body position with respect to the earth gravity.

Furthermore, it is possible to detect the changing of the cardiac output during the day and also the respiratory movements through impedance cardiography measure (ICG).

3.2 Technological key-point and main issues

The main objectives of this project deal with the creation of an industrial, compact, easy to use, automated solution designed with a special attention to elderly people. These demanding requirements are addressed by the different skills of the partners on yarns and textile solutions, electronic design and production, data collection and databases.

WEARABLE SENSORS

The t-shirts were designed in order to facilitate the integration of sensors during the industrialization and to assure the best sensors' positioning for ECG and ICG signals quality. The design of garments is a crucial point in the field of unobtrusive measures, in fact as previous research projects and studies have evidenced, it needs configurations able to reduce the effects of movements, without impacting the comfort. The testing phase for the t-shirt, their sensors and sensors' position has started with the ECG signal check, following a specific protocol. First of all the signals are recorded with the first prototype and standard electrode in the Einthoven's configuration, afterwards the device has to collect signals through the t-shirt. The last scheduled test requires to connect the prototype to standard electrodes but placed in the same positions of the wearable ones. Each recording is done 3 minutes at rest and 3 minutes into action.

ERGONOMIC and MECHANICAL ASPECTS

As far as the design of the t-shirts and the adherence of sensors affect the quality of the ECG and ICG signals, the enclosure of the device and its connection to the sensors pathways strongly impact on both the usability and the industrial sustainability. Our analysis of the production process and its related constraints evidenced the necessity to conceive custom boxes in order to create a real comfortable solution without renouncing to an appealing product. The enclosure will also include the visual signalling with yellow and green leds, compliant to the specifications for Holter medical devices (Fig. 2).
Moreover the custom case can be inserted in a docking station, directly sewed to the t-shirt and including the sensors connectors.
At this purpose, a custom solution is not a cost-effective one, while the use of the docking station as mating support can allow the choice of stable, reliable although simple and cheaper connectors.

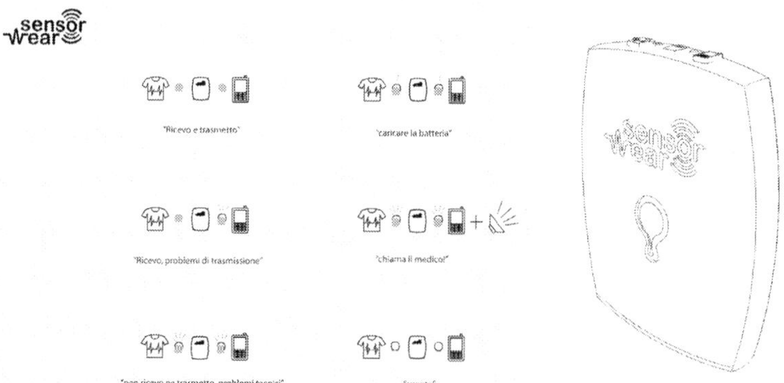

Fig. 2. The ergonomic study for the user interface and the device shape as regards wearability issues.

ELECTRONICS

As regards the electronic point of view the final objective is a scaled solution composed by a SIP for the analogue preconditioning and digital processing and a Bluetooth transmission system with a Dial-Up Network (DUN) profile. The latter specification faces the problem of long-range data transmission within the application model addressed to people who are not used or skilled to work with a PC, but usually are equipped with a generic mobile phone. The only constraint included in this scenario is the need of a Bluetooth connection, but nowadays we know it is easy to find it also in low-end mobile phones.
For what concerns the electronic design, the two main topics are the miniaturization of the circuitry and the reduction of power consumption in order to reach at least 5 days of continuous working with small, commercial batteries. Our technological partners already designed and developed products or prototypes able to collect the proposed signals through wearable sensors in a reliable way, but they need to be improved since all the solutions are not optimized in terms of power consumption and scalability. The design of a SIP solution requires the refinement of previous solutions and the research of new components that can be integrated with it. The choice of new elements is one of the strategies taken to achieve a low-power design, even if it implies to test again the performance of the system in terms of signal quality, signal-to-noise ratio, drifts and all the parameters influencing the compliance with the medical specifications. The final design, the list of components and the features of the system as output of the whole project will be released after the completion of the ICG tests. To date, the logical structure of the prototype in use is described in Fig. 3.
Signals are real-time recorded and processed in order to extract parameters relevant for the clinicians who will receive them through the remote server. Dialling, connection and authentication procedures are directly controlled by the wearable unit, thus excluding any user intervention. The processing output is directly stored in the remote database. The use of a new generation of 32-bit microcontroller unit (MCU) allows the management of the entire process, optimizing the power consumption at the same time.

Different strategies of power management are investigated for each working condition.
In fact there are two different situations:
- the normal one, when only brief parameters are transmitted, once in every minute;
- the "alarm" condition, during which also the raw signals are transmitted.
This latter configuration allows a prompt analysis of the ECG by the clinicians, who can decide to reject the alarm or to activate countermeasures.
This fully automated model of service is based on the possibility to identify different critical conditions from the biosignals applying the rules provided by the clinicians and embedded in the CPU. After the trigger of a possible critical situation has launched, the DUN Bluetooth profile tries to directly connect itself to the remote server and to transmit the raw signals, beginning from the past last minute, until the remote operator will decide to stop the "alarm condition". Its management implies the possibility to use also GPRS data transmission, because the 3G network coverage is still not ensured in all the neighbouring areas. As a consequence, we are also exploring data compression algorithms for raw signals transmission in case of poor mobile network coverage.

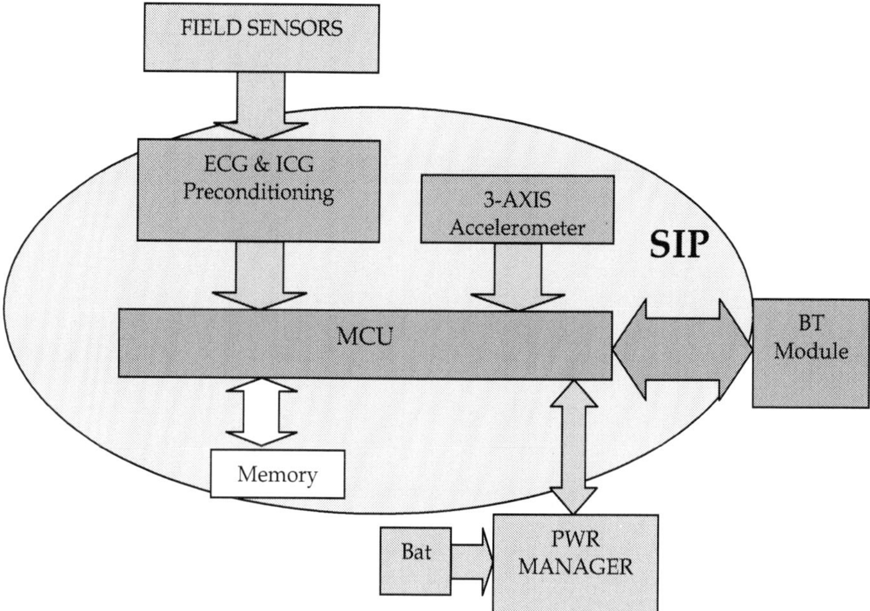

Fig. 3. The electronic device, the SIP components are evidenced.

SERVER and WEB-SERVICE

The hospital security model generally denies the possibility to directly connect a remote device to a local server, physically and logically placed inside the hospital, according to both the Italian and other countries regulation. On the same purpose, it is worth noting that it is not mandatory placing the main data collector inside the hospital network, in fact through a secure web-service application the operators can access data while being in the hospital, or more precisely, in a control room where the physiological parameters and alarms can be constantly observed by them. The use of different servers in order to cover the involved area in a better way and to create a local node to distribute the collision management overhead in case of multiple alarm conditions is thus made possible. The problem of priority management could not be faced at the mobile phone level because a typical mobile service provider can grant dedicated server resources only with business contracts. The mobile phone is just a transparent modem connected to the server. The policy in case of a coincidence of alarms is a matter of debate, but speaking from the informatics point of view, as soon as the connection mobile-server is established through the standard port, the link should be automatically turned on a specific port, in order to set free the common resource for the next alarm.

4. Preliminary results and conclusions

During one year and half of work the consortium faced the problems related to the industrialisation and certification of the product. Since some partners were already involved in such area of the market, preliminary operations like market survey or patent analysis were almost ready at the early stage of the project. This way it was possible to promptly release the main specifications for the system, although the industrialisation process is still a work in progress. In fact the targeted customers population, predominantly composed by not-or-less technology skilled people, requires a detailed analysis on specific components responsible for the usability and allowing a user-friendly system's management and handling.

As anticipated, we are currently addressing the testing phase on the t-shirts in terms of biocompatibility and clinical performances.

Regarding the hardware, we are testing the low-scaled device. The SIP will be the final result of the project because the design and production of a SIP system is an expensive and complex process, requiring a lot of efforts in order to reduce the risk of a major fault. For this reason we are carrying out specific tests collecting data on performances and trying to understand potential criticism before starting the first production.

	Current status	Industrialisation problems	Compliance with specifications [%]
T-shirt	Prototyping and validating 2nd release	Sensors embedding and connectors	70%
Hardware	SIP desing	Integration in the T-shirts	100%
Firmware	Testing and consolidation	Refine power management	80%
Algorithms	Testing	None	100%
System software	Developing	-	-

Table 1. Current project checkout list.

During the last months, the firmware has been tested on the same devices (MCU and Bluetooth module) in terms of power consumption and transmission throughput. Based on current measures, we forecast it will be possible to ensure a 5-days working time with a commercial Lithium-Ion or Lithium-Polymer battery with less than 500mAh of capacity with the transmission protocol already working.

Although there are still some critical aspects highlighted in Table 1, several problems related to the creation of a commercial unobtrusive and fully automated wearable monitoring solution have been solved. Moreover a great boost to the project has come from the introduction of a System in Package solution, the heart of the electronic device, which could probably have a deep impact also in next products and projects.

5. References

Andreoni G. (2008), *Sistemi di sensori indossabili per il monitoraggio: Dalla Ricerca al Mercato*, In: Bonfiglio A., Cerutti S., De Rossi D., Magenes G. (eds.), Sistemi Indossabili Intelligenti per la salute e la protezione dell'uomo, Patron, 2008

COM 689. (2008). Communication from the commission to the European Parliament, the Council, the European Economic and Social Committes and the Committee of the Regions on telemedicine for the benefit of patients, healthcare systems and society, *COMMISSION OF THE EUROPEAN COMMUNITIES*, Brussels.

David K. (2007), *Wearable Electronics Systems Global Market Demand Analysis: Health Care Solutions*, In: VDC Research Report # VDC6520.

Lymberis A. and De Rossi D. (2004). *Wearable eHealth Systems for Personalised Health Management. State of the Art and Future Challenges*, IOS Press, ISBN I 58603 449 9, Netherlands.

Lymberis A., Gatzoulis L. (2006), *Wearable Health Systems: from smart technologies to real applications*. Conf. Proc. IEEE Eng. Med. Biol. Soc.: 6789-92.

Lymberis A. and Paradiso R. (2008). Smart Fabrics and Interactive Textile Enabling Wearable Personal Applications: R&D State of the Art and Future Challenges, *Proceedings of 30th Annual International IEEE EMBS Conference*, pp. 5270-5273, Vancouver, British Columbia, August 2008, Canada.

Pantepopulous A. and Bourbakis N. (2008). A Survey on Wearable Biosensor Systems for Health Monitoring, *Proceedings of 30th Annual International IEEE EMBS Conference*, pp. 4887-4890, Vancouver, British Columbia, August 2008, Canada.

35

Neuro-Developmental Engineering: towards early diagnosis of neuro-developmental disorders

[1]Domenico Campolo, Fabrizio Taffoni, Giuseppina Schiavone,
Domenico Formica, Eugenio Guglielmelli and Flavio Keller
Università Campus Bio-Medico
00128 Roma - Italy
[1]*School of Mechanical & Aerospace Engineering*
Nanyang Technological University
639798 Singapore

1. Introduction

Neuro-Developmental Engineering (NDE) is a new and emerging interdisciplinary research area at the intersection of developmental neuroscience and bioengineering aiming at providing new methods and tools for: *i*) understanding neuro-biological mechanisms of human brain development; *ii*) quantitative analysis and modeling of human behavior during neuro-development; *iii*) assessment of neuro-developmental milestones achieved by humans from birth onwards.

Main application fields of NDE are:

- New clinical protocols and standards for early diagnosis, functional evaluation and therapeutic treatments of neuro- developmental disorders;

- New generations of educational, interactive toys which can provide adequate stimuli and guidance for supporting the physiological neuro-development process

This technology is expected to be also useful in the long term for developing new tools, e.g. toys, which can sustain, in *ecological* scenarios, the regular development of motor and cognitive abilities of the child, based on a rigorous scientific approach.

The long term goal is establishing standards against which development of infants at risk for neuro-developmental disorders, particularly autism, can be measured, with the aim of detecting early signs of disturbed development.

1.1 Sensori-Motor Integration Deficits in Neurodevelopmental Disorders

Neurodevelopmental disorders such as ASD, ADHD, Tourette syndrome and others are characterized by a genetic basis. In this case behavioral analysis, or behavioral phenotyping, will be instrumental for the analysis of the roles of genes in behavior (Gerlai 2002).

Autism is a behavioral disorder, with onset in childhood, which is characterized by deficits in three basic domains: social interaction, language and communication, and pattern of interests. There is no doubt that autism has a strong genetic component, and that biological disease mechanisms leading to autism are already active during foetal development and/or infancy, as demonstrated, for example, by the abnormal pattern of brain growth during late foetal and early postnatal life (see (Keller and Persico 2003), for a review). Autism is usually diagnosed at the age of 3 years, in many cases after a period of seemingly normal neurological and behavioral development. The diagnosis of autism is purely clinical, there are no laboratory tests to confirm or disprove the diagnosis. It has been recognized that, although typical autism is not associated with major neurological deficits, autism has characteristic manifestations in the *perceptual and motor domains.*

Deficits in the *perceptual domain* include altered processing and recognition of socially relevant information from peopleŠs faces (see (Grelotti et al. 2003), for a review), deficits in perception of motion cues (Milne et al. 2002), (Spencer et al. 2000), (Bertone et al. 2003), (Takerae et al. 2004), difficulty in disengaging attention (Landry and Bryson 2004) and alterations of auditory processing (Courchesne et al. 1984), (Boddaert et al. 2004). Studies based on analysis of home-made movies suggest that an impairment of spontaneous attention toward social stimuli is present already at 20 months (Swettenham et al. 1998), and possibly also as early as during the first 6 months of life (Maestro et al. 2002). Furthermore, an autism-like syndrome is frequently observed in congenitally blind children (Hobson and Bishop 2003). Taken together, these observations suggest that at least some individuals with autism are characterized by an early deficit of 'low-level' perceptual processing, which jeopardizes their ability to develop higher-level capacities, such as language and interpersonal skills.

Motor impairments in autism include deficits in postural reflexes (Minshew et al. 2004), (Schmitz et al. 2003), (Molloy et al. 2003), repetitive, stereotyped movements and awkward patterns of object manipulation, lack of purposeful exploratory movements (see e.g. (Pierce and Courchesne 2001)), gaze abnormalities (Sweeney et al. 2004), unusual gait pattern (Hallett et al. 1993), and alterations of movement planning and execution, which express themselves as 'hyper- dexterity' (Rinehart et al. 2001), (Mari et al. 2003). Motor abnormalities may be observed retrospectively in infants who later develop the autistic syndrome, on the basis of home-made movies made during the first year of life (Teitelbaum et al. 1998), (Teitelbaum et al. 2004). These clinical observations are consistent with a large body of evidence of subtle structural and functional abnormalities of cortical and subcortical neural systems involved in *movement planning and execution,* such as the prefrontal cortex, the basal ganglia and the cerebellum (see (Keller and Persico 2003), for a review).

1.2 Ecological Approach

The diagnosis of ASD is currently made at 3 years of age; Attention-Deficit Hyperactivity Disorder (ADHD) is always considered as an alternative diagnosis of "high functioning" autism; Tourette syndrome is diagnosed at age 7 or later. ASD is therefore a natural candidate for demonstrating the validity of novel approaches to early diagnosis. As shown in Fig. 1, infancy, i.e. the first 2-3 years of life before language development, represents an important temporal window for an early diagnosis of ASD.

The goal of our approach is twofold. On one hand, guided by neuroscientists, we develop technological platforms and methods to extract more information on perceptual and intersubjective capacities of human infants than is currently possible; this information could be later used for early diagnosis of developmental disorders. On the other hand, infancy provides us with an important window of opportunity to capture the mechanisms behind sensorimotor integration as these are just developing. Moreover, neurodevelopmental disorders are an important benchmark to highlight failures within such mechanism. Such a knowledge can be useful to neuroscientists to better understand the human brain functions involved in the

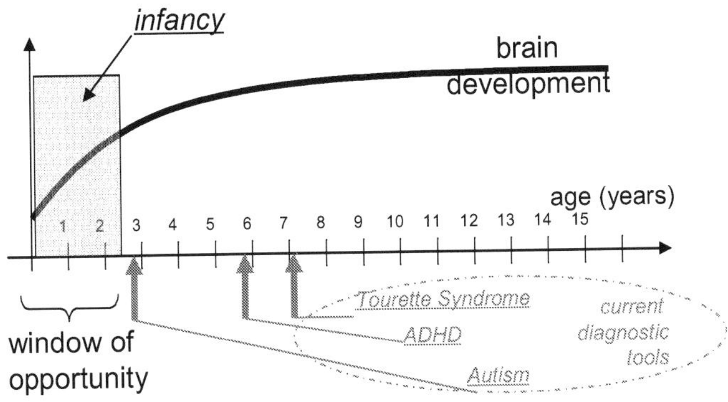

Fig. 1. Current diagnostic tools

sensorimotor integration but also to engineers, providing unique insights on how to build complex and adaptable artificial systems (Metta et al. 1999).

2. Technology for Assessing Movement and Gaze

2.1 Motion Tracking

Motion tracking can count on a host of different technological solutions, operating on entirely different physical principles, with different performance characteristics and designed for different purposes. As shown in (Welch and Foxlin 2002), there is not a single technology that can fit all needs. Each application defines the best technology to be implemented. In order to perform a selection, the main characteristics of available technologies are briefly summarized hereafter (see (Welch and Foxlin 2002) for details).

Mechanical sensing:
typically used for body motion capture; it uses angle and range measurements with the help of gears and bend sensors; very accurate but *bulky*, often limiting mobility.

Optical sensing:
several principles are available, typical systems are camera- based ones; position of markers in 3D space can be estimated very accurately within working volume (typically a few cube meters, depending on the number of deployed cameras); line-of- sight issues (i.e. the fact that body parts or other objects may occlude the visual scene of a camera, losing thus the sight of one or more markers) is a limiting factor; very expensive; often requires highly structured environments, at least when high accuracy is needed.

Acoustic sensing:
typically based on time-of-flight of ultrasound pulses between emitters and receivers; sound speed in air (about $340\,m/s$, resulting in sampling periods in the order of a few tens of milliseconds) is slow but still acceptable for sensing human (in particular infants) movements; line-of-sight issues are not as severe as for the optical technology; requires much less structured environments than optical trackers; suitable to be used in ecological conditions (e.g. kindergartens).

(Geo)Magnetic sensing:

a first method is based on electromagnetic coupling between a source and several trackers; main drawbacks are that signal decays as $1/d^3$ (where d is the source-tracker distance) and is affected by the geomagnetic field; these devices are quite expensive and require a certain amount of structuring of the environment. A second method is electronic compassing; estimates heading and solely relies on the *geomagnetic* field, i.e. it does not require any artificial source and is therefore *sourceless*; measurements can be altered by ferromagnetic influence of surrounding objects.

Inertial sensing:

highly miniaturized accelerometers and gyroscopes are used to sense, respectively, acceleration (comprising the gravitational field) and angular velocity; used as inclinometers, accelerometers can sense the gravity vector, i.e. the 'vertical' direction, in this sense they are also *sourceless*.

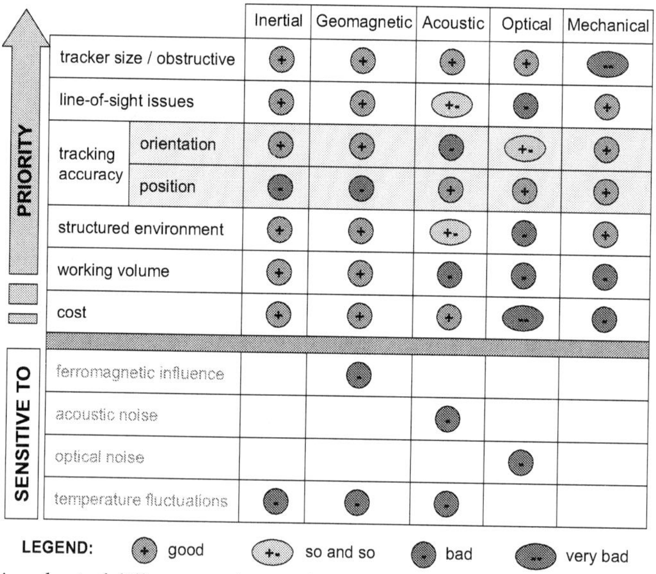

PRIORITY		Inertial	Geomagnetic	Acoustic	Optical	Mechanical
tracker size / obstructive		good	good	good	good	very bad
line-of-sight issues		good	good	so and so	bad	good
tracking accuracy	orientation	good	good	bad	so and so	good
	position	bad	bad	good	good	good
structured environment		good	good	so and so	bad	good
working volume		good	good	bad	bad	bad
cost		good	good	good	very bad	bad

SENSITIVE TO	Inertial	Geomagnetic	Acoustic	Optical	Mechanical
ferromagnetic influence		bad			
acoustic noise			bad		
optical noise				bad	
temperature fluctuations	bad	bad	bad		

LEGEND: (+) good   (+-) so and so   (-) bad   (--) very bad

Fig. 2. Selection chart of different motion tracking technologies

In Fig. 2, a selection chart for the different available technologies is provided. For each available technology (columns) its suitability with respect to the performance characteristics of interest (rows) is indicated. Since our main purpose is developing technological tools that are either wearable by infants or embeddable into toys, the highest priority is given to technologies which are unobtrusive. This directly leads us to discard solutions involving mechanical trackers.

The second element considered for selection are the line-of-sight issues, since we are going to deal with infants, it is extremely difficult to perform experiments with technologies that are limited by the line of sight, a peculiarity of the optical technology which is only suitable to experiments with collaborative subjects who are somehow willing to 'act' in front of a camera. Line-of-sight issues are much less severe for the acoustic technology which is thus still appealing for movements analysis in infants.

The third element of the selection criterion is performance with respect to tracking accuracy. Here a distinction is made between tracking positions and tracking orientations. Measurement principles such as the time-of-flight (typically deployed in acoustic measurements) or camera-based tracking are inherently suitable to measure the distance of points (markers) and the origin of the measurement system (e.g. the source of acoustic waves or a camera etc...). Orientations can be inferred indirectly by estimating distances between two or more markers and the source of measurement. The larger the distance between two markers, the better the estimation of orientation. As dimensions shrink, as in the case of infants, accuracy of indirect orientation measurements also decreases (e.g. accurate tracking of the orientation of an infant's wrist can be problematic even without considering line-of-sight issues). Other technologies allow a direct measurement of orientations (for example inertial sensors used as inclinometers can sense deviations from the vertical axis while magnetic sensors used as compasses can sense deviations from the horizontal geomagnetic north direction) without requiring the positioning of multiple markers.

As long as orientation is concerned, inertial and magnetic technologies appear to be very appealing since: are highly unobtrusive due the availability of miniaturized off-the-shelf devices; do not suffer from line-of-sight issues; can provide high accuracy in orientation tracking are *sourceless*: do not require any structuring of the environment; have virtually unlimited working volume; are low-cost.

The bottom half of Fig. 2 shows, for each technology, the main limiting factors to a correct operation. Besides temperature, which affects any electrical device and that can be compensated in most of the cases, the real limiting factor for the magnetic technology is the presence of ferromagnetic materials. Common ferromagnetic objects such as iron parts of doors, chairs, tables etc... can produce local distortions of the geomagnetic field, causing thus errors in the estimations of orientations. As discussed in (Kemp et al. 1998), some care should be taken, when conducting experiments, to avoid large ferromagnetic objects in the surroundings. We found that this can be easily done in environments such as day-cares where, for safety reasons, all metals are usually avoided and typical materials used with children are wood, rubber and plastic.

2.2 Gaze Tracking

Devices for measuring eye movements are commonly referred to as 'eye trackers'. In general there are two types of techniques for monitoring eye movement (Young and Sheena 1975):

- 'eye-in-head' measurement: the sensing device is fixed on the head and therefore the eye position is measured in craniotopic coordinates;

- 'point of regard' or gaze: the sensors are located in the external environment and the eye position is measured in spatial coordinates.

These two kind of measurements are coincident when the head is kept in a fixed position. When the head is free to move, measurement of the head orientation is also required to derive gaze from craniotopic coordinates. Eye tracking methodologies can be classified in four categories:

1. Magnetic Induction Method (Search Coil)

2. Electro-Oculography (EOG)

3. Photoelectric Methods: Infra-Red (IR) Oculography

4. Video-Oculography (VOG)

Each methodology is characterized by parameters such as range of measurement, sensitivity, linearity, accuracy, discomfort for the subject, interference with the field of view of the subject, tolerance to head movement.

Magnetic Induction Method (Search Coil):

The search coil technique has become the accepted standard for the measurement of 3D eye movement. This technique is based on the fact that a magnetic field induces a voltage in a coil (search coil) which is attached to the eye. The induced voltage has amplitude proportional to the sine of the angle between the coil axis and the magnetic field direction. The magnetic field is provide by coils mounted at the sides of a cubic frame. The dimensions of the sides of the frame can vary from few tens of centimeters to few meters, allowing to measure also other movements (i.e. eye-hand coordination). Robinson (Robinson 1963) was the first to apply this technique, using a coil secured to the eye by suction. Nowadays the search coil is embedded in a scleral contact lens. The lens is subject to slippage if the lens covers only the cornea. Eye movement is measured in absolute spatial coordinates. Head orientation can also be measured with a search coil mounted on the forehead, and orientation and movement of the eye within the head can be calculated from the orientation of the head and of the eye with respect to the magnetic field (Haslwanter 1995). Currently a number of different search coil systems are commercially available (e.g. by Skalar Instruments, C-N-C Engineering, Remmel Labs, etc.). Although the scleral search coil is the most precise eye movement measurement method (very high temporal and spatial resolution can be obtained with accuracy to about 5-10 arc-seconds over a limited range of about 5 deg), it is also the most intrusive method. Insertion of the lens requires care and practice and wearing the lens causes discomfort and risk of corneal abrasion or lead breakage. The requirements to stay in the center of the magnetic field precludes the use of search coils during many natural activities. Thus, this technique is mostly used for research purposes, it is not suitable for clinical routine.

Electro-Oculography:

First applications of electro-oculography are dated back to the '30s and are currently widely used both for clinical and research purposes. It relies on measurement of electrical potential differences between the cornea and the retina, discovered by DuBois-Reymond in 1849. Skin electrodes are positioned around the eye. The measured potential difference is proportional to the sine of the rotation angle of the eye. For small rotation the proportionality is almost linear; it decreases for higher angles of rotation (Byford 1963). The recorded potentials are in the range 15-200 μV, with nominal sensitivities of order of 20 μV/deg of eye movement. The eye movement is measured in craniotopic coordinates and head movement during recording does not affect the measurement. The discomfort for the subject is limited and the measurement range is wide both for horizontal movements (± 70 deg) and for vertical movements (± 30 deg), even if the sensitivity decreases for lateral position of the eye. The most important advantage of this methodology is the possibility of recording eye movement with closed eyes, which is relevant requirement during some experimental protocol (e.g.. during sleeping phases). The main drawback of this technique are related to the nature of the potential recorded and to the artifacts due to the electrodes properties. As concern the potential, the resting corneo-retinic potential (usually of the order of 0.4-1 mV) can be affected by lighting conditions of the environment and by the psycho-physical condition of the subject. The artifacts at the level of the skin electrodes relies on the contact resistance electrode-skin, on the oxidation and polarization of the electrodes.

Infra-Red Oculography:

Infra-red (IR) oculography is based on the recording of the light reflected by the eye when it is lighted with IR light beam. Since IR light is not visible, it does not interfere with the subject vision, moreover the IR detectors are not influenced by environmental lighting conditions. There are three categories of Infra-red (IR) oculography which use respectively: the corneal reflection, the Purkinje images and the track of the limb. Due to the construction of the eye, when a beam of IR light points to it, four reflections are formed on the eye, called Purkinje images (Cornsweet and Crane 1973): the first on the front surface of the cornea and it is called corneal reflection, the second image on rear surface of the cornea, the third on the front surface of the lens and the fourth on the rear surface of the lens. By detecting the corneal reflection and the pupil center and by using an appropriate calibration procedure, it is possible to measure the Point of Regard (gaze) on a planar surface on which calibration points are positioned. Two points of reference on the eye are needed to separate eye movements from head movements. The positional difference between the pupil center and corneal reflection changes with pure eye rotation, but remains relatively constant with minor head movements. The corneal reflection moves in the opposite direction of the eye respect to the pupil center. In other cases both the first and the fourth Purkinje images (Dual-Purkinje images eye trackers are detected. Both reflections move together through exactly the same distance upon eye translation but they move through different distances upon eye rotation. The third method based on photoelectric principle relies on the track of the limb (scleral-iris edge) of the eye by measuring the amount of scattered light. Most photoelectric systems must be mounted close to the eyes (i.e. EL-MAR tracking device), so they may restrict the field of view, moreover fast movements of the head can cause slippage of the device on the head leading to mis-alignment of the eye respect to the IR emitter and detector. There exist also external device and a support for keeping the head fixed is needed (i.e. Tobii eye tracker). The range of measurement of the photoelectric eye tracker is not higher then ±30 deg in the horizontal plane and ±20 deg in the vertical plane.

Video-Oculography:

Video systems for measuring ocular movements are based on the analysis of images recorded by cameras. This technique, introduced in the '80s, quickly improved in terms of performances and reliability thanks to the technological development of digital cameras and computer powerful. The Video Oculography (VOG) provides directly a digital output. Several algorithms are available for the pupil detection in an image frame and pupil centroid coordinates extraction, nevertheless environmental lighting conditions can affect the automatic detection (Eizenman et al. 1984) (Landau 1987). Thus, IR light is used together with video recording, so that the pupil appears brighter. This technique is called Pupil Center/Corneal Reflection (PC/CR) because the IR light produces also the Purkinje images, mentioned before. As in IR Oculography, also VOG can be realized both as wearable device (DiScenna 1995) and provides measurements in craniotopic coordinates or external device and provides measurements in spatial coordinates. Head-mounted system (i.e. EyeLink) can be worn without too much discomfort. High resolution and high frame rate CCD and CMOS cameras are used. Reduced dimensions and weight of the actual cameras allow to position them in such a way that they interfere as less as possible with the field of view of the subject (Babcock and Pelz

2004), (Pelz et al. 2000). The measurement range for VOG systems can exceed ± 30 deg in horizontal plane and ± 20 deg in the vertical plane; eye tracking can be executed both on-line and off-line. The drawback is that these systems have a low acquisition rate, in general 50-60 Hz, not suitable for recording fast eye movement such as saccadic movements, but suffices for smooth pursuit eye movements. External camera systems can go up to 1000-1250 Hz and have an accuracy of 0.01 deg. External camera are generally positioned under the screen of a computer, used for calibration and for specific visual stimuli. Head movements are tolerated if the eye is kept in the field of view of the camera. There are devices which include systems of pursuit of the subject and the camera orients automatically so that the eye of the subject is always in its field of view.

In Table 1 the relevant parameters of the eye tracking techniques presented are summarized.

3. Instrumented Toys and Wearable Devices

Virtually any toy, tool or piece of garment used by children could be a good candidate to host all sorts of technology and 'see what comes out' when the child wears it or plays with it.

Our approach is based on a closed-loop dialogue between neuroscientists and bioengineers. In the following, two platforms are presented which specifically address two domains of interest in child's development: spatial cognition and social behavior.

For both platforms, functional specifications are derived from protocols of experiments of interest for neuroscientists. The aim is twofold. On one side we wish to provide neuroscientists with novel technological platforms for the unobtrusive and ecological assessment of behavioral development in infants. On the other side, these platforms should enable/facilitate the transition from research to clinical practice.

3.1 Assessing Spatial Cognition Skills

By the end of the first year of life, infants start to pile-up blocks, put lids on cans and insert objects into apertures. Through these activities, the child learns to plan actions that involve more than one item. The ability to solve such problems reflects the child's spatial, perceptual and motor development. In particular, the representational ability to imagine objects in different positions and orientations must be in place before various objects can be fit into apertures. Recent studies by Ornkloo and von Hofsten (Ornkloo and von Hofsten 2007) show developmental curves, based on statistical rates of success of object-fitting tasks, relative to children aged 14-26 months old.

Specifically, the tasks consisted of inserting cylinders with different cross-sections into a box with similar holes on its lid, see Fig. 3 (top). All the objects had similar dimensions, 1 mm smaller than the apertures. Different cross-sections were used whose circumference was approximately the same but varied with respect to the number of possibilities they fit into a corresponding aperture, as also reported in Fig. 3 (bottom).

Based on visual inspection of video recordings, the data analysis consisted (among other things) in assessing horizontal and vertical pre-adjustments. In particular, the outcome was yes/no (i.e. successful or unsuccessful) based on the alignment errors between the object and the box. Both the vertical error (angular misalignment between the longitudinal axis of the object and verticality) and the horizontal error (angular misalignment between the orientations of the cross- section and the aperture) were estimated (from the videos). Results showed that successful solution was associated with appropriate preadjustments before the hand arrived with the block to the aperture; in particular it has been proved that the preadjustments can be considered appropriate for misalignments lower than 30 deg.

	Search coil	Electro-Oculography	Infra-Red Oculography	Video Oculography
Measurement Typology	Absolute spatial coordinate	Craniotopic coordinates	Head-mounted: craniotopic coordinates; External device: spatial coordinates	Head-mounted: craniotopic coordinates; External device: spatial coordinates
Range of measurement	±90 deg for all 3D space	±70 deg in horizontal plane ±30 deg in vertical plane	±30 deg in horizontal plane ±20 deg in vertical plane	±30 deg in horizontal plane ±20 deg in vertical plane
Temporal Resolution	linked to A/D conversion, 500-1000Hz (depends on software and hardware instrumentation)	linked to A/D conversion, 500-1000Hz (depends on software and hardware instrumentation)	linked to A/D conversion, 500-1000Hz (depends on software and hardware instrumentation)	Depends on camera frame rate: from 30Hz to 1000-1250Hz
Spatial resolution	0.01 deg	1-1.5 deg	0.1 deg	0.1 deg
Discomfort	High	Limited	Limited	Limited
Interference with the subject field of view	None	None	Head-mounted device can interfere with the field of view	Head-mounted device can interfere with the field of view
Tolerance to head movement	- Head has to be in the center of the magnetic field - Additional search coil on the forehead	Not affected by head movement	External device: low tolerance to head movements	- Head movements are tolerated when eye is kept in the field of view of the camera; - Additional sensors allow to re-orientate the camera
Other Notes	- limited recording time and risk of corneal abrasion or lead breakage - lens slippage	- Measurement with closed eyes (during sleeping) - Skin electrodes artifacts - Resting corneo-retinal potential variability	- Not suitable when the subject wears glasses or contact lens	

Table 1. Comparison of different gaze tracking technologies

3.1.1 Block-Box Platform

Inspired by such experiments and based on our previous experience with sensorized toys (Campolo et al. 2007), we developed a sensorized core, shown in Fig. 4 (top), for the cylindrical

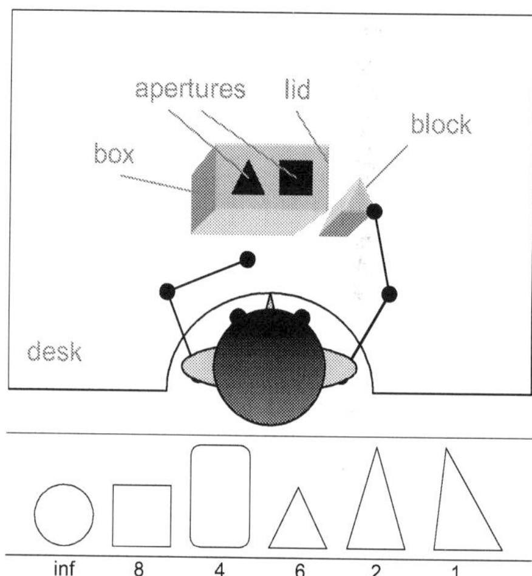

Fig. 3. Block-box experimental scenario (top). Different cross- sections (bottom) for the cylindrical blocks and the relative number of insertion possibilities ('inf' means infinite), readapted from (Ornkloo and von Hofsten 2007)

objects with various cross-sections, shown in Fig. 4 (bottom).

In particular, we found that from an *ecological* perspective, the *sourceless* estimation of objects orientation via inertial and magnetic sensors is especially suited to this application. Accelerometers can in fact be used to measure tilt while magnetometers can be used as compass to measure horizontal misalignments. Gyroscopes are required to compensate for non-static effects. Further details on the filter used to estimate orientation from the sensors raw data is described in (Campolo et al. 2008).

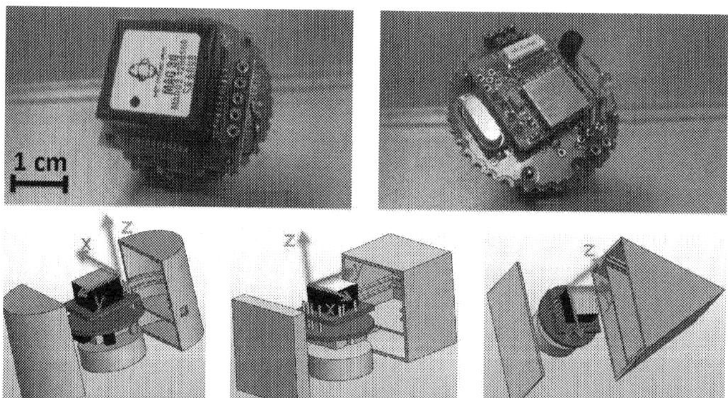

Fig. 4. Kinematics sensing unit (top left). Bluetooth transmitting unit (top right). Examples of assemblies of electronics and batteries for shells with different cross-section (bottom).

By considering the requirements of the experimental setup and protocol of the above mentioned study (Ornkloo and von Hofsten 2007), the functional specifications of the block-box platform can be resumed as follows:

- the device (electronic core and power supply) should be embeddable in solids with different shapes with a "grasping size" less than 5 cm;
- the sensor unit should consist of sourceless sensors for orientation tracking;
- the transmission unit should assure a bi-directional wireless communication to a remote workstation few meters far from the experimental scenario;
- the batteries should provide power supply for at least 2 hours of continuous use;
- the overall weight of the toy should not exceed the 50-60 grams.

According with these specifications, the block-box sensorized toys have been designed to be as compact and light as possible. In particular, the platform mainly consists of a compact (17.8mm × 17.8mm × 10.2mm), micro-fabricated 9-axis inertial-magnetic sensor (model MAG02-1200S050 from Memsense Inc.). The device is designed to sense ±2g accelerations, ±1200 deg/sec angular rates, ±1 Gauss magnetic fields, all within a 50 Hz bandwidth. The sensors are coupled with a multi-channel, 12 bits AD converter (model MAX1238 from Maxim Inc.) which can retransmit converted data over a 4-wires I2C bus. For our application, we sample each of the 9 channels at 100 Samples/sec rate. Such data are collected and rearranged in a specific message format by a microcontroller (PIC16F876A from Microchip Technology Inc.) and then retransmitted via a bluetooth module (Parani-ESD200 from Sena Technologies Inc.). Finally, two 3.6V Li-Ion Rechargeable batteries (LIR3048 from Powerstream Inc.) are used in series, in order to guarantee approximately two hours of autonomous operation. Data transmitted over the bluetooth interface are collected by a nearby PC, for later data analysis.

Fig. 5 represents the overall architecture of the block-box platform. As it can be noted, we decided to arrange the different components into two separate electronic boards (a sensor board and a transmission board), which are connected through the I2C bus. This solution makes the system modular, allowing us to easily change the sensor unit or put together several sensors that share the same bus.

In Fig. 6 the electronic CAD designs (left) and the real pictures (right) of the sensor (top) and the transmission (bottom) boards are shown. Fig. 7 reports the overall aspect of the electronic core of the Block-Box platform with the actual dimensions.

3.1.2 In-Field Calibration of Inertial-Magnetic Sensors

Magnetometers are meant to sense the geomagnetic field and provide its components $[b_x, b_y, b_z]^T$ along the $\hat{x}$, $\hat{y}$ and $\hat{z}$ axes of the sensing device itself (such axes move with the moving frame). Similarly, the accelerometers are meant, in static conditions, to read out the components of the gravitational field $[g_x, g_y, g_z]^T$ along the same axes.

Calibration of such sensors is straightforward when one can reliably count on precision alignment procedures, e.g. in a laboratory setting. In (Campolo et al. 2006), a procedure for in-field calibration of magnetometric sensors was presented which does not rely on previous knowledge of magnitude and direction of the geomagnetic field and which does not require accurately predefined orientation sequences. Such a method can be applied to accelerometers as well and is especially suited for clinical applications. The procedure relies on the fact the geomagnetic (or gravitational) field has constant components in the fixed frame. As the orientation of the sensors vary, the components in the moving frame also vary but the magnitude

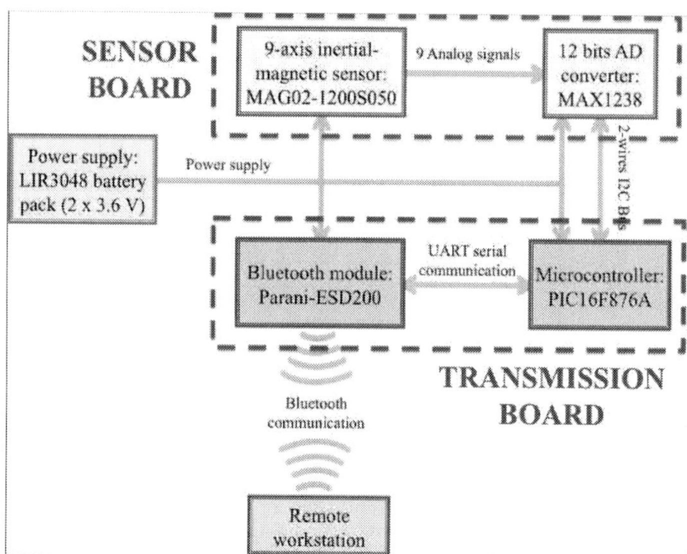

Fig. 5. Block-Box Platform architecture.

of the field keeps constant, i.e. the components are bound to lie on a sphere. Readouts from non-calibrated sensors are therefore bound to lie on an ellipsoid, see (Campolo et al. 2006) for details. Via the least-square method it is possible to robustly estimate the centroid and semi-axes length of the ellipsoid which coincide with the calibration parameters (gain and offsets for each axis).

Based on this method, a calibration protocol was devised to provide a sufficient number of measurements for the algorithm to robustly converge. The instrumented toy (of whatever shape) is secured inside a wooden box, shaped as a parallelepiped, so that the toy does not move as the box is displaced around.

Magnetometers:

as in Fig. 8-a, the box is placed on a table and an approximately 360 deg rotation (no need to be accurate) is performed by keeping one face of the box always parallel and in contact with the table. The same procedure is repeated for four different faces.

Accelerometers:

as in Fig. 8-b, the box is placed on a table and smoothly (i.e. avoiding shocks) tilted by 90 deg along one edge, this is repeated four times[1] until the box returns in the initial position. The whole procedure is repeated with a different initial position.

Gyroscopes:

the procedure is similar to the one deployed for the accelerometers.

---

[1] Each time on a different edge: once a 90 deg rotation is performed along one edge, the next edge is the non-consecutive one which also makes contact with the table.

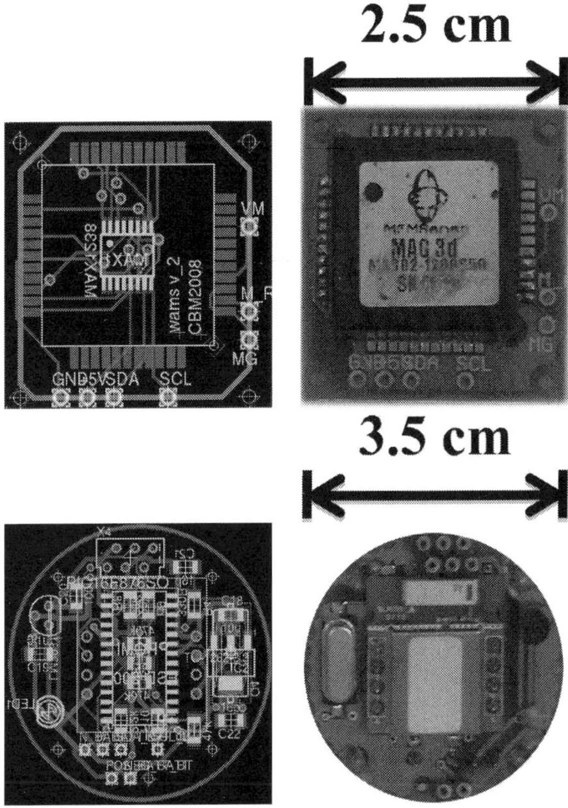

Fig. 6. The electronic CAD designs (left) and the real pictures (right) of the sensor (top) and the transmission (bottom) boards.

Measurements derived from a calibration sequence are shown in Fig. 8-c and Fig. 8-d, respectively for the magnetometers and for the accelerometers. The least-squares algorithm is then used to derive the best fitting ellipsoids (one for the magnetometers and one for the accelerometers) whose surfaces contain the two sets of measurements.

As previously mentioned, since the geomagnetic field is constant, its components in the moving frame are bound to lie on the calibrating ellipsoid, not only during the calibration sequences but for every possible movement. For this reason, also movements performed during the regular use of the toy, i.e. when the infants plays with it, can be used for updating the calibration parameters, or at least for an on-line check. Similar procedures apply to accelerometers, paying attention to consider only the quasi-static movements, i.e. when accelerations of the movement itself are negligible with respect to gravity. Details about 'in-use' calibration can be found in (Lotters et al. 1998).

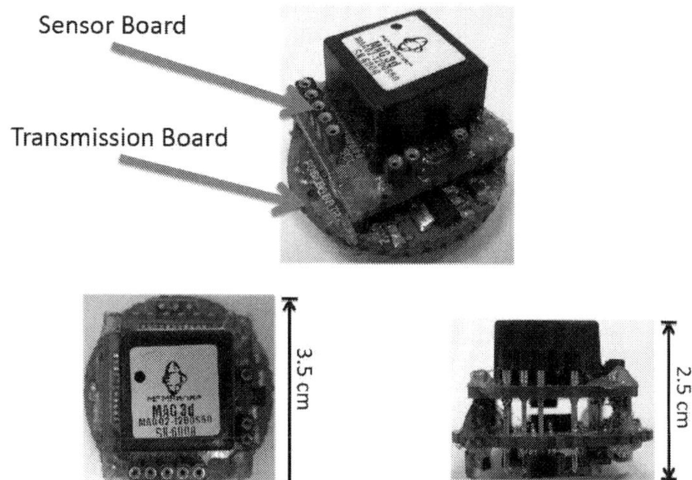

Fig. 7. Electronic core of the Block-Box platform with the actual dimensions.

3.2 Assessing Spontaneous Movements

Infants show a large variety of spontaneous movement patterns. Such movements are called spontaneous to tell them apart from reflex movements because they are endogenously generated by infantsŠ nervous system without any external sensory input.

While reflexive movements allow a detailed study of a stable, quantitative relationship between sensory input and reflexive motor output, spontaneous motility could be regarded as the expression of spontaneous neural activity, so it is an excellent marker of neural dysfunction caused by brain impairments during the first year of life (Prechtl and General 2001).

Among several spontaneous motor patterns, movements that appear to be more effective for functional assessment of infantsŠ nervous systems are complex sequential movements of arms, legs, neck, and trunk called General Movements (GMs): they are characterized by rotations along the axis of the limbs and slight changes in the direction of movements (see (Einspieler et al. 2005) for a review).

If the nervous system is impaired, GMs change their quality or even disappear: they lose their complex character and involve a reduced number of limbs in monotonous sequences; they appear to be rigid and less smooth because generated by the almost simultaneous contraction of all limb and trunk muscles. Such alterations are considered to be highly predictive for later neurological impairments like Cerebral Palsy (CP).

During the assessment phase, infants with bare arms and legs are videotaped in supine position. The duration of the recording depends on the age of the infant: to collect at least three GMs, 1 h recording is necessary with pre-term infants while 10 minutes are enough from term age onward. The same infant is videotaped at different ages: from 2 to 3 recordings during the pre-term period; one recording at term or early post-term age or both, and at least one recording between 9 and 15 weeks post-term. After each recording session, a trained clinician reviews the videotape looking for GMs sequences that are copied onto an assessment tape. The observed GM and the week of development are reported on a table called individual

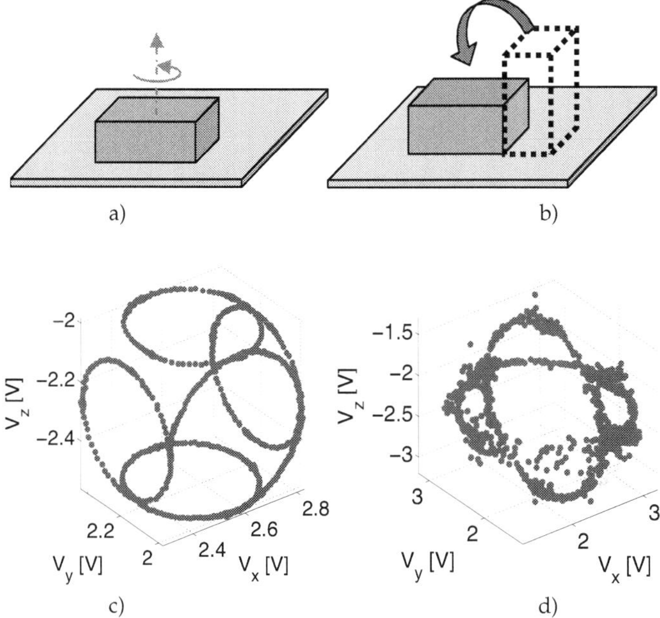

Fig. 8. Calibration sequences for magnetometers (a) and accelerometers (b). Plots of the measurements (i.e. voltages V_x, V_y and V_z from the triaxial sensors) derived from the calibration sequences for the magnetometers (c) and the accelerometers (d).

developmental trajectory. Such table is used to assess the risk of developing lateral neurological impairments. 11 studies on 358 infants assessed by 90 observers revealed an inter-rater reliability between 89% and 93% (Einspieler et al. 2005).

Wrist and Ankle Movement Sensor (WAMS)

GMs assessment protocol collects qualitative information on motor behavior of infants during their first year of life. In order to match the individual developmental trajectory with some quantitative objective information we proposed a magneto-inertial wearable device for ecological behavioral analysis of infants' motor behavior called Wrist and Ankle Movement Sensor (WAMS) (Taffoni et al. 2008). Such a device, which allows gathering objective information such as the angle of rotation along the axis of the limb, its velocity, smoothness, acceleration etc., could improve the predictive validity of GMs, thus reducing the inter-observer disagreement.

Because the target is assessing infants' movement, it is important to reduce size and weight of the device as much as possible. Although there are several commercial solutions, they are often exceedingly large and bulky. According to anthropometric data, the maximal linear length of a wearable device should not exceed 2.5 cm and should not weight more than 20 grams.

In order to estimate a proper scale range of the sensor, preliminary quantitative experiments have been conducted. A three-cameras (500 Hz) motion capture system was used (Qualysis

Motion Capture Systems Inc., SWE) to obtain position-time data from both arms of infants and evaluate frequency and dynamic content of their spontaneous movements. Three reflective markers were placed on the head and two on both hands. In Fig. 9-A data from one-week-old infant are shown.

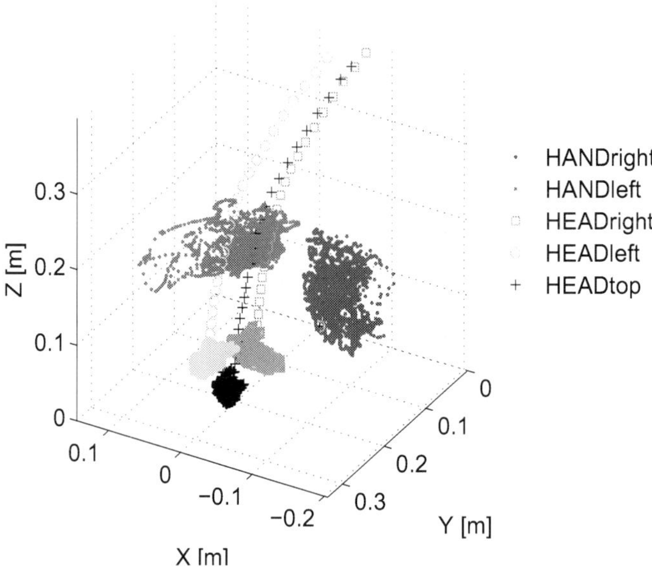

Fig. 9. Representative data relative to head-hands kinematics of a one week old infant

Probability Density Function (PDF) of several sets of experimental data was computed to estimate the dynamic range for the accelerometer sensors, showing that a $\pm 2g$ range would be sufficient to capture infants' kinematics. As for the magnetometers, since only the geomagnetic field (about 0.6 gauss) needs to be measured, the full measurement range should be in the order of ± 1 Gauss. Saturation of gyroscopes would result in a problematic loss of tracking and therefore, given several commercially available gyroscopes with full scale ranging from ± 150 deg/s to ± 1200 deg/s, the maximum scale range (± 1200 deg/s) was selected.

In line with such specification a sampling frequency of 250 Hz was selected. This frequency is between the sampling frequency of other magneto-inertial commercially available systems (typically 100 Hz) and the frequency of the optical devices (up to 500 Hz).

A preliminary analysis of commercial magneto-inertial sensors currently available highlighted a triaxial magnetometer, accelerometer and gyroscope analogue sensor from Memsense (MAG02-1200S050) that matches the technical requirements previously defined. Although there are several highly miniaturized components available off the shelf, we have chosen to use a microfabricated device integrating all the required sensing capability for two main reasons: 1) a more efficient packaging; 2) a more reliable axis orientation. Not orthogonal sensible axes directly translate in errors during orientation tracking. In order to simultaneously collect data from both arms and legs we propose a Body Area Network (BAN) of four sensors: two for arms and two for legs. Unlike common BAN (Jovanov et al. 2005) we chose to use a wired configuration in order to reduce the weight of each sensor: wired communication allows not to include the battery onboard, and therefore to reduce the weight. For such reasons each sensing unit is provided with a low power, 12-channels, 12 bits AD Converters with an I2C compatible two wires serial interface. In this way only 4 wires are required: 2 for data and 2 for supply, which is in a remote master station. In this station a microcontroller PIC16F876A collects data from each WAMS (identified by a unique address) and retransmits via RS232 to a PC where such data are stored. The electronic board is embedded into a soft silicon rubber structure used both for electrical passivation and for comfortable contact with the infant's skin. A Velcro strap is used to fix such sensors to the infant's limbs. Figure 10 shows the first WAMS prototype: total weight less then 14 grams and volume within $2.5 \times 2.5 \times 1.5 \text{ cm}^3$.

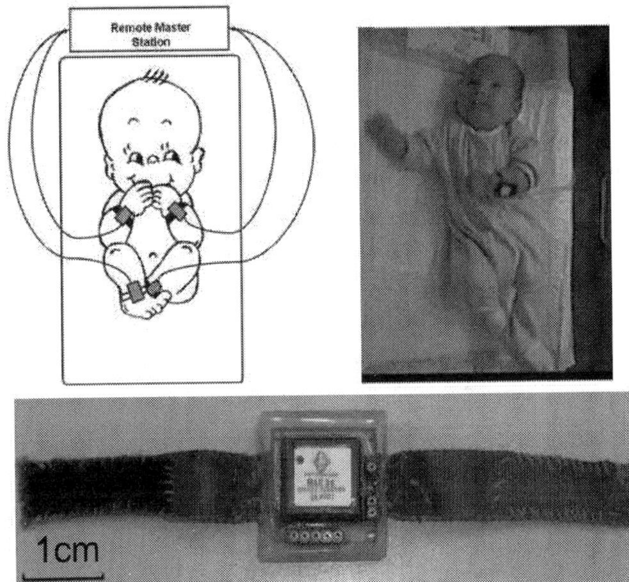

Fig. 10. Typical experimental scenario. (A). Example of use on a 3 months old baby (B). First WAMS prototype (C).

3.3 Assessing Social Attention

Poor sensorimotor integration has long been addressed as a cause of motor and social problems in developmental disorders such as ASD (Trevarthen and Daniel 2005). Failure in orienting towards occurring social stimuli (e.g. facial expressions, speech, gesture) represents one of the earliest and most basic social impairments in autism and may contribute to the later-emerging social and communicative impairments (Dawson et al. 2004). Early social exchanges require rapid shifting of attention between different stimuli. Impairments in social orienting can alter the developmental pathway of young children by depriving them of appropriate social stimulation (Mundy and Neal 2001).

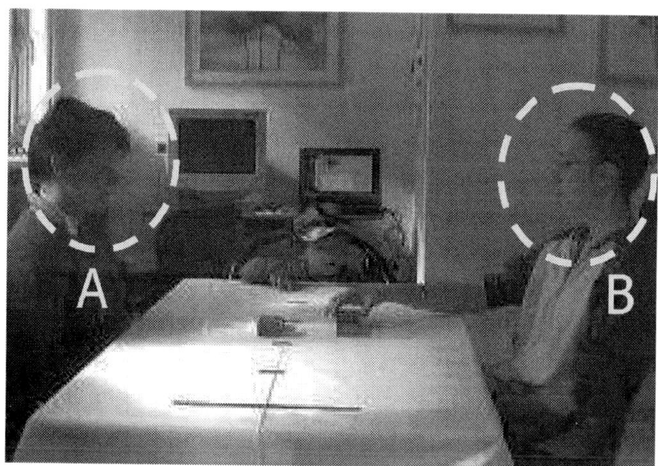

Fig. 11. Social situation.

A *social protocol* to study the response of a child to social stimuli was devised by G. Stenberg (Dept of Psychology, University of Uppsala, Sweden). As shown in Fig. 11 (top), a child sits at a table observing two adults sitting approximately 45 deg left and right. The adult subjects engage in a conversation while alternatively positioning blocks in front of the child. Observing the video-recordings, the psychologist would then take note (frame by frame) of when the child looks at the adult subjects, when at the blocks, whether the child can anticipate the 'next move' of an adult subject (based on the clues provided in the conversation). Indeed a lengthy process, requiring hours to rate a few minutes of an experiment.

3.3.1 Audio-Visuo-Vestibular Cap platform
Early diagnosis is also based on the possibility of screening a large number of children and automatic, or at least semi-automatic, methods would be very valuable.
To this end, we developed the *multimodal* Audio-Visuo-Vestibular Cap (AVVC) platform, shown in Fig. 12, specifically devised to assess sensorimotor integration in social orienting behaviors in very young children, from 6 to 24 months of age. In particular it allows monitoring the child's gaze and facial expressions, monitoring the head kinematics, localize in sound stimuli with respect to the child.

3.3.1.1 Gaze and facial expressions
in the current version, a lightweight eye-cam (1/4" CMOS sensor, 640 × 480 resolution, 30 frames/sec) is mounted on the beak of the cap monitors. A mini-objective (model RE-025S, 2.5 mm focal length, 84 deg diagonal field-of-view, 57 deg vertically and 71 deg horizontally) is used to keep the face of the child on focus. This provides still images of the face, independently of the head movements, and in particular allows monitoring the gaze.

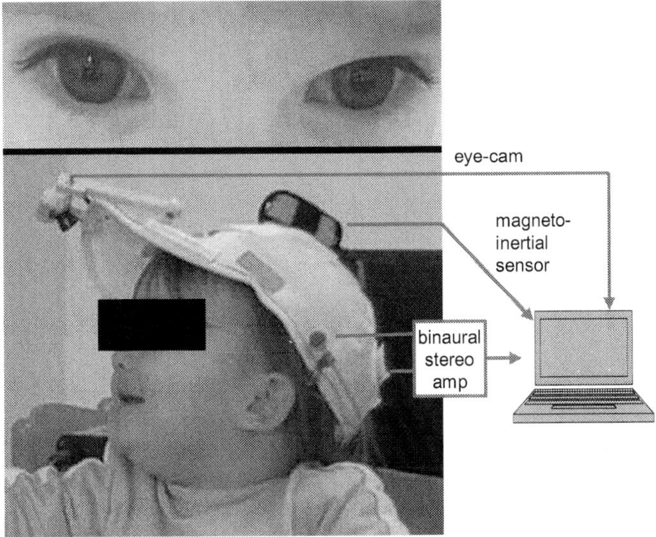

Fig. 12. Audio-Video-Vestibular-Cap (AVVC).

3.3.1.2 Head kinematics

is monitored via a commercial magnetic-inertial sensor (MTx-28A33G25 device from XSens Inc.; static orientation accuracy < 1deg; bandwidth 40Hz; sampling rate 100Hz). Similarly to the human vestibular system, the inertial sensors can be used to estimate tilt with respect to gravity as well as angular velocity of the head. Furthermore, the magnetic sensors, used as a compass, can determine the amount of head rotation on the horizontal plane.

3.3.1.3 Direction of sound stimuli

is an important clue in social behavior. Humans localize sound in space via interaural time differences (ITD) and intensity level differences (ILD), over various frequency ranges (Blauert 1997). To this end, we use a pair of microphones (MKE 2-ew Gold, Levalier, sampled in stereo audio quality at 44.2kHz) mounted on the cap in correspondence of the ears of the child. The ITD of sound arrival at the two microphones can be estimated based on the generalized cross-correlation algorithm (Rucci and Wray 1999).

3.3.2 Ecological Calibration of the Binaural Microphones for the AVVC

An ITD/angle relationship is required to determine the angular position of a sound source with respect to the head once the ITD is estimated. Typical calibration procedures involve relative positioning of a sound source with respect to a pair of binaural microphones. For various angular positions, the relative ITDs are estimated and the ITD/angle relationship is thus experimentally determined.

For the AVVC platform this is a challenging task as calibration can only be done after the child wears the cap, mainly for two reasons: *i*) the ITD also depends on how the sound propagates through the head of the child, therefore the cap must be worn; *ii*) the cap is manually fit onto the child's head and this procedure is neither accurate or repeatable, i.e. a calibration is required every time the child wears the cap.

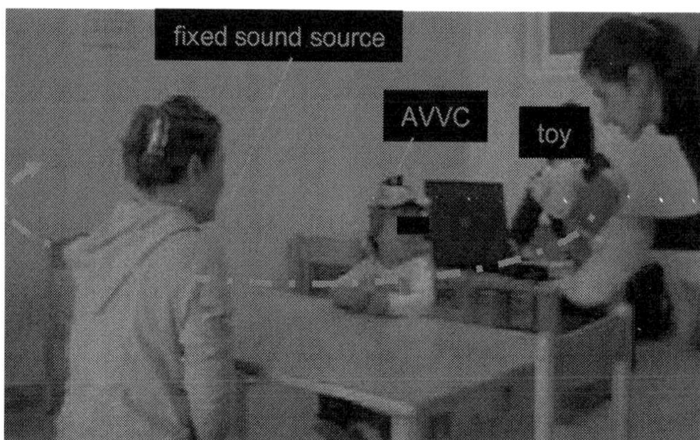

Fig. 13. Ecological calibration protocol for the binaural microphones of the AVVC platform.

An ecological calibration protocol was specifically devised to cope with these issues and considering that children are non-cooperative subjects (especially in the case of children with ASD). As shown in Fig. 13, an experimenter is sitting still in front of the child (already wearing the AVVC with the binaural microphones to be calibrated) and keeps talking, acting thus as a fixed sound source. Another experimenter (not talking) uses a colored toy to capture the child's attention. As the toy is moved around (see dashed line in the), the head of the child, who keeps looking at the toy, spans a wide range of orientations. It is worth noting that the position of the toy is not relevant, its only purpose is inducing the child to orient the head in different directions.

The magneto-inertial device, also mounted on the cap and fixed with respect to the binaural microphones, keeps track of the orientation of the head. In Fig. 14 the head orientation (in degrees) is plotted against the ITD (in milliseconds). The relationship is well fitted to a line ($R^2 = 0.98$). The slope of the fitting line is related to the physics of sound localization via ITD cues while the offset of the fitting line is mainly depended on how the cap is fit onto the child's head, which varies from trial to trial.

Clearly, the whole procedure relies on the hypothesis of 'fixed sound source'. Although the experimenter sitting in front of the child is instructed to remain still as much as possible while talking, the child's head is unconstrained and therefore free to translate while orienting towards the moving toy. These factors affect both resolution and accuracy. Nevertheless, preliminary in-field tests, presented in the next section, show how when used in combination with an experimental protocol it can still be used for data segmentation.

3.3.3 Calibration Procedure for the AVVC eye tracker

During calibration procedure movements of the pupil in pixels are transformed to eye position in degrees. Eye-tracking systems calibration usually consists of looking at several markers on a screen in order to collect enough data to modify the parameter of an adjustable model, often while keeping the head still. Also, this kind of calibration cannot be easily performed

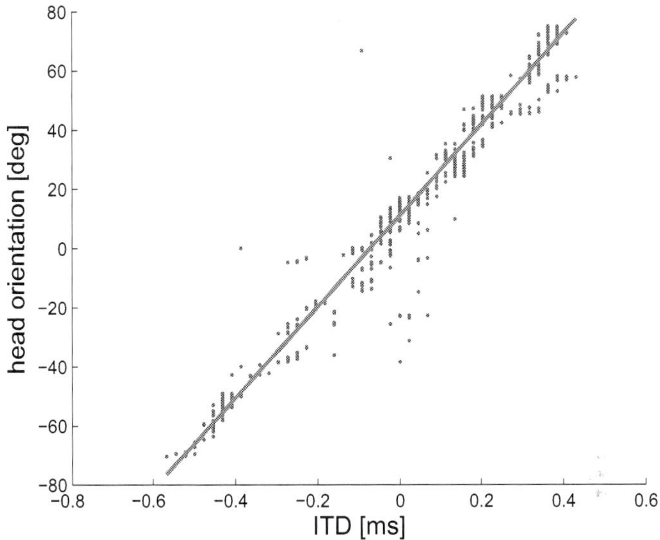

Fig. 14. Calibration curve for the binaural microphones. Fitting values: slope = 150 deg/ms; offset = 11 deg; R^2=0.98.

when the users are very young children. We propose a new calibration procedure, inspired by the vestibulo-ocular reflex (VOR) which allows generating compensatory eye movements in response to head motion as sensed by the vestibular organs in the inner ear.

When the head rotates about any axis (horizontal, vertical, or torsional) distant visual images are stabilized by rotating the eyes about the same axis, but in opposite direction (Crawford and Vilis 1991). The gain of the VOR (the ratio of eye angular velocity $\frac{d}{dt}\psi_e$ to head angular velocity $\frac{d}{dt}\psi_h$) is typically around -1 when the eyes are focused on a distant target.

During our calibration procedure, the child is asked to rotate the head to the left and to the right while keeping looking at the caregiver who is sitting in front of him. Head rotation movements are recorded at a frequency of 100 Hz by the magneto-inertial sensor mounted on the top of the cap. Given the relation between head and eye angular velocities, the head azimuth (ψ_h) correlates with the coordinates[2] of the pupil in the horizontal plane. Linear fitting can be applied to the calibration curve (see Fig. 15) to extract gain and offset. This allows expressing the eye orientation in degrees rather than in (normalized) pixels, as in Fig. 16

4. In-Field Testing

In this section preliminary experimental data relative to *in-field* testings of both the block-box and the AVVC platforms are presented. Such tests are significant as they prove usability of the proposed platforms in unstructured environments. In particular, the two platforms

---

[2] Coordinates of the pupil are derived from images and are typically in pixels, i.e. depend on factors such as resolution of the camera and its distance from the pupil. To avoid dealing with zooming factors, distances in pixels are normalized with respect to physiological features such as the width of the eye.

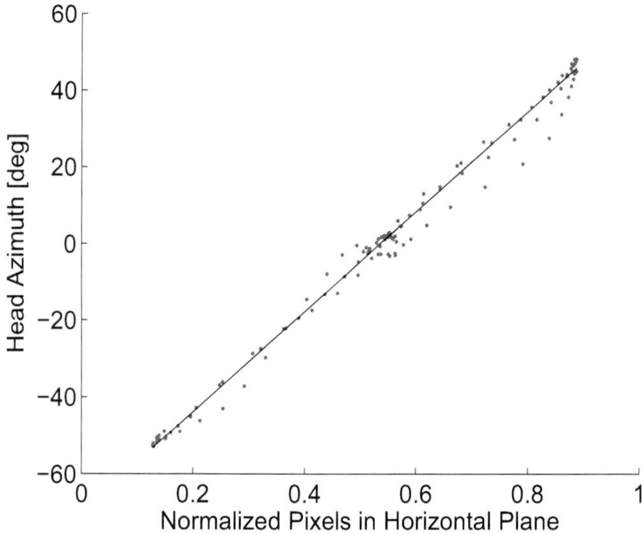

Fig. 15. Head-eye calibration curve: raw data (dots) and fitted line (solid) with $R^2 > 0.90$.

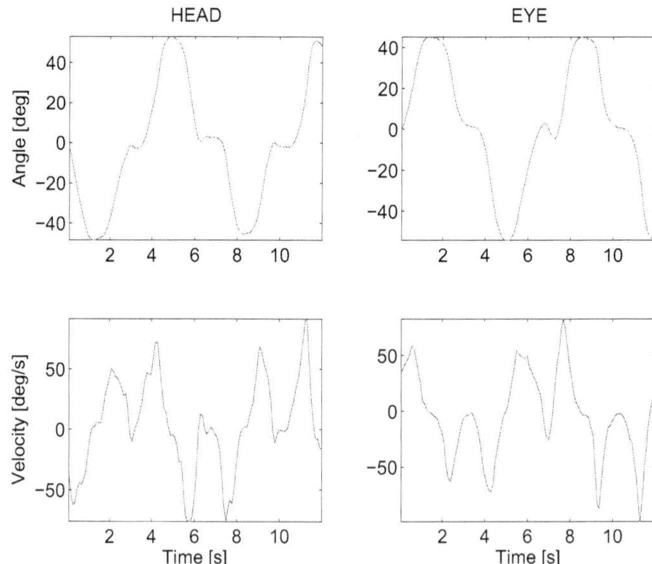

Fig. 16. Head and eye orientation and angular velocity as acquired during a calibration procedure.

were tested (separately) at our local day-care with typically-developing children aged 12-24 months. The experiments followed the two protocols described in Sec. 3.1 and in Sec. 3.3. Although tested separately, the two platforms could also be used in the same experiment or in conjunction with other devices. In fact, in every experiment, one or more video cameras are also present for recording purposes. A key aspect of multimodal assessment is *synchronization* among all devices. During the experiments we routinely performed simple actions such as 'tapping' on a switch button in order to trigger contemporaneous physical events, e.g. a flashing light, a buzzing sound, or a touch event. Each sensor present on the scene records the occurrence of at least one such physical triggers (e.g. cameras would capture flashing lights, microphones would capture buzzing sounds, accelerometers would capture 'tapping'). During off-line data pre-processing, the occurrence of such triggering events was then used as a time-stamp to synchronize movie files, with sound files, with kinematic data etc...

4.1 Experiments with the AVVC platform

To study sensorimotor coordination during attentional tasks, we need to correlate information coded relatively to different references: the operating space, the head, and the ears. A fixed sound source would appear as moving from the perspective of binaural localization unless the head of the child is held still. Since the child's head cannot be constrained, being able to sense the orientation of the head is crucial.

In particular, with reference to the experiment described in Sec. 3.3, the following relation holds:

```
sound-in-space = sound-in-head + head-in-space
```

where sound-in-head represents the direction of the sound stimulus with respect to the (moving) frame of the subjects's head, sound-in-space is the direction of sound stimulus in the (fixed) frame of the operating space (i.e. the coordinate frame in which the social protocol is planned), and head-in-space is the orientation of the head in the (fixed) frame of the operating space.

Sound-in-head can be estimated via binaural algorithms while head-in-space can be estimated via the inertial-magnetic device, therefore sound-in-space can be reconstructed by adding such two estimates.

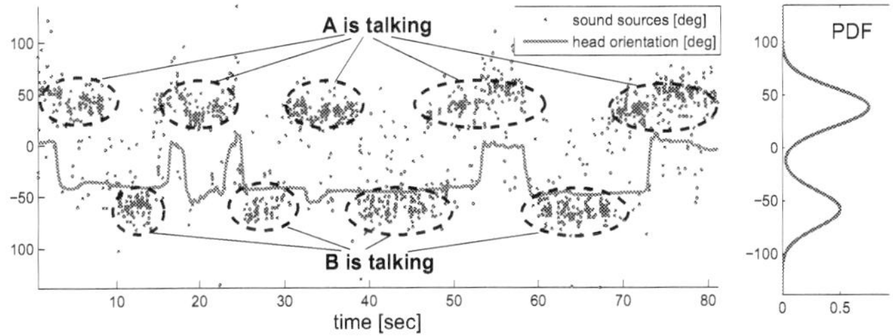

Fig. 17. Plots relative to the AVVC measurements

The data relative to a specific trial are reported in Fig. 17 which plots the head orientation of the child (solid line) as well as the direction of the sound stimuli in the operating space, i.e. sound-in-space (dots). The (fixed) angular position of the two experimenters in Fig. 11 can be identified by the clouds of dots. On the right side of Fig. 17 the distribution (PDF) of such dots is shown, the two peaks are relative to the angular position of the experimenters. This information can be used as a spatial filter, i.e. all dots far away from the two peaks can be ignored (despite all the care taken, day-cares remain noisy environments).

From Fig. 17 we can easily tell, at every time, which experimenter is talking and towards whom the child's head is oriented.

Note that the head never fully reaches either of the angular positions of the speakers. The reason is that orienting behaviors also involve eye rotations which should be added to the head orientation. This was confirmed by visual inspection of pictures taken by the eye-cam (e.g. see the details of a child's eyes in Fig. 12). Automatic detection of gaze is still work-in-progress.

4.2 Experiments with the Block-Box platform

The block-box prototype described in Sec. 3.1.1 was tested with several typically-developing children at our local day-care. Representative snapshots from one particular trial are shown in Fig. 18 in which the sensorized core was embedded into a cube. In the sequence of snapshots, the child (18 months old) first reaches for the cube with his right hand, than adjusts the orientation of cube with both hands and then successfully inserts the cube into the hole, after some final adjustment and pushing.

In the work of Ornkloo and von Hofsten (Ornkloo and von Hofsten 2007), two video cameras monitored the experiment providing respectively a top and a side view. From the videos, after determining the frame during which the object came into contact with the box, both vertical and horizontal alignment of the object with the aperture were evaluated from the specific frame, with a goniometer. Accuracy of the methods highly depends on the quality of the videos. As stated in the paper, the vertical and horizontal alignments were judged by two coders who disagreed on 31 out of 302 cases.

In our experiments, the raw data derived from the inertial-magnetic sensors were first fed into a complementary filter (Campolo et al. 2008) to derive the sequence of orientations of the cube (100 per second, for clarity only few are reported in the middle of Fig 18). Once the orientation of the cube is known, the vertical angular error (i.e. tilt with respect to gravity) and the horizontal angular error (i.e. misalignment between the horizontal projection of the cross-section axes of the object and the axes of the aperture) can be determined at any time, as shown in Fig. 18 (bottom). The time of contact with the box is determined by the peaks of acceleration produced by the shock and distinctively sensed by the accelerometers (2-3 times larger than g).

In the bottom plot of Fig. 18, the first 4 seconds are relative to the in-air manipulation of the block. Approximately at time $t = 4s$, the first impact with box occurs (detected by the accelerometers), since at this time both errors are below 30 deg, the pre-adjustment would be considered correct according to (Ornkloo and von Hofsten 2007). In the remaining 7 seconds, the child tries to insert the cube and only slightly before time $t = 11s$ both vertical and horizontal alignment errors drop to zero and the cube can be successfully inserted. As a final note, the exact time of dropping of the cube can also be determined from the accelerometers because for a body in free fall acceleration always drops to zero.

5. Conclusion

Although developmental milestones of children are largely described in literature, quantitative normative databases of sensorimotor integration skills in relation to increasingly complex

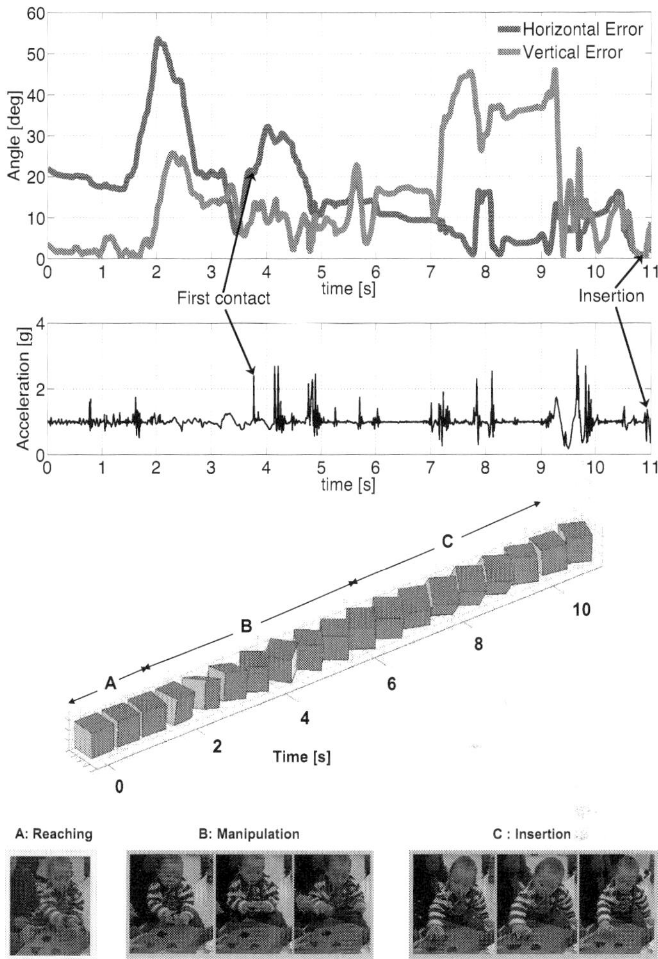

Fig. 18. Experiments with the block-box. Vertical and horizontal alignment errors (top). Reconstructed orientation vs. time (middle). Sequence of snapshots (bottom).

tasks are still lacking. On one hand this would extend the current knowledge on developmental mechanisms, with an impact on Developmental Sciences as well as on Robotics. On the other hand, it would allow early diagnosis of neurodevelopmental disorders such as Autism, with a major impact on society.

For this, technology plays a crucial role. Virtually any toy, tool or piece of garment used by children could host all sorts of technology. Our approach is based on a closed loop dialogue between neuroscientists and bioengineers. The functional specifications for the proposed platforms are derived from experimental protocols devised by neuroscientists. The selection of the technology strictly followed ecological requirements.

In this paper we present three technological platforms, an instrumented toys, a lightweight bracelet and a wearable cap, specifically devised to assess the development of social attention and spatial cognition in infants.

Deficits in *social attention* and abnormal social behavior are among the most typical traits of people with Autism. After a child is diagnosed with Autism, i.e. after the 3 years of age, parents retrospectively report failure to use gaze to regulate behavior and to engage in social games of infancy (Landry and Bryson 2004). Assessing social behaviors is *per se* challenging, due to the multitude of variables to take into account: multi modality is a must.

To this end, we developed the AVVC wearable device aiming at multimodal assessment of gaze and head kinematics in response to sound stimuli. Calibration procedures were also designed which would be appropriate to unstructured environments, appearing as a game to the child. Based on a protocol specifically devised to monitor the response of a child to social stimuli, experiments with the AVVC platform were carried out at a local day-care. These experiments proved that our approach to objective, quantitative and ecological assessment of social behavior is viable. Experimental results also show that, when combined with a structure protocol, semi-automatic segmentation of data is possible.

For *spatial cognition*, the scientific focus is on the ability of a child to mentally rotate an object in order to fit the appropriate hole. The experimental protocol is devised to assess the vertical and horizontal pre-adjustments of the block (with various levels of difficulty in relation to the different cross-sections) at the time of contact with the box. The 'traditional' methods rely on the (time-consuming) manual scoring of videos, frame-by-frame.

The block-box platform embeds magnetic-inertial sensors. The time of contact can be automatically determined from the large acceleration peaks due to the mechanical shock (i.e. when the block hits the box). For that specific time frame vertical and horizontal alignments are also available via the orientation reconstructed from the raw data (e.g. see values in Fig. 18 for $t = 4s$).

In fact, we can reconstruct the orientation *at any time*. Meaning that pre-adjustment kinematics can be assessed during the whole approaching trajectory. The studies of Mari et al. (Mari et al. 2003) have shown that children with ASD typically have difficulties in activating concurrent motor programs such as reaching for an object and pre- shaping the hand for grasping it. We expect similar findings to hold also for the block-box task, where reaching and pre-adjustment are concurrent motor programs.

In their study, Mari et al., used stereo-photogrammetry, assessing the pre-shaping of the hand via reflective markers on the index finger and the thumb. Although valuable for research, such a method is hardly applicable to clinical practice for screening purposes. The block-box platform is suitable to work in day-cares, or in the office of a pediatrician. In this way a large number of children may actually be objectively monitored.

Acknowledgement

This work was supported by a grant from the European Union, FP6-NEST/Adventure Programme, contract no. 015636.

6. References

[1] Babcock J. and Pelz J (2004) Building a lightweight eye-tracking headgear, in *ACM Eye tracking research and applications symposium*, San Antonio, TX, USA, 109-114

[2] Bertone A, Mottron L, Jelenic P, Faubert J. (2003) Motion perception in autism: a "complex" issue, *J Cogn Neurosci* 15: 218-225.

[3] Blauert J (1997) *Spatial Hearing*, revised ed. Cambridge, MA: MIT Press

[4] Boddaert N, Chabane N, Belin P, Bourgeois M, Royer V, Barthelemy C, Mouren-Simeoni MC, Philippe A, Brunelle F, Samson Y, Zilbovicius M (2004) Perception of complex sounds in autism: abnormal auditory cortical processing in children. *Am J Psychiatry* 161:2117-2120.

[5] Byford G.H. (1963) Non-linear relations between the corneo-retinal potential and horizontal eye movements, *J. Physiol.* (London), 168, 14P-15P

[6] Campolo D, Fabris M, Cavallo G, Accoto D, Keller F, Guglielmelli E (2006) A Novel Procedure for In-field Calibration of Sourceless Inertial/Magnetic Orientation Tracking Wearable Devices, *in Proc. of the first IEEE / RAS-EMBS Intl Conf. on Biomedical Robotics and Biomechatronics (BIOROB)*, pp.471-476, Pisa, Italy, Feb 20-22.

[7] Campolo D, Maini ES, Patane' F, Laschi C, Dario P, Keller F, Guglielmelli E (2007) Design of a Sensorized Ball for Ecological Behavioral Analysis of Infants, *IEEE International Conference on Robotics and Automation (ICRA)*, Pasadena, California, USA, pp. 1318-1323

[8] D. Campolo, L. Schenato, L. Pi, X. Deng, E. Guglielmelli (2009) Attitude Estimation of a Biologically Inspired Robotic Housefly via Multimodal Sensor Fusion, *RSJ Advanced Robotics Journal* 23:955-977

[9] Cornsweet T. N. and Crane H.D. (1973) Accurate two-dimensional eye tracker using first and fourth Purkinje images, *J. Opt. Sc. Am.*, 63, 921-928

[10] Courchesne E, Kilman BA, Galambos R, Lincoln AJ (1984) Autism: processing of novel auditory information assessed by event- related brain potentials. *Electroencephalogr Clin Neurophysiol* 59:238-248.

[11] Crawford JD, Vilis T (1991) Axes of eye rotation and Listing's law during rotations of the head. *Journal of Neurophysiology*, 65(3), 407-423

[12] Dawson G, Toth K, Abbott R, Osterling J, Munson J, Estes A, Liaw J (2004) Early Social Attention Impairments in Autism: Social Orienting, Joint Attention, and Attention to Distress, *Developmental Psychology*, 40:271-283

[13] DiScenna A. O., Das V., Zivotofsky A. Z., Seidman S. H., Leigh R. J.(1995) Evaluation of a video tracking device for measurement of horizontal and vertical eye rotations during locomotion, *Journal of Neuroscience Methods*, 58, 89-94

[14] Einspieler C. , Prechtl H. F. R. (2005), Prechtl̆s Assessment of General Movements: A Diagnostic Tool for the Functional Assessment of the Young Nervous System, *Mental Retardation and Developmental Disabilities Research Reviews*, 11:61-67.

[15] Eizenman M., Frecker R. C., and Hallet P.E. (1984) Precise non-contacting measurement of eye movements using corneal reflex, *Vis. Res.*, 24:167-174

[16] Gerlai R (2002) Phenomics: fiction or the future?, *in Trends Neurosci.*, 25:506-9

[17] Grelotti DJ, Gauthier I, Schultz RT (2003) Social interest and the development of cortical face specialization: what autism teaches us about face processing. *Dev Psychobiol* 40:213-225.

[18] Hallett M, Lebiedowska MK, Thomas SL, Stanhope SJ, Denckla MB, Rumsey J (1993) Locomotion of autistic adults. *Arch Neurol* 50:1304-1308

[19] Haslwanter T. (1995) Mathematics of three-dimensional eye rotations, *Vision Res.*, 42, 1053-1061

[20] Hobson RP, Bishop M (2003) The pathogenesis of autism: insights from congenital blindness. *Philos Trans R Soc Lond B Biol Sci.*, 358:335-344.

[21] Jovanov E., Milenkovic A., Otto C., de Groen P. C. (2005), A wireless body area network of intelligent motion sensors for computer assisted physical rehabilitation, *J. Neuroengineering Rehabil.*, 2:6
doi:10.1186/1743-0003-2-6.

[22] Keller F, Persico AM (2003) The neurobiological context of autism, *Mol. Neurobiol..* 28:1-22

[23] Kemp B, Janssen AJMW, van der Kamp B (1998) Body position can be monitored in 3D using miniature accelerometers and earth-magnetic field sensors, *Electroencephalography and Clinical Neurophysiology*, 109:484-488

[24] Landau U. M. (1987) Estimation of a circular arc centre and its radius, *Comput. Vis Graph. Image Process.*, 38:317-326

[25] Landry R, Bryson SE (2004) Impaired disengagement of attention in young children with autism, *J Child Psychol Psychiatry*, 45: 1115-22.

[26] Lotters JC, Schipper J, Veltink PH, Olthuis W, Bergveld P (1998) Procedure for in-use calibration of triaxial accelerometers in medical applications, *Sensors and Actuators A*, 68:221-228

[27] Maestro S, Muratori F, Cavallaro MC, Pei F, Stern D, Golse B, Palacio-Espasa F (2002) Attentional skills during the first 6 months of age in autism spectrum disorder. *J Am Acad Child Adolesc Psychiatry*, 41:1239-1245.

[28] Mari M, Castiello U, Marks D, Marraffa C, Prior M (2003) The reach-to-grasp movement in children with autism spectrum disorder, *Philos Trans R Soc Lond B Biol Sci.*, 358:393-403

[29] Metta G, Sandini G, Konczak J (1999) A developmental approach to visually-guided reaching in artificial systems, *Neural Networks*, 12:1413-1427

[30] Milne E, Swettenham J, Hansen P, Campbell R, Jeffries H, Plaisted K (2002) High motion coherence thresholds in children with autism. *J Child Psychol Psychiatry* 43:255-263.

[31] Minshew NJ, Sung K, Jones BL, Furman JM (2004) Underdevelopment of the postural control system in autism, *Neurology*, 63:2056-2061

[32] Molloy CA, Dietrich KN, Bhattacharya A (2003) Postural stability in children with autism spectrum disorder, *J Autism Dev Disord*, 33:643-652

[33] Mundy P, Neal R (2001) Neural plasticity, joint attention and a transactional social-orienting model of autism. In L. Glidden (Ed.), *International review of research in mental reterdation*, Vol. 23, Autism (pp. 139-168), New York: Accademic Press

[34] Ornkloo H, von Hofsten C (2007) Fitting objects into holes: on the development of spatial cognition skills, *Dev Psychol.*, 43:404-16

[35] Pelz J., Canosa R., Babcock J., Kucharczyk D., Silver A., and Konno D. (2000) Portable eyetracking: Astudy of eye movements, *in Proceedings of SPIE, Human Vision and Electronic Imaging*, San Jose, CA, USA, 566-582

[36] Pierce K, Courchesne E (2001) Evidence for a cerebellar role in reduced exploration and stereotyped behavior in autism, *Biol Psychiatry*, 49:655-664

[37] Prechtl H. F. R. General (2001), Movement assessment as a method of developmental neurology: new paradigms and their consequences, *Developmental Medicine & Child Neurology*, 43: 836-842.

[38] Rinehart NJ, Bradshaw JL, Brereton AV, Tonge BJ (2001) Movement preparation in high-functioning autism and Asperger disorder: a serial choice reaction time task involving motor reprogramming, *J Autism Dev Disord*, 31:79-88

[39] Robinson D. A. (1963) A method for measuring eye movement using a scleral search coil in a magnetic field, *IEEE Trans. Biom. Eng.*, 10, 137-145

[40] Rucci M, Wray J (1999) Binaural cross-correlation and auditory localization in barn owl: a theoretical study, *Neural Networks*, 12:31-42

[41] Schmitz C, Martineau J, Barthelemy C, Assaiante C (2003) Motor control and children with autism: deficit of anticipatory function?, *Neurosci. Lett.*, 348:17-20

[42] Spencer J, O'Brien J, Riggs K, Braddick O, Atkinson J, Wattam- Bell J (2000) Motion processing in autism: evidence for a dorsal stream deficiency, *Neuroreport*, 11:2765-2767.

[43] Sweeney JA, Takarae Y, Macmillan C, Luna B, Minshew NJ (2004) Eye movements in neurodevelopmental disorders, *Curr Opin Neurol.*, 17:37-42

[44] Swettenham J, Baron-Cohen S, Charman T, Cox A, Baird G, Drew A, Rees L, Wheelwright S (1998) The frequency and distribution of spontaneous attention shifts between social and nonsocial stimuli in autistic, typically developing, and nonautistic developmentally delayed infants. *J Child Psychol Psychiatry* 39:747-753.

[45] Takarae Y, Minshew NJ, Luna B, Krisky CM, Sweeney JA (2004) Pursuit eye movement deficits in autism, *Brain* 127:2584-2594

[46] Taffoni F, Campolo D, Delafield-Butt J, Keller F, Guglielmelli E, (2008) Design and assembling of a magneto-inertial wearable device for ecological behavioral analysis of infants, *IEEE/RSJ International Conference on Intelligent Robots and Systems (IROS)*, Nice, France, pp. 3832-3837.

[47] Teitelbaum P, Teitelbaum O, Nye J, Fryman J, and Maurer RG (1998) Movement analysis in infancy may be useful for early diagnosis of autism, *Proc Natl Acad Sci USA*, 95: 13982-13987

[48] Teitelbaum O, Benton T, Shah PK, Prince A, Kelly JL, Teitelbaum P (2004) Eshkol-Wachman movement notation in diagnosis: the early detection of Asperger's syndrome, *Proc Natl Acad Sci USA* 101:11909-11914

[49] Trevarthen C, Daniel S, (2005) Disorganized rhythm and synchrony: Early signs of autism and Rett syndrome, *Brain and Development*, 27:25-34

[50] Young L., Sheena D. (1975) Survey of eye movement recoding methods. *Behavior research methods & instrumentation*, 7(5), 397-429

[51] Welch G, Foxlin E (2002) Motion Tracking: No Silver Bullet, but a Respectable Arsenal, *IEEE Computer Graphics and Applications*, 22:24-38